R E A D I N G S

CONCEPTS FUNDAMENTAL TO NURSING

READINGS

CONCEPTS FUNDAMENTAL TO NURSING

Robert L. Ismeurt, RN, PhD
Assistant Professor
Arizona State University
College of Nursing

Elizabeth N. Arnold, RN, CS, PhD
Senior Year Chairperson
University of Maryland
School of Nursing

Verna Benner Carson, RN, MS
Assistant Professor
University of Maryland
School of Nursing

Springhouse Corporation
Springhouse, Pennsylvania

Staff

Executive Director, Editorial
Stanley Loeb

Director of Trade and Textbooks
Minnie B. Rose, RN, BSN, MEd

Art Director
John Hubbard

Acquisitions
Margaret Belcher, RN, BSN; Elizabeth Steinmetz

Editors
David Moreau, Nancy Priff

Copy Editor
Mary Hohenhaus Hardy

Designers
Stephanie Peters (associate art director), Matie A. Patterson

Art Production
Robert Perry (manager), Heather Bernhardt, Anna Brindisi, Donald Knauss, Robert Wieder

Typography
David Kosten (manager), Diane Paluba (assistant manager), Liz Bergman, Joyce Rossi Biletz, Robin Rantz, Valerie Rosenberger

Manufacturing
Deborah Meiris (manager), T.A. Landis, Jennifer Suter

Production Coordination
Aline Miller (manager), Joy Dickenson

Editorial Assistants
Maree DeRosa, Elizabeth McBeath

Printed in the United States of America

RF1-010190

Library of Congress Cataloging-in-Publication Data
Readings in concepts fundamental to nursing / [compiled by] Robert L. Ismeurt, Elizabeth N. Arnold, Verna Benner Carson.
p. cm.
Consists chiefly of reprints from various sources.
Includes bibliographical references.
1. Nursing. I. Ismeurt, Robert L. II. Arnold, Elizabeth. III. Carson, Verna Benner.
[DNLM: 1. Nursing—collected works. WY 5 R2868]
RT63.R4 1990
610.73—dc20
DNLM/DLC 89-26280
ISBN 0-87434-231-7 CIP

Table of contents

Foreword

The authors of *Readings in Concepts Fundamental to Nursing* have produced a uniquely valuable resource—a compilation of timely articles from a wide range of nurse practitioners and theoreticians who offer significant insights into the fundamental concepts that shape the profession. No other sourcebook provides such a comprehensive collection of informed views on the critical issues facing nurses today.

Articles are grouped by themes within units. Each unit establishes a historical context for the works it includes, defines abstract or difficult terms, and explains the relationships among the articles. Section introductions explain each article's importance, relate it to other articles in the section, and, where appropriate, refer to ideas or themes in other sections.

The 10 units in this book cover a range of topics of vital interest to all nurses and nursing students. Unit One, Nursing: The Science of Caring, presents a brief historical overview and current thinking about nursing's philosophy of caring for the individual, the family, and the self, from the origins of caring theory to contemporary applications of caring in practice. Unit Two, Unifying Concepts Basic to Nursing, investigates two irreducibly important concepts: client systems (therapeutic and interpersonal relationships) and environment (social, cultural, and spiritual).

Unit Three, Nursing as a Process, describes interactions within the profession and examines four ways in which nursing uses a process to provide care—(1) through the five-step nursing process, (2) while communicating with others, (3) during interactions with the law, and (4) while evaluating ethical options. Unit Four, Life Continuum in Health and Illness, examines the business of nursing as the improvement, promotion, and maintenance of client health from birth to death.

Unit Five, Diversity in Health Care Settings, examines nursing services offered in today's health care system: health promotion, illness prevention, illness diagnosis and treatment, and rehabilitation. Care settings include outpatient, community-based, volunteer, institutional, hospice, and health maintenance organizations. Unit Six, Psychosocial Concepts in Nursing, underscores the uniqueness of nursing in its emphasis on holistic care, which addresses the needs of the total client. The unit investigates common psychosocial concerns, including loneliness, fear, and grief, and psychosocial syndromes, such as drug dependence and neurotic behavior.

Unit Seven, Physiologic Concepts in Nursing, includes topics of universal concern in caring: pain, sleep pattern disturbances, and sexuality. Unit Eight, Professional Practice of Nursing, looks at appropriate education achievements for professional nurses (the pros and cons in the entry level controversy) and explores ways in which nurses can make the transition from theory to practice. Information on preceptorships and nursing management is also provided.

Unit Nine, Patterns of Nursing and Health Care, represents current thinking about nursing theories, nursing research, and contemporary nursing and health care. Unit Ten, Leadership for Change, examines leadership practices that can effect desired change.

Readings in Concepts Fundamental to Nursing includes practical aids that enhance the text's usefulness: introductions explain concepts, establish relationships, and provide historical contexts; glossaries define difficult concepts or unusual terms; and study questions at the end of each unit promote content recall and encourage critical thinking. The questions can be used by the professional nurse as a self-test, by the student as a study guide, and by instructors as independent student assignments. Further, this well-rounded selection of current articles provides a starting point for further reading, the development of papers, and topics for research. (Selected references refer to hundreds of original articles, chapters, and books.) In short, this convenient sourcebook, which bridges the gap between theoretical nursing and hands-on clinical practice, is ideal for nursing students, practicing nurses, or those in RN completion programs or refresher courses.

JEAN WATSON, RN, PhD
DEAN, SCHOOL OF NURSING
UNIVERSITY OF COLORADO MEDICAL CENTER

UNIT ONE

Nursing: The science of caring

CARING HAS BEEN an important part of life and health throughout the history of humanity. For hundreds of years, caring was practiced informally by medicine men, high priests, lay deaconesses, and others who managed the health care needs of their communities. Also, women cared for the day-to-day health needs of their families in the home. Eventually, as the science of caring for others became more sophisticated, the need arose for a more systematic form of caring — professional nursing care.

In the 19th century, Florence Nightingale responded to that need. She developed and promoted a philosophy of caring in nursing practice based on the principles of optimal wellness and health promotion. She emphasized the importance of cleanliness, fresh food, clean air, sleep, rest, and exercise to achieve the goal of nursing: "To put the patient in the best condition for nature to act upon him." (Nightingale, 1859)

Nightingale focused on environmental and physical care, especially for the sick. Although she never defined caring explicitly, it was fundamental to her view of nursing practice.

Today, the American Nurses' Association defines the goal of nursing as "the diagnosis and treatment of human responses to actual or potential health problems." At first, this goal may sound quite different from that proposed by Nightingale. Yet they share at least one thing in common: a philosophy of caring. Many of Nightingale's original principles still flourish in modern nursing practice. Her concept of caring helps the nurse understand how to use basic, effective nursing activities to promote health in our complex, high-tech world.

Nursing is a unique practice discipline with many specialties in various practice settings. Nevertheless, its fundamental concepts are bound together by a basic science of caring. Theorists differ in their definitions and views of caring, but all agree that caring is a key concept in the study of nursing practice. Leininger (1981) describes caring as the "central and unifying domain for the body of knowledge and practices in nursing." She and many others recognize caring as the defining characteristic that distinguishes nursing from other health care professions.

Watson (1987) takes a somewhat broader — almost transcendental — view. In a recent article, she used selected metaphorical passages from poetry and literature "to find a new language (literary rather than scientific) to express the covert, intangible, tacit, expressive dimensions of caring in nursing."

The following excerpt illustrates Watson's

belief that these aspects of caring can give the nurse a powerful, evolutionary edge toward personal and professional transformation.

SILVER BRIDGE

I am glad and sorry to give you this information
I see you know it already.
I want to tell you it is not your fault.
It is your fault.
So from now on you (we) are responsible.
This is what we mean when we say consciousness is a curse.
You see the Silver Bridge spanning a flood?
This is what we mean when we say consciousness is a blessing. [Ostriker, 1986]

> Nursing on the caring edge is the silver bridge spanning the flood in society with a new caring consciousness. Likened to Emerson's oversoul, caring acknowledges that there is a higher sense of spiritual wholeness. Caring affects healing and provides nurses with transforming perspectives on health, personality, and nature, and allows nurses to pursue notions of spirituality, energy fields, and new ethics of caring. Nurses grasp that the whole caring consciousness of the nurse can be in each caring instant; caring consciousness can transcend time and space and physicality. The silver bridge is the link between humanity and medical technology. (Watson, 1987)

In more practical terms, caring guides nursing practice. It helps the nurse differentiate between circumstances that one can control and those that one cannot. A caring commitment allows the nurse to develop a safe, healthful environment for the client and to sustain the conviction that care for the client and the nursing profession makes a difference in many people's lives, including one's own.

The nurse demonstrates caring through physical, psychosocial, and spiritual actions that strengthen the natural healing powers within each client. In nursing practice, caring behaviors can develop gradually through a therapeutic relationship, or they can occur spontaneously, as a simple, empathetic acknowledgment of a particular client's need. Whether planned or spontaneous, caring requires a commitment to enhancing the well-being of others, a willingness to experiment with different interpersonal strategies, and a professional respect for the basic human rights of the nurse and the client.

Because caring makes a unique and important contribution to nursing practice, *Readings in Concepts Fundamental to Nursing* begins with a unit about caring. After investigating the nature of caring, Unit One focuses on three major dimensions: caring for the individual, the family, and the nurse.

Caring for the individual

In its most basic form, caring for the individual means helping a client achieve or maintain optimal health. It requires the nurse to consider each client's needs, attributes, strengths, and disabilities.

Then based on these considerations, caring requires the nurse to individualize the client's care with commitment, enthusiasm, and creativity. As a client moves on the health-illness continuum, the nurse must modify caring activities to meet client's needs.

Caring for the family

When the client's family, loved ones, and friends become involved in care, the nurse must expand the circle of caring to include their needs, too. Any disruption in the client's health that affects roles and relationships can directly affect the psychosocial and physical health of the family and significant others.

The nurse provides care for these individuals not only because they need it, but also because the nurse wants to put them in the best possible condition to help the client and the nurse.

For the client, family members and significant others can form a vital network, providing essential emotional, physical, financial, social, and religious support. For the nurse, these people are an important resource. They can enhance the client's sense of security, especially if the nurse helps them cope with potentially overwhelming circumstances.

Caring for the family can be a complementary and adaptive part of the nursing process when the family gives and receives support and guidance from the nurse regarding the client's care. For example, the family can provide information about the client's likes and dislikes or bring the client's favorite personal articles from home, which the nurse can use to make the client more comfortable and to individualize the client's care. On the other hand, the nurse can give the family the social support, encouragement, and information they need to help care for the client at home after discharge.

Caring for the nurse

Finally, the concept of caring includes the nurse's self-care. This kind of care requires the same consideration, discipline, and commitment that a nurse would use when caring for a client.

This dimension of caring is essential to a nurse's effectiveness. Before a nurse can give freely to others, she or he must first practice self-care. To do this, the nurse must realize that assumptions about compassion, respect for dignity, and commitment for others also apply to oneself.

The rewards of caring

For the nurse and the client, caring offers many rewards such as deepened faith, hope, trust, and creativity. It also provides the experience of feeling cared for, which can lead to a greater understanding of oneself, a stronger sense of worth and dignity, and increased feelings of openness and compassion.

REFERENCES

Leininger, M. (1981). The phenomenon of caring: Importance, research questions, and theoretical considerations. In *Caring: An Essential Human Need* (Proceedings of Three National Caring Conferences) (pp. 3-15). Thorofare, NJ: C.B. Slack.

Nightingale, F. (1859). *Notes on Nursing: What It Is and What It Is Not.* London: Harrison & Sons. (Facsimile edition, Dover Publications, 1969.)

Ostriker, A.S. (1986). *The Mother/Child Papers.* Boston: Beacon Press.

Watson, J. (1987). Nursing on the caring edge: Metaphorical vignettes. *Advances in Nursing Science, 10*(1), 10-18.

SECTION ONE

The concept of caring

THIS SECTION PROVIDES a theoretical overview of the concept of caring. It prepares the reader to apply the concept to the individual, family, and nurse, as discussed in the other sections of this unit. It also provides a framework for understanding and using the rest of the fundamental concepts presented in this book.

The first article, "The Phenomenon of Caring: Importance, Research Questions, and Theoretical Considerations," views caring as the feature that most distinguishes nursing from other health disciplines. It provides specific definitions of *caring, professional caring,* and *professional nursing care*. Its author, Leininger, makes these distinctions to avoid the ambiguities that she feels are inherent in the professional and social use of the term *caring*.

Because Leininger believes caring is central to an understanding of nursing, she encourages the reader to study caring and its applications, especially from a transcultural perspective. Toward this end, she provides rationales for studying caring as well as assumptions, beliefs, and theoretical and hypothetical statements about caring. She concludes with a conceptual model for studying transcultural nursing care and preliminary findings that can help the nurse give more therapeutic care to each client.

Leininger's article is important for several reasons. Its author was one of the first nursing leaders to describe caring explicitly and assert its essentialness to nursing practice. In fact, her work prompted the development of National Caring Conferences (annual conferences that examine theories and research about caring). Also, Leininger's model is a foundation for much of the current thinking about caring.

In contrast to Leininger's concepts about caring, Benner and Wrubel (1989) make no distinction between professional caring and other types of caring. To them, caring "means that persons, events, projects, and things matter to people."

To provide an understanding of the nature and importance of caring in nursing and in life, Benner and Wrubel describes three ways in which caring is primary:
• Caring sets up what matters to a person, what counts as stressful, and which options are available for coping. It creates possibilities.
• Caring sets up an enabling condition of connection and concern.
• Caring sets up the possibility of giving and receiving help.

Although Benner and Wrubel might differ with Leininger about the scope of caring, they would all agree that it is essential to nursing.

In "The Ethic of Caring: Can It Survive in Nursing?," Fry affirms the importance of caring in nursing. She describes the influences that have helped caring develop into an ethic in nursing. Then, she points out certain trends, such as the nursing shortage, unsafe nurse-client ratios, and standardized (rather than individualized) care plans, that are threatening its survival. Finally, Fry challenges the nursing profession to protect this ethic of caring with deliberate, proactive strategies.

As this section will show, many nurses are accepting Fry's challenge. They are working hard to overcome these debilitating trends because, to them, nursing *is* caring.

REFERENCES

Benner, P., & Wrubel, J. (1989). *The primacy of caring*. Menlo Park, CA: Addison-Wesley.

The phenomenon of caring: Importance, research questions, and theoretical considerations

MADELEINE LEININGER, RN, PhD, LHD, FAAN

In the following excerpt, one of the nation's foremost nursing leaders reviews the importance and definitions of caring and shares her theories and research findings on this topic. With her writing, Leininger offers a framework that nurses can use to understand and apply the phenomenon of caring.

She encourages nurses to delve deeper into this phenomenon and highlights the transcultural aspects of care as needing further study. This, she believes, will enable nurses and others to know the full scope of the one characteristic that sets nursing apart from all other disciplines. Note: In this article, summaries (shown in bracketed italics) and excerpts (indicated by ellipses) condense extensive background material.

IT HAS LONG BEEN the author's position that *caring is the central and unifying domain for the body of knowledge and practices in nursing,* and a systematic investigation of caring could advance the discipline of nursing and ultimately provide better nursing care to people.[1] I hold that an in-depth knowledge of caring from diverse perspectives and from a historical, philosophical, and epistemological study will enable nurses and other caregivers to know the full nature of care or caring behaviors, patterns, and processes. Most importantly, as nursing moves toward full disciplinary status, it will be essential for nurses to know the nature, scope, and distinguishing features that characterize nursing from other health disciplines. I hold that caring behavior and practices *uniquely* distinguish nursing from the contributions of other disciplines. Thus the critical and essential challenge is for nurses to systematically and rigorously explicate and analyze caring phenomena in depth and breadth, and from a cross-cultural viewpoint....

Undoubtedly, caring has long been expressed by human cultures throughout the history of humankind. Care, I believe, was *essential* for human growth, development, and survival. This anthropological and nursing position makes one pause to consider the importance and significance of caring for the human race and for the lifeways of *homo sapiens* as a species. If this major assumption can be investigated, then nurses and others should give more attention to this phenomenon. Such research would be especially pertinent to nursing as a profession since they have laid claim to nursing care for many decades. Caring appears to be an extremely important and generic construct in human services. It appears to be at the heart of all health care services. It is the largely unknown ingredient for helping humankind in wellness, illness, and stressful situations. Why then, has so little attention been given to caring by humanistically-oriented scientists and caregivers? This question is an intriguing one that has yet to be answered, and one which deserves more thought than it has received in the past. It is a question that could lead to many fascinating research lines of inquiry about human be havior in health and illness states.

[World view: An anthropologic approach to study care and caring

Redfield introduced the term world view *to refer to the way individuals or cultures grow, perceive, and know their world. The world view approach requires the nurse to learn about and experience the client's world.*

A world view and ethnoscientific approach to caring emphasizes similarities and differences among client needs. It can help the nurse conceptualize theories and models of holistic caring, which will advance knowledge through revolution and evolution. It provides cross-cultural paradigms (models) of caring that identify the universal aspects of caring and offers a method for studying the broad humanistic and scientific aspects of caring.

Ambiguities about caring

Nurses and many other health professionals have used the terms care, caring, health care, and nursing care *for many years, without any knowledge base for them. These terms are often used interchangeably or in a vague and nondiscriminatory manner. So when nurses discuss* nursing care, *ambiguities exist regarding the meaning, function, and therapeutic usage of the term.*

Yet all nurses are expected to know about care *and* nursing care *and use them in practice. Unfortunately, many nursing schools do not provide in-depth instruction on caring behaviors, processes, and patterns; and their curricula contain more information about medical conditions and regimens than about nursing care or caring behaviors.*

Nevertheless, concepts and theories about caring are essential links with ideas related to nursing care. Therefore, nurses must focus on caring in research, teaching, and practice to bring credence and legitimacy to a major implied and claimed concept that has been used in nursing for more than 100 years.

Rationale for studying care

Nurse researchers and others should pursue caring research for four main reasons:

1. To determine the importance of care to human growth, development, and survival throughout the years. Caring appears to be a distinctly human act, separating us from animals. It also seems to be a mode of action and interrelatedness since the beginning of time . Although anthropologists have not proven the connection between human caring and existence, the need for caring seems logical for human survival through the millenia. Cultures presumably have depended on care and caring for their survival and cultural evolution.

2. To explain caregiver and care recipient roles in living and survival. Currently, we know little about these roles and the ways nurses and nonnurses provide care in different cultures. Yet caregiving behaviors in health and illness must have helped people overcome trauma and illness since prehistoric times.

3. To preserve and maintain caring for current and future cultures. Today, many forces seem to devalue human life, such as human depersonalization with technological equipment and economic, political, and legal constraints that reflect a lack of human caring. Caring could become extinct if we do not recognize and value it in our lives. Without caring, the human race could destroy itself.

4. To determine the relationship between caring and nursing care. Although Florence Nightingale used the term care, *she never explained it or discussed its function. Her ideas focused primarily on environmental and physical care of the sick. Her ideas helped nursing evolve as a profession, but did not define* care *per se.]*

Definition of care/caring

Since the days of Florence Nightingale, the word *care* has been used in nursing as a verb, as in *to be cared for, caring for others, or to manifest care* with concern, compassion, and interest in another human being. Care and caring appear to have multiple conceptualizations and characterizations. Although care has a common and recurrent usage by nurses, definitions of care are needed to include strangers who give care by comfort, alleviation of distress, and other human ways. While definitions of *nursing care* can be found in the literature, there are few that define the *generic concept of care*. For example, in Henderson's work (frequently used by nurses), she speaks of nursing and implies care activities:[2]

> ...Nursing is primarily helping people (sick or well) in the performance of those activities contributing to health, or its recovery (or to a peaceful death) that they would perform unaided if they had the necessary strength, will, or knowledge.

For heuristic purposes, I define *care/caring in a generic sense as those assistive, supportive, or facilitative acts toward or for another individual or group* with evident or anticipated needs to ameliorate or improve a human condition or lifeway. I define *professional caring* as those cognitive and culturally learned action behaviors, techniques, processes, or patterns that enable (or help) an individual, family, or community to improve or maintain a favorably healthy condition or lifeway. And finally, I define ***professional nursing care*** *as those cognitively learned humanistic and scientific modes of helping or enabling an individual, family, or community to receive personalized services* through specific culturally defined or ascribed modes of caring processes, techniques, and patterns to improve or maintain a favorably healthy condition for life or death.[3]

In the above definitions, one will note the emphasis is on *helpful* and *enabling* activities of individuals, social, and community groups based upon culturally defined, ascribed, or sanctioned modes of helping people. I believe that caring acts can be culturally identified through the beliefs, values, and practices of cultural groups. From a cross-cultural study of caring behaviors, one can then identify what caring acts, processes, and techniques are culturally specific, and those that are universal. Other theoretical and philosophical positions will be discussed later with the focus on discovering transcultural nursing care phenomena.

In Mayeroff's work, he speaks about caring with some general attributes:[4]

> ...Caring is the antithesis of simply using the other person to satisfy one's needs. The meaning of caring I want to suggest is not to be confused with such meanings as wishing well, liking, comforting and maintaining, or simply having an interest in what happens to another. Also, it is not an isolated feeling or a momentary relationship, nor is it simply a matter of wanting to care for some person. Caring, as helping another grow and actualize himself, is a process, a way of relating to someone that involves *development,* in the same way that friendship can only emerge through mutual trust and a deepening and qualitative transformation of the relationship.

Rollo May also offered some ideas about care in his discussion about man living and relating to the world in which he lives:[5]

> ...Care is the necessary source of eros, the source of human tenderness....Care is given power by nature's sense of pain; if we do not care for ourselves we are hurt....In care one must, by involvement with the objective fact, do something about the situation, one must make some decisions. This is where care brings love and will together....

From cursory review of the philosophy and the social, biological, and health science literature, the terms *care* and *caring for others* are frequently used. Many diverse ideas are associated with care, such as being used analogously with love, tenderness, compassion, and empathy. Accordingly, in the dictionary the verbs *care, caring,* and *cared* mean: to have an interest in, to be concerned for, to provide or look after, and to be disposed to help others.[6] One could then infer that *to not care* for someone would reflect indifference, antipathy, disregard for another, lack of attention, or no interest in helping another human being. Noncaring behaviors are of equal interest to study.

During the past decade I have found in studying nearly 30 world cultures through interviews, structured questionnaire guides, literature sources, and direct observations, that there are many concepts associated with care or caring. Intercultural variations clearly exist with no universal ethnoscience definition or social usage of care by cultural representatives. While the data are still under analysis and being checked for validation of what informants *said* with the *actual* cultural practices, the following constructs are associated closely with care/caring (varying in cultural usage with respect to which terms are used in different cultures): support, tenderness, touch, compassion, empathy, stress alleviation, presence, loving acts, comfort, direct and indirect helping behaviors, enabling, facilitating, nurturance, succorance, surveillance, protection, restoration, instructive acts, coping, concern, interest in, trusting, and need fulfillment.[3] With each of these constructs, there are many embedded ideas associated with the concepts of care or caring. And there are some constructs that may not be found in designated cultures. For example, the nurse as a caregiver is not permitted by cultural roles to touch a patient in the Yap culture. How would an Anglo-American nurse provide care to the Yap people in the Micronesian cultural area? Many extremely fascinating data are coming from my investigation, which should throw new light on old conceptualizations of nursing care and the need to use transcultural caring knowledge in culturally specific ways.

Some assumptions and beliefs about human caring

In pursuit of knowing the nature of humanistic and scientific caring, and based upon my preliminary research findings, I have identified several assumptions to guide nurses' deliberations about caring. The following assumptions may challenge nurses to discover in depth the phenomenon of caring:

1) Human caring is a universal phenomenon, but the expressions, processes, and patterns vary among cultures.
2) Every nursing care situation has transcultural caring behaviors, needs, and implications.
3) Caring acts and processes are essential for human development, growth, and survival.
4) Caring should be considered the essence and unifying intellectual and practice dimension of professional nursing.
5) Caring has biophysical, psychological, cultural, social, and environmental dimensions which can be studied, and practices to provide holistic care to people.
6) Transcultural caring behaviors, forms, and processes have yet to be verified from diverse cultures; when this body of knowledge is procured, it has the potential to revolutionize present-day nursing practices.
7) To provide therapeutic nursing care, the nurse should have knowledge of caring values, beliefs, and practices of the client(s).
8) Caring behaviors and functions vary with social structure features of any designed culture.
9) The identification of universal and non-universal folk and professional caring behaviors, beliefs, and practices will be important to advance the body of nursing knowledge.
10) Differences exist between the essence and essential features of caring and curing behaviors and processes.
11) There can be no curing without caring, but there may be caring without curing.

Some theoretical statements and hypotheses about caring

The following theoretical statements or hypotheses are offered to stimulate research studies on caring behaviors, processes, and patterns. A few nurses are already investigating aspects of these hypotheses.[3]

1) Intercultural differences in beliefs, values,

and practices of caring would reflect differences in nursing care practices.
2) Self-care practices will be valued and practiced in cultures that value individualism and independence in social structure features, whereas group care practice will be valued and practiced in cultures where interdependency and high individualism *is not* espoused.
3) Congruence between caregiver and care recipient's behaviors and goals is important for therapeutic practices to occur.
4) The greater the differences between folk caring values and professional caring values, the greater the signs of cultural conflict and stresses between professional caregivers and non-professional care receivers.
5) Technological caring acts, techniques, and practices differ in cultures and have different outcomes for health and nursing care practices.
6) The greater the efforts of professional nurses to blend the folk caring practices with professional care practices, the greater the signs of clients' satisfactions.
7) The nurse as a professional caregiver may produce unfavorable stresses and conflicts with the client due to lack of knowledge about cultural beliefs, values, and practices of caring.
8) Symbolic forms of nursing care behaviors have referent meanings in different cultural groups and necessitate that nurses study the meaning and functions of symbols in cultures to give efficacious nursing care.
9) The greater the signs of technological caregiving, the less the signs of interpersonal care manifestations.
10) Caring behaviors and patterns are closely linked to social structure features.

A conceptual model for studying transcultural nursing care theories and practices

During this time I have been investigating the definitions, nature, and scope of care and caring, using an ethnoscientific approach. (Leininger M: unpublished data, 1964-1981.) The study of the cultural usages, meanings, and functions of caring in different cultures appears closely related to the social structure and cultural beliefs of people. Essentially, my research is focused on explicating and studying caring phenomena from different cultural viewpoints. A body of ethnocaring knowledge is being sought. I am interested in how people perceive, know, and experience caring behaviors in different cultures so that nurses can use this knowledge in providing both cultural-specific and cultural-universal nursing care practices. *The ultimate goal is to improve health care to people*. Transcultural health care should become more manifest, along with the new generation of nursing care theories and practices.

To date, approximately 30 cultures have been studied by direct interviews, structured questionnaires, library data, and direct observations focused upon beliefs and practices related to caring. From these data, a taxonomy of caring constructs, theories, and hypotheses are being developed. The conceptual framework is offered in Figure 1.1.[3] In the model one can identify a dynamic process to cross-cultural caring phenomena. It is a process model to show how the knowledge of caring is obtained and validated. On the left side of the model, Phase I, are the major sources from which I derived ethnocaring data that have been identified; namely, by doing an ethnography (or lifeways of the societies), studying the social structure features, cultural values, and in identifying the health-illness caring behaviors and practices in a designated culture. Phase I is followed by Phase II, which focuses upon the identification of the major enthnocaring constructs from data obtained from Phase I domains, and examples of these constructs are offered. Several subsets of ideas are found within each construct. These constructs have been prioritized and defined by the people. Phase III reflects the next step in ethnocare study by analyzing the data and developing theories that will be tested in subsequent research. The model

FIGURE 1.1 Leininger's conceptual and theory generating model to study transcultural and ethnocaring constructs

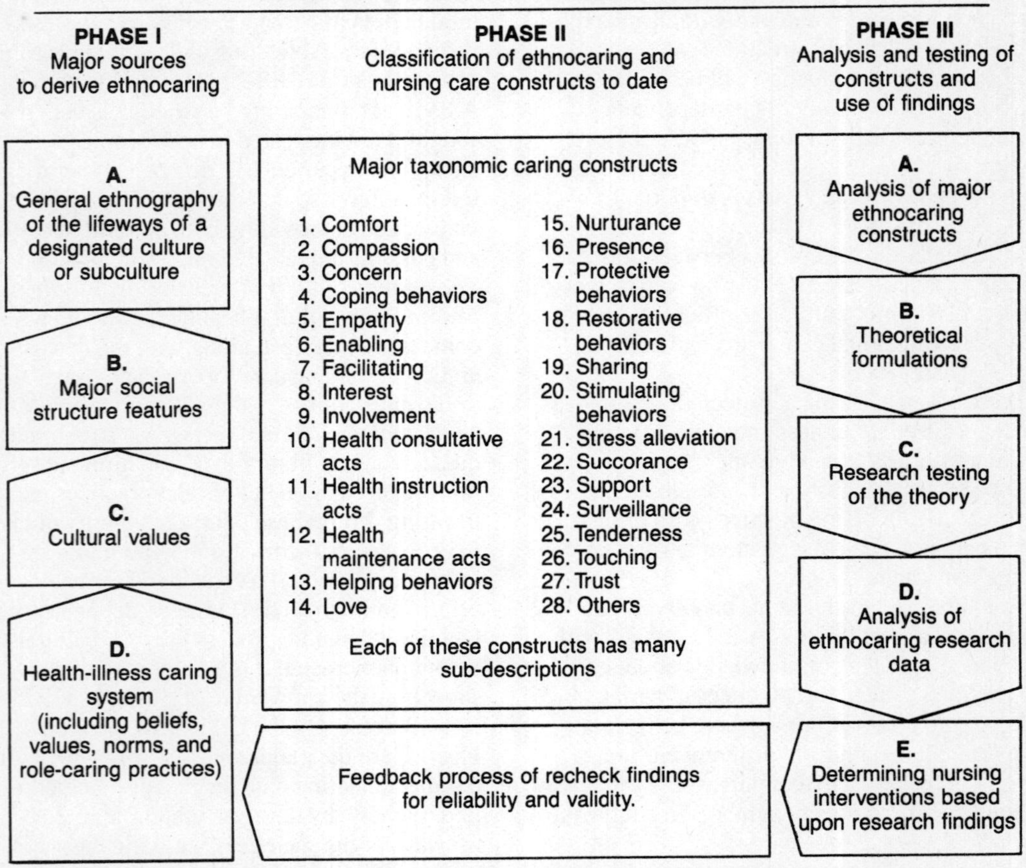

*Model was developed in 1968 and reflects revisions and additions since that time. (The ethnocaring definitions are not presented here.) Data come from 30 cultures using a modified ethnoscience and ethnonursing research approach.

also shows ways to recycle findings to check for reliability and validity of the data.

From the research work to date, there are several common principles or guidelines which have become evident and could be used to help nurses focus on and further refine caring behaviors and processes. They are as follows:
1) Caring behaviors and processes can be identified in cultures to help guide nursing care decisions and actions.
2) Caring behaviors appear closely related to the social structure features of designated cultures and can help to predict nursing care behaviors of the culture groups.
3) Caring rituals may be therapeutic and nontherapeutic depending upon how closely the caregiver links activities with cultural values and beliefs.

4) Caring behaviors vary transculturally in priorities, expressions, and need satisfactions.
5) Westernized nurses tend to rely heavily on technological and psychophysiological stress alleviation activities to help clients; whereas nurses in non-Westernized cultures tend to rely more frequently on non-technological and more sociocultural expressions of behaviors.
6) Caring behaviors appear more important than curing in recovery of clients, but receive less economic and social reward than curing by physicians.
7) Efficacious caring tends to be humanistically oriented and reflects professional care concepts of concern, compassion, stress alleviation, nurturance, comfort, and protection, and especially by female caregivers.
8) Caring behaviors have important symbolic referents which need to be identified and used in therapeutic care practices.
9) Care-giving and care-receiving behaviors require signs of reciprocal behavior satisfactions for such activities to continue over time.
10) Professional nursing care values, beliefs, and practices tend to follow more medical and curing model attributes in the United States than caring attributes as perceived by the clients.
11) Self-care is gaining emphasis in the United States, but has less credence and relevance in other parts of the world — especially non-Western cultures — where other care is emphasized.

Such preliminary findings (and others yet to be identified) indicate the enormously rich data found in a cross-cultural focus on caring. From such data come guides to help nurses and others give therapeutic care. Knowledge of the values, beliefs, and practices of a culture regarding caring opens the door to culture-specific care and universal caring practices. The close interrelationships of care, culture, and social structure are clearly apparent from my cross-cultural work on caring behaviors, patterns, and processes. It appears essential that professional nurses know variations in cultural caring and the ways caring is linked with specific value systems. Future and ongoing research on caring and its relationship to nursing care appears highly promising and encouraging. I believe a new breakthrough in nursing has occurred with the focus on caring and its relationship to nursing and health care practices. Nurses should build upon such research findings, and other theories and research studies of caring.

In summary, caring should be the central, critical, and unifying domain and focus for nursing care knowledge. The generic construct of caring is essential to explicate nursing. The possibilities for developing a scientific and humanistic body of nursing knowledge related to caring appear favorable. However, too many nurses are still following medicine and focusing on their medical model of diagnosing and curing largely physical illnesses, rather than on the caring phenomenon. The transcultural nursing approach provides a highly promising mode for studying universal and non-universal aspects of caring in all areas of nursing for all cultures. This knowledge can then be linked to nursing care practices and to essential changes for a humanistic and scientific body of caring knowledge. This contribution will not only serve nursing, but other disciplines and human groups. I believe we are on the threshold of some new discoveries in nursing that will make nursing's contribution visible, substantive, and distinctive in the near future.

REFERENCES

1. Leininger M: Caring: The Essence and Central Focus of Nursing. American Nurses' Foundation (Nursing Research Report), Vol 12, No 1, February 1977, p 2.

2. Henderson V, Nite G: Principles and Practice of Nursing. New York, Macmillan Publishing Co, Inc, 6th ed, 1978.

3. Leininger M: Transcultural Nursing Concepts, Theories, and Practices. New York, John Wiley and Sons, 1978, p 35-38, 39.

4. Mayeroff M: On Caring. New York, Harper & Row Publishers, 1971, p 1.

5. May R: Love and well. New York, Norton, 1969, pp 286-8.

6. Oxford English Dictionary, p 339.

The ethic of caring: Can it survive in nursing?

SARA T. FRY, RN, PhD

A RECENTLY RELEASED VIDEO...claims that one of the reasons why one should enter the profession of nursing today is to have the opportunity to expand the quality of caring in health care.[1] Indeed, by portraying nursing practice as the major source of caring within the health care system, the video effectively uses this "ethic of caring" as a major recruitment device and public relations message about nursing. How well established is the ethic of caring in nursing? Can it survive the nursing shortage and changes in health care delivery created by prospective payment systems?

Caring is often considered a universal phenomenon.[2] Although its expression, processes, and patterns vary among cultures, all caring apparently includes direct or indirect nurturant activities, processes, and decisions that are designed to assist people.[3]

Caring, however, is not necessarily a moral value. It is possible to speak of *natural caring* simply as an attitude that exists between individuals in certain relationships (say, between mother and child).[4] To have moral content, caring must be viewed as "good" or "right" for specific reasons. First, caring must be viewed as an ultimate or overriding value to guide one's actions. Second, caring must be considered a universal value, and, hence, applied to all persons in similar circumstances. Third, caring must be considered prescriptive in that certain behaviors (empathy, support, compassion, protection, etc.) are preferred. Last, caring must be other-regarding; it must consider the human flourishing of others and not just one's own welfare (or care). When our view of caring has these characteristics, it is a moral value and can serve as an ethical standard for the practice of nursing.[5]

Within nursing, caring has developed into an ethic as a result of several influences. The primary influence is the nature of nursing practice itself. As defined by Nightingale, nursing is taking "charge of somebody's health...to put the patient in the best condition for nature to act upon him."[6] The very nature of nursing requires and reinforces the ethic of caring.

A second influence on the development of the caring ethic in nursing has been the work of the National Caring Conferences, conducted since 1976, and the research and literature supporting transcultural nursing. Based on the assumption of care as "the essence of nursing," these conferences and research results have propelled care into a central concept within nursing curricula. The most recent National Caring Conference, which was held in April 1987, specifically focused on the ethics and morality of caring and identified issues that are critical to the further development of caring as a central concept of nursing.[7]

These efforts have been matched by a third influence on the caring ethic — the development of theories of human care and care behaviors within nursing and within the discipline of ethics.[4,8-11] Viewing caring as a moral ideal, nursing theories have created conceptual frameworks of caring within the science of nursing. Viewing caring as a fundamental moral concept, theories in ethics have focused on metaethical questions such as the relationship of care to other moral concepts or the justification of judgments based on care. Both approaches have contributed to the moral and theoretical foundations for an ethic of caring within nursing.

However, the survival of the caring ethic within nursing requires: the opportunity to see persons as having certain duties and rights, in a nonhypothetical manner, within health care delivery,[11] and the continued potential for reciprocity and mutuality within the nurse-patient relationship.[4] This means that values held important to nursing (caring, advocacy, respect for persons, etc.) must have the opportunity to be realized and fostered in health care *and* that nurses and patients must have ample time to connect as ones who care (nurses) and ones who are cared for (patients). The nursing shortage, unsafe staffing patterns, and payment-directed nursing care plans have all tended to undercut the opportunity and/or potential for the realization of an ethic of caring in nursing. Its survival is in question. Nursing must now decide whether or not it is important enough to fight for.

REFERENCES

1. American Journal of Nursing Company. Educational Resources Division. *Nursing: Expanding the Quality of Caring* (video). New York. The Company, 1987.

2. Leininger, M.M. *Care: The Essence of Nursing and Health.* Thorofare, NJ, Slack, 1984.

3. Leininger, M.M. *Transcultural Nursing: Concepts, Theories, and Practices.* New York, John Wiley and Sons, 1978.

4. Noddings, N. *Caring: A Feminine Approach to Ethics and Moral Education.* Berkeley, University of California Press, 1984.

5. Veatch, R.M. and Fry, S.T. *Case Studies in Nursing Ethics.* Philadelphia, J.B. Lippincott Co., 1987.

6. Nightingale, F. *Notes on Nursing: What it Is and What It Is Not.* London. Harrison & Sons, 1859. (Facsimile edition, Dover Publications, 1969).

7. Leininger, M.M. *Care: Discovery and Uses in Clinical and Community Nursing.* Detroit, Wayne State University, 1988.

8. Watson, J. *Nursing: Human Science and Human Care: A Theory of Nursing.* Norwalk, CT, Appleton-Century-Crofts, 1985.

9. Duldt, B.W., and Giffin, K. *Theoretical Perspectives for Nursing.* Boston, Little, Brown and Co., 1985.

10. Paterson, J.G., and Zderad, L.T. *Humanistic Nursing.* New York, John Wiley and Sons, 1976.

11. Frankena, W.K. Moral-point-of-view theories. In *Ethical Theory in the Last Quarter of the Twentieth Century,* ed. by N.E. Bowie. Indianapolis, IN, Hackett Publishing Co., 1982, pp. 39-79.

SECTION TWO

Caring for the individual and the family

WHEN PROVIDING CARE for others, the nurse puts caring concepts into action. The readings in this section demonstrate how to apply the concepts in Section One to clients and their families. Although these types of caring differ somewhat, they require a basic commitment that directs the nurse's practice and gives a distinctive pattern to caring actions.

Individual care

Over time, the nurse develops a unique ability to care for all types of individuals. Caring becomes a personal act manifested through such activities as physical assistance, client education, emotional support, social support, advocacy, and positive regard for the client. Each of these activities shows respect for the client's individuality and demonstrates the nurse's integrity as a professional caregiver.

In "The Primacy of Caring," Orlick and Benner show how one nurse used caring concepts in her practice. In the first part of this article, Orlick describes a real-life example in which her caring was instrumental in an individual's recovery.

In the second part, Benner comments on the example. She identifies two aspects of nursing that are vital to expert practice: the primacy and power of caring in making cure possible, and the way that the nurse becomes a participant in the client's community.

The second article, "Advocacy in Nursing" by Nelson, focuses on the nurse's advocate role (client representative role) in caring for a client. Through advocacy, the nurse helps the client become an autonomous, informed decision maker, which enhances the client's self-care abilities and speeds the healing process. Advocacy is especially important when a client cannot act in his or her own best interest because of illness or a lack of information.

Nelson traces the development of advocacy in nursing, which some view as "a natural outgrowth of nursing's traditions of holism and 'care more than cure.'" (Winslow, 1984) Then she explores its issues, prerequisites, and significance, pointing out that advocacy offers the nurse an opportunity to show one's integrity and professional commitment.

Family care

Throughout a nurse's education and practice, client care takes the first priority. Yet family care can be almost equally important because it can help determine the effectiveness of nursing care. Every client exists within a larger context of a family, and that family can support or hinder the nurse's efforts to care for the client. Also, the current trend toward early discharge forces families to provide more care for ill members. This means that families will need more extensive nursing and social support to care for the ill family member and to prevent undue stress and health problems in other family members.

To help the nurse understand the nature of family social support, Kane developed a conceptual model. Her model assumes that family characteristics (social network, family structure, esteem, and stability) and interactional factors (reciprocity [reciprocal helping relationships], advice and feedback, and emotional involvement) affect family social support. Based on this model, Kane (1988) developed the following propositions about family social support:

- The larger the family's social network, the greater the opportunity for reciprocity, advice and feedback, and emotional involvement.
- The more flexible the family structure, the more reciprocity, advice and feedback, and emotional involvement.
- The more esteem the family has within its social network, the more reciprocity, advice and feedback, and emotional involvement.
- The more stable the family, the more substantial the reciprocity, advice and feedback, and emotional involvement.
- The more reciprocity occurring, the greater the family social support.
- The more advice and feedback occurring, the more family social support.
- The more emotional involvement, the more family social support.

A family with strong social support will-function with versatility and resourcefulness and will be exposed to more information, goods and services, and help in a crisis. This increased exposure should lead to improved health.

According to Kane, the nurse can use this model to assess a family's social support. If the family is lacking in reciprocity, advice and feedback, or emotional involvement, the nurse can initiate strategies for building family processes and can provide appropriate resources in the interim.

In "Caring for Julie" by Garbett, Allen, and Bennett, the nurses focus on meeting the needs of a family facing a potentially overwhelming situation. Although the family's problems are complex and troublesome, each nurse's individualized care helps the entire family cope and grow. The care is successful because the nurses have commitment, compassion, and strong relationships with the client and her family. They help the husband, wife, and son deal with their problems by considering the unique needs of each family member in their nursing care.

REFERENCES

Kane, C. (1988). Family social support: Toward a conceptual model. *Advances in Nursing Science 10*(2), 18-25.

Winslow, G.R. (1984, June). From loyalty to advocacy: A new metaphor for nursing. *Hastings Cent. Rep. 14*:32-40.

The primacy of caring

SHEILA ORLICK, RN, PhD; PATRICIA BENNER, RN, PhD, FAAN

GERALD, A 39-YEAR-OLD construction foreman, was admitted to our hospital to have surgery for a bleeding gastric ulcer. He was married and had two children, aged five and nine, with whom he was very close. His family lived about 200 miles away and could visit only on weekends. The rest of Gerald's family lived in the East.

Gerald was outgoing and charming in a down-home, country sort of way. He was used to being in charge of his life and carried this with him as a patient. I was Gerald's primary nurse and developed a close relationship with him. We would laugh and joke and Gerald would confide in me about his personal problems. His relationship with his wife was strained at the time and he had little outside support from family and friends.

Gerald's hospital course was very rocky. He developed multiple complications after his gastrectomy, including an enterocutaneous fistula, recurrent gastointestinal bleeding, and an esophageal stricture. Because of these complications, Gerald had two more operations and made two trips to the ICU, where he almost died.

After his second stay in intensive care, Gerald was noticeably withdrawn. He refused to get out of bed, turn, or use his incentive spirometer. His affect was flat and he would not make eye contact with me. I felt frustrated with his uncharacteristically passive behavior because I realized it meant that Gerald was giving up hope of ever getting better.

Various strategies to get him to talk about his feelings didn't work; all he would do was nod his head or stare blankly at the wall. Finally, I said to him: "You just don't care anymore, do you?" He only shook his head no in response.

At that point my emotions got the best of me. I had worked with this man for two months, knew his family, and had developed a relationship with him. Because I felt he was shutting me out, it made me feel sad, frustrated, and angry all at once. At that moment, all the therapeutic interventions I knew deserted me and I responded to Gerald on a gut level. I yelled at him, "Well damn it, Gerald, we care."

A little shaken by my outburst and by his lack of response to it, I left the room, saying that I would return later to take his vital signs. When I did return after an hour, I noticed that he had been crying. I asked gently, "Gerald, are you OK?" He just reached for my hand, squeezed it, and said "Thank you."

Not long after that incident, Gerald began to act more like his "old self." He started to take more interest in his care and eventually he recovered and went home.

I've lost touch with Gerald, but the lesson I learned from my experience with him has served me well. To show your feelings for a patient is not unprofessional. It is human.

Commentary

In this example, Sheila Orlick demonstrates two aspects of nursing that I have repeatedly found in my study of expert practice: the primacy and power of caring in making cure possible, and the way that nurses as helpers place themselves *inside* the patient's community as members and participants in a common humanity. Both aspects deserve commentary.

The primacy and power of care as necessary to cure. In our technological era, we tend to separate the means from the end. But as Albert Borgmann points out, we do violence to the meaningfulness of things when we separate the means from the end.[1] In health care, this separation can be seen in the ideological divison between nurses and physicians, where nurses provide the care and physicians attend to the cure. There can be, however, no recovery — no "end"— without both.

Sheila Orlick's "emotional outburst" is an example of care that is an integral part of Gerald's cure. In the ravages of his serious illness, Gerald lost his sense of connection to others, his sense of hope, the sense that he mattered and that his recovery was important. Sheila Orlick's caring reminded Gerald that he mattered, that his response to his illness mattered, that he was cared for. Her words reawakened his connection to his world. Elsewhere, I have referred to this as the integrative power of caring, because caring reintegrates the sick person with his or her world.[2]

Sheila Orlick also withdrew from Gerald at a most propitious time; her intent was to regain her composure, but Gerald probably needed time alone to reflect on what had just occurred.

Sheila Orlick first tried the standard "therapeutic communication" practices, but these were ineffective. Therapeutic strategies help people gain insight and clarify feelings, allowing them to gain rational control over their feelings; these strategies are not aimed directly at enhancing involvement. Gerald's problem was not a lack of clarity or an inability to express his feelings. The problem was he *had* no engaged feelings. Gerald no longer "cared" nor felt cared for.

Sheila Orlick learns that "therapeutic technique" alone will not work in all cases. Nursing is more than mere technique. Central to effective nursing care is communicating that the nurse cares. This communication is necessarily contextual and relational. You cannot extract the action from the relationship. Had Sheila Orlick been a stranger, or had she not cared, her expression of care would not have had the same positive outcome.

Nurses are understood as members and participants in the patient's community. In this exemplar Sheila Orlick's "distant professionalized" image of expert nursing care gives way when she realizes that she must respond first as a human being. In our culture, nurses are viewed as insiders. Patients expect nurses to be able to listen to and provide care for patients' intimate physical and personal concerns.

Nursing is the most intimate of the helping professions. Expert caring requires that the "expert" not be set apart; rather, expert caring means one is approachable and available. The goal of expert caring is empowerment rather than domination and control.

Orlick describes how she had listened to the patient's innermost concerns about his personal life and had seen him through a rocky course. She was committed to his recovery. She cared. This may be the essential ingredient to any patient's recovery.

Patients are not persuaded to return by a world that is cold, impersonal, and technical. They are persuaded by care, and often that care must be expressed in ways that run counter to convention and hospital routine. This is why caring is often described in the language of making exceptions, of "individualizing" care.

REFERENCES

1. Borgmann, Albert. *Technology and the Character of Contemporary Life.* Chicago, University of Chicago Press, 1987.

2. Benner, Patricia. *From Novice to Expert: Excellence and Power in Critical Nursing Practice.* Menlo Park, CA, Addison-Wesley Publishing Co., 1984, p. 211.

Advocacy in nursing

Margot L. Nelson, RN, MS

In this article, Nelson discusses the evolution of advocacy and its implications for nursing practice. As Nelson shows, advocacy plays an important role in caring, especially for an individual. Note: Summaries (shown in bracketed italics) condense extensive historical information.

The concept of advocacy has been an integral part of nursing since the founding of the profession, although the intent of the nurse advocate has changed immensely as the profession has evolved. Advocacy has moved from a posture of interceding, supporting, or pleading a case for the client to acting as guardian of the client's rights to autonomy and free choice. A number of factors have impeded nurses in their implementation of advocacy. Chief among them is the perceived obligation of loyalty to an employing institution and the physician, which may at times conflict with loyalty to the client. Despite this and other strong counterforces, however, nurses have been able to serve as advocates to clients, both as individuals and as groups.

As Brower declares, advocacy is a "neologism originating out of social concern" for one's fellow human beings.[1] As such, it has fit well with nurses' tradition of concern for health care recipients and for the health of society generally. Speaking of it as a popular "buzz-word," Kohnke asserts that advocacy, an act of loving, is neither something we are born with nor something we acquire automatically, nor even something we all claim or practice.[2] Instead, it involves an act of free will and a studied choice to view ourselves in a particular way in our relationship to others.

Kosik represents the advocate as someone who intercedes on behalf of groups of people as well as individuals. She identifies goals of the nurse advocate as "humane and just treatment and equality of opportunity (for everyone) to obtain food, clothing, shelter, jobs, health care, respect and dignity."[3] This view captures the social mission of nursing, which concerns health, but also addresses the entirety of the human condition.

[Acting for or on behalf of another

Although early nursing leaders did not use the word advocacy, *many of them — including Florence Nightingale, Lillian Wald, and Lavinia Dock — viewed the nurse as someone who acted for or interceded on behalf of the client or the community.*

Some nursing leaders have objected to this view of advocacy because it implies an active role for the nurse and a passive role for the client. Others objected that this view of advocacy placed the nurse in a "mothering" role.

Loyalty and obedience

In the early 20th century, nurses were expected to give client advocacy the highest priority unless *it conflicted with their loyalty and obedience to the physician or employer. Most health care professionals held a military view of medicine in which disease was the enemy and nursing students were soldiers trained to follow orders without question. In this context, nurses were not allowed to criticize their hospital or school, other nurses, or physicians. By 1910, some nursing leaders began to ques-*

tion this view of advocacy. One asked, "Is a nurse required to be untruthful or practice deceit to uphold the reputation of the physician at her own expense or that of the patients?"[6] Others suggested that nurses owed a higher loyalty to the client and the community than to the physician or employing institution.

Nurse as mediator

Slowly, the nurse's advocacy role evolved into one of mediator. In this role, the nurse coordinated services, described the relationships between different health care providers, and clarified communication by others to the client. The mediator role became dominant in the 1970s when the public lost confidence in medicine and began to view it as a large, impersonal institution that resisted change. Clients expected nurses to help them through the maze of the American health care system.

To do this, nurses needed personal commitment to clients as well as skill and knowledge. They were expected to resolve and balance the conflicting interests of the client and the health care providers. Unfortunately for many nurses, they were hampered in the mediator role by insufficient power and positions in institutions that restricted their autonomy and accountability to the client.

Nurse as protector of self-determination

This new version of advocacy emphasizes "the client's rights as the unconditional first priority." It values the client's right to make decisions autonomously. When protecting this right, the nurse performs two essential tasks: "informing *clients adequately so they can make knowledgeable decisions, and* supporting *them in whatever decisions are made."*[2] *This type of advocacy requires open-mindedness and a broad knowledge base.*

In 1985, the American Nurses' Association reflected on the nurse as a protector of self-determination in its "Code for Nurses:"

> *Since clients themselves are the primary decision makers in matters concerning their own health, treatment, and well-being, the goal of nursing actions is to support and enhance the client's responsibility and self-determination to the greatest extent possible*
>
> *Truth telling and the process of reaching informed choice underlie the exercise of self-determination, which is basic to respect for persons.*
>
> *The nurse's primary commitment is to the health, welfare, and safety of the client. As an* advocate *for the client, the nurse must be alert to and take appropriate action regarding any instances of incompetent, unethical, or illegal practice by any member of the health care team or the health care system, or any action on the part of others that places the rights or best interests of the client in jeopardy.*[8]

Patient rights advocate or representative

Some institutions have developed a new position of patient representative (or patient rights advocate) to provide clients with an advocate. The patient representative may or may not be a nurse. However, the basic duties remain the same: to provide information objectively, and to offer anticipatory guidance about such things as consent forms, tests, and treatments.

A nurse who chooses to become an advocate must be prepared to make waves and take risks. The Tuma case is an example of the kind of risk an advocate may take. Nurse Jolene Tuma discussed alternatives to cancer chemotherapy with a client and family members at the client's request. The client opted to continue chemotherapy, but the physician sued Tuma for interfering in a physician-client relationship. Tuma lost her job and license to practice nursing, although the Idaho Supreme Court later restored her license.

Tuma's experience raises some important questions about advocacy: Do nurses have the right to help clients toward full, informed con-

sent? Do nurses have the authority to fulfill their responsibilities as client advocates?[9]*]*

Issues related to advocacy

Several issues need resolution before nurses can fully embrace a commitment to client advocacy. The traditional public view of the physician as sole authority and decision maker in health care is an obvious obstacle and also lends strong support to the *need* for advocacy. Physicians tend to view patients as their exclusive domain, and as Leddy points out, there is a definite foundation for this view in the real world, given that the patient's admission, diagnosis, treatment, and discharge are physician controlled in most settings.[4] In such a scheme, the would-be nurse advocate may be viewed as a troublemaker rather than a meaningful contributor to patients' welfare.

A second, related issue is that nurses are not recognized by consumers, by physicians, or often by nurses themselves as active initiators of health care, but rather as caregivers or implementers of the physician's plan of care.[10] Patients and families may be unprepared to accept the nurse as advocate because the nurse has not been selected by them as such. Nurses may, therefore, find themselves offering a service that has not been chosen and may not be expected. Colleagues may also view client advocacy by the nurse as a problem. Patients who have had a nurse advocate may ask too many questions, want to do things their own way, and even be "noncompliant."[2] Nurses may, with fair accuracy, perceive that they must go against the entire system to function in the role of advocate.

Lack of authority or power is a further deterrant. Probably most nurses would identify the client as the first priority, but there are strong competing loyalties to physicians and employing institutions. The nurse is often cast as a "double agent" attempting to represent both patient and physician.[11] Furthermore, patients come and go while employing institutions and colleague relationships remain, and loyalty to the latter is acknowledged by most persons (including nurses) as a virtue.[5]

The question of sufficient power for advocacy is addressed by Miller et al. in three categories of power: personal, invested, and delegated.[7] Personal power is defined as the nurse's competence, currency, and self-esteem. Invested power is that conferred via trust and confidence to an agent or an institution. Delegated power is that which is formally delegated by means of policies, rules, regulations, and/or job descriptions. All of these kinds of power are amenable to change and augmentation; for example, measures to encourage consumer investment of power in nursing could potentially add viability to the role of patient advocate. However, the hierarchical health care system and the traditionally subserviant role of the nurse have been highly effective influences against nurses' acquisition of authority.

Prerequisites for effective advocacy

What would be necessary for nurses to become more effective advocates? A radically different health care system wherein the nurse is employed by the client rather than an institution? Perhaps. A system in which collegial respect and mutuality are the underpinnings rather than a hierarchical system in which physicians are viewed as gods or kings over consumers and health care providers alike? Helpful, but not realistic in the near future.

There are, however, some realistic starting points. First, the meaning of advocacy and the degree of nurses' commitment to its practice must be clarified. Once a definite commitment is made, nurses can begin to project to the public a clearer, more integrated image of the nurse as advocate.

For the sake of advocacy as well as other crucial issues, nurses also need to broaden their sociopolitical knowledge base to achieve a better understanding of the bureaucracy in which they function. Based on this knowledge, nurses must seek more viable individual and collective roles in social and political spheres. This includes speaking out on consumer issues, continuing and expanding attempts to influence legislation, and increasing nurse membership on governmental health policy-making boards and councils.

Winslow suggests that efforts also be directed toward revising nurse practice acts to safeguard nurses' obligations as client advocates.[5] Such revisions should be directed toward making advocacy a less dangerous activity. Murphy's account of a situation in which a medical resident's incompetence caused the death of a patient serves as a dramatic example of the need for such protection. Report of the resident by Murphy (a nurse) resulted in a threat from the medical director that she not pursue the matter further without hiring a lawyer. As she stated, "Dr. X kills the patient and I need a lawyer!"[12]

Significance of advocacy

Winslow, among others, views nursing's adoption of advocacy as a "hopeful paradigm of the future."[5] He sees it as a natural outgrowth of nursing's traditions of holism and "care more than cure." Aiken identifies the following societal changes as significant indicators of the need for nurses to address themselves to advocacy:

1. An increase in the proportion of the population over age 65. (These people have "special" needs related to choices about their health-related goals and how to achieve them.)
2. Increased "sophistication" of the public with the rapid diffusion of scientific knowledge and cultural emphasis upon self-care.
3. Consumer outrage at the escalating costs of health care.
4. Technological advances and the accompanying need to distribute scarce and expensive resources in a "just" manner.[13]

These and other needs of consumers and the developmental level of the profession combine to form a receptive climate, perhaps even an imperative, for the nurse to act as client advocate. Perceptions of the concept, however, are ambiguous, the risks to the nurse are immense, and a multitude of questions and challenges remain as to the wisdom and even the possibility of implementation.

Is advocacy a question or an answer? Is it a response in keeping with a professional evolution or a risk to be avoided? Does it put nursing's values (the individual's health, autonomy, self-determination, and free choice) into practice or is it a challenge circumvented because of its hazards? Although many obstacles and questions remain, advocacy is an...opportunity for nurses to demonstrate integrity and professional commitment.

REFERENCES

1. Brower, H.T. Advocacy: what it is. *J. Gerontol. Nurs.* 8:141-143, Mar. 1982.

2. Kohnke, M.F. *Advocacy: Risk and reality.* St. Louis, C.V. Mosby, Co., 1982.

3. Kosik, S.H. Patient advocacy or fighting the system. *Am J. Nurs.* 72:694-698, Apr. 1972.

4. Leddy, S., and Pepper, J.M. *Conceptual Bases of Professional Nursing.* Philadelphia, J.B. Lippincott Co., 1984.

5. Winslow, G.R. From loyalty to advocacy: a new metaphor for nursing. *Hastings Cent. Rep.* 14:32-40, June 1984.

6. Where does loyalty end? (editorial) *Am.J.Nurs.* 10:230-231, Jan. 1910.

7. Miller, B.K., and others. Patient advocacy: do nurses have the power and authority to act as patient advocate? *Nurs.Leadersh.* 6:56-60, June 1983.

8. American Nurses' Assocation. *Code for Nurses with Interpretive Statements.* Kansas City, MO, The Association, 1985. (Publ. No. G-56)

9. Tuma, J. Professional misconduct (letters). *Nurs.Outlook* 25:546, Sept. 1977.

10. Weiss, S.J. Role differentiation between nurse and physician: implications for nursing. *Nurs.Res.* 32:133-139, May-June 1983.

11. Bandman, E.L. and Bandman, B. The nurse's role in protecting the patient's right to live or die. *Adv.Nurs.Sci.* 1:21-35, Apr. 1979.

12. Murphy, P. Deciding to blow the whistle (Dilemmas in Practice). *Amer.J.Nurs.* 81:1691-1692, Sept. 1981

13. Aiken, L.H., ed. *Nursing in the 1980s: Crisis, Opportunities, Challenges.* Philadelphia, J.B. Lippincott Co., 1982.

Caring for Julie

JANE ALLEN, SRN; MAUREEN BENNETT, ENROLLED NURSE;
MARGARET GARBETT, EN(G), RGN, RM, NDN CERT., ENB 930

JULIE'S DIAGNOSIS of inoperable carcinoma of the cervix coincided with other immense domestic and social problems. Then a 31-year-old, with a husband, Michael, 28, and a son, John, aged almost five, Julie's medical history is tragic. Until July 1984 she had been healthy, happily married for eight years....

In July, she had a routine cervical smear which proved negative. In December, she developed an offensive vaginal discharge that was treated by her GP with creams and pessaries but which persisted. At this stage, Julie felt she had no support from her GP and changed to a female doctor from whom she requested a vaginal examination.

On examination, the doctor felt a large, hard, irregular cervix, and referred Julie immediately to a gynecologist who performed a dilatation and curettage, the histology of which confirmed a carcinoma of the cervix. Subsequently, Julie underwent 27 treatments of radiotherapy, and in May the following year had a radium implant.

In June everything appeared satisfactory; Julie's vaginal discharge had stopped and her main concern was Michael's involvement in a court case on an embezzlement charge. He was convicted and sent to prison for six months. Needless to say, this caused a tremendous strain on the family. Julie came from a stable background and Michael was the only child of a good working-class family who had never been in trouble before.

In July, Julie noticed a further discharge and was referred back to her gynecologist, who diagnosed postradium vaginitis. She was admitted to [the] hospital for treatment — creams and pessaries again.

While an in-patient, Julie discussed the merits of chemotherapy with her consultant [physician], who said he would use it only as a last resort and advised surgery which, in Julie's case, would be extensive as her tumor had infiltrated all the pelvic organs. It would entail hysterectomy, bilateral salpingo-oophorectomy, and probably partial removal of the bladder and sigmoid colon. Although shocked at this news, Julie agreed to the operation and returned home to make arrangements for her family to care for John while she was in [the] hospital.

However, while at home, Julie hemorrhaged quite severely and was readmitted for a blood transfusion and to be prepared for surgery on November 1, 1985, John's fifth birthday. Unfortunately, Julie's consultant [decided that] she was too sick to undergo such drastic surgery, and he decided instead to start chemotherapy, just six weeks after Julie had been told it was worthless.

She was devastated at this and suffered greatly because Michael was still in prison and John was refused permission to visit her on his birthday, as he had been in contact with measles.

Julie underwent two chemotherapy treatments, developing severe nausea and vomiting and feeling very poorly. Subsequently her blood count remained too low for further treatment. She was discharged home to be reunited with Michael on his release from prison.

Michael was extremely supportive but feeling guilty, and he began to keep other family members at a distance, wanting to be Julie's sole carer.

It was at this stage, at the beginning of December 1985, that I became involved. On my first visit, I was greeted by Michael; he was pleased that I was visiting but extremely wary of me. He knew I had come from the hospice, but did not want to discuss this. He knew Julie's diagnosis but would not accept it and certainly could not accept that she was in the terminal stage of her illness. However, he let me in to see her and we discussed her problems, which at that stage were pain in the lower pelvic area radiating around her back and down her legs, a vaginal discharge, poor appetite, constipation, a urinary tract infection, and generalized weakness....

We discussed Julie's illness and her goals. At that moment her one desire was to see her son open his Christmas presents. We did not really talk about dying, other than she knew that she had cancer and would die. No time was put on it, but she asked what I could do to improve her quality of life. My priority was to control the pain, so I began a pain chart with her. From this she kept a daily diary and let me know exactly how she was, how well the pain was controlled, and if and when she had any pain breakthroughs. I contacted her GP who agreed to start...prednisolone...to improve her appetite and increase her sense of well-being.

I visited three times each week. Michael, who had initially been a little distant, gradually came to lean on me for support. Often I would spend half-an-hour with Julie and one to two hours with Michael. He could not accept what was going on and, although he discussed Julie's illness and future death, he desperately sought for some relief and felt that my presence was admitting the inevitable.

When Julie became drowsy, he wanted [her morphine] to be discontinued. [He] sought the help of a hypnotherapist in Liverpool and insisted she...see him. After one session, Julie was advised to throw away her tablets and use meditation to relax. When I visited the next day, Julie was in extreme pain, so we had to sort the situation out quickly. We reached a compromise. I referred them to a local hypnotherapist who proved to be very supportive while Julie continued with her medication.

We carried on in this vein. Some days Julie was quite well and Michael was able to take her out shopping for John's Christmas presents....On one or two occasions she was well enough to meet John from school. She fought hard to be a mother and have normality in her house. We achieved this by [having] her remain...in bed until the afternoon so she could be with John when he came home until his bedtime.

But the situation was breaking down: Michael still refused help from his and Julie's families. Although Julie needed more care, Michael was still feeling guilty and was determined to nurse her alone. He did agree, however, to get the family together on Christmas Day. Julie fought hard for a happy Christmas. She got up early to help John unwrap his presents and played with him, returning to bed while Michael prepared lunch.

Over the next few days, Julie's condition deteriorated. It was as though she had achieved her goal, and now pain breakthroughs and bouts of vomiting developed. Michael was finding it harder and harder to cope and would ring up sometimes two or three times a day for advice or a visit.

I discussed the possibility of her admission to the hospice. Michael was very, very angry; he did not want anyone else to nurse his wife. However, Julie herself asked to come in and admission was arranged for January 3, 1986.

The problems had been discussed with the hospice staff, including the family problems and Michael's need to nurse Julie himself. We arranged a four-bed room to be used as a family unit where Michael and John could stay and help with Julie's care, but with the support of the hospice staff.

However, at 8:30 p.m. on January 2, Michael telephoned in tears. Julie had been vomiting, and he felt he could just not cope any longer. An ambulance was hurriedly arranged, two beds were pushed together in the family room, and Julie and Michael were installed at the hospice. John [went] to stay with his grandparents.

The hospice team's first impression of Julie was of a young, pale, thin girl, in obvious distress from persistent nausea and who appeared very anxious. She was accompanied by Michael who seemed equally anxious and very protective.

We settled them into our family room and reassured Michael that he could continue to care for Julie and that we would help in any way we could.

Shortly afterwards, they were seen by one of the GPs who provided medical cover for the hospice. He chatted to Julie and Michael, taking a full history, examining Julie, and prescribing her drugs accordingly.

A nurse is present, whenever possible, during the admission procedure and assesses any nursing problems at the same time, so that patients will not have to answer the same questions twice, and so that we hear what they understand about their illness. Julie's nursing problems were assessed and a care plan was devised to meet these needs.

Her main problem was her nausea and vomiting, which could have been caused by a partial obstruction owing to tumor spread throughout the pelvis, involving the rectum. Our aim was to relieve her nausea and vomiting as much as possible. So her antiemetics were changed....This did not really improve the problem....So on January 10 a syringe-driver [syringe pump] was set up with cyclizine...;this greatly improved her vomiting, and she rarely complained of nausea afterwards.

Another problem was pain, mostly in the abdominal area, which was already well controlled by [morphine]. She had occasional pain breakthroughs during the first week of admission, requiring diamorphine injections, however. So when the syringe-driver was instituted, diamorphine...was prescribed instead of the [morphine].

Julie's other nursing problems were a sore, coated mouth with signs of oral thrush, which responded to nystatin applications. Michael was taught how to clean Julie's mouth, and he reminded her to have frequent drinks and mouthwashes. She ate small pieces of fresh pineapple which stimulated saliva production and moistened the mouth.

Julie also had a slight vaginal discharge, which was not offensive. [It] needed no care other than to wear a pad, keep the area washed and clean, and observe for any signs of skin soreness.

Constipation was another problem....Rectal examinations were occasionally done if she became very uncomfortable, and suppositories were given if needed, but once her obstruction had become complete, no treatment was given at all.

Julie was already very thin and weak on admission and so a potential problem was that she could develop pressure sores, although her skin was healthy and intact. She was nursed on [a special] mattress, and Michael was taught the importance of helping her to lie on alternate sides at least every two hours. Her generalized weakness meant that she was unable to manage her own personal hygiene, so Michael would help her to wash or bedbath every day. He would ask for help with this and in turning her when she became weaker.

She had a very poor appetite, which was more of a problem to Michael than Julie, [because] he became very upset if she did not eat as much as he thought she should. So we repeatedly explained to him that Julie did not feel like eating because of her illness, her sore mouth, nausea, and obstruction, and he gradually accepted this.

Julie's last problem...was one of poor communication. It was very hard to assess how much she had understood of her illness and how far she had come to terms with it, as at first she was reluctant to talk about her feelings.

Michael was fully aware of Julie's diagnosis and had been told that she would not recover, but he was still hopeful that she might get well....Julie was aware that she had cancer, but did not talk much about this and gave the impression that she did not realize she was dying.

Michael was protective towards her and was worried that we would tell her she was dying, as he felt she would then "give up" and stop fighting. We told him several times that we would not force knowledge on Julie but that if we felt that she really wanted to know what was happening, we would answer her questions honestly.

In fact, about a week after admission, Julie was chatting on her own to one of the nurses while Michael had gone to collect John. We had begun to feel that Julie did want to know more and to talk about her illness, so the nurse took the opportunity to ask Julie what her aim was regarding her illness and her reply was: "To go home on Friday, but it doesn't seem as though I will." She then asked to be told more about her illness and how much longer she had to live.

She had obviously realized...that she was not getting better and needed to have her fears confirmed. She was told that we felt she had only a few weeks left to live and she was able to talk openly about this. She said she was not afraid to die, and that now she knew she had only a few weeks left to live, she could see her family and friends and say her goodbyes.

She asked if Michael knew she was dying, and we told her that he did know but had been very worried about her knowing. Julie told Michael herself that she now knew she could not be cured. His initial response was one of anger towards the staff for telling her and anxiety about her feelings, but Julie immediately reassured him that she would not stop fighting yet, and told him that she was glad she now knew where she stood.

They decided they would tell John the truth....The next day, [they] gently told him that his Mummy was not going to get better and was going to die, but that his dad and grandparents would still be here and would look after him.

They were both anxious about telling their parents, especially Julie's parents and brother, who were also unaware that she had such a short time to live, and hopeful that the chemotherapy she had had would cure her. Julie wanted to chat with her mother alone, which she was able to do, and they discussed her death openly.

The day after Julie was told her prognosis, she began to suffer frequent breakthroughs of abdominal pain, requiring injections of diamorphine. Her syringe-driver was increased almost every day to control the pain....It was obviously physical pain, but we felt it was worsened by fear. Also, Julie sensed Michael was anxious and this in turn increased her anxiety, leading to more pain.

After a few days she appeared to become more settled and accepting of her situation, and the pain breakthroughs became less frequent, but it was noticeable that each time Julie became anxious and frightened her pain increased.

Once Julie knew that she was not going to recover she was able to talk openly about her coming death. She realized that she should make the most of the time left to her and asked Michael to arrange visits from her family and a few close friends so that she could talk to them again before she died.

She enjoyed John's visits, and Michael would fetch him several times a week to see her while she was well enough to enjoy them. He appeared to be quite happy and settled with his grandparents, which was a relief to everyone. Julie and Michael decided that John would not be there when Julie died as they felt he would not understand what was happening and Julie wanted him to remember her when she was well and able to play with him. As her condition deteriorated, Julie would often comment that she hoped she would die quickly, because she did not want her family to have to watch her "going downhill."

Michael was slower in coming to terms with her deterioration. He was still hoping that she would recover and that a miracle would happen, and commented several times that "Nobody could say it wouldn't." He tried hard to make Julie fight and not accept her death.

He was anxious about her poor appetite and tried hard to make her eat more. He asked once why we did not set up an infusion to feed her, but was able to understand and accept the reasons why this would be unfair to her.

He said he just felt so helpless watching her illness get worse without being able to help her. He needed a lot of time spent with him, listening to him talk about Julie and his feelings about her illness. He felt that he had had to stay cheerful and hopeful because "life wouldn't be worth living for Julie" if everyone was pessimistic.

He said that as long as she did not realize how ill and near death she was she would not give up, but really it seemed to be Michael rather than Julie who was not ready to accept her coming death. He could accept that she would die in the future, but as her state slowly deteriorated he found it much harder to face the fact that her death was drawing much nearer. He continued to talk about how she would die — whether she would be unconscious or aware, if it would be sudden, how he would know that she was about to die, and we told him that she would probably become more and more drowsy and weak and should remain very peaceful.

He talked about what he wanted to do when she did die, to lay her out himself and put on her a dress he had bought her. He and Julie had decided that John should have her wedding ring when he was older, and Julie had decided she would be cremated.

Michael planned to have her body brought to their home the day before the funeral and to keep her overnight with him. He was also thinking about John and his future and how to bring him up, and he talked a lot about Julie, their past life together, and how happy they had been.

Gradually, Julie's condition deteriorated and she became much weaker, needing more physical care which Michael was able to carry out, requesting help as he needed it. By now, her pain and vomiting were well controlled with her syringe-driver, which was increased as required. She had been catheterized because she had problems in passing urine and had also developed a urinary tract infection. She was so weak that it exhausted her to get out of bed to a commode, and so a catheter was a great relief.

Julie was now occasionally becoming confused, which caused a lot of distress both to her, as she realized she was not making sense, and to Michael, who had to watch her distress. But these episodes of confusion did not last long, and she could usually be calmed by being told that she was safe and that we were with her and would not leave her.

For most of the time, though, she remained quite lucid and well aware of how ill she was. She would ask occasionally why she had to continue like this and why she could not die immediately.

Paul, our chaplain, had become involved with Julie and Michael and he seemed able to give Julie some measure of comfort about this, but she commented several times that she should have died by now. Her deterioration was very, very slow and both she and Michael and the staff found this hard to cope with. They had both now accepted that she was dying but it took such a long time to happen. Each time her condition worsened, Michael prepared himself for her death, and then she would brighten up slightly. This happened several times and was very stressful for him.

He desperately wanted to be with Julie when she died and was very reluctant to leave her for more than a few minutes at a time, but was himself exhausted by now, and occasionally we could persuade him to go and have a sleep while a nurse sat with Julie.

He asked once if the doctors would give him something to keep him awake while Julie needed him, and it seems very ironic that when Julie did die, it was while Michael was asleep beside her. Michael was naturally very distressed at Julie's death and felt guilty that she had died alone while he slept.

He was too upset to lay Julie out himself as he had wished, but she was dressed as he had requested and her wedding ring removed for John. Michael did have her body brought home the day before her funeral as he had planned.

John appeared to accept Julie's death fairly well. Michael asked him if he wanted to attend the funeral, but John said he did not want to because "Everyone will be crying, and I don't want to cry anymore." He moved back from his grandparents to live with Michael and he had settled down again at school.

Michael continued his close contact with the hospice for several months after Julie's death. He returned two or three times each day until after the funeral and often telephoned at night to chat with the staff. He would give us a progress report on John, on how well he was doing at school, and how "He must get his brains from Julie." Michael then got a job as a milkman so that he could spend more time with John, collecting him from school and spending the rest of the day with him.

About six months later, he began trading on a market stall, often accompanied by John during his school holidays.

John appeared quite content, spending weekends with both sets of grandparents and enjoying life with Michael. Michael slowly seemed to come to terms with Julie's death, knowing he had done all he could to ensure that she died peacefully, with dignity, and that he was now fulfilling his promise to Julie to care for John always. He has now settled into a new relationship.

SECTION THREE

Caring for the nurse

AT FIRST, MANY STUDENT NURSES think that caring for the nurse sounds selfish—not at all the purpose of nursing. With experience, however, they begin to realize that they cannot care for others properly unless they care for themselves first.

This is true because nursing is a demanding and challenging profession. Not only is a nurse expected to use — and constantly upgrade — highly technical skills, but she or he also is expected to care for clients and families who face pain, suffering, and death.

The demand of caring deeply for others can cause a nurse to lose the balance needed to sustain caring. Caring for others can become so consuming that the nurse loses any sense of self. When this happens, the meaning of caring becomes clouded, and the nurse suffers detachment and burnout.

To help prevent burnout, Arnold (1989) has identified its causes, symptoms, and cures. She defines burnout as "exhaustion of physical and emotional strength...the end result of prolonged stress." She believes that "most nurses enter the profession with a healthy dose of idealism and commitment," which puts them at high risk for burnout if their "professional commitment becomes too one-sided and there is no room for other types of social and spiritual development."

Arnold cites many frustrations that can lead nurses to chronic stress and burnout. Such frustrations include: inadequate staffing, inadequate compensation, angry physicians, lack of recognition, client deaths, educational demands, improper equipment, unrealistic schedules, inappropriate assignments, frightened clients, interdisciplinary conflicts, rigid or unfair policies, unreasonable families, personal illness, and peer competition or conflict.

When dealing with these frustrations, some nurses show no outward signs of a stress reaction. Others, however, may develop such symptoms as anxiety, generalized tension, fatigue, confusion, inability to concentrate, and lack of energy.

According to Arnold, "In all cases of potential or actual burnout, there is a need to make whole, to reunite opposites, and to draw life back into balance." She sees burnout as an assault on the nurse's inner spirit, which makes life seem fragmented and meaningless. To help restore meaning and balance to the nurse's life, Arnold suggests the ABCs of healing spiritual burnout:

- Awareness. Development of an awareness of the strengths and limitations of personal coping skills.
- Balance. Achievement of balance by setting priorities that allow time for all aspects of living — family, work, education, and leisure.
- Choice. Making a deliberate choice to view a situation or oneself in a different way.
- Detached concern. Expression of detached concern by avoiding ego involvement or ambition and "doing the best one can at the moment," without worrying about the past or the future.
- Egoism. Development of altruistic egoism by discharging duties responsibly while accepting human frailties and limitations.
- Free will. Exercise of free will by directing personal actions and being responsible for — and persistent about — them.
- Goals. Establishment of goals that are designed to achieve inner harmony.

• Hope. Fostering of hope by building relationships, changing old ways of encountering life, and making a leap of faith.

By using these techniques, Arnold explains, the nurse will be able to expand the capacity to care. This, in turn, will promote personal involvement and a sense of connectedness with a larger community, giving greater meaning to the nurse's life.

The first article in this section, "Caring Comes First" by Benner and Wrubel, echoes some of Arnold's concepts and expands on others. The authors define burnout as a "loss of human caring." They describe several factors that make nurses feel vulnerable and suffer a diminished sense of self in caring for clients. They point out that some nurses withdraw emotionally and distance themselves from clients to avoid being hurt. Then they explain why this is a destructive way to cope with caregiving.

Based on some of the principles described in Section One, this article points out that caring is not the cause of burnout. Instead, it is the cure. Caring is the one characteristic that consistently gives meaning to life.

To help the nurse cope with caregiving, the authors suggest:

• acknowledging the pain — and possibilities — of caring for clients who are suffering, dying, or facing other difficulties.
• sharing secret fears about making mistakes and falling behind in the job's knowledge demands, and organizing educational sessions to prevent these fears.
• working to empower all nurses so that they can shape their own practice.
• understanding the ability of caring to liberate and enrich the client and the caregiver.

The next article, "Helper Secrets: Internal Stressors in Nursing" by Larson, takes a closer look at the dangers of "helper secrets," which Benner and Wrubel addressed briefly. Because nursing is demanding and emotionally complex, it can arouse self-doubts and emotions that may be embarrassing or difficult for the nurse to share with others. These disturbing thoughts and feelings — and the nurse's reactions to them — represent helper secrets. Such secrets can place additional stress on the nurse, which may lead to burnout and poor health.

Larson investigates nurses' secrets and uncovers the inner dilemmas nurses face in caring for clients. His study reveals nine categories of helper secrets that range from feelings of inadequacy and anger to descriptions of emotional and physical distancing. These common responses to chronically high-stress situations usually originate from self-blame, unrealistic self-expectations, and discrepancies between real and ideal self-images.

To help dissolve helper secrets and prevent burnout, Larson offers several antidotes that can promote growth and help nurses meet the challenge of caring. This article may be especially valuable to student nurses as they attempt to reconcile the ideals of their education with the realities of their practice.

REFERENCES

Arnold, E. (1989). Burnout as a spiritual issue: Rediscovering meaning in nursing. In V. Carson. (Ed.), *Spiritual Perspectives in Nursing Practice* (pp 324-353). Philadelphia: W.B. Saunders.

Caring comes first

PATRICIA BENNER, RN, PhD, FAAN; JUDITH WRUBEL, PhD

CARING, AS WE use the word, means persons, events, projects, and things *matter* to people. Because caring sets up what matters, it also sets up what counts as stressful. The risks and vulnerability inherent in caring can lead to the temptation to create safe places of "controlled caring" where the person dictates what matters and exercises the freedom to stop caring when the person or project is threatened.

Many stress-management strategies are designed to increase distance and control. However, if they are inappropriately used or understood to mean that detachment is always preferable and least "stressful," such distancing strategies can render the person unavailable to the possibilities and meanings inherent in caring, as this story by Mary Culnane, a clinical nurse specialist at NIH, shows.

> Jim Smith was 45 years old when I met him. He was happily married, had no children, worked in a bar, and was busy on weekends playing banjo in a country band. Because he had had an eight-hour period of slurred speech and blurred vision, he was admitted for a diagnostic workup to the unit where I worked.
>
> He and his wife had a lot of questions about the diagnostic tests. To help answer them, I took him to visit the procedural laboratories and introduced him to patients who had recently completed those particular tests.
>
> Two days after he went home with a negative workup, he was readmitted because of a seizure. I was on vacation at the time. By the time I returned, he had a diagnosis of metastatic lung cancer.
>
> I do not know how he responded to the initial diagnosis. When I returned, I didn't see him for a couple of days because I was really frightened—I did not know what to say or do. He made it easy for me and I began working with him again, teaching him about his chemotherapy and radiotherapy.
>
> I felt I was teaching him a lot, but actually he taught me. One day (probably after I had "delivered" some well-meaning technical information about his leukopenia), he said to me, "You are doing an OK job, Mary, but I can tell every time you walk in that door you are walking out."
>
> After this, clinical experiences were different for me. One Sunday when I was returning from lunch I heard some angry screaming. I recognized the voice. It was a man named Dave, in his early forties with a diagnosis of lung cancer. I can't remember all the treatments he had been through, although at the time he was going to receive a phase I agent.
>
> He was yelling that he wanted everything packed up. I felt a panic among the staff. It was a very disruptive outburst. It was apparent to me that he wanted to communicate. I went into his room and he yelled at me: "Are you listening?" Pretty calmly, I said, "Yes." He began crying softly and talking. He knew I was listening.
>
> For about an hour he told me about the first time he went to the oncologist, about his biopsy, waiting for results, the first time he had chemotherapy, what it was like to have a "recurrence." He reviewed his relationship with his family and friends. Ironically, he said what Jim Smith had said: "They are walking out when they come through that door." It was great that he wasn't saying that to me. I knew that I did not relate like that anymore.

The enabling condition of connection and concern is what we mean by the primacy of caring. Caring enables people to discern problems, to recognize possible solutions, and to implement those solutions. Caring makes the nurse notice which interventions help, causes the nurse to notice subtle signs of patient improvement or deterioration. In fact, caring — implementing a certain level of involvement — is required for any expert practice.[1]

Caring is primary because it sets up the condition of trust where help can be given and help can be received. This is why nursing can never be reduced to mere technique. The way medicines are given and the way patients are taught all have different effects when they are done in a context of care.

From analyzing the practice of expert nurses, it becomes clear that one cannot simply transfer effective interventions intact from one situation to another. The flexibility and diversity of expert practice depends on making the interventions unique through care and involvement. And so, caring is a concept that is central to our theory of nursing practice, as well as to our theory of stress and coping.

Tracey White describes the first two hours on an acute med-surg unit in a community hospital:

> I am in charge tonight with five nurses and 30 patients. Two of my nurses are floats who have never been on the floor; one will be an hour late so I will have to cover her patients.
>
> Our medical-surgical patients have diagnoses ranging from system failure of the kidney, stroke, diabetes, cancer, sickle-cell disease, hepatitis, AIDS, pneumonia to Alzheimer's disease. The average age of our patients is 79.
>
> We have five fresh postoperative patients and one going to surgery in two hours. As I come out of report, one of our stable patients who transferred from CCU yesterday is having chest pain. A doctor on the phone wants to give admission orders and the anesthetist for our preoperative patient wants the old chart *now*.
>
> Down the hall an elderly confused patient has just crawled over the side rails and fallen. Two of our fresh postop patients are vomiting as a side effect of anesthesia, their families are very tense and need reassuring.
>
> One of the patients I am covering for has just pulled out his IV; another wants something for pain; another needed the bedpan and I got there too late. The lab has called with a critically low hemoglobin level on the patient who pulled out his IV; he'll need a few units of blood as soon as possible.

In acute care, nurses daily confront life-threatening situations and complicated treatment regimens that have little margin for error. Moreover, the knowledge explosion in highly technical health care adds to the fear of failure. Nurses who work in hospitals must also confront the problems inherent in working in a complex organization where they lack the authority and recognition commensurate with the life-and-death responsibility of nursing care.

Furthermore, the demands of working in complex organizations are increased by chronic nursing shortages, ill-advised reductions in nursing staff to save money, and compressed salaries.

Coping with caregiving cannot be addressed without addressing the meanings and context of nursing care in society.

A major source of stress and a major stumbling block lie in society's devaluation of caring and the lack of social recognition and rewards accorded to caregiving. As long as society overvalues technology's heroic promises of freedom from pain and fails to recognize the care required to support the technology, those who provide care will feel the stress of being invisible and undervalued by society.

During the past 20 years, science and technology have become central to nursing practice. Nurses now have the only resident knowledge of administering and monitoring a wide range of diagnostic tests and treatments.[2,3] Nurses could make their claims for enhanced recognition, rights, and status simply on the basis of their highly specialized knowledge and ignore the battle to gain legitimacy and status for caring. But in the best of nursing schools, science and technology are only the tools for caring.

The modern epidemic: Burnout

The separation of caregiving and caring is a good definition for the modern epidemic of "burnout," which is defined as the loss of human caring.[4] When one is burned out, the world ceases to have meaningful distinctions. What once gave pleasure can feel like a demand.

It is a peculiarly modern mistake to think that caring is the *cause* of the "disease" of burnout, and that the cure is to protect oneself from caring. In fact, the loss of caring is the sickness. And the return of caring is recovery.

While pain may be numbed through disengagement, one is also numbed to the resources and support of others in the situation. Recovery from burnout requires rest and respite but it also requires the reintegration of concern and involvement.[2]

The right level

It is an art to know what to offer in a situation without overextending or assuming more responsibility for the situation than necessary. Weisman recommends that caregivers make the "least possible contribution":

"A little goes a long way; the least possible contribution is the one with the least strain but with the best chance of making a difference, however small. Having made this contribution, which may be very insignificant against the background of need, one can make another contribution, and still another, until something quite unanticipated but substantial results. Morale in everyone seems better, care is effective, one's plight is less painful. 'Least possible contribution' does not, of course, mean doing as little as possible, but doing only a little bit beyond the ordinary, something that most closely reflects the caregiver at his or her best."[5]

The art reflected by the maxim "least possible contribution" is offering what you can without dictating the results and recognizing that you are not the only one to contribute. It takes courage to be involved and to offer what you can even though it may not be enough.

Acknowledge the pain

Health care workers are repeatedly exposed to breakdown, tragedy, and death. Even with the best defenses, the nurse must confront the limits of control, the inevitability of death, and, in the case of violence, the very real presence of cruelty.

Health care workers may cope by using laughter, bravado, detachment, and elaborate self-protective maneuvers to feel immune to the calamity they confront, but these are temporary "Band-Aids." Acknowledgement, on the other hand, allows one to come to terms with feelings and move on.

Acknowledgement of threat and pain involved in caring for the suffering, the dying, and those confronted with major disability or disfigurement also opens the nurse to the possibilities in the situation as well as the pain. Nurses learn from patients and families the unimaginable courage and resilience of the human spirit.

In the final analysis there can be no magical reassurances or bravado, only the acknowledgement that the suffering is real, that it cannot be completely erased, and that we all would be imperiled if nurses were not there to care.

Keeping it a secret

Given the knowledge explosion in medicine and nursing, it is not surprising that many nurses fear making a mistake and fear not being able to keep up with the knowledge demands.[6] This understandable fear is rendered more stressful, according to Larson, because nurses often keep their fear of making mistakes a secret from colleagues. Pennebaker found that failure to express thoughts and feelings about a stressful event heightens the probability of obsessing about the event, as well as the probability of illness.[7]

The fear of making mistakes in patient care, where there is little margin for error, is reasonable and helpful if the fear causes the person to seek information. The fear becomes destructive if the person views it as a personal deficit and experiences isolation and shame.

Staff meetings need to be organized for the purpose of assessing educational needs and discussing the fear of mistakes, along with troubleshooting and debriefing after mistakes are made.

Knowledge workers

Nurses are the front line of defense for the patient and the contact point for all other departments and services. Providing care around the clock makes nurses the ones to fill in and substitute for all other departments that do not have the same level of continuity.

Despite the many demands nursing administrators and the hospital structure place on nurses, nurses have not uniformly been treated as knowledge workers. Instead, administrators have too often set up extensive rules, guidelines, and protocols inappropriate to the level of discretionary decision making required by professional nurses.

A new vision of the nurse as knowledge worker is needed. Programs of clinical promotion and participatory management, with nurses sitting on governing boards and central committees, are required so that nurses can have more power to shape their own practice. Empowering the practicing nurse is the best remedial action for the organizational stress that nurses confront in hospitals.

Caring intent

Expert caring has nothing to do with possessing privileged information that increases one's control and domination of another. Rather, expert caring unleashes the possibilities inherent in the self and the situation.

Expert caring liberates and facilitates in a way that the one caring is also enriched in the process.

When nurses are permitted to care for patients and families to the best of their knowledge and ability, the stresses in nursing are reduced to those legitimate to the realm of caring.

We do not seek to sentimentalize the difficulty and pain inherent in liberated caring. But we do want to point out the power, the challenge, and the stunning human victory when the difficulties are met with a caring intent....

REFERENCES

1. Dreyfus, Hubert L., and Dreyfus, Stuart E. *Mind Over Machine, The Power of Human Intuition and Expertise in the Era of the Computer*. New York, The Free Press, 1985.

2. Benner, Patricia. *From Novice to Expert: Excellence and Power in Clinical Nursing Practice*. Menlo Park, CA, Addison-Wesley Publishing Co., 1984.

3. Benner, P., and Tanner, C. Clinical judgment: how expert nurses use intuition. *Am.J.Nurs.* 87:23-31, Jan. 1987.

4. Maslach, C. *Burnout: The Costs of Caring* Englewood Cliffs, NJ, Prentice-Hall, 1982.

5. Weisman, A.D. Understanding the cancer patient: the syndrome of caregiver's plight. *Psychiatry*. 44:161-168, May 1981, p. 167.

6. Larson, Dale G. Internal stressors in nursing: helper secrets. *Psychosoc.Nurs.* 27:20-27, Apr. 1987.

7. Pennebacker, J.W. Traumatic experience and psychosomatic disease: exploring the roles of behavioral inhibition, obsession, and confiding. *Canadian Psychology*. 26:82-95, 1985.

Helper secrets: Internal stressors in nursing

DALE G. LARSON, PhD

To determine the nature of helper secrets, Larson asked 495 nurses from diverse clinical specialties to share their "secret behaviors, thoughts, and feelings related to their work by writing them on uniform sheets of paper." After the responses were used in an exercise, they were analyzed and assigned to one of the nine categories described in this article.

When reading this article, keep in mind that these secrets represent difficult, embarrassing thoughts and behaviors about work that the nurses in the study would not want to discuss openly. They required much soul searching and were gathered with the assurance of anonymity. They deserve your compassion and respect. Note: Excerpts (indicated by ellipses) condense extensive descriptions and examples.

THE SELF-DISCLOSURES of the nurses [below] reveal troubling thoughts and feelings about themselves and their work situations that are difficult to share with others. When these thoughts and feelings are kept inside and not confided, they can become "helper secrets" (Larson, 1985), and can act as invisible, internal stressors affecting the health and the job performance of the nurse. This article reports an initial investigation of the content — the major themes and issues — of nurses' helper secrets. A conceptual framework for thinking about helper secrets and recommendations for reducing their harmful impact are also presented....

> There are times when I'd like to shake some of the people I work with until they scream and cry. I hate detachment as a coping mechanism. I can't reach them and I don't feel like they can *hear* me. So how on earth can we deal deeply with patients, families, and each other?

> If I had been more knowledgeable and insistent about having a doctor come in for a late deceleration [a fetal heart rate pattern indicative of fetal distress], that baby would be about four years old today.

> Sometimes I feel as if I'm just barely getting by—my knowledge and skills are not enough for the job I am currently doing and there are big mistakes just waiting to happen.

"I feel inadequate"

One of the most frequently occurring themes inthese nurses' secrets is the feeling that "I am incompetent" or that "I am inadequate." Twenty percent of the secrets were assigned to this category. A feeling of being almost an imposter — someone posing as a competent professional, but lacking the expertise to do the job — is common.

> I feel I can't keep up with the fast pace of change in medicine and stay *current and safe* in my practice and lectures. As an educator and part-time worker in L&D, I'm presumed "on top," "most current," and "best read"— never makes mistakes. I'm human too.

> I feel I've really fooled the world. That I'm in this position and people think well of me... I'm not that great....

The prevalence of this kind of helper secret in this sample is not surprising for two reasons.

First, it is consistent with other research findings. Feelings of inadequacy and incompetence are also frequent themes in the secrets of other helper and non-helper populations (Larson; Norton, 1974). Second, feelings of inadequacy and strong self-doubt are understandable given the many challenges facing today's nurse, not the least of which are staying current with rapidly changing medical technologies and negotiating complex psychosocial tasks on a daily basis.

When a mistake can make the difference between life and death, these self-doubts can mushroom into what might be called a "terror of error" experience:

> I'm afraid of being caught in a crisis (life/death) situation of mother and/or baby when no doctor is around and other staff are too busy to help me — I'll do something wrong or fail to do the right thing.

"Errors" inevitably occur and, as the next secrets illustrate, the emotional consequences for the caregiver can be quite powerful and persistent.

> Sometimes I feel that I've been careless, giving the wrong IV and rate to a patient. Instead of helping him, I'm making things worse. God! I feel so guilty and I have sleepless nights worrying what the consequences can be.

> I made an error once and never told anyone and have always worried about it.

One-way giving: "What about me"

One-way giving is built into the practice of nursing. Of course, there are moments of reciprocity — a deeply felt thank you from a patient or family member, an award, unsolicited caring from a co-worker — but these events do not change the fundamental reality that in nursing, as in other human services professions, the focus is on the recipients of care (Pines, 1982) and there is no guarantee that helpers will receive anything more in return for their services than a paycheck and the intrinsic satisfaction of helping others.

A small but significant group of secrets contain direct expressions of a desire to receive — as well as to give — caring and appreciation from patients, patients' families, and staff. Although these secrets represent only 3% of the total secrets, they poignantly highlight an important stressor in nursing practice.

> Sometimes I wish I weren't a nurse — because I don't want to give anymore and don't want to have to keep constantly learning. I resent it. I want to be taken care of — me.

> I sometimes get to the point where I can't pick up a baby and hold and cuddle him/her because I can't "give" anymore. I'm the one that needs to be held and rocked!

These secrets usually include a voice from within that is asking "What about me?" as well as critical feelings toward oneself for not being assertive in getting one's own needs met. Nurses holding these secrets are...burnout-prone....

Too many demands

Another theme, one closely related to that of one-way giving and found in 5% of the disclosures, is difficult feelings associated with emotional and physical demands at work and at home:

> Trying to be supermom, supernurse, and superwife sometimes burdens me so. When I fail in one area, there is a domino effect. I hate to fail.

> Sometimes I feel like too much is expected — janitor, counselor, maid, mother, sister, etc. It makes me feel like I'm being manipulated and drained. I feel resentful.

These self-disclosures underline the fact that even the most common stressors encountered by nurses, such as being overburdened by multiple roles at work and at home, have the potential to create an inner turmoil that is then kept concealed from others. These nurses would probably feel relatively comfortable confiding about the excessive demands they face. However, the experiences that are more difficult for these nurses to discuss openly —those that are kept concealed — are the feelings of "hating to fail," the pain when the "domino effect" occurs, "feeling manipulated and drained," and the "resentment." These are their secrets.

"I'm angry"

Unspoken anger, frustration, and impatience—with patients, family members, co-workers, physicians, and hospital administration — is one of the most frequently occurring themes in the secrets.

> There are times when I feel like screaming or kicking or hitting something — like I'm about to lose control — but I usually just make tight fists, breathe, and then return to the situation looking and hopefully acting calm, in control, and like a nurse. It's very hard, often painful.

Sometimes this anger can have an extremely traumatic impact:

> A couple of weeks ago, I was feeling really burned out and I had a newborn who wouldn't eat, and when I gavaged (tube-fed) him, he spit all the formula back up, and I gritted my teeth and became so angry at the baby, it really scared me because I felt like I could have hit him or something for not eating. I waited about 15 minutes and then tried to feed him again, feeling much better, but I really felt guilty for a *long* time.

Not only patients but doctors, fellow nurses, and administration are targets of the nurse's unexpressed anger and frustration:

> Sometimes I feel like I'd really like to tell a few certain arrogant doctors to stop feeding their egos through their ill patients, and that their patients aren't the only sick patients in the hospital.

> Why does it seem to take a disastrous event to make the "powers that be" initiate change? It puts the staff in a very bad situation of waiting for some terrible event to happen so change for the better is mandatory.

"I'm in over my head"

Another central theme was reflected in descriptions of being emotionally overly involved in work situations — a kind of empathic overarousal. Nurses are constantly moving back and forth on a continuum of emotional involvement, from highly-involved to less-involved stances, and vice versa. The "I'm in over my head" secrets describe experiences at the extreme high-involvement end of this continuum. These secrets often included feelings of helplessness or fear and conveyed the message "I'm really hurting" or "That situation is really difficult for me because of the emotional buttons it pushes in me."

> I hate coming to work because I feel once I'm here it engulfs me like fire.

> The very worst times are the ones when I have felt so much and hurt so long for a family that finally I can't feel anything at all.

Every nurse — every helper, for that matter —must find a way to be emotionally involved with patients and families that is helpful, congruent with one's unique helping style, and not overwhelming. The desire to help others and the capacity to be deeply empathic are probably a nurse's greatest assets — but they can also be liabilities. Stotland and his colleagues (1978) found that student nurses scoring highest on a measure of empathic capacity were the first to leave the rooms of dying patients. The nurses could imagine what it was like to be in that bed, feeling that pain, and dying, and they were overwhelmed. Later, after receiving supervision and support, these nurses proved to be the best helpers. They had to learn how to use that extra empathy, how to be empathic without burning out. This task, a central challenge for every nurse, might be called the challenge of caring.

Emotional and physical distancing

More than one out of every five helper secrets in this sample contained descriptions of wanting to or having actually emotionally or physically distanced oneself from patients, patients' families, staff, or personal family members. This distancing took many forms: becoming "emotionally distant," "ignoring patients' needs," "avoiding visiting the difficult patient," "withdrawing," "holding a part of myself back," and "feeling cold and unsympathetic" are just a few examples.

These experiences might be placed at the low-involvement end of the continuum discussed above. Here the difficulty is that the nurse, often in an effort to avoid getting "in over her head," moves toward the other end of the emotional involvement continuum. However, the paradoxical reality for the nurse is that these attempts to distance him or herself emotionally or physically often raise, not lower, stress levels. Efforts to decrease emotional involvement through emotional distancing and avoidance lead to feelings of self-doubt, guilt, and personal and professional inadequacy that augment distress and make this an untenable long-term stance (Kolotkin, 1981). This stress-avoidance-guilt sequence is reflected in many of the following disclosures.

> Sometimes when caring for a critical baby, I shut myself off from the parents and avoid them at all costs—sometimes I also avoid that patient if possible. I feel like I'm abandoning the parents and I'm dumping the patient on someone else (especially if it is a baby I took care of continuously when he/she was well).

> I feel guilty that my caregiving has become more emotionally distant. Seems I'm protecting myself. I don't want to give so much of my energy to others' lives or my work.

Wishing for a patient's death

When patients are enduring agonizing suffering, with no hope of recovery, or when the prognosis for a reasonable quality of life is poor, continuing life-saving interventions can become a highly conflicted arena for the nurse. Another theme in these nurses' disclosures is strong emotion — empathic distress, guilt, and anger — experienced in these trying situations:

> I have felt relieved and thankful that a baby with multiple anomalies did not survive long enough for the transplant team to arrive. The entire family needed support, and I felt guilty about my thankfulness and tried not to let that show.

> Sometimes I wish I could pull the plug on someone I know will have a poor quality of life.

The frequency of such thoughts and feelings in this secrets sample suggests that greater efforts to discuss staff feelings surrounding care of terminally-ill patients are sorely needed.

"I want out"

This final group of secrets (3% of all secrets) contained direct expressions of a desire to leave the nursing field or one's job:

> This is too much. I don't want to work in this place anymore.

> I wish I could earn money equivalent to nursing so I could quit right away.

Other

Eleven percent of the secrets were assigned to the "Other" category. Secrets coded as Other included multiple-secret responses, philosophical comments, personal secrets unrelated to the work situation, and other responses not meeting the criteria for inclusion in any of the above eight categories.

The self-concealment/stress connection

The helper secrets presented here reflect a wide range of traumatic and personally distressing experiences endured by these nurses as part of their everyday work. By inhibiting processes of healing communication and promoting cognitive obsession, helper secrets can increase the likelihood that these difficult experiences will result in long-term stress-related illnesses and burnout. Designing appropriate interventions to prevent these health consequences requires a better understanding of the origins of helper secrets.

Origins of helper secrets

Tendency toward self-blame. People approaching burnout often misperceive its cause. They tend to think that their exhaustion or conflicts or "failures" reflect a lack of competence. Even though they know their work is stressful, they tend to blame themselves for their problems, struggles, and undesirable outcomes. They tend to look for some inadequacy in themselves when they fail with a patient, when they do not reach their goals, or when they are dissatisfied. Maslach calls this tendency the "mea culpa reaction." This kind of self-doubt and lowered self-esteem was a major theme in the secrets gathered here.

Unrealistic self-expectations. Unrealistic self-expectations are another major cause of the self-doubt, self-blame, and lowered self-esteem that characterize helper secrets. Questioning oneself and the work one does is inevitable when helping others. Self-examination is an important skill; however, blame and guilt can destroy this process. Expecting too much of oneself is a formula for defeat; controlling that tendency is essential.

Discrepancies between real and ideal images of self as a helper. The inner struggle reflected in many of these secrets can be viewed as a conflict between the nurses' idealized self-concepts as helpers and the thoughts, feelings, and behaviors revealed in their secrets. For example, nurses expressing secrets containing the theme of "one-way giving" could be comparing their actual experiences of overload and lack of appreciation with an idealized image of the nurse as totally other-oriented and all-giving. Because feelings of "what about me" are not congruent with these idealized (and internalized) images of the "good nurse," they are concealed and not openly confided. Similarly, the "I'm angry" secrets presented earlier express an inner conflict between the nurses' experiences of intense anger and their images of the "good nurse." We can infer that for these nurses the "good nurse" is in control and doesn't have strong negative feelings such as these, or if they do, they don't let others know about them.

Thus, the internal process of the nurse might go something like this: "I am a caring and giving person. That's why I got into this work in the first place. How can I feel such strong anger toward patients, distance myself, and ignore patients' needs? Why do I have to pretend to be interested? Is there something wrong with me? If my peers knew this about me they would also think less of me."

This negative self-talk becomes an internal stressor that can make even the brightest of helping flames at least flicker, if not burn out.

The fallacy of uniqueness

Again, what is so intriguing about many of these helpers' secrets is the very fact that they are kept secret. Of course, the secrets gathered here ranged from those that had been discussed with many people to those told to no one. However, the comments of many participants suggested that their helper secrets were actively concealed from others—that they had considered discussing them but had not, or had done so only once. How can we explain this pervasive phenomenon of self-concealment? The social psychology concept of the "fallacy of uniqueness," as described by Pines and Aronson, adds to our understanding:

> In our society it is often undesirable to admit one's limitations, vulnerabilities, ignorance, and problems, especially in one's work. A professional is expected to be impeccable and in control. When problems do arise, most people feel at fault and hide the problems from others, feeling that "everybody else" is coping effectively and they alone are failing. The result is what social psychologists call the "fallacy of uniqueness" or "pluralistic ignorance"; the individual's false assumption that he or she is the only one responding in this way.

The irony is that some, maybe all, of the nurse's co-workers are probably feeling the same way, but most likely no one talks about it. When helpers do talk about their stress and learn to see it as an inevitable part of the work, constructive action can take place.

Antidotes to helper secrets

Both research and our informed intuitions suggest that the best antidote to self-concealment is self-revelation, and that the choice of confidants and of the context for this self-disclosure are important considerations. Friends, family, and other members of one's social support network can provide one arena for these disclosures. However, helper secrets are perhaps best shared with someone else who does the same kind of work, someone who can have "instant empathy" with these difficult feelings....

Assuming that an atmosphere of trust and support exists, regularly scheduled staff support meetings can be highly facilitative contexts for these disclosures. Here, each of the factors contributing to the development and persistence of helper secrets is met with an opposing force. Group members go from "I'm the only one having a difficult time with this" to learning that they are "all in the same boat"— that everyone has difficulty with the stressful and sometimes seemingly impossible situations encountered in nursing work. Unrealistic self-expectations and images of oneself as a helper are tempered and corrected through dialogue with peers. Difficult feelings are shared, worked through, and normalized. Once this occurs, the bias toward self-blame can be corrected, and one's energies can be directed toward developing better coping and problem-solving skills and strategies (Maslach).

A good illustration of what can happen when helper secrets are communicated in a safe and supportive context is provided by the experiential exercise conducted during the data gathering phase of this research. In each of the large groups from which the secrets were gathered the cards with the secrets and no other identifying information on them were randomly redistributed so that no one knew whose secret they held. All the secrets were then read out loud and the other participants were asked to share feelings and thoughts of their own similar to those expressed in the secret being read.

The listening group members could always find some part of the experience conveyed in the secret with which they could self-disclose in response. Sometimes the entire room was filled with nodding heads. A tremendous sense of relief — for both the author of the secret and the listeners — came in knowing that one is "not alone" in having these thoughts and feelings. Many nurses indicated that what had just ten minutes earlier been a well-kept secret had now become a topic they could discuss with others.

Conclusion

Helper secrets alert us to our inner crises as helpers. The Chinese pictograph for crisis is composed of two characters, one signifying danger, the other opportunity. Helper secrets have a similar twofold nature. Though frequently quite painful, they contain information vital to the nurse's survival as a helper by pointing to difficult areas of experience that demand greater attention and signaling a need to make some changes. When kept concealed, helper secrets can corrode from within; when revealed to empathic listeners, they can promote personal and professional growth and aid the nurse in meeting the challenge of caring.

REFERENCES

Budd, R.W., Thorp, R.K., Donohew, L. *Content Analysis of Communications*. New York: Macmillan, 1967.

Goodman, G. *SASHAtapes: Self-led Automated Series on Help Intended Alternatives*. New York: BMA Audiotapes, Guilford Press, 1979.

Kolotkin, R.A. Preventing burn-out and reducing stress in terminal care: The role of assertive training, in Sobel, H.J. (ed.): *Behavior Therapy in Terminal Care: A Humanistic Approach*. Cambridge, Massachusetts: Ballinger, 1981.

Larson, D.G. Helper secrets: Invisible stressors in hospice work. *American Journal of Hospice Care* 1985; 2:35-40.

Maslach, C. *Burnout: The Cost of Caring*. Englewood Cliffs, New Jersey: Prentice-Hall, 1982.

Norton, R., Feldman, C., Tafoya, D. Risk parameters across types of secrets. *Journal of Counseling Psychology* 1974; 21:450-454.

Pennebaker, J.W. Traumatic experience and psychosomatic disease: Exploring the roles of behavioral inhibition, obsession, and confiding. *Canadian Psychology* 1985; 26:82-95.

Pines, A., Aronson, E. *Burnout: From Tedium to Personal Growth*. New York: Free Press, 1981.

Steiner, C.M. *Scripts People Live*. New York: Bantam, 1974.

Stotland, E., Mathews, K.E. Jr., Sherman, S.E., et al. *Empathy, Fantasy, and Helping*. Beverly Hills, California: Sage Publications, Inc., 1978.

UNIT ONE

Study questions

1. In "The Phenomenon of Caring: Importance, Research Questions and Theoretical Considerations," Leininger describes several types of caring. How is professional nursing care different from generic care or caring? How is it similar?

2. According to "The Ethic of Caring: Can It Survive in Nursing?" factors such as the nursing shortage, unsafe staffing patterns, and payment-directed nursing care plans threaten the survival of caring. How do these factors interfere with caring? How great an impact do you think they will have on the ethic of caring? Why?

3. In "The Primacy of Caring," Orlick and Benner discuss two aspects of nursing that are common to all expert practice: the primacy and power of care as necessary to cure, and the way that nurses establish themselves as members and participants in the client's community. Describe a clinical experience that portrays caring behaviors. How would you compare the nursing aspects of your experience with the ones described in the reading?

4. "Advocacy in Nursing" offers several definitions of the term *advocacy*. Choose one definition and discuss how it relates to caring.

5. A client's family can be a resource or a limitation in planning the client's care. Based on the article "Caring for Julie," how did Julie's family affect her care? What techniques did Julie's nurses use to care for her and her family?

6. In the reading "Caring Comes First," Benner and Wrubel suggest that nurses should make the "least possible contribution." What does this mean? What is the value of this practice? How does it reflect expert caring?

7. According to "Helper Secrets: Internal Stressors in Nursing," nurses frequently suffer from bottling up their thoughts about emotional and physical distancing, feelings of inadequacy, anger, and other concerns. Select a helper secret and discuss its possible origins and cure.

UNIT TWO

Unifying concepts basic to nursing

THIS UNIT BUILDS on the caring described in Unit One by providing important information and insights into the concepts of client systems and the environments that influence those systems. These interrelated concepts are common to the practice of all nurses.

Client systems

The term *client system* refers to the recipient of nursing care and the factors affecting that recipient. To be meaningful, caring must have a recipient. So the nurse directs care to the self or the client system, which can be an individual, family, small group, or community. The client system concept helps unify a profession that is rich in diversity. For regardless of the specialty or practice site, the nurse always focuses on a client or client system.

The nurse is concerned with the factors that place the client at risk for illness. Such factors may include physiology (as in Unit Seven), psychosocial concerns (as in Unit Six), lifestyle, age, or family history. The nurse is also concerned with the client's strengths and available supports that can help promote a positive response to illness.

Environment

The client system does not exist in a vacuum: It constantly interacts with the environment (all factors that affect the client's life and survival). Therefore, the nurse must be concerned with the effects of environmental factors. Because the environment interacts with every client in every setting, it represents a unifying concept that is fundamental to nursing.

The environment can be divided into external and internal. The external environment includes factors outside the client, such as the physical environment (air and water quality, for example) and social and cultural factors.

Social factors include the presence or absence of a support network of relationships, access to health care, and the availability of jobs, finances, and housing. These factors can help or hinder a client in times of need, such as loss of income, or in personal crises, such as death of a loved one.

Also, these factors can affect the client's ability to use the nursing help that is offered. For example, an individual who lives in a rural area and has limited access to health care may not be able to come to a downtown clinic for follow-up visits. A family with a limited income may not be able to afford costly treatments for a sick child.

The client's cultural traditions may influence such things as the definition of health and illness, the family's role in promoting care, and the type of health care sought. For in-

Glossary

Client system: recipient of nursing care (which may be an individual, family, small group, or community) and all of the internal and external factors affecting that recipient.

Culture: all learned and shared values, beliefs, customs, and behaviors of a group of interacting people; the "personality" of a people. Cultural factors represent an important part of the external environment.

Environment: all factors that affect the client system's life and survival. The environment may be divided into external and internal environments. The external environment includes factors outside the client, such as the physical environment (air and water quality, for example) and social and cultural factors. The internal environment includes factors within the client, such as physical (genetics, physiology, and disease), mental (intelligence, creativity), and spiritual factors (beliefs, sense of meaning or purpose).

Social factors: an aspect of the external environment that includes such things as the presence or absence of a support network of relationships, access to health care, and the availability of jobs, finances, and housing.

Social relationships: a client's interactions with others, which may involve birth, friendship, marriage, stress, economic hardship, and personal crises such as loss of a loved one.

Spirituality: a client's relationship with a supreme being as well as his or her beliefs about the meaning of life. Spirituality, which is not necessarily related to organized religion, is an important factor in the internal environment.

stance, a client from a minority group may seek health care from a cultural healer who specializes in remedies that are outside traditional medicine. The nurse must recognize and accept these practices. Otherwise, the care provided by the health care team can conflict with that of a cultural healer, possibly leading to client noncompliance and to unresolved or increased health problems.

A nurse who understands cultural differences can respond to the client with respect — rather than intolerance or derision — for beliefs that differ from those held by the health care establishment. This approach will promote trust, facilitate a good nurse-client relationship, and may help the client supplement cultural healing practices with more traditional medical procedures, if necessary.

The internal environment includes factors within the client, such as physical factors (genetics, physiology, disease), mental factors (intelligence, creativity), and spiritual factors (beliefs, sense of meaning or purpose). The nurse can obtain information about internal environmental factors by observing the client system's actions and interactions. For example, an individual who speaks well and has an extensive vocabulary may have above-average intelligence. A family that prays together daily may have a strong sense of spirituality.

Internal environmental factors can directly affect the client system. For example, the client system's spirituality can interact with and give meaning to all other experiences, including illness. In fact, the psychologist Carl Jung (1933) believed that, in all illness, at the heart of healing is a quest for spiritual meaning.

When individuals, families, small groups, and communities can find opportunities for spiritual sustenance and growth in illness, death, and other misfortunes, healing is greatly facilitated. With its emphasis on caring and its holistic approach to the client system and the environment, nursing can assist in this process.

REFERENCES

Jung, C. (1933). *Modern Man in Search of a Soul.* New York: Harcourt, Brace, & Co.

SECTION ONE

Client systems concept

SECTION ONE EXAMINES the ways that nurses use themselves with client systems in therapeutic (professional helping) relationships. To develop a therapeutic relationship with a client system, the nurse can use personal qualities, such as caring, compassion, empathy, humor, and problem-solving and communication skills. The ability to use these personal qualities is often referred to as "therapeutic use of self."

Although experts differ on the exact definition of this term, they all agree that the abilities it implies are essential to all therapeutic relationships. For when the nurse extends these abilities — the very essence of his or her being — to help the client system, the nurse places that individual, family, small group, or community at the heart of caring and healing.

Whall (1988) views therapeutic use of self as an important concept, especially in geriatric nursing where an elderly client may be cut off from former interpersonal relationships and forced to establish new ones. Whall offers the following description of this vital skill:

> Although the critical attributes of this concept are not agreed upon, it has been discussed at length in nursing. To many, it means using oneself as an instrument or a means wherein the "other" [patient] may experience a healing force or a corrective emotional experience and thus, may grow and change. Although the limits of this relationship must be delineated by professional norms, the term implies becoming an important healing source to the patient. Rather than applying or simply using techniques or procedures, therapeutic use of self implies more of a reaching out...to others.
>
> When attempting to use oneself as a therapeutic agent, the nurse should ask, (1) Why am *I* doing this? (2) Who will benefit *most* from these actions/activities? and (3) Will the patient experience positive growth and change from the relationship?

The answers to these questions provide concrete direction to an important — yet sometimes elusive — nursing task.

"Conceptual Components of the Therapeutic Relationship" by Arnold and Boggs investigates the four basic elements in a therapeutic relationship: caring, trust, empathy, and mutuality. The nursing student and the professional nurse must understand these concepts and be able to use them in interactions with client systems. In addition to the nurse's ability to apply therapeutic use of self, these concepts are at the core of therapeutic relationships. For without caring, trust, empathy, and mutuality, relationships are sterile and devoid of healing power. The student will benefit from the authors' explanations of these concepts and the clinical examples that bring the concepts to life.

The other article in this section, "The Family as the Unit of Care in Nursing: A Historical Review" by Whall, looks at nursing's past and current therapeutic relationships with the family as the client system. Based on an extensive literature review, the author reports great support for the notion that the family unit was — and continues to be — a focus of nursing care. Whall also identifies several trends in family nursing care, from the earliest efforts of the first public health nurses to the most recent work of nursing leaders who focus on the family as a unit of nursing care.

A student nurse will benefit from Whall's summary of the ideas of several 20th-century nursing theorists about the family as a client system. She also discusses the family as a context within which the client exists because, although the client is an individual, he or she is linked to a family in ways that can dramatically affect health and health care.

REFERENCES

Whall, A.L. (1988). Geropsychiatry: Therapeutic use of self. *Journal of Gerontological Nursing, 14*(2), 38-39.

Conceptual components of the therapeutic relationship

ELIZABETH ARNOLD, PhD; KATHLEEN BOGGS, RN, PhD

This article, taken from Interpersonal Relationships: Professional Communications Skills for Nurses *by Arnold and Boggs, focuses on the most important components of therapeutic relationships. It provides theoretical information about these components and useful techniques for their application in nursing practice. Note: Excerpts (marked by ellipses) have removed student exercises and shortened some clinical examples.*

...THE ESTABLISHMENT OF a therapeutic relationship relies upon the comprehension and application of the concepts of caring, trust, empathy, and mutuality. Other concepts such as anxiety, stereotyping, personal space, and confidentiality add dimensional qualities to the relationship. Although these concepts may be easily understood, much practice is needed to implement techniques that convey feelings of caring, warmth, accepting, and understanding to the client....

Caring

Caring is a commitment by the nurse to become involved. The caring is relational in character. Nurses enter the experience with their whole being. It involves clients in their struggle for health rather than simply doing for clients those actions they cannot perform for themselves. It includes the act of giving freely and willingly of oneself to another through warmth, compassion, concern, and interest. Nurses care for others during times of physical discomfort, emotional stress, and health maintenance. According to Gault (1983), nurses express caring as a concern for others, as exemplified in the statement, "I care about your health," as a responsibility, as in the statement, "I will be caring for you today," and as a fondness or attachment, as in the statement, "I like you and care for you."

Caring includes treating others with respect out of kindness and consideration. Caring individuals recognize others as separate and unique persons with various needs. Through caring, nurses identify client needs, implement appropriate nursing actions, make knowledgeable decisions, and bring about positive changes in clients (Gault, 1983).

Trust

According to Eric Erikson (1963), trust is the reliance on the consistency, sameness, and continuity of experience that are provided by an organized combination of familiar and predictable things and people. Trust is based on past experiences and begins in infancy through consistent and continual care by the same caregiver. It allows the infant to believe in self, in others, and in the external world. Through trust, one learns how to cope with the world and resolve frustrations and problems. Characteristics of a trusting relationship include respect, honesty, consistency, faith, and hope.

A therapeutic relationship begins with trust. The nurse begins the relationship with a genuine sense of caring. The client accepts help from the nurse and moves toward changes in lifestyle and behaviors. Certain techniques will promote a trusting relationship (Table 4-1).... Once a sense of trust is established between two people, a sharing of feelings and emotions occurs.

Trust, however, can be broken. For example,

an alcoholic or abusive parent may be gentle one minute and explode with anger the next, leaving children and others unsure of how the parent will behave. The community-health nurse who is always late for client appointments and interviews and the pediatric nurse who indicates falsely that an injection will not hurt are at risk of jeopardizing their therapeutic relationships. In order for a trusting relationship to continue, trust must be reinforced. Otherwise, trust may be destroyed during a negative experience.

Clients can also jeopardize the trust a nurse has in them. Sometimes, clients may "test" a nurse's trustworthiness. They may try to send the nurse on unnecessary errands or talk endlessly about superficial topics. As long as nurses recognize testing behaviors and set clear limits on their roles and the client's role, trust will ensue....

Empathy

Empathy is the ability to accurately perceive another's emotions and communicate the meanings of feelings to the other through verbal and nonverbal behaviors. The goal of empathy is to communicate hidden emotions and their meanings of which the client is unaware. Objective and nonjudgmental nurses feel the emotions that a client feels, but at the same time maintain their own separate identities. The nurse should not overidentify with or internalize the feelings of the client. If internalization occurs, objectivity is lost, along with the ability to empathize. It is important to recognize that the client's feelings belong to the client, not the nurse.

Attaining high levels of empathy, although difficult, is rewarding to both nurse and client. Carkhuff (1969) identifies five levels of empathy. From least to most empathic, they are:...

1. *Unawareness of client's message or feelings.* Unawareness is the lowest level of empathy. Since there is no evidence of active listening or understanding of the client's feelings, the nurse's response communicates significantly less than the client's.

> *Client* (frantic): "Bobby (10 months old) has had a terrible cold for more than a week."
> *Nurse* (hurriedly, not looking at client): "Is he up-to-date on his immunizations?"

In this example, the nurse ignores the feeling tone of the client and changes the subject to serve the desire for information. The nurse's insensitivity may arise from boredom, uninterest, bias, or differing reasons for communication.

TABLE 4-1. Techniques designed to promote trust

Convey respect	Be flexible
Consider the client's uniqueness	Provide for allowed preferences
Show warmth and caring	Be honest and open
Use the client's proper name	Give complete information
Use active listening	Provide consistency
Give sufficient time to answer questions	Plan schedules
Maintain confidentiality	Follow through on commitments
Show congruency between verbal and nonverbal behaviors	Set limits
Use a warm, friendly voice	Control distractions
Use appropriate eye contact	Use an attending posture: arms, legs, and body relaxed; leaning slightly forward
Smile	

2. *Superficial acknowledgment of client's message; minimizes client's feelings.* The nurse shows awareness of superficial feelings but responds in a way that detracts noticeably from the emotions expressed by the client.

> *Client* (frantic): "Bobby has had a terrible cold for more than a week."
> *Nurse* (casually glancing briefly at client): "This is the time of year for colds. Everyone has one. He'll get over it."

This example shows that the nurse responds to the client's concern, the content of the statement, but not to the feeling tone of the client. The nurse minimizes and degrades the client's feelings.

3. *Recognition of client's message and some of client's feelings.* This level is minimally facilitative, unlike the first two levels, which do not foster a therapeutic relationship. In level three, the nurse responds to the same meaning of emotions as the client. Verbal and nonverbal behaviors are congruent. The nurse's words are interchangeable with the client's.

> *Client* (frantic): "Bobby has had a terrible cold for more than a week."
> *Nurse* (tone of voice same as client's, making eye contact, leaning forward in chair): "You're upset that Bobby has had this cold for more than a week." [Level 3]
> *Client* (crying): "Yeah. He's so little, and I want him to get better."
> *Nurse* (breaks eye contact and leaves): "He'll get better. The doctor will be in momentarily to examine him." [Level 2]

The nurse's first response shows a level-three empathy. The nurse accurately interprets this superficial feeling tone of the client. The nurse then reverts to a level-two response, however, and essentially ignores the client's tears. Level-three responses are often a beginning to higher-level responses, which reflect the client's hidden emotions. Nurses who are unable to cope with deep feelings are unable to develop empathy beyond levels two and three.

4. *Acknowledgment of message and obvious feelings.* Level four responses add to the client's feelings and their meanings somewhat. There are still deep hidden meanings of which the nurse is unaware.

> *Client* (frantic): "Bobby has had a terrible cold for more than a week."
> *Nurse* (same voice tone as client, making eye contact, with attending, open posture): "You are quite upset about this, aren't you?"
> *Client* (softly spoken with tears): "Yes. He's so little, and he just has to get better."
> *Nurse:* "You're afraid it might develop into something worse?" [Level 4]
> *Client*: "Could he have pneumonia?"
> *Nurse:* "I don't know. The doctor will examine him soon. How would you feel if he had pneumonia?" [Information—asking]
> *Client:* "Oh, I couldn't stand to have him in the hospital away from me."
> *Nurse:* "You feel anxious about the possibility of hospitalization, in which the two of you would be separated and it's so important at Bobby's age to preserve your close relationship." [Level 4]
> *Client:* "Yes, being separated would be awful."

In this example, the nurse begins responding on Level 3, and then moves to Level 4 responses. The nurse reflects slightly hidden feelings but has not accurately perceived deeper feelings. Level 4 responses increase the client's awareness of his or her own feelings. Often, Level 4 responses build upon Level 3 responses, as well as information-gathering questions, which increase the nurse's knowledge about the client and increase the probability of an accurate assessment of emotions.

5. *Full therapeutic acknowledgment of client's*

hidden message and meaning. Level 5 empathy includes therapeutic responses, which add significantly to the meanings behind the feelings. Because the nurse has a clearer, more objective view than the client, the nurse is able to state deep, hidden feelings unknown to the client.

Review the example from level 4 and begin with the client's response:

> *Client:* "Oh, I couldn't stand to have him in the hospital away from me."
> *Nurse:* "What is it about the hospital separation from Bobby that makes you so anxious? [Reflects hidden feelings, asks for more information.]
> *Client:* "It's just his being in a *hospital*."
> *Nurse* (questions, still same feeling tone): "Have you or anyone else ever been hospitalized?"
> *Client:* "My brother when he was young."
> *Nurse* (question again): "And what was he there for?"
> *Client:* "Pneumonia. And then he died there of complications!"
> *Nurse:* "So now you're frightened that if Bobby has pneumonia and is hospitalized, he will die, too, like your brother." [Reflects deep feelings]

The nurse, then, goes on to give information about pneumonia and some reassurance of its treatment. She communicates the client's feelings to the physician so that the physician can discuss Bobby's diagnosis and treatment with the client to lessen the client's anxiety.

In this example the nurse is able to communicate deep feelings after gathering information and using lower levels of empathy. Often, clients are unable to voice deep feelings of fear, loneliness, emptiness, sadness, grief, anger, rejection, hurt, betrayal, vulnerability, helplessness, uselessness, and worry. By communicating empathy, the nurse assists the client in understanding hidden feelings. The understanding can then mobilize energy to cope with the feelings and solve the problem.

Empathy is an essential skill for competent nursing care. It allows for a more accurate needs assessment of the client and a more thorough care plan. Imagine the difference in outcomes between a nurse's responses on levels 2 and 3 as compared with responses on levels 4 and 5. The quality of care increases directly with the levels of empathy. Attaining high degrees of empathy requires practice and self-evaluation....

Levels of nursing actions. Nursing actions that facilitate empathy are classified by Clay (1984) into four major hierarchical categories: accepting, listening, clarifying and informing, and analyzing. *Accepting behaviors* are those that recognize the client as a unique individual. The nurse identifies the client by name, maintains an attentive open posture, responds to verbal and nonverbal cues through appropriate gestures and facial expressions, uses intermittent eye contact, and allows self-expression by the client.

The second level of empathic nursing actions is *listening behaviors*. These responses encourage client participation. They include head nodding, smiling. Also included are the use of verbal prompts, such as "Hmmm," "Uh-huh," "I see," "Tell me more," and "Go on" to facilitate expression of feelings. Repeating phrases and using silence are also useful responses.

Clarifying behaviors indicate that the nurse seeks to understand the client's perceptions. The nurse uses open-ended questions to validate perceptions and invite opinions. Furthermore, the nurse acknowledges confusion and seeks to resolve it by restating the problem. Informing behaviors relate to clarifying on the same level because they, too, seek to understand the client's perceptions. The nurse in-

TABLE 4-2. **Empathy: levels of nursing actions**

LEVEL	CATEGORY	NURSING BEHAVIOR
1	Accepting	Uses client's correct name Maintains eye contact Adopts open posture Responds to cues
2	Listening	Nods head Smiles Encourages responses Uses therapeutic silence
3	a. Clarifying	Asks open-ended questions Restates the problem Validates perceptions Acknowledges confusion Provides honest, complete answers
	b. Informing	Provides honest, complete answers Assesses client's knowledge level Summarizes
4	Analyzing	Identifies unknown emotions Interprets underlying meanings Confronts conflict

forms by providing honest and complete answers in language the client understands. The nurse also assesses the client's knowledge level and uses summarization to highlight important points.

The final set of nursing behaviors designed to facilitate empathy is *analyzing behaviors*. When analyzing behaviors are used, high levels of empathy, levels 4 and 5, are reached. In this group of behaviors, the nurse identifies unknown emotions, which are communicated by the client. The nurse interprets the meanings behind the feelings and confronts conflicting verbal and nonverbal behaviors. Levels of nursing actions to facilitate empathy are depicted in Table 4-2.

Research has shown that empathy can be learned and knowledge transferred from simulated experiences to real clinical situations (Smith and Walker, 1984). Empathy skills, so important to the art of caring, improve through practice, feedback, and self-evaluation.

Mutuality

In developing mutuality, the nurse, through the therapeutic use of self, maximizes the client's involvement in all phases of the nursing process. Mutuality includes shared communication and collaboration in problem-solving between the nurse and client. The extent of mutuality within a relationship grows as the nurse-client relationship matures. Only when a trusting relationship has been initiated by the nurse through a sense of caring can a fully mutual relationship exist and continue to develop.

The attainment of mutuality is enhanced by several factors. The nurse exhibits a caring attitude, is trustworthy, and uses a high degree of empathy to facilitate understanding of the client. These are concepts basic to a therapeutic relationship. Without the establishment of such a firm foundation, a sense of mutuality becomes an unattainable goal.

To foster mutuality within the relationship, the nurse needs to remain cognizant of her own feelings, attitudes, and beliefs. Negative, unresolved attitudes surrounding typical stereotypes may quickly halt or damage mutuality already attained and may actually jeopardize the relationship if the client suddenly views these attitudes as threatening. The client who has entrusted the nurse with specific confidential information may feel betrayed if the nurse is unaccepting of the client's decision not to change aspects of an "unhealthy lifestyle," one that involves smoking, drug abuse, or sedentariness, for example.

Nurses who are truly sensitive to others' feelings and accepting of differences between their own lifestyles and those of others have the capacity to develop and attain mutuality in relationships. Such caring nurses involve clients in the decision-making process and they do not belittle decisions made by clients. In addition, effective use of values clarification assists clients in decision making. As clients clearly identify their own values they are better able to solve problems effectively and arrive at decisions that have a higher chance of being successful.

Mutuality does not end with decision making. The nurse and client must now implement the decisions, perhaps even difficult ones that require commitment, time, and patience for successful outcomes. As the client implements changes, regression to old behaviors and habits may occur temporarily. The nurse monitors for expected changes and confronts the client about regressive behaviors.

Another aspect of mutuality is that of shared communication. Mutuality is an important part of an I-thou relation. The client never becomes an "it" in the nurse's eyes. Sharing feelings and emotions forms a stronger therapeutic relationship. Not only does the client express feelings through assistance by the nurse, but the nurse expresses feelings about the relationship. For example, a nurse, feeling proud of a client who has quit smoking, should communicate this pride to the client. Sharing feelings, whether happy or sad, enhances mutuality.

Mutuality encompasses all phases of the nursing process and enriches nurse-client relationships. Evidence of mutuality is seen in the development of individualized client goals and nursing actions that meet a client's unique health needs. A mutual relationship is terminated with both parties having a sense of shared accomplishment and satisfaction. Evaluating mutuality is not easy and may reveal insightful information about oneself that can enhance one's mutuality skills in future relationships....

REFERENCES

Chapman, J., and Chapman, H. *The Psychology of Health Care: A Humanistic Perspective*. Monterey, Calif: Wadsworth Health Sciences, 1983.

Gault, D.A. "Development of a Theoretically Adequate Description of Caring," *Western Journal of Nursing Research* 5:313, 1983.

Erikson, E. *Childhood and Society*, 2nd ed. New York: W.W. Norton, 1963.

Carkhuff, R.R. *Helping and Human Relations*, Vol. 1. New York: Holt, Rinehart, and Winston, 1969.

Meize-Growchowski, R. "An Analysis of the Concept of Trust," *Journal of Advanced Nursing*, 9:343, 1984.

The family as the unit of care in nursing: A historical review

ANN L. WHALL, PhD, FAAN

The following article was published several years after it was presented as a paper at the Nursing Theory Think Tank in 1983. It reviews literature from Florence Nightingale's time to the present to evaluate nursing's emphasis on the family as the recipient of care over the years. The author found that the early literature used family position terms (such as mother *and* child*) instead of the term* family, *but that later works used* family *and considered it a single entity or unit of care. The author also identified important trends in nursing care of the family. Note: Excerpts (shown by ellipses) shorten an extensive literature review and methodological description.*

CURRENT DISCUSSIONS OF theory in nursing make reference to the metaparadigm [archetypal example] of nursing as being focused upon person, environment, health, and nursing (Fawcett, 1983). Not explicit is the understanding that the family as well as individuals may be recipients of care. A review of the literature was conducted to determine the emphasis on the family as the recipient of care....

Definitions

Present definitions of family were identified and compared with the historical evolution of the concept....The two definitions examined were "family" and "family unit."

Reisner (1980, p. 8) defined the family as a relational group that consists of two or more individuals who are associated with each other and whose association is characterized by such terms as parent, mother, father, sister, brother, and grandparent. In Logan's (1979, p. 9) definition, the family is a "social system" and "a set of components interacting with each other"; the sense of a whole is both implied and explicit. In this perspective, the family member is responsive to the larger whole or family system, and changes in patterns between persons result in changes in the entire system. Gillis (1983) defined the family as a complex unit with attributes of its own, but containing component parts that are significant as individual units. According to Roberts (1983), there are several ways in which to define a family but all have some negative features. For example, definitions based on bloodlines and law exclude groups that consider themselves to be a family but who are not related by bloodlines or law (p. 8).

Examination of discussions of the family and family unit in major reviews led to several conclusions. The family is a self-identified group of two or more individuals whose association is characterized by special terms, who may or may not be related by bloodlines or law, but who function in such a way that they consider themselves to be a family. A unitary approach is one in which the wholeness of the unit is recognized. With these definitions in mind, the literature was reviewed to identify important instances in which the family or family unit was discussed as a focus of care....

Nightingale

A biography of Florence Nightingale (Tooley, 1905, p. 153) was one of the earliest texts examined. Tooley stated, "Miss Nightingale found the wives of soldiers, respectable women, without decent clothing, living in three or four rooms of the damp basement of a hospital. There by light of rushlight, measures were taken, the sick attended, and their babies born and nourished." In all, 22 babies were born to this group. In winter, due to a broken drain in the basement, a fever broke out. "Miss Nightingale procured a house, had it cleaned and furnished; she organized a plan to give employment to soldiers' wives...she started a school for the children and got a chaplain to visit them and help them." Nightingale wrote later (according to Tooley) that as improvements in the system were made which the war suggested, care should be taken that the wives and the children of soldiers not be forgotten. Florence Nightingale "was...possessed by the idea of the district nurse as a health missioner ...[these missioners were to] introduce to village mothers particular knowledge [such as in the area of] sanitation and skillful hands" (Cook, 1913, p. 383). "The movement for district nursing was always dear to Miss Nightingale's heart." She regretted "that once district nursing came, it was too late for her to help" (Cook, 1925, p. 340).

The quotation from Tooley contains all the elements of the concept of family: Nightingale recognized family members, husbands, wives, and children; she mentioned needs of both mothers and infants, and in her own words she used the relationship terms wife and child, and implied (as soldier) husband and father. The last quotation hints at a regret on the part of Nightingale that she had not further developed the branch of nursing, which at that time dealt mostly with families....

1890-1910

...In the *Trained Nurse*, Brooks (1890) stated, "Caring for the insane in their homes will relieve their families" and Stewart (1908) made note of a nurse who "ministered to three ill children and two who were not stricken" with diphtheria. Stewart also noted that in one family the parents were very frightened by the children's illness, and it was two hours before they "could decide what was best to do." After seeing the older boy successfully treated, "the parents decided I should treat the baby."

Wald (1904) set forth general principles as to how to "nurse in the home," including advice about how to enter the family; that is, before removing "children lying upon the bed of the sick mother" and "washing their faces," the nurse should first "establish herself" (p. 430). Wald recommended evaluating whether a family can care for "an invalid" without becoming "demoralized." She also discussed the relationship of the family to their neighbors and to service agencies. Several case studies were given in which the nurse assessed the ability of the family to care for the ill member, wherein the nurse taught a family member to give care and/or put the family in touch with community agencies (pp. 603-606).

1910-1930

...By 1917 Beard...stated that the public health nurse must have as "her conviction, that upon her observation and foresight depends the health of their whole family." The family "as a unit more than any other individual member of it must be her thought...the correction of defects may be the pivot upon which family health turns" (p. 247). Beard described several cases in which the family was approached as a unit by the public health nurse (pp. 249-250).

The 1917 *Standard curriculum for schools of nursing* was prepared by the committee on Education of the National League for Nursing Education (NLNE). In the outline of the subject matter, it stated that students were to receive instruction in "Household Science," which pertained to "housekeeping problems of an industrial family." The overall objective of this course was to prepare "pupils who intend to go into families either as a public health or as a private duty nurse" (p. 62). The most satisfactory teaching method was to "have the pupil study individual families" (p. 62).

Laird (1923) was primarily concerned with the control of communicable disease, when she identified that "any plan of health education which does not include the whole family is not adequate" (p. 40). While a patient was hospitalized, she wondered, "What about the other members of the family? Even though the patient is adequately cared for...may not his progress be dependent on the condition and attitude of his in the home?" (p. 40)....

1930-1950

The NLNE (1937) published a third curriculum guide in which "The Modern Family" was a major unit of study....On the subject "Nursing and Health Services in the Family," the text declared, "The entire program outlined in this curriculum is based on the assumption that the participation in health conservation and prevention of disease is inherent in the whole concept of nursing...also that the patient should not be considered as an individual only, but as a member of a group" (p. 510). In addition, courses that were directed toward family health care were not "specific preparation for public health nursing." It was intended to round out the nursing students' "experience, to meet more common situations found in family health" (p. 510). This theme continued in the statement that "the nurse must consider the family as a unit. This may involve making study of the family" (p. 513). Thus the increased discussion of the family and the analysis of the family as a unit was well established by 1937....

A textbook that dealt primarily with medical-surgical nursing (Harmer, 1935) stated, "Very often patients although pronounced cured, require further care. When this is the case, the nurse in charge of the social service department will see that patients are properly cared for. As previously stated the patient can never be rightly understood or adequately cared for considered apart from the family...in the homes of rich and poor alike, rural or army nursing includes all of this" (p. 367)....

Bean and Brockett (1937) titled an article "The family as a unit for nursing service." They noted that when going into a home, the public health nurse should not only give nursing care to individuals, but address the health needs of the entire family and work out a health plan for its members. The authors also identified ways to ascertain if nurses were carrying out the commitment to care for the entire family. They described a one-year survey by the United States Public Health Service (USPHS) conducted at three county health departments....A review of over 3000 records revealed that in 62 percent of the cases, nurses addressed problems other than those for which they first came into the home. The authors concluded, however, that the visits tended to be confined to services for just a few family members on any one visit. This did not meet their criteria for total family service.

1950-present

...Beasley (1954) reported on service to families who had a mentally ill member, stating, "It was this concept of supportive services to the families of the mentally ill that became the basis for an experimental program" (p. 482). The function of public health nurses in this regard was in part to help the family accept the patient's illness and understand the patient's need to be hospitalized, to help the patient to be accepted back into the home, and to arrange for several families to meet together to discuss common problems. Beasley noted that the emphasis of service was placed purposefully on the family needs rather than on the patient.

Garside (1958) stated, "The home visit provides for a closer observation of intangibles such as family relationships and intergroup personality reactions" (p. 153). She also indicated that school nurses tended to address the needs of school-age children and thereby unintentionally neglect family health. She stated further that the health of individual family members must be addressed "in order to protect the family as a whole" (p. 155). The need to approach the family unit as the client was found in many other articles (Kvarness, 1959; Reinerston, 1963; Hess, 1966; Mereness, 1968; Smiley, 1973). The issue at this time was not whether the family was the client, but how to address a multiperson group.

Standards of practice

As one might expect, the interest in the family was evident in the American Nurses' Association's (ANA) *Standards of community health nursing practice* (ANA 1973). The opening statement said, "Nursing practice is a direct... service to the individual, the family, and the community during health and illness." Consumers may be "individuals or families," and "active involvement of the individual, family, and community is necessary in attainment of positive health."...

Nursing models

King's 1981 edition of "A Theory of Nursing: Systems, Concepts, Process" indexed the family extensively. On the first page she stated that most persons begin life as a part of a family and learn ways to meet basic needs in families, and that the family constitutes one of the groups in which one performs a certain role. King noted that the family demonstrates the features of a social system; that is, structure, status, role, and social interaction. King later noted that the family as a social system, as well as health as a goal for nursing, are two major concepts in her framework (1983, p. 178). She discussed "family-nurse interactions" as well as the need to assess "the family's perceptions," thus treating the family as a unit.

In 1979 Newman did not index or discuss the family as such; however, in 1983 she restated the assumptions of her earlier work in terms of families, noting that health could be described as "fluctuating patterns of energy exchange...that are part of the developing consciousness of the family" (p. 169).

She discussed the family unit in terms of a whole or single entity and focused on the interactions of all members and how this related to family health. Newman's focus in her discussion of families is thus definitely a family unit in terms of the nurse approaching the family as a unit of care.

Although Orem's 1971 text did not index the term family, she did indicate that the nurse "learns how to work in cooperation with patients and their families" (p. 119) and that in terms of achieving goals "one had to be aware of family implications" (p. 71). In the 1980 edition of this work the term family is indexed as appearing on several pages. Orem stated in this later edition that, "In search of valid ways to provide health care to families...it has been recognized that it may be essential to work with all members of the unit" (p. 200). Orem (1983) extended the discussion of family as a unit of analysis, stating, "First, accept the family as a system...and the family culture as basic conditioning factors for all family members....The system of family support should be examined and adjusted as needed and then incorporated into the family system of living" (pp. 367-368). This last statement indicated that family interactions and the family system as a whole are a unit of analysis.

In 1970 and 1980 Rogers did not reference or discuss the family as such. In 1983, however, she stated, "The proposed paradigm is as applicable to families as it is to individual human beings...an irreducible, four dimensional ...family energy field becomes the focus of study" (p. 226). Rogers continued the point that the family could logically be the focus of analysis in her model by applying to the family as a unit the concepts of pattern and organization and energy fields. She stated that families may or may not live in the same household, and may or may not be related by blood or by law (p. 226).

Roy in 1976 addressed the family primarily as it related to the individual. Roy and Roberts in 1981 stated, however, "The client of nursing may be a person, a family, a group, a community, or society" (p. 42).

In 1983, however, Roy explicated the family as the client or unit of analysis: "Nursing may focus on an individual person, the family, and group, a social organization, or a community" (p. 262). Families are an adaptive system with input, output, and internal processes (p. 273), and just as nurses assess the person as an adaptive system, so too do they assess the family when a family is the focus of care (p. 275).

Summary

The conclusion is drawn that the family as a unit of care in nursing is by now well established. The historical and current literature is clear in terms of this conclusion.

The literature review verified the position taken at the outset that the discussion of family proceeds from discussion of family position terms to the discussion of the family as a whole or as the unit of care. The review also identified several trends: (1) public health or district nursing was the first practice area that clearly focused on the family as a unit of care; (2) later, other practice areas reflected this focus; and (3) certain nursing models tended to focus less on family in their initial statements.

REFERENCES

American Nurses' Association. (1973). *Standards of community health nursing practice*. Kansas City, MO: Author.

Bean, H., & Brockett, G. (1937). The family as a unit for nursing service. *Public Health Report, 52*, 1923-1931.

Beard, M. (1915). Home nursing. *Public Health Nursing Quarterly*, 7, 44-51.

Beard, M. (1917, October). The family as the unit of public health work. *Modern Hospital*, (1954). 247-251.

Beasley, F. (1954). Public health nursing services for families of the mentally ill. *Nursing Outlook, 2*, 482-483.

Brooks, J. (1890). Nursing the insane. *Trained Nurse, 4*, 10-12.

Cook, E. (1913). *The life of Florence Nightingale* (Vol. 2). London: Macmillian.

Cook, E. (1925). *The life of Florence Nightingale* (rev. ed.) London: Macmillian.

Fawcett, J. (1983). Hallmarks of success in nursing theory development. In P.L. Chin (Ed.) *Advances in nursing theory development*. Rockville, MD: Aspen Systems, pp. 3-18.

Garside, A. (1958). The school nurse as a family counselor. *Journal of School Health, 28*, 153-157.

Gillis, C. (1983). The family as a unit of analysis: Strategies for the nurse researcher. *Advances in Nursing Science, 5*, 50-59.

Harmer, B. (1935). *Textbook of the principles and practice of nursing*. New York: Macmillian.

Hess, G. (1966). Family nursing experience. *Nursing Outlook, 14*, 51-53.

King, I. (1981). *A theory for nursing: Systems, concepts, process*. New York: John Wiley & Sons.

King, I. (1983). King's theory of nursing/analysis and application of King's theory of goal attainment. In I. Clements & F. Roberts (Eds.), *Family health: A theoretical approach to nursing care*. New York: John Wiley & Sons.

Kvarness, M. (1959). The patient is the family. *Nursing Outlook, 7*, 142-146.

Laird, M. (1923). The value of follow-up work in the family. *American Journal of Nursing, 24*, 4043.

Logan, B. (1979). The nurse and the family: Dominant themes and perspectives in the literature. In K. Knafl & H. Grace (Eds.), *Families across the life cycle: Studies for nursing*. Boston: Little, Brown.

Mereness, D. (1968). Family therapy: An evolving role for the psychiatric nurse. *Perspectives in Psychiatric Nursing, 6*, 259.

National League for Nursing Education. (1917). *Standard curriculum for schools of nursing*. Baltimore: Waverly Press.

National League for Nursing Education. (1937). *A curriculum guide for schools of nursing*. New York: Author.

Newman, M. (1979). *Theory development in nursing*. Philadelphia: F.A. Davis.

Newman, M. (1983). Newman's health theory. In I. Clements & F. Roberts (Eds.), *Family health: A theoretical approach to nursing care*. New York: John Wiley & Sons.

Orem, D. (1971). *Nursing: Concepts of practice*. New York: McGraw-Hill.

Orem, D. (1980). *Nursing: Concepts of practice* (2nd ed.). New York: McGraw-Hill.

Orem, D. (1983). The self-care deficit theory of nursing: a general theory/analysis and application of Orem's theory. In I. Clements & F. Roberts (Eds.), *Family health: A theoretical approach to nursing care*. New York: John Wiley & Sons.

Reinerston, B. (1963). The patient is part of a family. *American Journal of Nursing, 63*, 106-107.

Reisner, W. (1980). The historical development of the conceptualization of family within the context of nursing care of well children.

Unpublished master's thesis, Francis Payne Bolton School of Nursing, Case Western Reserve University, Cleveland, Ohio.

Roberts, S. (1983). The American family. In I. Clements & F. Roberts (Eds.). *Family health: A theoretical approach to nursing care*. New York: John Wiley & Sons.

Rogers, M. (1970). *An introduction to the theoretical basis of nursing*. Philadelphia: F.A. Davis.

Rogers, M. (1980). Nursing: a science of unitary man. In J. Riehl & C. Roy (Eds.). *Conceptual models for nursing practice*, 2nd ed. New York: Appleton-Century-Crofts, 1980.

Rogers, M. (1983). Science of unitary human beings: A paradigm for nursing. In I. Clements & F. Roberts (Eds.). *Family health: A theoretical approach to nursing care*. New York: John Wiley & Sons.

Roy, C. (1976). *Introduction to nursing: An adaptation model*. Englewood Cliffs, NJ: Prentice-Hall.

Roy C., & Roberts, S. (1981). *Theory construction in nursing: An adaptation model*. Englewood Cliffs, NJ: Prentice-Hall.

Roy, C. (1983). Analysis and application of the Roy adaptation model. In I. Clements & F. Roberts (Eds.). *Family health: A theoretical approach to nursing care*. New York John Wiley & Sons.

Smiley, O. (1973). The family-centered approach—A challenge to public health nurses. *Int Nurs Rev, 20*, 49-50.

Stewart, H. (1908). In quarantine with diphtheria. *Trained Nurse, 41*, 92-94.

Tooley, S. (1905). *The life of Florence Nightingale* (2nd ed.). London: Macmillian.

Wald, L. (1904). The treatment of families in which there is sickness. *American Journal of Nursing, 4*, 427-428, 515-519, 602-606.

SECTION TWO

Environmental concepts

THIS SECTION ADDRESSES the external and internal environmental factors that may influence a client system's health. The external environment includes the physical environment and social and cultural factors; the internal environment includes physical, mental, and spiritual factors. (For more information, see Unit Two Introduction.)

To help the nurse understand the external environment, Section Two begins with "Social Risk Factors: Impact on Elders' Perceived Health Status" by Cox et al. This article identifies three social risk factors that elderly individuals typically face in the United States: income adequacy, education, and social isolation. It also discusses how these factors can affect an elderly individual's perceived health. For example, it suggests that an elderly client with a large social network is likely to feel healthier than one with a small social network.

The social risk factors cited are quite common. Many elderly clients must adjust to an income reduction caused by retirement and a shrinking social network caused by the death of friends and loss of family members who move away. Therefore, these risk factors are the ones most likely to threaten an elderly client's health.

This article is especially relevant today because the number and proportion of elderly Americans is increasing. This phenomenon, sometimes called "the graying of America," has prompted nursing to focus more attention on the issues of the elderly population. To provide effective care, nursing students and practicing nurses will have to be aware of the social risk factors and health needs of these clients.

The next article presents information about culture — another aspect of the external environment that can affect a client system's health practices. In "Home Remedies: A Cultural Study," Roberson investigates the health practices of a rural black community in Virginia. Based on interviews, observations, and participation in community life, she reports that the community's residents rely on a wide range of home remedies to cope with common ailments, home emergencies, and chronic illnesses. She states that, in many cases, the residents are more comfortable with their cultural remedies than with the practices suggested by the nurse. So to promote client comfort and compliance, the author advocates a nursing approach that considers and incorporates the cultural health practices, customs, and values of the community.

Roberson's advice is particularly relevant for American nurses. Some experts call the United States "a nation of immigrants" because, except for the Native Americans, the entire population has come here from other countries. Because of this unusually rich mixture of people from many different origins, a nurse is likely to care for clients from many different cultures. To work with them effectively, the nurse should take a transcultural approach. (For more information on transcultural nursing, see Leininger's article in Unit One.)

Just as culture influences health practices, it can also affect sexuality. This, in turn, can affect the client's reproductive health, roles, and relationships. Brink (1987) explains how culture influences sexuality:

> ...the rules for sexual behavior are developed for each society and are taught to its members. Every culture exerts an enormous amount of social pressure on individuals to conform to accepted norms. Every society has an inherent social structure or hierarchy of valued roles, and the behaviors that are permissible or even required for one role may not be permissible for other roles. What is allowed for the privileged class may not be allowed for the common person. Every society sets rules of conduct that express the range of permissible behaviors and the range of punishments associated with sexual conduct. Pressure is always brought to bear to conform to those rules. In some societies, young boys are taught to hold their erections and ejaculations until the woman is ready. In other societies, something is wrong with a young boy who refuses to participate in homosexual activities. In some societies, members are taught that biting and scratching by both partners during intercourse is erotic while others believe this is simply aggressive behavior. In some societies, there are severe restrictions on premarital sexual exploration, while in others it is encouraged.

For these reasons, Brink advises the nurse to evaluate a client's sexuality according to the client's cultural values, not the nurse's. This assessment approach helps the nurse maintain a nonjudgmental role and intervene effectively. The nurse can take a similar approach to other culturally determined aspects of a client's life.

The last article in this section, "Responding to the Spiritual Needs of the Chronically Ill" by Soeken and Carson, examines spirituality, a vital part of the client system's internal environment. After defining the nature of spirituality, the authors look at the effects of chronic illness on the individual's spirit. They note that pain, low self-esteem, feelings of isolation, powerlessness, hopelessness, and anger are common spiritual and emotional reactions to illness.

Then the authors suggest the appropriate spiritual care for nurses to provide when addressing each of these reactions in a chronically ill client. Their suggested nursing interventions rely on therapeutic use of self and appropriate communication skills to help the client examine the impact and meaning of the illness. By describing how to provide spiritual care, this article helps prepare the student for holistic nursing practice.

REFERENCES

Brink, P. (1987). Cultural aspects of sexuality. *Holistic Nursing Practice, 1*(4), 12-20.

Social risk factors: Impact on elders' perceived health status

CHERYL L. COX, RNC, PhD; MARTHA SPIRO, RNC, MSN; JUDITH A. SULLIVAN, RN, EdD

Researchers have identified the general physical, behavioral, and life-style risk factors that can threaten a client's health. Many health care professionals believe, however, that the complete list of risk factors should include social characteristics, such as poverty, isolation, and ignorance, which are especially critical to the health of elderly clients.

Although many studies have examined the connection between social risk factors and mortality, few have investigated the relationship between these factors and the health status of elderly clients. This article fills that knowledge gap by studying social risk factors and providing guidelines for their nursing assessment and related interventions. Note: An introductory summary (in bracketed italics) and excerpts (marked by ellipses) condense extensive methodological information.

[TO DETERMINE THE CORRELATION between social risk factors and perceived health status, the authors began with a literature review. Then they conducted personal interviews with 379 healthy elderly individuals in four different apartment complexes (not specialized residences). The questions evaluated each client's self-perceived health status and three social risk factors: income, education, and social isolation (both objective and subjective).

After analyzing the information from these interviews, the authors developed a model that indicated the effects of the social risk factors on the elderly individuals' perceived health status. A discussion of the study's findings follows.]

Income adequacy. Income adequacy demonstrated a pronounced independent impact on health status. These effects were not significantly diminished even when the variation in health status attributed to all the other variables was considered. In addition to this direct impact on health, income adequacy also exerted effects on loneliness. Feelings of loneliness increase as perceptions of income adequacy decrease. This finding is increasingly significant in consideration of the demonstrated health impact of loneliness. Congruent with previous mortality research in this field, perceived income is clearly implicated as a clinically significant health risk as well. The sample demonstrated adequate socioeconomic variability to lend confidence to these results.

Education. Education was shown to have a direct impact on the elders' perceived health status. Again the findings in this study were congruent with the mortality data findings of earlier research (Kitagawa & Hauser, 1973); the health effects attributed to education are independent of income. These findings support the position that lack of education alone can be considered a health risk.

Education demonstrated some significant indirect effects on both the social network size and the elders' perception of loneliness. Lack of education is associated with a more limited social network and greater loneliness. More education potentially may foster one's ability to better manipulate or interact with the social environment, which in turn supports an improved health status.

Social network and loneliness. The findings from this study indicate that health status is indeed affected by merely the size of the social network. A breakdown of network components indicates that contact with friends, relatives (other than children), and church membership or activities were the significant objective network predictors of health status. Congruent with Blazer's study (1982), however, perceived loneliness was the strongest predictor of perceived health status when all the social variables tested were considered. Although actual network size and perceived loneliness are strongly associated, they exert their effects on health independently. This suggests that a person who has a limited social network but who does not express feelings of loneliness may in fact still be at risk for a decreased health status; similarly, a person who feels lonely despite a large social network may also be at risk....

Implications

Community health nurses have always recognized the importance of a client's social environment; however, the quantification of the impact of the social environment on health has not been a part of our knowledge base. Therefore, although community health nurses have traditionally informally assessed the adequacy of a client's social resources, our assessments and interventions have been inconsistent and primarily based on each...nurse's perspective and interest. The primary goal...should be to educate community care givers about the role of structural social factors in determining health status and the assessment of social risk. These social assessments can then be incorporated into preventive and screening efforts at both the individual and community levels. Although we do not know yet the extent or the exact mechanisms of these effects, we can be more alert to these clients as being "at risk."

Social considerations in nursing interventions are not new to the profession. Community health nurses have intuitively known that social contact and support were essential to the client's health and have provided a variety of services and resources to address these very issues. However, these nursing services are not reimbursed and therefore exist only when "justified" by the presence of a medical diagnosis. This study begins to provide the data to substantiate the claim that nursing services focused on strengthening the social contact and social support network — alone — are significant and justifiably reimbursable. Investment in preventive nursing services such as these is perhaps more sound than awaiting illness in order to financially justify services.

Finally, the observed relationships [among] education, income, and health immediately suggest a more global preventive approach. The knowledge that elders' health is at risk due to lack of education or due to poverty is not easily addressed in a preventive manner at the individual level. Health professionals and policy makers must therefore shift from an individual focus to consider the larger and more dramatic implications of these findings for the aggregate. "Ensuring economic health must be considered a fundamental prerequisite to more conventional health promotion efforts" (Minkler & Pasick, 1986, p. 40). Although the efforts of health care providers are essential, those who determine health policy have a more critical role in creating or not creating healthy environments. Nurses need to present such information to local and national health and social policy makers. In this way, we can begin to effect broader change in the structural base of our clients' health....

Summary and conclusions

Physical factors alone do not account for all the variation in health among individuals. Social factors also have an impact on health status: Poverty, lack of education, an inadequate social network, and perceived loneliness all pose additional health risks for the elderly. By identifying relationships such as those proposed here, new and perhaps more appropriate nursing interventions can be developed to decrease health risks in the elderly populations.

As the research base that elaborates these relationships grows, the need for research that would expand the theoretical understanding of these relationships becomes even more apparent. Studies are needed to determine (a) What are the essential elements of the relationships observed here? (b) By what mechanism do these "risk factors" exert their effects, and how can community health nurse clinicians and researchers quantify these effects? (c) What are the modifiable aspects of the social risk factors? and (d) What are the results of nursing interventions directed at social risk factors?

REFERENCES

Blazer, D.G. (1982). Social support and mortality in an elderly community population. *American Journal of Epidemiology, 115*, 684-694.

Kitagawa, E.M., & Hauser, R.M. (1973). *Differential mortality in the United States: A study in socioeconomic epidemiology*. Cambridge, MA: Harvard University Press.

Minckler, M., & Pasick, R.J. (1986). Health promotion and the elderly: A critical perspective on the past and future. In K. Dychtwald (Ed.), *Wellness and health promotion for the elderly* (pp. 39-54). Rockville, MD: Aspen.

Home remedies: A cultural study

MILDRED H.B. ROBERSON, RN, PhD

WHEN PEOPLE DEVELOP a health problem or need, they secure relief by means of a variety of options, one of which is the use of home remedies. All cultural groups use home remedies, but the mode of use, substances used, and associated beliefs differ.[1-6] Community health nurses need to be knowledgeable about their clients' use of home remedies so that they can provide culturally sensitive and meaningful quality care.

The study

The data reported here form one aspect of a comprehensive ethnographic study of the health culture of rural black Virginians. An ethnographic study utilizes the techniques of anthropologists to analyze the health beliefs and behaviors of a cultural group. A more recent study of the health culture of rural black Georgians in a comparable community supported the findings of the Virginia research. During one year of field work, intensive interviews and participant observation were carried out in a rural community of 10,000 persons. The formal interviews focused on 46 households whose 138 members had diverse demographic characteristics. Many informants were interviewed multiple times. Informal interviews were conducted with these people as well as other informants during chance meetings, drop-in visits, and telephone conversations. Data were also gathered during participant observation, which included attendance at church services and other church functions, visits to places of work, social functions, participation in meetings, as well as living in the community.

The findings

The study participants used a wide variety of home remedies to obtain relief for their health problems and needs. These remedies will be classified here according to the clinical situation for which they were used.

Common ailments. Table 1 lists some of the home remedies used by the participants for such common health problems as colds, coughs, sore throats, fever, stomach or intestinal problems, boils, rashes, and aches.

An individual's favorite remedy for a particular ailment often depends upon his family's customs or prior experience, and it is not unusual for people to combine treatment modalities. For instance, a person with a cold might drink hot tea with lemon, take onion syrup, rub the chest with tallow, cover up, go to bed to "sweat it out," and also take a patent drug.

Home emergencies. Home remedies are often used for emergency health problems because they require immediate attention. Particularly in rural areas where medical assistance may be some distance away, where transportation may be limited, and where telephones may not be readily available, people often rely on their own resources to handle a problem. Some of the home remedies reported by the study participants for these emergencies are given in Table 2. Again, it is not unusual for people to combine remedies. Thus, a person might rinse a cut with cold water, apply fatmeat, and then bandage it.

Chronic health problems. The participants also used home remedies to treat chronic illnesses or their symptoms; these remedies may either supplement an allopathic medical regi-

TABLE 1. **Home remedies for common ailments**

COMMON AILMENTS	REMEDIES
Internal remedies	
	Teas
Colds, upset stomach	Tansy
Colds, rash	Ginger
Upset stomach	Peppermint, nutmeg, Jerusalem oak, or clove
Colds, rash, "wind colic" (babies)	Catnip
Constipation	Comfrey or sage
Diarrhea	Black pepper, cinnamon, or nutmeg
	Syrups
Colds, cough, fever	Onion and sugar (whiskey) or lemon and honey
Cough, sore throat	Horehound leaf and sugar
Cough	Wild cherry bark and sugar
	Oral remedies
Colds	Turpentine, kerosene, or coal oil
Cough, chest cold	Vaseline and sugar
Colds, constipation	Castor oil
Fever	Niter, quinine
Upset stomach	Calamus root (chew) or soda and vinegar
Headache	Coca-Cola
Diarrhea	Flour water or blackberry juice or wine
Colds, headaches	Patent medicines
External remedies	
	Poultices
Fever, headache	Cabbage leaf (bruised)
Fever	Raw onion (cut and bind in place) or raw potato (slice and bind in place)
Swellings	Mullein weed
	Topical
Chest colds	Mutton or beef tallow (cover with flannel)
Toothache	Lemon extract, perfume, tobacco, red pepper seed, heat, or hot salt bag
Rash	Vaseline, oatmeal, or burned flour
Thrush	Vaseline, urine, or boric acid
Boil or "rising"	Membrane of an egg, flaxseed, tansy, jimsonweed, or tobacco
Boils, splinters	Fatback, salty meat
Earache	Molasses, honey, sweet oil, warm chamber water, or pipe smoke (blow into ear)

men or may constitute the primary therapy. These remedies may be used on an ongoing basis as part of a total therapeutic approach or may be employed only when the symptoms seem to dictate the need. Table 3 lists some of the remedies described by the participants.

Health promotion. Home remedies are also relied upon to promote health or to prevent illness. Various teas may be imbibed to help ward off colds; tea may also be prepared as a spring tonic to rid the body of impurities built up over the winter months. Informants frequently mentioned the use of sassafras tea for this purpose; this tea has long been used in the United States as an aid to health.[1,5,7]

Many people believe that cod liver oil helps to build or strengthen the bones as well as prevent colds. It may be used in conjunction with such dietary practices as including lots of fruit, juice, and fresh vegetables in the diet. Ingestion of cod liver oil is one folk practice that is consistent with the teaching of medical science; doctors value this oil for its vitamin A and D content which helps to prevent such nutritional deficiency problems as rickets.

Besides ingesting certain substances, people sometimes wear garlic, asafetida, silver, copper, or other materials to ward off sickness.

Related factors

Social, cultural, and personal factors all affect the ways in which a client chooses to meet his health needs, including his use of home remedies.

Alternative approaches to health. Health professionals sometimes mistakenly assume that there is only one health care system—allopathic medicine. Since nursing education is largely based upon allopathic medicine, nurses may overlook the fact that alternative sources of health care are available and embraced by many people.[3,6,8-12] There are organized approaches, such as naturopathy, homeopathy, acupuncture, and naprapathy, and individual approaches, such as spiritual advisers, lay healers, or root doctors.[3,13-15]

People may also utilize such health resources as family, friends, neighbors, home medical books, and the public media. Any of these sources of health information may be

TABLE 2. Remedies for home emergencies

HOME EMERGENCIES	REMEDIES
Burns, cuts	Aloe vera, sulfur and vaseline, or cold water
Stings, burns	Baking soda
Burns	Butter or other grease, linseed oil, raw potato (cut), toothpaste
Cuts, stings, bites	Chlorox, ammonia, kerosene, comfrey (bruised)
Burns, cuts, spider bites	Cobweb
Cuts, stings	Flour or mud (pack on)
Cuts, punctures	Fatback poultice, turpentine, epsom salts in hot water, soot, ashes, or tobacco
Bee stings	Honey
Burns, poison ivy	Milk
Cuts	Salt, alcohol, peroxide, or iodine
Stings, bites	Tobacco (chewed)
Nosebleed	Fatmeat or hang cold keys down back and put brown paper under upper lip
Nail punctures	Burn nail causing wound
Sprains	Mullein poultice

TABLE 3. Home remedies for chronic illness

ILLNESS	REMEDIES
Internal remedies	
	Teas
Bladder/kidney problems	Jerusalem oak
High blood*	Oak leaves (boiled down)
Low blood,† sugar‡	Peach branch or leaves
Sugar	Wild cherry bark
Oral remedies	
Low blood	Beets, raisins, black molasses, blackberry or red wine, liver or other meat (rare), or fish (raw)
Sugar	Brewers yeast or molasses and sulfur
Arthritis	Castor oil, lemon juice and baking soda, lemons or lemon juice
High blood	Pickles, sweet pickle juice, epsom salts, garlic, garlic salt, onions, vinegar, or lemon juice
Asthma	Asafetida (rolled into pill)
Arthritis, high blood	Potato, white (sliced in 1 quart of water)
Bladder/kidney problems	Vinegar
External remedies	
Arthritis	Pennyroyal (make salve); mullein, pine bark, and pokeweed poultice; dry mustard (make paste); heat (dry or moist); "gold eye" needles (dissolve nine in bottle of white vinegar); or snake oil liniment
	Other
Asthma	Jimsonweed (smoke) or rabbit or life-everlasting tobacco (smoke)
Low blood	Support hose (wear)

*Often refers to hypertension. †Often refers to anemia. ‡Usually means diabetes.

tapped when an individual wants to resolve a health problem. Any of the self-care practices, including the preparation and administration of home remedies, may draw on one or more of these resources. The availability and choice of a particular health care strategy will depend upon cultural norms and values.

Contextual issues. In order to understand the use of home remedies by Southern blacks or others, one must consider the influence of political, economic, social, and historical factors. Those who belong to disadvantaged groups are acutely aware of the politics of health care delivery. For many Southern blacks, for example, there is no doubt as to who controls the formal health care system. Since it is dominated by whites, this has a significant impact on the blacks' trust and confidence in allopathic medicine. The informants in this study cited countless examples of discrimination in health care. In situations where people have had more positive experiences with alternative measures (such as home remedies), they will probably be more inclined to rely on these for their health needs.

The economics of health care is also an important determinant of people's health choices. Health care is costly. Medications are expensive and not always covered by insurance, even for those who have it. Many of the study informants were not fortunate enough to have health insurance through their places of employment. Thus, home remedies were able to help them reduce the cost of health care.

Social norms and values, social roles, and religious beliefs may all affect health-seeking behavior. If the use of home remedies is socially acceptable to a given cultural group, then members of that group may feel comfortable in adhering to this practice. Certain family and/or community members may be viewed as knowledgeable in health matters and thus consulted for advice. Many study participants indicated that they had great respect for such persons and their wisdom. Grandmothers were often cited as important sources of information for home remedies. Religious beliefs may also support health practices. The participants pointed out that the Bible speaks of the use of herbs for healing; many people also believe that God — not man — determines the success of healing.[14,16]

The history of a group may include reliance on home remedies. Certainly, Chinese or American Indian herbal medicine practices have a long tradition. Historically, for both social and economic reasons, American blacks needed to rely on black healers and the transmission of therapeutic advice through the black community. The origin of many Southern black home remedies dates back at least to the era of slavery.[17,18] Some remedies have even been traced back to the home medical books of an earlier period.[16,19]

Therapeutic approaches

Since people frequently combine treatment modalities, healing approaches may complement, supplement, or conflict with one another. An individual may be taking home remedies and prescription drugs concurrently. This medical syncretic approach can lead to outcomes viewed as successful by both the client and the health professional.

Moreover, in the folk belief system described by the study participants, there is a blending of spiritual, mental/emotional, and physical aspects of health. These people do not limit themselves to treatment of the physical body; rather, they take a more holistic view of health. Thus, a home remedy is not likely to be the sole strategy used in addressing a health problem. An individual might also focus on building a positive outlook and faith in successful results, pray for God's assistance, and enlist the support of the family, the pastor, or others.

Community health applications. The findings of this study have several implications for home and community health nurses. Since America is a multicultural society, effective nursing practice means that nurses need to know about various health cultures as well as the individual client's beliefs and practices.

Cultural sensitivity. Nurses need to show respect for health beliefs and practices that differ from their own. If a client senses that his health practices may be ridiculed or chastised by the nurse, he may never reveal that he is taking home remedies or following an alternative to allopathic medicine.

People adopt health practices that they perceive to be helpful. A client's reason for using a home remedy may be just as convincing to him as the nurse's reason is to her for advocating an allopathic approach. For example, in the case of a client who believes that a rash indicates that impurities are being expelled from the body, the use of catnip to help bring out the rash is more logical than use of an ointment applied to dispel the rash.

Health choices are an aspect of cultural norms, values, and customs. The tradition of using home remedies for healing is a more established norm in some groups than in others. Among the study participants, such a tradition was more prominent in some families than in others, although all of the participants had occasionally used home remedies. The role of the family, the nature of leadership, the position of elders, and the networking of a cultural group all affect health practices. All of the participants valued the family highly and had great respect for elders both in the family and in the black community. They also described many instances of networking in the sharing of information and resources.

A nurse who is working to improve health in a given community must recognize the cultural norms, customs, and values of that community. It may be more meaningful to a client to have the approval of a parent, grandparent, pastor, or community member who is respected for his health knowledge and wisdom than to have the approval of a nurse or physician. For the nurse to be successful, therefore, she may find it beneficial to involve those who are important to the client in the client's care, to accept their wisdom on some aspects of care, and even to treat them as colleagues, when feasible.

Compliance. The issue of compliance is of great concern to health professionals. However, the emphasis has usually been on what the client is or is not doing rather than on problems with the health care system or with the providers. It is assumed that if a client does not follow the health professional's recommendations, there must be something wrong with the client and/or family.[20,21]

Perhaps it would be more accurate to recognize that both cultural factors and barriers within the formal health care system affect compliance. As mentioned earlier, clients do not necessarily view allopathic medicine as the only or the most effective way to resolve health problems. My research and that of others show that black clients are resourceful in meeting their health needs by means of various therapeutic modalities.[8,11,13,16]

It would be helpful for the nurse to realize that people often consider natural home remedies to be generally more beneficial (and less harmful) than the chemical products of pharmaceutical laboratories.[22] Informants expressed grave concern about the side effects of drugs and the possibility that such effects could be worse than the original symptoms the drugs were expected to alleviate.

Individuality. Although it may be tempting for nurses to assume that all members of a given ethnic or cultural group have certain beliefs and practices, this is not a helpful approach. Within any cultural group, there is a wide variation among individuals or subgroups. Particularly in the United States, where a person may be exposed to multiple influences in developing his belief system, the end result may reflect borrowing from other cultures.

Also, within any group, there will be intergenerational differences. The elders are likely to share more beliefs among themselves than they share with the young people. Since culture is a dynamic process, one would expect cultural changes over generations as well as over time. New ideas and products may totally replace the old — the adoption of holistic health beliefs, published health advice, and certain products.

Client plan of care. In working with clients, nurses may assume that many of them utilize home remedies and that this practice relates to their total health belief system as well as the context in which that system exists. In order to incorporate the client's beliefs into the plan of care, nurses must include cultural components in making their assessment. The research reported here suggests that data on the client's beliefs in the areas of preventive health, concepts of body function, the etiology of sickness, and health restoration should be useful to the nurse. More specific information may be important for such specialized needs as the care of pregnant women. (Beliefs about childbirth itself comprise a very large field.[23-25])

As mentioned earlier, in order to make an accurate assessment and ensure the success of a plan of care, nurses need to have respect for and be open to the client's beliefs. The plan of care should perhaps incorporate the family, the pastor, or others who are a part of the client's approach to care. It may also be necessary to accept the client's use of home remedies and to include this in the plan of care. If the nurse believes that a particular remedy is harmful, she may need to develop a strategy for encouraging the client to change. Modification of that remedy or substitution of another which is not harmful may resolve the problem. It is also helpful to give the client credit for past successes in health matters and to treat him as an essential partner in both present and future health care.

In conclusion, home remedies are one approach to meeting health needs. The research reported here suggests that home remedies and other self-care practices are frequently part of a holistic health framework, which includes physical, psychosocial, and spiritual elements. Since community health nurses tend to be the most holistically oriented group of caregivers, they are ideally suited to incorporate cultural considerations into their client care.

REFERENCES

1. Aikman L: *Nature's Healing Arts*. New York, National Geographic Society, 1977.

2. Clark M: *Health in the Mexican-American Culture*, ed 2. Berkeley, University of California Press, pp 163-183.

3. Moore LG: Van Arsdale E W: Glittenberg J E: et al. *The Biocultural Basis of Health*. St. Louis, CV Mosby, 1980.

4. Spindler GD: Volksheilkunde, in Klein N: (ed). *Culture Curers and Contagion*. Novato, Calif., Chandler and Sharp, 1979.

5. Vogel VJ: *American Indian Medicine*. Norman, Okla., University of Oklahoma Press, 1970.

6. Weisberg ME: Graham J R: *A Barefoot Doctor's Manual*. Oceanside, NY, Cloudburst Press, 1977.

7. Angier B: *Fieldguide to Medicinal Wild Plants*. Harrisburg, Pa., Stackpole Books, 1978.

8. Hill C, Mathews H: Traditional health beliefs and practices among Southern rural blacks, in Black M, Reed J: (eds). *Social Science Perspectives on the South*. New York, Breech Science, 1981.

9. Powers BA: The use of orthodox and black American folk medicine. *Adv. Nurs. Sci.*, 1982; 4(3):35-47.

10. Scott CS: Health and healing practices among five ethnic groups in Miami, Florida. *Public Health Rep* 1974;89:524-532.

11. Snow LF: *The Medical System of a Group of Urban Blacks*, thesis. University of Arizona, Tucson, Ariz, 1971.

12. Strauss AL: Glaser B G: *Chronic Illness and the Quality of Life*. St. Louis, CV Mosby, 1975, chap. 2.

13. Roberson MH: *Folk Health Beliefs and Practices of Rural Black Virginians*, thesis. University of Utah, Salt Lake City, Utah, 1983.

14. Roberson MH: The influence of religious beliefs on health choices of Afro-Americans. *Top Clin Nurs* 1985;7(3):57-63.

15. Semmes CE: African-Americans seeking non-medical health care. *West J Black Studies* 1981;5(4):254-263.

16. Hill CE: *A Study of Folk Medical Beliefs and Practices in Rural West Georgia*, thesis. University of Georgia, Athens, Ga, 1972.

17. Genovese ED: *Roll, Jordan, Roll*. New York, Pantheon Books, 1974.

18. Savitt TL: *Medicine and Slavery*. Chicago, University of Illinois Press, 1978.

19. Melenday MR: *The Ideal Woman: For Maidens, Wives, and Mothers*. JR Peper, 1911.

20. Sackett DL, Haynes RB: (eds). *Compliance with Therapeutic Regimens*. Baltimore, Johns Hopkins University Press, 1976.

21. Zola IK: Structural constraints in the doctor-patient relationship, in Eisenberg L, Kleinman A: (eds). *The Relevance of Social Science for Medicine*. Boston, D Reidel: 1981, pp 241-253.

22. Capra F: *The Turning Point*. New York, Bantam Books, 1982, pp. 155-156.

23. Frankel B: *Childbirth in the Ghetto: Folk Beliefs of Negro Women*. San Francisco, R and E Research Association, 1977.

24. Kay MA: *Anthropology of Human Birth*. Philadelphia, FA Davis, 1982.

25. Murphree AH: A functional analysis of Southern folk beliefs concerning birth. *Am J Obstet Gynecol* 1968;102(1):125-134.

Responding to the spiritual needs of the chronically ill

KAREN L. SOEKEN, PHD; VERNA J. CARSON, RN, MSN

Chronic illness can have a dramatic effect, altering a client's physical, mental, and spiritual well-being. Although information about physical and mental care abounds, data about spiritual care are sparse. Yet these data suggest that "spirituality can be a mediator in times of stress for the chronically ill," indicating that spiritual care is a vital component of holistic nursing care.

To help the nurse become familiar with spiritual care, Soeken and Carson address spirituality and provide a framework for assessing the chronically ill client's spiritual needs and for implementing a plan to meet those needs. Note: Portions of the article have been excerpted (marked by ellipses) to condense extensive background material.

NURSES HAVE TRADITIONALLY adopted a holistic perspective, viewing the patient as a balance of mind, body, and spirit. These parts cannot be separated, but rather function as an integrated unit with the whole person more than the sum of the parts. Each dimension — mind, body, spirit — affects and is affected by the others. Consequently, healing or illness at any one level reverberates throughout the other levels. Responding to the needs of the chronically ill patient, then, requires the nurse to understand and care for the total person, including the spirit.

Spirituality

The spiritual dimension of a person is broader than institutionalized religion, although for some persons spirituality is expressed and developed through formal religious activities such as prayer and worship services. Spirit refers to humanity's "inner resources especially...ultimate concern, the basic value around which all other values are focused, the central philosophy of a life...which guides a person's conduct."[8] This ultimate concern is a generic or basic faith that positively affirms life, as distinguished from tradition or particular faith with its doctrine, dogma, and rituals. Although spirituality need not be expressed through these more traditional channels, it is always expressed.

Stoll[11] refers to the spiritual dimension as "the part of a person that allows God-consciousness and the possibility of relatedness to God, however God is defined." ...Banks[1] has characterized the spiritual dimension as involving four aspects. First, the spiritual dimension is a unifying force that integrates and transcends the physical, emotional, and social dimensions. Second, it enables and motivates one to find purpose and meaning in life and to relate to God, however God or an Ultimate Other is defined. Third, because the spiritual dimension transcends the individual, it provides a common bond [among] individuals, enabling them to share themselves with others. Fourth, the spiritual dimension is based on individual perceptions and beliefs that will guide behavior.[1] Thus spirituality can be considered a conscious or unconscious belief that relates the individual to the world and gives meaning and definition to existence....

Spiritual care in chronic illness

Chronic illness can affect each component of spiritual well-being, the harmonious interconnectedness with God, others, nature, and self. Pain, low self-esteem, feelings of isolation, powerlessness, hopelessness, and anger — all possible consequences of chronicity — impact on one's ability to affirm life to its fullest. Jourard[5] has discussed the nurse's role as an "inspiriting" one, providing a sense of identity, worth, hope, and purpose in existence. Although the concept of inspiriting encompasses approaches that are customarily viewed as affecting psychologic and affective processes, to inspirit someone is consistent also with providing spiritual care.

Because spiritual care occurs over time and within the context of a relationship, probably the most effective tool at the nurse's disposal is the use of self. Self can be a means of healing, support, and affirmation to another. The offer of self serves as a conduit whereby the inner strength and hope of the nurse flow to the patient. Through the nurse's presence, touch, and attempts to understand the patient's feelings, the nurse may transmit the message that the patient is worthy and accepted. The message may come at a time when the patient is having difficulty accepting and recognizing self-worth and dignity.

Hand in hand with the use of self is the use of effective communication skills. A patient with chronic illness has many feelings to deal with — anger toward God, guilt because of feeling angry, and a sense of loneliness. These feelings are so powerful and potentially all-encompassing that for the patient to affirm life in any relationship, they must be acknowledged, accepted, and dealt with so that the patient can move on with life. The nurse needs to be able to communicate warmth, respect, and empathy. Warmth conveys the nurse's caring for the patient; respect conveys the nurse's belief in the patient; and empathy conveys the nurse's understanding of the patient's situation.[3] In addition, the nurse needs to be able to deal with confrontation and immediacy — skills that characterize a relationship that is working on change, but skills that are not as comfortable nor as easy to use.

In the following discussion, specific consequences of chronic illness will be considered along with suggestions for intervention. Appropriate to each of the individual consequences, however, is the use of self and the effective use of communication skills.

Pain. Pain is a subjective phenomenon determined by many psychologic variables in addition to sensory input. The expression or display of pain that varies from one patient to another and may change over time directs the patient's attention inward, sapping vitality and a sense of aliveness. The patient often feels powerless and controlled by the amount and quality of pain. Some of the responses to pain frequently seen are depression, irritability, withdrawal, and hostility. When intense pain occurs, it becomes difficult for the patient to relate effectively to God, self, or others; as a consequence, spiritual well-being is affected.

The nurse providing spiritual care can explore with the patient the meaning of suffering and the patient's beliefs about God. Such feelings and beliefs can help the patient come to terms with the pain. One concept that applies here is that of finitude or limitation. Humans are not divine but limited. God is in ultimate control and can provide relief from suffering. In most religious traditions, health and lack of pain are believed to be gifts from God, and suffering often is viewed as part of the condition of humankind and not as a punishment from God.[13]

Communication with God also is a part of all traditional faiths. Such communication, prayer, or supplication helps the patient to remember God and for many is a source of strength in enduring pain. In the Judeo-Christian tradition there is also the promise that God will not send more pain than the person can bear.[9] Thus, the nurse can discuss with the patient his or her feelings about God, and the meaning and meaningfulness of prayer.

As the health care team explores methods of pain relief, alternatives to pharmacologic methods also can be considered. The use of imagery, relaxation, meditation, and self-hypnosis, all akin to prayer and for some a spiritual discipline, could be offered as potential avenues to decrease the patient's suffering.

Self-concept. Chronic illness, depending on the consequences to the patient, can produce varying degrees of feelings of self-denigration and low self-esteem. The patient may actually look different because of disability or may just feel different because of the limitations imposed by the illness. In any event, the person sees himself or herself as different and out of step with the rest of the world. The patient may lose sight of unique personal worth, abilities, gifts, and talents. The nurse needs to: (1) be cognizant that the patient may be feeling very low; (2) be willing to discuss these feelings with the patient; and (3) be able to help the patient see strengths as realistically as weaknesses.

A person's spirit is uplifted when feeling good about oneself. The ability to love oneself is inextricably connected to the very edge of Love itself (love with a capital L); we come very close to the mystical slendor of God. It is only with a positive self-concept that a person is able to relate to God in a way that provides support and sustenance. One who feels very bad about oneself has difficulty believing that God could love him or her, and does not perceive that there is anything personally appealing to others. A lack of self-regard, then, affects all relationships and reflects the state of spiritual being.

The nurse's acceptance of the patient can communicate that at least to the nurse the patient is worthwhile. It is also helpful for the nurse to share beliefs about God's love and concern for each of us (that is, if the nurse holds such beliefs). As the patient affirms beliefs about creation and that God cares about what is happening to each person, the patient begins to trust in God's faithfulness and to accept oneself. For those in the Western tradition there is a doctrine that theologians refer to as *imago Dei:* each is created in the image of God, and each mirrors God in some way.[9] This belief may provide the patient with a deep sense of joy and self-esteem. Through the rituals and practices of traditional faith, the patient also can enhance self-esteem. Sacraments such as communion or confession and ceremonies of the community of faith are avenues for one to experience the unconditional love and concern of others.

Isolation and loneliness. Feeling different from and inferior to others can lead to a desire to retreat from all interactions and from all social activities. This can be exacerbated if the chronic illness itself decreases mobility and independence. Long periods of hospitalization can further remove the patient from others. Isolation can be so complete that the patient feels cut off from the support of God, loved ones, social interaction, and even superficial contact with others. Left in this state, a person can sink lower into a morass of self-pity, feelings of worthlessness, utter loneliness, and spiritual deprivation. Research has [documented] this inverse relationship between loneliness and spiritual well-being.[7] Among both chronically ill and healthy adults, those with higher levels of spiritual well-being experience less loneliness.

The nurse needs to be aware of signs that the patient is becoming increasingly isolated and discuss this openly with the patient, family, and other support people. The nurse can help the patient and family mutually devise a plan in which the patient's needs for companionship, diversion, and support are recognized and met. The nurse also can explore ways that the patient can be assertive and reach out to others to get the support that is needed. This approach also enhances the patient's belief of being in control of personal destiny and not being buffeted about by the whim of others.

The patient's reaching out can take many forms: letter writing, telephone calls, participation in self-help groups, contact with church groups, and volunteer work.

The notion of shared traditional rituals and practices (such as worship and sacraments) also can be useful in overcoming loneliness. Participating in rituals handed down over centuries gives persons the feeling that they are part of something immortal rather than transient, and connected to others across time and space. Religion affirms that we are not alone, but that we are connected to all (nature and others) that participate in life through God. This connectedness also can be experienced through art, music, and literature.

Powerlessness. Chronic illness with its constant demands on the patient can result in a feeling of powerlessness. The patient no longer feels able to affect personal destiny, but rather is controlled by the vagaries of the disease process. Powerlessness is a pervasive feeling that undermines the person's sense of self, self-efficacy, decision-making abilities, and efforts to control the illness. Those who experience powerlessness no longer feel empowered by God. They lose sight of God's presence in their lives and feel unprotected and defenseless. If God was once believed to provide support, power, and protection, the loss of this assurance may leave the person feeling naked and exposed, buffeted about by the illness itself.

Spiritual well-being is an empowering state wherein life has meaning in the secular as well as the eternal sense. When that sense of power is gone, so too is the sense of spiritual well-being. This is an issue that should be confronted early with the patient. Efforts need to be made to involve the patient in mutual planning about his or her care. The patient needs to live with illness and to do so effectively must participate in the plans that are made to enhance coping. Even when people are very debilitated, there are always areas where choice and decision-making are still possible. Retaining a sense of power and control enhances the patient's ability to see meaning in life's events and particularly in the illness. Without that sense of power, life is without meaning. God has no power.

Traditional rituals and practices often are empowering for the patient....Prayer is often a coping method for the chronically ill. Through prayer and other rituals such as communion, the patient feels the power of God and adopts that power in the fight against the disease. Exploring these beliefs with the patient can be very important.

Hope. Hope has several components: future orientation, the setting of goals, the taking of action to meet those goals, and the importance of interpersonal relationships.[4] Each of these components has implications for spiritual well-being and consequently for nursing interventions. Hope is derived from relationships with others, oneself, and the world where a person believes that what is desired is possible. Ultimate hope resides in God and the belief that the Supreme Being will impart meaning to individual lives and sufferings. Both components of hope are important for the patient with chronic illness. The patient still needs to hope for future-oriented goals, even if it means changing aspirations to be consistent with the limitations imposed by illness. Patients still need to hope for the support, love, and constancy provided by the important relationships in life and to take action to meet the goals that are set. If God is a reality for the patient, then the patient needs to hope in God. This hoping in God surpasses all the aspirations that are transitory. The hope in God is an eternal abiding hope that keeps the others alive.

Anger. Anger is a common reaction during chronic illness. The patient may direct anger on himself or herself for having the disease or may direct it at others for being healthy. Anger toward God also can emerge if God is blamed for the disease. To overcome the anger, the patient must be able to receive and accept forgiveness and, in turn, to forgive others. If not, the anger and guilt become destructive to the spirit, destroying the relationships among self, others, and God. The nurse needs to be willing to allow the patient to express feelings of anger and to explore the patient's image of God. By so doing, the nurse can assist the patient in experiencing the freedom offered in unconditional forgiveness.

Summary

The steps of the nursing process apply to needs of the spirit as well as body and mind. Several nurses have provided guidelines for assessing spirtual needs. Stoll,[12] for example, considers four areas of concern: the person's concept of God; source of strength and hope; significance of religious practices and rituals; and perceived relationship between spiritual beliefs and state of health. In approaching the patient about these four areas, it is important for the nurse to clearly articulate the purpose in seeking such information. For instance, a nurse might explain to a patient that research has demonstrated the positive relationship of spiritual concerns to a patient's ability to cope with chronic illness. Because the nurse is interested in assisting the patient to identify, strengthen, and develop a variety of coping strategies, spiritually related data are relevant to the patient's care. Having collected data from the patients, a nursing diagnosis can be made. Spiritual concerns, spiritual distress, and spiritual despair have been included in the accepted classification system.[6]

Meeting the spiritual needs of patients can be uncomfortable for the nurse. Several reasons for such discomfort include embarrassment, the belief that it is not the nurse's role, lack of training, and the lack of [one's] spiritual resources. Experience with an elective course in spirituality for undergraduate nursing students would support the value of offering training. Discussing God-related issues can assist a health care professional to clarify a personal spiritual position.[2] There also is research suggesting that nurses with higher levels of spiritual well-being have a more positive attitude towards providing spiritual care for patients and view potential intervention as appropriate for meeting spiritual needs of their patients.[10]

REFERENCES

1. Banks R: Health and the spiritual dimensions: Relationships and implications for professional preparation programs. J Sch Health 50:195, 1980

2. Carson V, Winkelstein M, Soeken K, et al: Altering students' spiritual attitudes through an elective course on spirtuality. Image 18:161, 1987

3. Gazda G, Asbury FS, Balzer, FJ, et al: Human Relations Development. Boston, Allyn and Bacon, 1984

4. Grimm P, Soeken KL, Carson V: Hope and its relationship to spiritual well-being. Presented at the Seventh Biennial Eastern Nursing Research Conference, Yale University, April 1986

5. Jourard S: The Transparent Self. New York, Van Norstrand Reinhold, 1971

6. Kim MJ, McFarland G, McLane A (eds): Classification of nursing diagnoses: Proceedings of the Fifth National Conference. St. Louis, CV Mosby, 1984

7. Miller JF: Assessment of loneliness and spiritual well-being in the chronically ill and healthy adults. J Prof Nurs 1:79, 1985

8. Moberg DO: Spiritual Well-Being: Background and Issues. Washington, D.C., White House Conference on Aging, 1971

9. Sevensky RL: The religious foundations of health care: A conceptual approach. J Med Ethics 9:165, 1983

10. Soeken KL, Carson VJ: Study measures nurses' attitudes about providing spiritual care. Health Prog 67:52, 1986

11. Stoll RI: Emotional and spiritual support. *In* Kravis TC, Warner CG (eds.): Emergency Medicine: A Comprehensive Review. Rockville, Maryland, Aspen, 1983, pp 575-583

12. Stoll RI: Guidelines for spiritual assessment. Am J Nurs 79:1574, 1979

13. Vanderpool HY: Religion and medicine: A theoretical overview. J Rel Health 19:7, 1980

UNIT TWO

Study questions

1. According to "Conceptual Components of the Therapeutic Relationship," a nurse can facilitate empathy by using four levels of nursing actions: (1) accepting, (2) listening, (3) clarifying and informing, and (4) analyzing. List two examples of actions for each level. How does a level 4 action contrast with a level 1 action in establishing a therapeutic nurse-client relationship?

2. In "The Family as the Unit of Care in Nursing: A Historical Review," Whall describes the views of several modern theorists: King, Newman, Orem, Rogers, and Roy. How does King's view of the family as a unit of nursing care differ from that of another theorist? (Pick one.)

3. Based on the research findings discussed in "Social Risk Factors: Impact on Elders' Perceived Health Status," in what ways can income, education, social network, and perceptions of isolation affect an elderly client's health?

4. In "Home Remedies: A Cultural Study," Roberson argues that a nurse should be sensitive to cultural differences in a client's health beliefs and practices. Why? How can a nurse exhibit cultural sensitivity?

5. Soeken and Carson, in "Responding to the Spiritual Needs of the Chronically Ill," tell how a chronically ill client may experience pain, low self-esteem, isolation, powerlessness, hopelessness, or anger. How can these consequences of chronic illness affect a client's spirituality? Which nursing interventions can help the client overcome these consequences? (Give three examples.)

UNIT THREE

Nursing as a process

By investigating client systems and their interactions with the environment, Unit Two answered the questions "For whom is nursing practiced?" and "With whom is nursing practiced?" This unit will build on the previous material by answering the question "How is nursing practiced?"

Nursing is an interactive profession: the nurse regularly engages in reciprocal relationships with client systems. Because client systems interact with their internal and external environments and are always in a state of change, nursing too is constantly in process, growing and evolving to meet the health care needs of individuals, families, small groups, and the community.

This unit examines four ways in which nursing is a process: in providing care via the five-step nursing process, in communicating with others, in interacting with the law, and in interacting with ethical standards.

Nursing process

A method of organizing and delivering nursing care, the nursing process involves interactive problem solving between the nurse and the client and forms the basis for nursing actions and decisions. This cyclical process continually adapts to the client's changing needs.

The nursing process consists of five steps:

1. assessment of the client's health by gathering, verifying, and documenting health-related information
2. diagnosis of the client's health care needs through the use of nursing diagnoses that identify actual or potential client problems
3. planning of nursing strategies to achieve the mutually established goals for the client
4. implementation of the plan of care
5. evaluation of the plan's effectiveness in achieving the client's health care goals. When goals are not met, the nurse reassesses the client and begins the process again. When the goals are met, the nurse may apply the process to achieve different goals.

The nursing process itself has changed and grown since 1955 when Lydia Hall first described nursing as a process. In 1959, Dorothy Johnson described a three-step method that included assessment, decision, and action. Later, Ida Orlando (1961) and Ernestine Wiedenbach (1963) introduced similar three-step approaches.

Throughout the 1960s, nursing leaders

modified the nursing process. In 1967, after intense study with the Western Interstate Commission of Higher Education, the School of Nursing at the Catholic University of America divided the nursing process into four phases: assessment, planning, intervention, and evaluation (Yura & Walsh, 1983).

Finally, the nursing profession accepted the current version of the nursing process in 1973 when Kristine Gebbie and Mary Ann Lavin organized the first conference on the classification of nursing diagnoses. This conference was the impetus for adding the nursing diagnosis step to the nursing process, making it a five-step method.

Today, the nurse can use the nursing process effectively in any setting (as described in Unit Five), with any client system (as described in Unit Two), and with individuals of any age (as described in Unit Four). In fact, use of the nursing process is an important part of the nurse's independent role. It allows the nurse to develop nursing care plans that focus clearly on nursing responsibilities. It helps the nurse identify health care problems that fall within the scope of nursing practice, and it clearly links the nurse's actions to expected client responses. In these ways, the nursing process helps nurses define their roles, increase their autonomy, and demonstrate their accountability (responsibility to themselves and to the client, profession, health care facility, and society for the effectiveness of their nursing care).

Communicating with others

As part of the process of nursing, the nurse not only interacts with individual clients, but also with families, small groups, communities, other nurses and health care professionals, administrators, and many other individuals. For these interactions to be effective, the nurse must communicate well.

For example, the nurse must communicate effectively to help a client acquire or maintain healthful behaviors. To do this, the nurse must speak and act in ways that facilitate client change. The nurse builds collaborative relationships (equal working relationships with other members of the health care team) through effective communications. Such relationships depend on the nurse's ability to express observations about clients clearly and articulately.

The nurse can improve communication skills by eliminating factors that can hinder communication, such as cultural or emotional biases, and by developing self-awareness and acceptance of different life-styles. Through self-awareness of personal perceptions, values, feelings, internal and external environmental factors, and biases, the nurse can communicate more effectively with individuals from different backgrounds.

Additionally, the nurse must understand verbal (spoken or written) and nonverbal (physical) messages. In verbal communication, the nurse must realize that words can have different meanings; that vocabulary can affect understanding; that the intonation, speed, and clarity of a message can greatly affect its meaning; that short, simple messages are more effective than long, complex ones; and that the timing of a message can influence its reception.

With nonverbal communication (sometimes called body language), communication occurs continually even when verbal communication stops. Nonverbal messages help assess the validity of — and usually are more reliable than — verbal messages. For these reasons, the nurse should pay close attention to a client's appearance, posture, gait, facial expressions, eye movements, and gestures. Discrepancies between a client's or coworker's actions and words may give the nurse important insights.

Moreover, the nurse can use personal and technical skills to facilitate communication.

Personal skills include the ability to be genuine, empathetic, and warm with a client. Technical skills include the ability to use silence effectively, listen actively, ask pertinent questions, aid in clarification, maintain the focus of a conversation, paraphrase, and share information.

Interacting with the law

Like nursing, the law is in process, constantly changing and redefining its parts. It touches the nurse in three major ways: It differentiates nursing practice from that of other health care professionals, protects the client's rights, and describes the nurse's responsibilities. Because of the law's changing nature and its effect on nursing, the nurse should stay abreast of legal issues throughout her or his career.

The law guides nurses in their professional practice in several ways. The nurse practice act (a state or provincial law that defines nursing activities) requires licensure by the state or province in which the nurse plans to practice. To obtain this license, the nurse must meet educational requirements and pass an examination. After receiving a license, the practicing nurse must adhere to standards of care specified in the nurse practice act and must follow the guidelines of professional organizations and the employer's policies and procedures.

The nurse practice act also governs the nursing student's actions. It stipulates that a nursing student should be assigned only to nursing tasks for which she or he is prepared and should be adequately supervised during the learning process. If a nursing student's actions harm a client, the student, instructor, and health care facility usually share the liability.

Through the nurse practice act and the laws that protect clients' rights, the courts can find a nurse legally liable for negligence (care that does not meet legal standards), invasion of privacy (such as improper release of confidential information or gossiping about a client), defamation of character (harm to the reputation of another by libel or slander), or assault (an attempt or threat to physically injure another) and battery (unauthorized touching of another).

Because the laws can vary from state to state and because policies differ among health care facilities, the nurse should be aware of specific local requirements that apply to practice. This is especially important for nursing activities with a high legal risk, such as obtaining informed consent (permission from a client for a physician to perform surgery or for a health care professional to perform a procedure after the client has been fully informed about it), witnessing a written will or an autopsy consent form, handling a deceased client with dignity, carrying out physician's orders (unless the orders are incorrect or would harm the client), and caring for more clients than is reasonable and safe.

Some national laws also affect the nurse's professional duties. For example, the 1970 Comprehensive Drug Abuse Prevention and Control Act stipulates that the nurse may administer drugs such as narcotics, depressants, stimulants, and hallucinogens only under the direction of a licensed physician. Under this law, the nurse also must ensure that these drugs are securely locked up and that only authorized personnel have access to them.

A nurse who works in critical care, obstetrics, or another specialty is legally accountable for performing additional duties, which are determined by professional organizations and the nurse practice act. Such a nurse, therefore, requires advanced training and ongoing in-service education.

No matter what a nurse's setting or specialty, nurse-client interactions can raise legal questions. If a situation poses a potential legal problem, the nurse should seek guidance from nursing administration. If the administration cannot provide a satisfactory answer, the nurse should seek legal counsel, which is available in most hospitals.

Glossary

Accountability: responsibility. In nursing, accountability refers to the nurses's self-responsibility and responsibility to the client, profession, health care facility, and society for effective nursing care.

Assault: attempt or threat to injure another physically, as when a health care professional coerces a client to take unwanted medication.

Battery: unauthorized touching of another, as when a health care professional injects medication after the client has refused it.

Collaborative relationships: equal working relationships with other members of the health care team based on joint communication and decision making.

Communication: activities that transfer meaning from sender to receiver. Communication may be verbal (using spoken or written language) or nonverbal (using body language).

Defamation of character: harm to the reputation of another by libel or slander.

Ethics: principles of appropriate conduct that govern an individual or group.

Informed consent: permission obtained from a client to perform surgery or a procedure, after the client has it fully explained.

Legal issues of nursing: aspects of the law that differentiate nursing practice from the practice of other health care professionals, protect the client's rights, and describe the nurse's responsibilities.

Liability: legal responsibility for failure to act or for actions that fail to meet standards of care and cause harm to another.

Malpractice: a professional's wrongful conduct, improper discharge of duties, or failure to meet standards of care that causes harm to another.

Negligence: failure to exercise the care that a prudent individual would exercise normally. In nursing, negligence is a form of malpractice; it refers to nursing care that does not meet legal standards, such as performing a procedure without proper training or causing a burn.

Nurse practice act: state or provincial law that defines the scope of nursing activities.

Nursing process: systematic, five-step method for assessing a client's health, diagnosing health care needs, planning the necessary care, implementing the planned care, and evaluating the effectiveness of that care.

Interacting with ethical standards

With the rise of high-tech care, the shortage of nurses, and the reduction in health care resources, the nurse increasingly faces dilemmas that challenge the mind and wrench the soul. Dilemmas such as artificial prolongation of life, involuntary hospitalization, and refusal to care for individuals who cannot pay demonstrate the nature of ethics: confrontation of problems that require a choice between two equally desirable or equally undesirable alternatives. In such dilemmas, the nurse may base decisions on ethics — principles of conduct — that are formed by personal and professional values, philosophies of life and nursing, and cultural, emotional, and spiritual beliefs.

When making such decisions, the nurse needs to differentiate among moral, ethical, and legal issues. Moral issues reflect a belief that something is absolutely right or wrong in all situations. Individuals usually do not compromise or negotiate about their moral beliefs. For instance, some individuals believe that abortions are morally wrong and that no circumstances could make them acceptable.

An ethical issue is present when no clear

choice exists between right and wrong. For some people, abortion is an ethical issue because they would accept it under some circumstances, such as a risk to the mother's life or the needs of the woman seeking the abortion. Therefore, a moral issue for some is an ethical issue for others.

Ethical and legal issues also differ. Legal issues refer only to those situations covered by the law. Ethical issues cannot be settled by the law, but must be resolved in the hearts and minds of those making the decision. For example, the law may permit abortions in some states under some circumstances, but the woman who has a legal abortion may have to resolve her own ethical issues about termination of life. Parents may have the legal right to withdraw life-support for an anencephalic infant who will not benefit from therapy, but they may wrestle with the ethical issue of hastening the death of another human being.

As the nursing student becomes a professional nurse, personal values and beliefs may intertwine with professional ones. Ideally, the student's increasing experience will help personal values complement professional ones, making it easier to resolve ethical dilemmas. Nevertheless, the nurse always must be willing to dedicate the time and personal energy required to arrive at logical, fair, and humane ethical decisions.

REFERENCES

Gebbie, K., & Lavin, M.A. (1974). Classification of nursing diagnosis. *American Journal of Nursing, 75, 250.*

Hall, L.E. (1955). Quality of nursing care, address given at the Department of Baccalaureate and Higher Degree Programs of the New Jersey League for Nursing. *Public Health News,* New Jersey State Department of Health.

Johnson, D. (1959). A philosophy of nursing. *Nursing Outlook, 7,* 198.

Little, D.E., & Carnevali, D.L. (1969). *Nursing care planning.* Philadelphia: J.B. Lippincott Co.

Orlando, I. (1961). *The dynamic nurse-patient relations.* New York: Putnam.

Western Interstate Commission of Higher Education. (1967). *Defining clinical content, graduate nursing programs, medical surgical nursing.*

Wiedenbach, E. (1963). The helping art of nursing. *American Journal of Nursing, 63,* 64.

Yura, H., & Walsh, M. (1983). *The nursing process: Assessing, planning, and evaluation* (4th ed.). New York: Appleton-Century-Crofts.

SECTION ONE

The nursing process

By using the nursing process, the nurse can determine which health problems to try to alleviate, which potential problems to try to prevent, what kind of and how much assistance the client requires, and which desired outcomes are realistic. The nurse can use this process with clients of all ages in any setting.

To illustrate the practicality of the nursing process, the articles in this section focus on its application to two very different groups: depressed elderly clients in hospitals and at home, and developmentally disabled children and adults in a long-term care setting.

The first article, "Therapy for Depression" by Ronsman, demonstrates effective application of the nursing process and Maslow's hierarchy of needs to depressed elderly clients.

Maslow's hierarchy states that individuals have five levels of needs from the most basic to the most elevated. The needs are:

1. physiologic
2. safety and security
3. love, belonging, and affection
4. esteem and self-respect
5. self-actualization.

Because these needs are hierarchical, an individual will seek to satisfy them in order, first gratifying physiologic needs, then safety and security needs, and so on.

As Ronsman shows, the nurse can use Maslow's hierarchy of needs to establish priorities within the nursing process. For example, if a nurse's assessment and diagnosis reveals that a depressed client has a nutritional deficit (a physiologic need) and a sense of social isolation (a love, belonging, and affection need), the nurse should develop, implement, and evaluate a plan that addresses the client's physiologic need first.

The author provides details for using the five steps of the nursing process for each type of need. She believes that nurses are well-prepared to meet all five levels of needs. She explains that nursing interventions related to basic needs (levels one, two, and three) are often simple and uncomplicated, such as providing reassurance and assisting with activities of daily living. Then she describes nursing interventions for addressing higher needs (levels four and five), which include counseling, problem solving, and client education — the forte of nurses.

In the second article, "The Impact of Nursing Diagnoses in a Long-Term Care Setting," Miller et al. examine the effects of using the nursing process — including nursing diagnoses — with developmentally disabled clients.

After detailing the implementation of nursing diagnoses in the facility, the authors discuss its impact. They attribute several benefits to this step of the nursing process: clear identification of the nurse's roles and functions, a uniform taxonomy, improved communication among nurses, population-specific care guides, a written system for nursing orders, and organized nursing standards.

Therapy for depression

KAYE RONSMAN, RNC, GNP, MSN

In this article, the author suggests that nurses already have the skills to relieve much of the pain and suffering of depression. Here, she describes how to apply these skills to depressed elderly clients and shows how to use the nursing process and Maslow's hierarchy of needs to identify their problems and set priorities. Note: Summaries (shown in bracketed italics) and excerpts (marked by ellipses) condense extensive background material.

DEPRESSION IS THE MOST common mental illness in the elderly. Approximately 10% to 15% of people over 65 have clinically significant depression and probably twice that number have mild depression.[1] There is a great disparity between the number of elderly with a *diagnosis* of depression (5%)[2] and the number of elderly with *symptoms* of depression (20% to 50%).[3,4] Symptoms of depression are the same as those of several other conditions, thus making diagnosis difficult.

Depression at any age may present with symptoms in four areas: emotional, cognitive, physical, and behavioral. In the elderly, vague physical complaints and preoccupation with bodily function may be the only symptoms....

The main feature of clinical depression is change — change from usual patterns, habits, or moods. The second feature of depression is that it persists — changes may last months or even years. Depression can be differentiated from normal blue days in that the symptoms last at least two weeks. A summary of signs and symptoms of depression is found in Table 1....

[Traditionally, physicians have treated depression in elderly clients with hospitalization for those who are suicidal and with medications for moderately to severely depressed outpatients. When the client's symptoms are mild to moderate or unrecognized as symptoms of depression, they are typically ignored.]

Treating depression in the elderly only by administering medications is a practice that should be challenged. Other treatment options should be considered, in combination with medications, for the severely depressed and instead of medications for the mild to moderately depressed. Research indicates that mild to moderate depression frequently responds to supportive care, increased activity, counseling, or psychotherapy [5-7] and only requires medication when these other measures do not result in a favorable response. Normal grieving following a loss can also be helped by these same nondrug treatments.

Supportive care includes such measures as: 1) assistance with activities of daily living; 2) good nutrition; 3) promoting comfort; 4) relief of physical and emotional pain; 5) giving information and encouragement; 6) encouraging the person to talk about feelings; 7) encouraging physical and mental activities; 8) advocacy; 9) ongoing interest; 10) encouraging involvement of family and friends; and 11) environmental adjustments. These measures are the forte of nurses. With guidance in choosing the appropriate supportive measure for each individual, many more depressed elderly could be helped.

Most nurses are familiar with both the nursing process and Maslow's hierarchy of needs. The nursing process includes assessment, iden-

TABLE 1. Summary of signs and symptoms of depression in the elderly

Emotional or mood symptoms
Sadness
Crying
Apathy (lack of feeling)
Feeling blue
Feeling depressed
Being "down in the dumps"
Being unhappy
Decreased pleasure or enjoyment
Lack of interest
Decreased life satisfaction
Cognitive (thinking) changes
Pessimism
Hopelessness
Rumination about past failures
Sense of worthlessness
Feeling of uselessness
Low self-esteem
Memory disturbance
Disorientation
Decreased attention span
Suicidal thoughts
Somatic delusions
Physical symptoms
Sleep disturbance
Loss of appetite
Weight loss or weight gain
Fatigue
Loss of sexual interest
Constipation
Hypochondriasis
Headaches
Backaches
Muscle/skeletal pain
Stomach distress
Behavioral changes
Reduction in activities
Slowing of physical movements
Agitation
Handwringing
Obsessive worrying
Restlessness
Angry or hostile behavior
Irritability

tifying problems, establishing goals, intervention, and evaluation. This problem-solving process is very helpful in organizing thinking into a logical format that leads to a specific, measurable approach to care planning. An essential part of the nursing process is problem identification or nursing diagnosis. "Once the problem is clearly identified, the solution is evident. The nursing actions to be taken also become evident when the problem is recognized."[8]

Maslow's hierarchy of needs naturally groups data into categories that nurses recognize and remember easily. It also establishes priorities for intervention from more basic needs to higher needs. Nursing process begins with assessment, the gathering of data, and includes history taking and physical assessment. The goal of assessment is to uncover symptoms of depression previously discussed.

Critically important to assessing depression is a careful history. Emphasis should be placed on the psychosocial history and should include both the person's normal characteristics and those the person is now exhibiting. In order to be significant, symptoms must be new to differentiate from life-long characteristics and must persist for at least two weeks to differentiate from normal "blue days."

Once the data are gathered, they must be analyzed to identify problems. This is probably the most critical step and to be effective must include the elderly person. "The nurse must be careful that problems identified are perceived as problems by the client."[8] Problems can be arranged in terms of Maslow's hierarchy of needs which are: 1) physiologic needs; 2) safety and security needs; 3) need for love, belonging, and affection; 4) need for esteem and self-respect; and 5) need for self-actualization. Table 2 shows the interaction between the nursing process and Maslow's hierarchy of needs.

Maslow made it clear when developing his theory that people are not likely to be moti-

TABLE 2. The nursing process and Maslow's hierarchy of needs

MASLOW'S HIERARCHY OF NEEDS	ASSESSMENT	IDENTIFYING PROBLEMS	ESTABLISHING GOALS	INTERVENTION	EVALUATION
1) Physiologic Needs Food/Fluid Shelter/Warmth Air Rest/Sleep Avoidance of pain Sex	Usual and present nutritional, elimination, sleep and sexuality patterns Physical activity–exercise pattern Emotional pain and discomfort Suicide potential Physical health Medications	Nutritional deficit Dehydration Constipation Sleep pattern disturbance Sexual dysfunction Self-destructive behavior Medications or physical illnesses that may cause depression	Establishing and maintaining adequate biological functioning in areas of sleep, nutrition and elimination Relief from emotional pain and discomfort Elimination of drug or disease-induced depression	Assist with ADLs Support of self-care abilities Encouragement to start a physical activity regimen Teach side effects of antidepressants Treat medical problems under poor control Change medications that may cause depression	Feelings of physical satiation Homeostasis Optimal physical health
2) Safety and security needs Feel free from danger Need for a predictable, lawful, orderly world Need to feel in control	Home environment assessment Mental status exam Assessment of visual acuity and hearing Knowledge of disease process Physical mobility	Perceived inability to control feelings or behavior Perceived powerlessness Translocation syndrome Cognitive impairment Alteration in sensory perceptions Impaired physical mobility	Establish predictability and structure in environment Maintenance of a safe environment Realistic understanding of disease course and expected outcome Reversal of treatable confusion	ECT, hospitalization, antidepressive medications for the severely depressed Avoid relocations when possible Correct environmental hazards Encourage a structured daily routine Instruct about disease course and prognosis	Feeling in control of one's disease and optimistic about the future Confidence in the future Feelings of safety, peace, security, protection, lack of danger and threat

TABLE 2. **The nursing process and Maslow's hierarchy of needs** *continued*

MASLOW'S HIERARCHY OF NEEDS	ASSESSMENT	IDENTIFYING PROBLEMS	ESTABLISHING GOALS	INTERVENTION	EVALUATION
3) Need for love, belonging, and affection Need for contact and intimacy Need for friends Need for a feeling of having a place, "belonging" Need for interactions with others	Family relationships and members Friends that are supportive Recent losses Present and past social interactions	Disruption in significant relationships Social isolation Lack of contact with or absence of significant others Alterations in socialization with reduced social interactions	Maintenance of significant relationships with family and friends Establish community support system Resumption of previous level of social activity	Encourage social interactions that have been enjoyed in the past Encourage interactions with family members, friends, and health care givers Provide reassuring, supportive atmosphere	Feelings of loving and being loved, of being one of a group, of acceptance
4) Need for esteem and self-respect Need for achievement, mastery, and competence Need for reputation or prestige, appreciation, and dignity Need for love of self	Number of pleasurable pursuits Emotional or mood assessment Role patterns Coping–stress tolerance pattern Attitude about self, the world, the future	Negative feelings or conception of self Loss of significant roles Unrealistic self-expectations Anxiety Life-style change Dependency on others	Acceptance of realistic limitations Establish appropriate roles Achieve self-acceptance Accept consequences of one's own behavior	Teach problem-solving skills Cognitive therapy Promote self-care Counseling Behavior therapy Relaxation techniques	Feelings of self-confidence, worth, strength, capability, adequacy, and of being useful and necessary in the world
5) Need for self-actualization Need for beauty Need for self-expression Need for new situations and stimulation	Occupation, job history Value-belief patterns	Distress of human spirit Loss of zest for life	Expression of self through meaningful recreational activities Exploring new interests	Encourage a nonrestrictive environment Provide beauty in environment Read to the sick or hard of hearing Music	Autonomy Freshness of appreciation Creativeness Spontaneity Feelings of self-fulfillment

vated to satisfy higher needs until lower ones are somewhat satisfied.[9](p 98) The elderly with the most severe symptoms must have their most basic needs met first. Elderly persons with only mild symptoms of depression are likely to be able to take care of their most basic needs independently and will require assistance only in fulfilling higher needs. To look at treatment for depression in this kind of framework will focus on symptoms and provide relief for many depressed elderly now being ignored or "lost in the cracks."

[Physiologic needs

The most basic needs—for food, fluids, warmth, air, shelter, rest, sleep, sex, and avoidance of pain—must be met first. A severely depressed client will have severe emotional pain, which is likely to be a main motivator. A suicidal client, who is motivated to end the pain, will need immediate attention and treatment with electroconvulsive therapy, hospitalization, or medication.

For a client who is taking antidepressant medication, the nurse may need to intervene to prevent or help cope with common anticholinergic adverse reactions, such as constipation, dry mouth, and urine retention. The nurse may also need to advise the client, that these medications may take two weeks before becoming effective, to prevent noncompliance during this period.

Safety and security needs

After satisfying the client's physiologic needs, the nurse can move to the physical and psychological safety and security needs. For a client whose limited mobility or altered sensory perception increases the risk of accidents at home—and heightens insecurity—the nurse should suggest ways to make the environment safer, such as removing loose rugs, adding night lights and a telephone with volume control, or using a walker, cane, or other adaptive equipment.

If confusion adds to the client's sense of insecurity, the nurse should explain that the confusion will lessen as the depression improves and explain the disorder's progression and prognosis. The nurse also may minimize confusion and insecurity by helping the client establish a structured routine in stable surroundings with familiar people.

Love, belonging, and affection needs

After physiologic and safety needs are met, the nurse can address the client's need for contact, intimacy, friends, and a feeling of belonging. One of the best ways to intervene in this area is to let the client know that he or she is "unconditionally accepted as a fellow human being." The nurse should develop a trusting, nonjudgmental relationship with the client and should encourage the open expression of feelings. Allied health professionals can assist in this endeavor by spending time talking with and listening to the client.

The nurse also may help the depressed client by suggesting attendance at social activities and participation in favorite hobbies. In addition, the nurse can encourage family and friends to spend time with the client and can provide them with information and support so that they can become a stronger support to the client.

Esteem and self-respect needs

These higher level needs include the desire for strength, achievement, mastery, competence, reputation, status, recognition, appreciation, and dignity. They include "love of self as well as recognition that one is...unique...."[9] However, many depressed clients hold negative opinions of themselves, belittle their past achievements, and feel they have nothing to look forward to.[13]

The nurse is well equipped to meet these needs with problem-solving skills, counseling, and patient education. As a skilled observer, the nurse can provide feedback that may help the client define the problem. Then the nurse can provide information or teach problem-solving skills that may help the client resolve the problem.

The nurse may find counseling skills invaluable in helping the client deal with minor symptoms or normal grief. However, if the client does not respond, the nurse should refer the client to a specialist.

Self-actualization needs

Because depression interferes with satisfaction of many basic needs, most depressed clients do not have the energy to attempt self-actualization. Therefore, it is rarely a priority in a depressed client. The nurse should help the client overcome depression, leaving the self-actualization level for later.]

Discussion of Maslow's hierarchy of needs as it relates to treatment of depression may be helpful to nurses by demonstrating that to attempt to do patient education or problem-solving with a person whose basic needs are unmet is probably unrealistic. When an elderly person is institutionalized for depression, there is a tendency to try to solve all problems before the patient leaves the institution. This cannot always be done.

In this era of DRGs, it is conceivable that a person may be discharged from the hospital or nursing home once the threat of suicide has abated. The elderly person may still be suffering from one of the physical symptoms of depression such as insomnia, constipation, and anorexia and may also be suffering emotional symptoms of sadness and discomfort.

To insist that a patient participate in patient education and problem solving is likely to be fruitless and frustrating until lower level needs are satisfied. It may well be that only the first three levels of the needs hierarchy can be addressed while a person is in the hospital; counseling sessions may have to wait for the home situation or an outpatient clinic.

Nurses often feel insecure around depressed persons, see themselves as unable to help, and believe treatment is only in the hands of physicians and psychiatrists, who consider medications the single treatment mode. In fact, most depressed elderly persons need nursing therapeutics as much if not more than medical therapeutics. The first three basic needs of Maslow's hierarchy must, however, be met before the higher needs can be tackled. All nursing personnel are equipped, without further training, to help the elderly depressed person fulfill these basic needs. It is just a matter of thinking logically through each specific case, observing individual needs, and making an appropriate health care plan.

The interventions themselves are not difficult or complicated. They simply need to be correctly identified and emphasized. Nurses, and nurse's aids with guidance, can be instrumental in relieving much of the pain and suffering associated with depression. Good nursing therapeutics are not restricted to any environment. Hospitals, nursing homes, nurse-run clinics, home health-care services, or any environment where nurses care for the elderly can be the right environment in which to assist the 10% to 15% of the elderly who are clinically depressed.

REFERENCES

1. Gurland BJ, Toner JA: Depression in the elderly: A review of recently published studies in *Ann Rev Gerontol Geriatr,* vol 3. Eisdorfer C (ed). New York, Springer Publishing Co, 1982, p 229.

2. Gurland BJ: The comparative frequency of depression in various adult age groups. *J Gerontol* 1976; 31(3):288.

3. Weissman MM: The psychological treatment of depression. *Arch Gen Psychiatry* 1979; 36(10):1261-1269.

4. Rosenfeld AH: *New Views on Older Lives.* US Dept. of Health, Education, and Welfare Publication No. 76-687, 1978.

5. Bames R, Veith RC, Raskind MA: Depression in older persons: Diagnosis and management. *West J Med* 1981; 135(6):466.

6. Raskind M: *Depression in the Elderly*. Roche Products Inc, 1982, p 5.

7. Finlayson RE, Martin LM: Recognition and mangement of depression in the elderly. *Mayo Clinical Proceedings*. February 1982, p 118.

8. Ebersole P, Hess P: *Toward Healthy Aging*. St. Louis, CV Mosby Co, 1984, p 25.

9. Maslow AH: *Motivation and Personality*. New York, Harper and Row, 1954, p 98.

10. Brown RS, Ramirez DE, Taub JM: The prescription of exercise for depression. *Physician and Sportsmedicine* 1978; 6(12):35-45.

11. Martinsen EW, Medhus A, Sandvik L: Effects of aerobic exercise on depression: A controlled study. *British Medical Journal* 1985; 109.

12. Mellion MB: Exercise therapy for anxiety and depression. *Postgrad Med* 1985; 77(3):59-66.

13. Emery G: Cognitive therapy of depression in the elderly, in Crook T, Cohen G (eds): *Physicians' Guide to the Diagnosis and Treatment of Depression in the Elderly*. New Canaan, Connecticut. Mark Powley Assoc Co, 1983, p 67.

The impact of nursing diagnoses in a long-term care setting

JACKI MILLER, RN, MS; KATHLYN STEELE, RN, MS; AND ALICE BOISEN, RN, MS

This article describes how the Central Wisconsin Center for the Developmentally Disabled used nursing diagnoses in its care of mentally retarded children and adults. The authors demonstrate the versatility of the nursing process in problem resolution and in the promotion of change. Note: Summaries (shown in bracketed italics) condense extensive background information.

IN THE 1960s, little was known about the needs of individuals with multiple handicaps, and care techniques were primarily custodial in nature. The recruitment of registered nurses was difficult, due in part to societal attitudes toward this unique population. An administrative decision was made in 1961 to recruit licensed practical nurses to administer medication and treatments. The release of registered nurses from task-oriented, time-related duties allowed a greater focus on role definition.

The early years were a time of learning about the care needs of this complex population. Selected nursing theories were reviewed to identify a framework for developmental disabilities nursing. Many nursing theories relied upon active client participation. The population characteristics (nonverbal and nonambulant, with cognitive and sensory impairments) restricted the application of these theories. Orem's self-care concept, while the most appealing, had limited application, since clients were unable to fully participate in the care-planning process.[5] The criteria for "patienthood" as defined by most nurse theorists would seldom be met by persons who are developmentally disabled. To date, nursing service has not adopted a specific theory. The emerging philosophy supports the belief that persons with disabilities can learn self-care skills.

To explore this concept further, developmental theorists were studied. Expertise in the stages of human development from conception to age 3 years was critical. The developmental models of Piaget and Erikson were appealing and applicable to this population.[1,6] Normal human growth and development were the basis for learning about a population with deficits in gross and fine motor skills, communications skills, psychosocial development, and social skills. This view of the developmentally disabled persons as capable of growth and change provided an optimistic model for the delivery of services, including nursing. An organizational realignment from a medical to a developmental model throughout the Center created a program-focused, multidisciplinary, unit-based system. The team participation model was put into practice. Care practices based on a developmental model were incorporated into staff education programs.

[Organizational changes in nursing service

After the reorganization, nursing service focused more on quality assurance in nursing practice. Each living unit was assigned a primary nurse who maintained nursing assessments and care plans for that group of clients. The director of nursing and six other nurses completed master's degrees in nursing, which enriched and added diversity to the Center. To prepare the registered nurses for more ex-

tensive use of the nursing process, the Center held four workshops in 1974 and 1975 that highlighted such topics as decision-making, change theory, and the steps of the nursing process.

Assessment

One nursing committee established health care standards and an audit system. Another committee, directed by clinical nurse specialists, developed a format for nursing assessment, which was presented at the annual nursing workshop.

Planning

The annual workshop emphasized team process and goal writing. It included a review of nursing standards, which were considered valuable to care planning and evaluation.

Diagnosis

Center nurses closely followed the national conferences on nursing diagnosis. They joined committees, read books and journals on the topic, and studied the application of diagnostic labels. In 1981, the Center adopted North American Nursing Diagnosis Association (NANDA) diagnostic labels.

Implementation

The Staff Development and Nursing Service Departments joined forces to teach Center nurses about nursing diagnoses and their application to practice, the nursing process, and documentation.

The Center established a goal of performing a nursing assessment of each client annually. To reach this goal, guidelines were developed for the assessment form, a survey was done to evaluate nurses' assessment skills, and physical assessment workshops were held in 1979 and 1980.

As needed, Center nurses increased their understanding of the nursing process through lectures, self-study modules, workshops, clinical problem-solving sessions, practice laboratories, and care conferences. Then the nurses began to use NANDA diagnostic labels with etiologies and other information appropriate for developmentally disabled clients.

Nursing orders system

Because the Center had no formal procedure for ensuring that delegated tasks were performed, a committee started to research and develop a nursing orders system in 1981.[4] *By 1984, the system was finalized, and inservice programs were planned to support the regular use of nursing diagnoses and to implement the written nursing orders system.*

To assess the new system's effectiveness, the Center conducted a survey of nursing orders. The survey revealed that nurses wrote orders for acute and chronic care needs, their orders emphasized the primary nurse's accountability, the staff complied satisfactorily to the orders, and documentation had improved. It also identified barriers to implementation of the nursing orders system: limited time, lack of a storage area for nursing orders, nurses' apprehension about order writing and defending their rationales for decisions, and general resistance to change.

Evaluation: Nursing diagnosis audits

One year after the decision to use NANDA labels, the Center audited all care plans to evaluate NANDA terminology use and determine the most frequently used labels.]

Data indicated that nurses were using diagnosis as follows: NANDA labels, 42 per cent; incomplete NANDA labels, 24 per cent; the remaining 34 per cent did not meet criteria — that is, medical diagnoses, surgical procedures, signs or symptoms, or staff goals.

The audit identified the five most frequently used NANDA diagnostic labels: (1) Ineffective Breathing Pattern, (2) Alteration in Bowel Elimination: Constipation, (3) Alteration in

TABLE 1. Recommendations to assist with implementation of nursing diagnosis

1. Use a common assessment tool to collect data and formulate nursing diagnoses.
2. Establish a collaborative relationship between nursing service and training departments to share resources and reduce duplication of effort.
3. Form nursing committees to establish and evaluate policies and procedures related to nursing diagnosis.
4. Develop self-study materials for nurses to build on current knowledge and skill levels.
5. Present mandatory annual workshops to update nurses on current information and trends related to nursing diagnosis.
6. Encourage and support nursing staff in presenting professional papers at conferences, meetings, and conventions.
7. Promote attendance of nurses at educational offerings on nursing diagnosis as available within the facility and the community.
8. Develop bibliographies and route selected articles on nursing diagnosis to all nursing staff.
9. Schedule frequent meetings with nurses and nursing service representatives to facilitate sharing of clinical expertise.
10. Establish a monitoring system to evaluate the quality of nursing documentation, including nursing diagnosis.
11. Include nurses in the decision-making process when change is being considered.
12. Support nurses with tuition reimbursement or paid time (or both), for career development, including university course work.

Nutrition: Less than Body Requirements, (4) Fluid Volume Deficit, and (5) Impairment of Skin Integrity: Actual-Potential.

For the five identified diagnoses, independent study materials and prototype care guides were developed (see Appendix). These resources are used in orientation and continuing education for Center nurses. Two of these care guides have been published.[4]

[Evaluation: Nursing standards revision

In 1985, the Center revised its nursing standards for developmental disabilities from a body-system format to a nursing-diagnosis format. This change facilitated the use of standards that were directly related to areas of nursing accountability.[2]

In 1986, a survey found that the nurses understood the standards and their use and that they enthusiastically supported the nursing-diagnosis format of the revised standards.]

Summary

Nursing diagnosis as a critical component of the nursing process provides a common taxonomy to describe problems that nurses can treat and is a convenient, logical way to reference nursing standards. Theory is translated into practice with the use of population-specific prototype care guides and a written orders system.

Nurses in leadership are responsible for providing the necessary resources to promote professional growth and facilitate desired change. Recommendations to assist with the implementation of nursing diagnosis are identified in Table 1. The system is dependent on staff nurses' professional commitment to learning and willingness to actively participate in change. Involvement of staff nurses continues to be a critical factor in the improvement of nursing practice.

REFERENCES

1. Erikson EH: Childhood and Society. New York, Norton, 1950

2. Gordon M: Nursing Diagnosis: Process and Application. New York, McGraw-Hill Book Co, 1982, pp 276-277

3. McCloskey JC: Nurses' Orders: The next professional breakthrough? RN 80:99-113, 1980

4. Miller J, Steele K: Nursing care of patients with development disabilities. In Kim MJ, McFarland GK, McLane AM (eds): Pocket Guide to Nursing Diagnoses. St. Louis, The CV Mosby Co, 1984

5. Orem DE: Nursing: Concepts of Practice. New York, McGraw-Hill Book Co, 1971

6. Piaget J: The Origins of Intelligence in Children. New York, Norton, 1963

APPENDIX: Population-specific NANDA diagnosis*

Central Wisconsin Center for the Developmentally Disabled, Madison, Wis. 53704

Nursing diagnosis
Ineffective breathing pattern

Definition
The state in which an individual's inhalation or exhalation pattern, or both, does not enable adequate pulmonary inflation or emptying

Etiologies
CNS pathology
Neuromuscular impairment
Chest trauma
Discomfort-pain
Fear-anxiety
Immobility
Inactivity
Skeletal deformities
Congenital facial anomalies
Frequent upper respiratory infection (URI)
Chronic asthma
Pneumonia (viral-bacterial-aspiration)
Food-fluid aspirations
Excessive pooling of mucus
Inadequate fluid intake
Abdominal distention (constipation, air swallowing)
Chest-abdominal surgery

Defining characteristics
Cyanosis
Slow, irregular respiratory movements
Respiratory rate greater than 30/minute or less than 5/minute
Diminished breath sounds
Asymmetric chest expansion
Increased expiratory phase
Use of accessory muscles
Increased AP diameter (chest)
Shortness of breath
Air hunger
Hyperventilation
Mouth breathing
Pursed-lip breathing
Periods of apnea
Nasal flaring
Cough
Fatigue

Expected outcomes and goals (samples)
Expected outcome
Decrease incidence of URI to prevent changes in breathing pattern.

Goal
Will have less than one URI per month within 3 months (current baseline two URIs per 3 months)

Expected outcome
Improve daily hydration level to prevent mucus stasis

Goal
Will consume 1,200 ml of fluids per 24 hours for 1 week

Expected outcome
Will increase ability to cough and expectorate pooled secretions to prevent URI.

Goal
Will cough each time assistive breathing techniques are implemented (twice per shift for 7 days).

Other expected outcomes (goals to be developed)
Decrease in frequency of pneumonia over established time period
Decrease mucus production
No episodes of food or fluid aspiration
Increase expansion of chest as measured with tape measure
Increase ease and depth of respirations
Reduce number of asthmatic episodes
Absence of rales, rhonchi, and laryngeal stridor
Decrease heart rate
Able to clear airway of secretions

Interventions
Perform a comprehensive assessment including:
1. Physical examination of respiratory system p.r.n.
2. Visual observation of breathing pattern.
3. Need for p.r.n. medications (pain control, fever).
4. Fluid intake to prevent dehydration.
5. Significant factors and events that might have precipitated the change in breathing pattern.

General interventions
1. Prepare for mealtime—speak in soft tone, explain events while feeding.
2. Sleep on two foam pillows.
3. Avoid exertion activities on hot and humid days.
4. Monitor frequency of bowel movements—may decrease chest expansion ability.
5. Avoid restrictive clothing.
6. Perform oral hygiene and tooth brushing p.r.n.
7. Give 4 oz of unsweetened lemonade before meals to decrease mucus production.

*Format includes definition, etiologies, defining characteristics, expected outcomes and short-term goals, interventions, and process standards for planning and evaluation.

APPENDIX: Population-specific NANDA diagnosis* *continued*

Central Wisconsin Center for the Developmentally Disabled, Madison, Wis. 53704

Specific respiratory interventions

1. Monitor breath and lung sounds p.r.n.
2. Suction nasopharynx p.r.n.
3. Increase cough through assistive breathing (firm, steady pressure to base of ribs on expiration).
4. Jaw-thrust technique to open upper airway when stridor is audible.
5. Use of chin strap as directed.
6. Raise head of bed with shock blocks.
7. Position changes every 1 to 2 hours as directed.
8. Active and passive postural drainage as directed.
9. Saline nose drops p.r.n. for nasal congestion.
10. Passive postural drainage position before meals p.r.n.
11. Use nasal airway p.r.n. per doctor's order.
12. Use of oxygen for persistent or acute episodes of ineffective breathing.
13. Referral to respiratory therapist for evaluation and treatment program.

Process standards

The client with an ineffective breathing pattern is provided with planned nursing and medical measures to optimize oxygen and carbon dioxide exchange needed for body function. These measures include:

1. Ongoing assessment of respiratory status/breathing patterns.
  A. Monitoring rate, character, and depth of respirations; and noting presence or absence of rales, rhonchi, and laryngeal stridor.
  B. Monitoring associated responses, such as presence of secondary muscle retraction of the abdominal, chest, and neck muscles; evidence of circulatory insufficiency or cyanosis; increased heart rate; and changes in blood pressure.
  C. Monitoring client's level of available energy through observation of motor activity and level of awareness.
  D. Monitoring the production of secretions; the density, color, and amount of mucus; and the ability of the client to clear the airway of secretions.

2. Provide an environment that (1) is well ventilated, (2) has adequate humidity level to assist in keeping mucous membranes moist and mucus consistency thin, and (3) contributes to the reduction of physical and emotional stress.

3. Clients with limited respiratory function are observed and vital signs are monitored carefully when (1) oxygen is being administered to avoid overadministration of oxygen with resulting respiratory depression and (2) when receiving medications known to depress respirations (such classes of drugs as sedative-hypnotics [barbiturates], tranquilizers [Valium], and narcotics [opium derivatives]).

4. The health care plan describes schedule for observing and documenting effects of specific medications, measures of intervention to relieve those effects, and client responses.

5. Clients with limitations in independent mobility are provided with care measures to prevent respiratory problems, including:
  A. Frequent opportunity to be in upright position to facilitate increased lung expansion.
  B. Daily exercise to increase ventilation capacity.
  C. Turning assistance at least every 2 hours whenever in recumbent position to prevent stasis of secretions.
  D. Special interventions, individually planned, to maximize eating, chewing, and swallowing abilities to reduce the danger of aspiration.
  E. Provision of adequate hydration to keep mucous membranes moist and secretions easily cleared.
  F. Suctioning nasopharynx to remove pooled mucus to prevent potential aspiration of secretions, as needed.

6. Oral hygiene is provided three times daily for every client who is experiencing either an upper or lower respiratory tract infection to reduce bacterial flora in the mouth.

7. Clients experiencing respiratory congestion and difficulty in cleansing thick tenacious mucus from the respiratory tract are provided with a humidified atmosphere. (Refer to Nursing Procedure for specific information regarding tracheostomy humidification.)

continued

*Format includes definition, etiologies, defining characteristics, expected outcomes and short-term goals, interventions, and process standards for planning and evaluation.

APPENDIX: Population-specific NANDA diagnosis* *continued*

Central Wisconsin Center for the Developmentally Disabled, Madison, Wis. 53704

8. Clients experiencing problems in breathing patterns are provided with:

A. Continuous observation for evidence of acute respiratory distress.

B. Positioning to maximize potential for chest expansion and comfort (that is, head of bed elevation between 30 and 45 degrees, shock blocks on bed, and so on).

C. Active intervention to clear mucus, open airways, and expand ventilation, including such measures as postural drainage, vibration and cupping, deep-breathing and coughing, and turning every hour.

D. Light coverings and avoidance of restrictive clothing or ties across chest.

E. Provision for oxygen therapy and mechanical suction in care of acute respiratory distress.

F. Monitoring of adequate hydration and nutrition levels through recording of intake and output and observation of client's physiologic status.

G. The application of medical orders to relieve the symptoms of respiratory distress.

9. During recovery from anesthesia, measures taken to prevent pulmonary complications include:

A. Direct supervision by professional nurse, doctor, or dentist until fully conscious.

B. Client is kept dry and warm.

C. Position is changed at least every hour.

D. Position allows for drainage of secretions and prevents obstruction of airway by soft tissues.

E. Rate and quality of respirations are closely monitored.

F. Stretching, deep-breathing, and coughing are encouraged when the client is able to cooperate.

10. Direct care staff is knowledgeable and will perform, when necessary, emergency measures for oxygen and carbon dioxide exchange. Such measures include manual removal of object, positioning for maximum opening of airway and drainage of secretions, suctioning, and use of the Heimlich maneuver.

11. Direct care staff recognize indicators of respiratory obstructions due to aspiration and seek nursing and medical assistance as needed.

12. Clients who experience respiratory arrest are provided mouth-to-mouth (nose) emergency ventilation by the direct care provider until professional assistance can be obtained.

*Format includes definition, etiologies, defining characteristics, expected outcomes and short-term goals, interventions, and process standards for planning and evaluation.

SECTION TWO

Interactive process

COMMUNICATION REPRESENTS the core of the interactive process of nursing. It allows the nurse to relate to all client systems, including individuals, families, small groups, and communities. It facilitates sharing of information and beliefs, understanding of emotions and needs, and expression of pain, sorrow, support, and caring. Ultimately, communication can produce changes in behavior, attitudes, feelings, or values. For the nurse, its usual purpose is to improve the client's health or the nurse's caregiving ability.

The nurse can use communication skills in many work-related situations. Obviously, the nurse employs them when caring for clients. But the nurse may also apply communication skills in daily interactions with other members of the health care team, during counseling and teaching sessions with small groups, when sharing information with other nurses, and while addressing a community group on health topics.

In this section, the articles provide examples of two situations in which the nurse's communication skills play a vital role: in a therapeutic conversation with a client and in a working relationship with an interdisciplinary team.

The first article, Burnard's "Meaningful Dialogue," discusses the communication skills a nurse needs to engage in therapeutic conversations. The nurse may find these skills especially useful when communicating with psychiatric clients, clients who are anxious about surgery, family members who are worried about the client's disorder, and even colleagues who are under stress.

The author presents five "minimum requirements" for a therapeutic conversation:

- emphasizing the "here-and-now"
- focusing on feelings
- employing empathic understanding
- using nonprescriptive conversation
- focusing on the client.

According to Burnard, if every nurse-client interaction contained these five elements, the resulting dialogues would be consistently more meaningful and therapeutic. This article unites several concepts from previous units. In its discussion of empathic understanding, it draws on Leininger's concepts of transcultural caring (from Unit One) and Arnold and Bogg's description of the conceptual components of a therapeutic relationship (from Unit Two). It also expands on the notion of therapeutic use of self, which was discussed in Unit Two.

In the next article, "No Longer a Silent Partner," Katzman and Roberts demonstrate how a nurse can interact as part of an interdisciplinary training team. They describe a program held for caregivers from day-care centers to explore causes and consequences of child abuse. The nurse-trainer used highly developed communication skills to interact with the other team members, to develop reciprocal relationships with the trainees and the other team members, to facilitate the sharing of ideas and experiences, to increase the trainees' knowledge, and to modify their attitudes.

The interdisciplinary approach helped the nurse-trainer demonstrate her autonomy and gain greater visibility and respect for her professional skills. A similar approach may help display and gain recognition for the nurse's talents at work and in other settings.

Meaningful dialogue

Philip Burnard, RGN, RMN, DipN, CertEd, RNT, MSc

Therapeutic conversation is an important part of nurse-client interaction and communication. According to the author, however, merely talking to a client cannot achieve a therapeutic effect. The nurse needs to conduct a structured, meaningful dialogue using the elements of a therapeutic conversation described in this article. Note: Excerpts (marked by ellipses) condense extra examples and references.

As interpersonal skills training becomes a regular feature of nurse education and learners discover more about social skills, counseling, and group skills, so they take part increasingly in "therapeutic conversations" with patients....

The five aspects of the therapeutic conversation are:

- An emphasis on the "here-and-now"
- A focus on feelings
- The nurse needs to develop empathic understanding
- The nurse should be nonprescriptive
- The client should remain the central focus of the conversation.

These are the minimum requirements for a therapeutic conversation but they are not exhaustive.

First, an emphasis on the "here-and-now." In a sense, what is happening now is all there is. The future has yet to happen and the past is history. If the conversation focuses too much on the future, it may be unrealistic and contain much fantasy. Interestingly, a conversation which focuses too much on the past may be the same. Our memories are rarely accurate, and there is no conclusive evidence that past personal events necessarily affect the present. Many people find the present painful to live in. The past, however inaccurate our recollection, often feels more comfortable. Notice, for instance, how much time is spent in "ordinary" conversation discussing how things used to be. In the therapeutic conversation, however, it is rarely useful to dwell much on the past. It is more therapeutic if the nurse stays with the client's moment-to-moment phenomenology and notes his changing verbal and nonverbal cues as they occur.[1]

Such attention to the present means considerable effort by the nurse. It requires concentration, close awareness of subtle changes, and the ability to "stay awake" and remain focused on the client. There are a number of ways to develop the necessary skills to do this.[2,3]

How is such concentration on the here-and-now therapeutic? First, if we agree that we live in the here-and-now, it is in the here-and-now that we make decisions. Clearly we cannot make decisions in the past and future; we decide now. Therefore, if the therapeutic conversation is to have practical value, it is important that the client is able to express choice and make decisions. As this can only be undertaken now, it is important that the main thrust of the therapeutic conversation is on the present.

Second, it can be argued that we are dynamic, evolving beings. We are not exactly as we were yesterday and will be different again tomorrow. If the therapeutic conversation concentrates on the present, it becomes more "realistic." It is dealing with the person as he is, not as he was or may be. Nurses can be trained in methods of staying in the here-and-now, and a report of such developments is described by Faugier and Reilly.[4]

In learning to focus on feelings, it is helpful to contrast them to thoughts. Feelings are concerned with our emotions and include a wide spectrum such as happiness, sadness, anger, and disappointment. Thoughts, however, are mental considerations. Thinking is rational or irrational, pondering, or conceptualizing. Clearly, thinking is a valuable activity. But if we spend much time thinking about how we feel we do nothing but build theories about our feelings: we never address the feelings themselves.

Consider the following "thinking" conversation between a nurse and a client.

Client: I feel really upset at the moment — sort of bottled up.

Nurse: What do you think has caused that?

Client: I don't know really. I've got a lot on my plate at the moment. I suppose I'm a bit of a worrier by nature.

Nurse: So you think you're a born worrier?

Client: Yes, I think I am.

Here, the conversation has become a conversation about feelings. It does not explore the feelings themselves. No attempt is made to help the client express the feelings he talked about. Instead, a theoretical debate takes place about *why* the client is feeling this way. Arguably, a more fruitful approach may be:

Client: I feel really upset at the moment — sort of bottled up.

Nurse: upset and bottled up...?

Client: I feel as though I want to cry and yet I can't.

Nurse: You seem very close to tears now.

Client: (begins to cry) I've been wanting to do this for ages; it's as though I've been holding on to this for years.

Here, the accent is clearly on the feelings themselves, as they occur. The nurse uses reflection and empathy building to convey that she understands what the client is feeling. She also tacitly gives the client "permission" to cry. Arguably, such expression of feeling is therapeutic in itself[5] and the release of pressure following such expression of emotion can lead to clearer thinking and increased problem-solving ability.

To develop the basic skills involved in focusing on feelings, the nurse requires training in fundamental counseling techniques. There is a considerable literature on counseling training[2,6,7] and there is no reason why it cannot be incorporated into courses for all learner nurses. The techniques are easily learned and need to be absorbed by the nurse: that is, they need to become more than just techniques. They need to become a natural part of the nurse's conversational ability. We cannot leave such learning to chance but need to ensure that learners are given adequate training.

The nurse needs to develop empathic understanding because we all look at the world differently. Our culture, education, perception, and thinking affect the way we view the world, and we tend to build up a series of beliefs about how the world is and act accordingly.

Sometimes as we do this we realize that our belief system is inaccurate and we seek to change it. Thus we may progress and develop. We develop a "frame of reference," a particular and reasonably consistent view of the world. Empathy consists of attempting to enter the other person's frame of reference. It involves attempting to understand and "see" the world as he sees it.

Empathic understanding involves entering and moving in the other person's frame of reference. If we are to understand another person — if this is possible — we must develop such understanding. It is through such empathy that we begin to appreciate why this person is experiencing this set of feelings at this time.

Empathic understanding, therefore, requires that we set aside our own belief and value system and give ourselves freely and openly to the other person. Again, the development of empathy is demanding and requires training, but the available literature is comprehensive.[8,9,10]

To be prescriptive is to make suggestions or offer opinions about what the client should do next, and there are clearly times when this is appropriate [such as] when buying a house.... In the domain of personal concern, however, such prescription is rarely valid. How can we prescribe for others? How can we suggest what others do in their lives? What qualifies us to attempt to put other people's lives right for them? Because of this, the nurse should be nonprescriptive.

Given that we all view the world differently and all live "separate lives," it would seem more appropriate if the client is helped to make his own decisions and draw his own conclusions. The nurse can act as a trouble shooter or problem poser but should not offer direct advice. This approach to the therapeutic conversation is in line with the principles of non-directive or client-centered counseling, laid down by Carl Rogers many years ago.[11] There seems little evidence that Rogers' basic arguments are any less valid today than in the 1950s. People still need to choose for themselves.

The final element of therapeutic conversation, that the client should remain the central focus, is the basis of the philosophy outlined in the other four elements. That the client must remain the central focus of the therapeutic conversation may seem obvious yet it is easy, in everyday conversation, for the focus to move back and forth between the two people involved. Take, for example, the following piece of conversation between two nurses:

1st nurse: I'm enjoying working in [surgery]: there's always a lot going on.

2nd nurse: I never liked [surgery] — it's too impersonal.

1st nurse: Anyway, I'll be back in school soon — it will all be over in a week or so.

2nd nurse: I'm not back in school for over six weeks: it seems ages, really.

Here, the focus of conversation shuttles back and forth. It is possible that neither is really giving her full attention to the other. It is possible, too, that such to-ing and fro-ing is acceptable in a social conversation — we expect to hear the other person's point of view. In the therapeutic situation, however, the conditions are different. It is the client's world that is important and it is the nurse's role to listen. It can be argued that it is the quality of listening that makes the conversation therapeutic. In a therapeutic conversation, the client is telling his story and the nurse is hearing it. In many cases the nurse does not have to respond to what she hears: she is often only required to listen. If she does this and offers minimal intervention, she can ensure that the locus remains with the client.

It is the telling of the story that is important for the client. It is listening to that story that is important for the nurse. If we realize that we are not duty bound to respond or react to everything that is said, we can become more patient, more empathic, and more understanding. Finally, we are free really to listen. If we are not rehearsing our responses while we listen, we can give ourselves over completely to the task of hearing what the client says.

Such skills need to be learned experientially and explored through personal involvement. If we are to become good listeners, we need to experience what it is like to be heard. If we are to develop skills in reflection and empathy building, we need to practice those skills with other people and experience their value ourselves....

The climate in nursing is changing. There is greater emphasis on the need for nurses to demonstrate their caring. The therapeutic conversation offers one such vehicle. To listen to another person is perhaps the most caring action of all. We can all learn to listen and be better nurses as a result.

REFERENCES

1. Shaffer, J.B.P. *Humanistic Psychology.* New Jersey: Prentice Hall, 1978.

2. Burnard, P. *Learning Human Skills: A Guide for Nurses.* London: Heinemann, 1985.

3. Ernst, S., Goodison, L. *In Our Own Hands: A Book of Self Help Therapy.* London: The Womens Press, 1981.

4. Faugier, J., Reilly, S. Towards a communication breakthrough. *Nursing Times* 1986; **82**:41, 60-62.

5. Heron, J. *Catharsis in Human Development.* Human potential research project. Guildford: University of Surrey, 1977.

6. Nelson-Jones, R. *The Theory and Practice of Counselling Psychology.* London: Holt, Rinehart & Winston 1981.

7. Tschudin,V. *Counselling Skills for Nurses.* London: Bailliere, Tindal, 1982.

8. Rogers, C.R. *On Becoming a Person.* London: Constable, 1967.

9. Egan, G. *The Skilled Helper.* Brooks/Cole: Monterey, 1982.

10. Tschudin, V. *Beginning with Empathy.* Sheffield: ENB Learning Resources Centre, 1986.

11. Rogers, C.R. *Client-Centred Counselling.* London: Constable, 1952.

No longer a silent partner

Elaine Menter Katzman, RN, PhD; Joan I. Roberts, PhD

In this article, the authors show how a nurse's skills contribute greatly to the work of an interdisciplinary team assigned to train caregivers from local day-care centers. Note: Summaries (shown in bracketed italics) and excerpts (marked by ellipses) condense extensive background material.

Professionals in various disciplines — psychology, sociology, nursing, social work, medicine — have often joined to address the problems of child abuse, adolescent sexuality, and adolescent pregnancy. But while nurses have been included on interdisciplinary teams, their participation has seldom been thoroughly described in the literature.

Not only are nurses natural members of such teams, but are, by virtue of their experience, vital contributors to them. Nurses, for example, are educated in adolescent sexuality, pregnancy and parenting, community health, and family problems in a community context, and can perform prenatal, perinatal, and neonatal risk assessments. Nurses also help teams maintain a holistic perspective.

In 1980, an interdisciplinary team that included a nurse specialist formed the Model Caregiver Training Project (MCTP) at Syracuse University. Their aim was to design a program about the causes and consequences (short- and long-term) of child abuse and adolescent pregnancy and to teach it to caregivers of children. Trainers and trainees alike evaluated the program as successful. Its success was attributed not only to the knowledge and expertise of the trainers, but to their emphasis on a feminist approach (placing high value on the abilities of the women involved) and a nonhierarchical framework. The nonauthoritarian structure of the group enhanced the working ideology; the members were all women and were all selected by the project director for their feminist philosophy.

[The problem: One group's solution

National statistics indicate that more than one million cases of child abuse are reported. In addition, 6.5 million more children are abused, but show no physical injury.[1,2] Such abuse is associated with emotional and learning difficulties,[4] teenage pregnancy,[5] and abuse in succeeding generations.[3]

Although many children are cared for outside the home, few of their caregivers are aware of the causes and effects of abuse or of strategies for helping parents alter abusive behaviors. To remedy this situation, the MCTP organized a program that involved community day-care and university employees. It responded to the growing number of abused children and adolescent parents among day-care clients and to the caregivers' need for accurate information and interventions.

The project director chose trainers with diverse backgrounds in nursing, family studies, child development, psychology, and social work. Because of their backgrounds, the trainers could discusss the physical, social, and psychological aspects of child-adult interactions, family interactions, and the connection between social and family violence.

Goals and process

The MCTP used group dynamics, a feminist approach,[6,7] and a nonhierarchical structure that encouraged the participation of the 16 trainees who were all caregivers at local day-care centers.

The trainers' goals were to:

- *facilitate trainee involvement and development, rather than to impart information*
- *build on each trainee's interests and strengths*
- *develop trust and respect with trainees and among the trainees to promote communication*
- *help the trainees develop a teaching style that would allow children to interact with adults and their environment for maximum growth and development.*

Pretraining. *After the trainees were tested on their knowledge and attitudes toward child abuse and related topics, the training team prepared program content and materials to meet their needs.*

Training. *In Module One, child development specialists covered the normal physical, social, and emotional development of children. In Module Two, social-work specialists highlighted child abuse, sexual molestation, and neglect in families and in society. In Module Three, the nurse-trainer discussed parental involvement in child care centers, highlighting the needs of adolescents and others at high risk for child abuse.*

After showing the group an instructional film about adolescent sexuality,[8] the nurse helped the trainees examine their feelings about this topic and discuss it openly. One trainee shared her personal experience as a teenage mother, helping the group gain greater empathy for women in similar situations.

Under the nurse-trainer's guidance, the group then discussed parenting. The trainees learned that young mothers who undergo maturational and situational crises are most likely to abuse or neglect their children. Then the nurse-trainer explained how to detect signs of neglect or abuse and investigate the situation. A role-playing session helped the trainees learn intervention techniques and replace punitive attitudes toward abusive parents with more constructive ones.

Trainee evaluation. *Generally, the trainees hailed the MCTP as a valuable experience. Their post-tests showed significant increases in their knowledge and attitude scores. The nonhierarchical structure allowed trainees and trainers to learn from one another and develop mutual trust and respect. The trainees' involvement was high, as evidenced by 92% class attendance and no dropouts.]*

Teaching caregivers of children about family violence has many benefits. Primarily, it heightens the awareness of the caregivers about the family backgrounds of those they serve. This information can lead to a new understanding of the behaviors they observe in children and their parents. The result can be predicted to be improved relationships between caregivers and parents, increased involvement of the parents in the center's activities, and more successful interventions with the children attending day care programs.

Interconnecting family and societal violence with adolescent sexuality and pregnancy presents another new perspective to caregivers. Moreover, discussing the sexual initiation that some teenagers experience provides a forum for caregivers to explore their own sexual values. While caregivers learn about the children and parents they serve, they also learn about themselves....

The sources of success

One often hears people who are not nurses say, for example, that nurses can only do what physicians tell them. Many people are unaware of the autonomous roles of nurses, such as in health promotion and assessment; prevention of illness and other health problems; advocacy; and consulting. When nurses work in interdisciplinary teams, their expanded roles are visible to a wide range of people.

The training project provided many opportunities for nurses' involvement yet, ideally, they could do even more. For example, nurses could initiate and direct such projects. Nurses could suggest other health-related topics for inclusion. They could also bring in other nurses with different areas of expertise. Increased exposure through community service has great potential for promoting the image of nursing.

The MCTP's success had many sources, but a unique aspect of the program was that more than lip service was given to the nurse's place on the team; there was power in her role, encouraged by the project director and acknowledged by the rest of the team; for example, nurses were given the opportunity to use their health-teaching skills. Health teaching is an important part of nursing education, but too few nursing positions allow for its use.

Further, research, although taught in many nursing programs, is difficult for nurses to integrate into their clinical practice. However, in the MCTP, research was built into every component of the intervention to document what worked and what did not work.

Finally, the outstanding factor that made the MCTP work was that the personal "chemistry" among the trainers was facilitated from the start. This dynamic was a product of the careful selection of trainers, the early encouragement of cooperation, the delineation of roles and responsibilities, and the demonstrated respect for each participant's ability. Clearly, the MCTP was a model program.

REFERENCES

1. STRAUS, MURRAY, AND GELLES, R.J. *Behind Closed Doors: Violence in the American Family,* New York, Anchor Press, 1980.

2. STACEY, W.A., AND SHUPE, ANSON. *The Family Secret: Domestic Violence in America.* Boston, Beacon Press, 1983.

3. BALDWIN, W., AND CAIN, V. The children of teenage parents. In *Teenage Sexuality, Pregnancy and Childbearing,* ed. by Frank Furstenburg and others. Philadelphia, University of Pennsylvania Press, 1981, pp. 265-279.

4. WILLIAMS, GERTRUDE, AND MONEY, JOHN. *The Traumatic Abuse and Neglect of Children at Home,* Baltimore, Johns Hopkins University Press, 1980.

5. KATZMAN, E. AND PURDY, T. *Adolescent Fertility: Concerns for Present and Future.* Syracuse, NY, Syracuse University, 1980. (Unpublished manuscript).

6. MILES, M.B. *Learning to Work in Groups,* 2nd ed. New York, Columbia University, Teachers College Press, 1981.

7. CULLEY, MARGO, AND PORTUGES, CATHERINE. *Gendered Subjects: The Dynamics of Feminist Teaching.* New York, Methuen, 1985.

8. ADOLESCENT SEXUAL CONFLICT. Film New York, McGraw-Hill Book Co., 1976.

SECTION THREE

Legal aspects and accountability

NURSES ARE INCREASINGLY vulnerable to work-related lawsuits. This is true partly because of today's legal climate, which encourages resolution of grievances through the courts, partly because of nurses' growing autonomy and expanded responsibilities, and partly because of the growing complexity of client care, which increases the risk of errors. That is why each nurse must understand how nursing interacts with the law and must learn how to minimize legal risks while providing optimum nursing care.

The first article, "The Legal Significance of Charting" by Creighton, does just that. Documentation or charting is becoming increasingly important because "the medical record is often a lawyer's chief source of information and evidence in a courtroom," especially in a negligence or malpractice suit. As the author explains, whether the client's "medical record is an ally or enemy depends on how the nurse uses it."

To ensure that the medical record is a nurse's ally, Creighton suggests these rules for charting:

- Chart accurately and concisely.
- Chart objectively.
- Chart promptly.
- Make no mention of an incident report in the chart.
- Write legibly and use only standard abbreviations.
- Keep charting free of criticism or complaints.
- Do not destroy or attempt to obliterate documentation.
- Do not leave vacant lines, and sign every entry.
- Record the date of each return visit, cancelled or missed appointment, and telephone conversation; specify all follow-up instructions.

These rules will protect the nurse from lawsuits, promote positive resolution of disputes, ensure accurate communication with other members of the health care team, and promote high-quality care for the client.

Legal responsibility is just one aspect of a nurse's overall accountability (professional responsibility). Unfortunately, *accountability* sometimes is used to indicate blame, as when an *accountable person* is held solely responsible for a problem. However, *accountability* means much more: Nurses are answerable to themselves as well as to the client, profession, institution, and society for the effectiveness of their nursing care. Accountability should be a source of professional pride and a reflection of the nurse's power.

In the next article, "Nurse Accountability Program Improves Satisfaction, Turnover," Ethridge examines accountability in this positive context. She begins by describing the implementation of a seven-point nurse accountability program in a southwestern health care facility. Then she reviews the program's effects, which include increased feelings of professionalism and job satisfaction for the nurses and decreased employee turnover and operating costs for the facility.

This article has another significance. The program it describes may serve as a model for other health care facilities that hope to beat the nursing shortage by attracting and retaining top-flight nurses and making nursing a higher paying, more widely respected profession.

Legal significance of charting

HELEN CREIGHTON, RN, JD

Part I

AS THE NURSING PROFESSION becomes more autonomous and patient care grows more complex, nurses find themselves increasingly vulnerable to malpractice suits. Whether the patient's medical record is an ally or enemy depends on how the nurse uses it.[1] As the Ohio Nurses' Association so aptly states: *"Charting documents the professional surveillance of the patient, the nursing action taken in the patient's behalf, and the patient's progress with regard to illness."* [2] This article will point out the legal significance of medical records and identify some important points in charting. To facilitate the plan of care and to coordinate treatment, medical records are the principal means of communication. In addition, the medical record is often a lawyer's chief source of information and evidence in a courtroom. The patient's chart is almost always introduced into evidence at the trial of a negligence or malpractice suit.

Chart accurately and concisely. [3] The medical record is an account of what happened to a patient during a stay in the medical care facility.[4] Since it is written as a matter of policy and routine, it is a "business record of the facility and admissible in court as evidence and the information contained in the chart is presumed to be true. Any omission is presumed not to have taken place." In *Collins v. Westlake Community Hospital,* [5] the first recorded entry about the condition of a boy's leg reported a darkening of the toes and that a doctor had been called. However, the entry was made at the sixth hour of the nurse's shift. The nurse at trial testified that she had previously observed the boy's leg. However, the jury found her negligent for failing to observe the condition of the leg until it was too late.

In *Kenyon v. Hammer,*[6,7] during the course of pregnancy, a routine blood test revealed that Mrs. Kenyon had Rh negative blood, but one of Dr. Hammer's nurses erroneously charted that the patient's blood was Rh positive. A normal, healthy child with Rh positive was later delivered. If Dr. Hammer had known Mrs. Kenyon had Rh negative blood, he would have administered RhoGAM, a drug which suppresses the immune response which Rh negative mothers may develop to the Rh positive blood cells of their children. The drug must be administered within 72 hours after delivery of an infant with Rh positive blood, if the drug is to be effective. Since Dr. Hammer was misled by the incorrect information on the chart, the RhoGAM was not given and the risk of the immune response and risk to subsequent pregnancy is increased about ten times. About six years later, a second baby of Mrs. Kenyon was stillborn as a result of the destruction of its blood cells by the mother's Rh antibodies, and Mrs. Kenyon had a tubal ligation to prevent such future tragedies and to protect her own health. The Kenyons sued Dr. Hammer for damages for the wrongful death of the second baby and for damages for Mrs. Kenyon in conjunction with her second pregnancy, tubal ligation, and consequent sterility. The doctor was sued for vicarious liability for the negligence of his nurse in incorrectly recording Mrs. Kenyon's Rh factor during the 1971-72 pregnancy. The Supreme Court of Arizona held that the wrongful death claim and bodily injury were both governed by the three-year statute of limitations applicable to medical malpractice actions and that it commenced to run on the date of injury rather than the date of the negligent act. Here, the nurse's incorrect charting was the basis of the lawsuit. For accuracy of charting in the operating room, see Murphy's list of 14 points in "Documenting OR Nursing Care" in the May 1983 issue of *Today's OR Nurse*.[8]

Deliberate inaccuracies impugn the author's credibility and expose the nurse to charges of fraud. In the well publicized case of *People v. Smithtown General Hospital*,[9] the surgeon and OR supervisor were criminally indicted for falsifying business records when they failed to include the presence and extent of involvement of a manufacturer's sales representative during an operation. In *Hiatt v. Groce*,[10] a woman who sustained injury during and immediately after delivery by a nurse recovered damages where the nurse testified she had been advised by her supervisor never to state in the records that she had delivered a baby. The nurse recorded that the physician who had been passing in the hall was called and had delivered the child.

Chart objectively. An Oregon court allowed the jury to consider the recovery room nurses' failure to record the rate and depth of respirations as evidence that the nurses had not monitored the respirations despite other entries that the patient was "doing well."[11] The phrases "appears to be" and "seems to be" which nurses were routinely taught 30 or 40 years ago (when nurses supposedly were not making a judgment or decision about what was happening to the patient) are out of place in today's nurses' charting. Today, it is important for nurses to record what they see, hear, feel, and smell. Many times nurses chart "Patient doing well." — which means nothing at all. Rather one might chart: "Patient eating all of prescribed diet, tolerates activity of walking the length of the unit's corridor three times at least three times daily, no complaints of pain at operative site, and enjoys visits from his family and minister." In one chart I reviewed, the patient was having a "good day." The patient was a 70-year-old on bedrest with cancer of the breast which had metastasized to the sternum and the patient was terminal. The next chart I reviewed the patient was also having a good day. This patient was a 34-year-old foundry worker who was recovering from a hernioplasty and was receiving intravenous antibiotics and was ambulatory. The difference between these patients is not evident from the notation that each was having a good day.

Chart promptly. Notify the physician of significant changes in the patient's condition. In *Thomas v. Corso*,[12] a widow and administratrix of her deceased husband's estate recovered almost $10,000 in a malpractice action where a doctor testified that he might have helped the patient and arrested the shock if he had been notified promptly of the vital signs indicative of shock. In a similar situation in *Goff v. Doctor's General Hospital*,[13] where a woman was bleeding excessively following a delivery, the evening nurse did not take any vital signs and failed to notify the doctor when she assessed the woman as going into shock. The physician was not notified until the night shift. The woman died from blood loss, and the nurse and hospital were held liable in damages. In another case, *Ramsey v. Physician's Memorial Hospital*,[14] an emergency department nurse was held liable for failing to convey to the physician information given by the mother about the removal of ticks from the children. As a result two different physicians made incorrect diagnoses and one child died from Rocky Mountain spotted fever.

Nurses also should carry out physicians' orders promptly, and in case of doubt, they should make certain that the order is correct. In *Norton v. Argnot Insurance Company*,[15] a nurse and physician were held liable when a nurse administered a fatal dose of Lanoxin by injection, because she did not realize that the order was for an oral dose. A nurse from the nursing office was making rounds and stopped to help an overworked unit nurse. When she came to the Norton order it seemed incorrect to her; however, as a nursing office nurse she was unfamiliar with pediatric medications. While the nurse questioned two physicians about the order written by a third physician and the order itself was ambiguous, the nurse failed to question the attending physician and this provided the basis for holding her liable for negligence.

Make no mention of an incident report in the chart. The nurse's notes are not a proper place for reporting an incident report. If an untoward event occurs, the nurse should document the facts (e.g., a patient's fall or the failure of a piece of equipment) and what was done. The purpose of an incident report is to provide a record of the facts and circumstances of untoward events happening to patients, and to protect the patients, nurses/employees, and the hospital/nursing home/health agency. It is made as near as possible to the time that the event occurred, states facts (no opinions, no admissions of error), and names and addresses of witnesses. The incident report should be prepared by the person having knowledge of the facts, should be processed expeditiously through required hospital/agency channels and filed with the hospital/agency lawyer for his action. Incident reports, properly completed and timely filed, enable the hospital or agency to make necessary investigations of untoward events to protect patients from any preventable consequences and the hospital or agency and its employees from potential liability. They also enable management to institute any needed corrective measures. Failure to complete and file incident reports savors of a "cover up" — with which the judicial system and public have little patience. It is important to state only facts, the minimum needed for a true picture — no embroidery and no speculation and no elaborate explanations. Facts only!

Write legibly and use only standard abbreviations. Printing nurse's notes is no longer necessary but legible, easily read writing is. Only abbreviations listed in a standard medical dictionary or a printed hospital list are to be used. Consider the following entry: Pt. complains of Hs SOB — S 3 pk d., HA 73, Apd. 75, ANK, PN 78, 80. No NVDV, FRT 81, Ac 83 R 7, 8, and 9 FR. BL Dia; M-Ty/AR. Would you know that it means — Patient complains of a history of shortness of breath — smokes three packs of cigarettes daily. Heart attack in 1973. Appendectomy 1975. Allergies — none known. Pneumonia in 1978 and 1980. No nausea, vomiting, diarrhea, or vertigo. Fractured tibia in 1981. Accident in 1983 with fracture of ribs seven, eight, and nine. Borderline diabetic. Currently taking Tylenol for arthritis? Nurse's notes are to record and communicate information to the physician and other members of the health team and hence they must be readily readable to serve such purpose. Further, since court actions are usually brought to trial several years after the cause of the action occurred, the notes must be readable after such period of time if they are to serve the purpose of refreshing the nurse's recollection of the material.

Calloway cites the case of *Rogers v. Kasdam* where in 1981 the Kentucky Supreme Court ruled against the doctor and hospital nurses based on the medical record. The patient had been in an automobile accident, was admitted to the hospital, and died seven days later. The emergency room record was incomplete, the I&O sheet was incorrectly tallied, and the records contained a number of discrepancies. Several records were illegible while others contained incomplete notations.[16] While brevity is desirable, clarity is essential.

Legal significance of charting

HELEN CREIGHTON, RN, JD

Part II

Keep charting free of criticism or complaints. As Bailey-Allen states, "A nurse's note that couldn't get Dr. Jones to see the patient does not release the nurse from responsibility, but it does clue the attorney to a problem."[3] The nurse still has the responsibility to continue to attempt to locate a physician even if this means calling the Chief of the Staff or the Director of Nursing Service and the hospital administration.

Far too frequently, a physician will write an order for a nurse to "Make out an incident report," and this is inflammatory and aggravates an already large malpractice problem.

If a nurse has criticism of the work performed by another nurse, it is not appropriate to record this in the nurse's charting. Tell the nurse about the problem, report it to the supervisor, or make out an incident report if there is adequate cause. For example, in a recent chart, the following nurse's note appeared: "...7 a.m. Patient's toes on right foot beyond the cast are blue and cold. Night shift apparently never checked the circulation in them." The assessment of the condition of the toes is appropriate but the gratuitous remark about the nurses on the night shift serves only to stir up trouble. If, in fact, the nurses on night shift did not properly check the circulation of the patient's toes, this evidence will come out upon investigation and it is certain to be inquired about by a patient's attorney at trial.

Bernzweig states that "the medical records should not include remarks concerning 1) the patient's personality traits or idiosyncracies, unless pertinent to his case, 2) the physician's personal views to the effect that the patient is a malingerer, a troublemaker, or a potential litigant, or 3) gratuitous admissions of liability with respect to untoward medical events."[17]

Do not destroy or attempt to obliterate documentation. [3] If a nurse makes an error in charting, the acceptable way to correct it is to draw one line through the incorrect material, initial it and date it, and write the correct entry above it or in the next available space on the chart with a note identifying the correct entry. To black out, white out, or use ink eradicator or an erasure gives the appearance of an attempt to hide a mistake....

In *Ahrens v. Katz,* [18,19] a petition in equity alleges white-outs in the nurse's notes were part of a fraudulent scheme to hide relevant facts concerning Gary Ahrens' treatment, or alternatively, the cause of a mutual mistake concerning Gary Ahrens' treatment. The nursing notes and other documents were, in fact, x-rayed to determine exactly what had been stricken. In court the nurse stated that the white-out/white-over procedure was not in accordance with correct nursing standards, and that the proper procedure would have been for her to line through the erroneous material, mark it "error," and then make a correct entry beneath it. She said that she could not remember why she used the white-out fluid instead. The court found the white-out procedure was improper but from the nurse's testimony was unable to infer a fraudulent or guilty intent.

In *Carr v. St. Paul Fire and Marine Insurance Co.,*[20] where a patient with severe pain entered an emergency room and was sent home without the opportunity to see a physician and the nurses testified they had taken the patient's vital signs but the records had been destroyed, the federal district court allowed the jury to infer [that the records] would have shown an emergency situation existed. The court held that the jury could find the hospital negligent.

In *Pisel v. Stamford Hospital,* [21] when a 23-year-old schizophrenic patient was admitted to a psychiatric hospital, she was placed in a quiet room and all furniture was removed. On the fourth day, the bed frame and mattress were placed in the room for no explained reason. A few days later the nursing staff failed to record an ordered antipsychotic medication, so she received none for three days. Later the patient was found semicomatose with her neck wedged between the mattress and siderails of the the bed. Some days after the injury, the director of nursing ordered the nursing staff who had charted the patient's care to rewrite and change the records. Without the knowledge of administration and in violation of hospital policy, the revised record was substituted for the original one. A $3.6 million verdict was upheld when the court observed, "An allowable inference from the hospital's bungled attempt to cover up the staff inadequacies...was that the revision indicated a consciousness of negligence." It is important that a nurse never let anyone pressure her into concealing the truth about something that happened during the course of nursing care or treatment. [17]

Do not leave vacant lines, and sign every entry. It is important for a nurse not to leave vacant lines as this opens the way for others to vary the chart by adding material at a later date. To be sure, a nurse's charting is often interrupted and sometimes this is unavoidable. However, if notations are made after the fact, they should be noted in the record as a notation made not at the time of actual occurrence, but as an after-the-fact notation. For example:

> 1:00 p.m. 9 a.m. range of motion exercises and morning care given on time. Due to rounds and CPR emergency it is charted now.

The above entry is believable but does not purport to have been charted on time. When four lines of vital information is squeezed on two lines, it signals that the charting was done at a later time; otherwise the four lines of vital information would be charted on four lines. Late charting is always "suspect." It may be received as evidence or it may not be. We all know from experience that given enough time to think about it, any nurse can chart what should have been done rather than what was done at the moment of occurrence.

Unless your institution has a policy that specifies a method of signing charts, sign every entry and take credit for the nursing care that you gave. In both nursing school and in hospital/agency orientation, nurses are taught how to sign an entry correctly. Most institutions permit nurses to sign with their first initial, last name, and title. Many nurses draw a line through any blank spaces to prevent others from adding information to their nursing notes.

Do record date of return visit, cancelled/ failed appointments, all telephone conversations, and all follow-up instructions. When a patient is examined and/or treated, the date the patient is to have a follow-up appointment should be documented in the record. By recording it immediately on the record, it will protect physician, nurse, and the hospital or agency against a patient's claim that he or she was not told to return. Since patients often suffer adverse effects as a result of their failure to follow medical advice, a documented record of missed appointments is quite helpful to the nurse's defense if a patient sues later. Where there is an apparent problem of missed appointments, it may be worthwhile to send follow-up letters, return receipt requested — to be certain the patient is aware of his or her failure to keep medical appointments. Both nurses and physicians should exercise caution in giving any advice or prescribing any treatment over the telephone without seeing the patient. In any telephone conversation in which advice is given or a drug refill prescribed, the substance of the conversation should appear in the chart. Increasingly, malpractice suits revolve around disputes concerning the contents of a telephone call. *Thomas v. Corso,*[22] previously discussed, contains a dispute by a nurse and doctor over the contents of a telephone call. The nurse denied telling the doctor he need not see the patient and the doctor said the nurse wanted only a pain medication order.

Cortez v. Chi[23] also illustrates the risk of telephone orders. The baby was delivered by Dr. Chi on June 5. On June 18, the baby was seen in Dr. Chi's office for a well-baby visit. On June 19, since the child was crying a lot, the mother took the baby back to Dr. Chi's office and received several prescriptions. The baby had a fever and continued to be ill and after two telephone conversations with Dr. Chi, the mother told him she would take the baby to the hospital. When the mother took the baby to La Casuta Hospital where he had been born, they refused to admit him. The mother then took the baby to the emergency room at the Indio Community Hospital at about 7:30 a.m. At that time the nurse recorded the baby's rectal temperature of 104.8 degrees and called the doctor at 7:45 a.m. to report the baby's temperature and that he was in the emergency room. Although he lived only two blocks from the hospital, the doctor prescribed some medications including Dipuron and also told the nurse to send the baby to his office at 9:00 a.m. When the nurse rechecked the baby at 8:30 a.m., his temperature was 106.4 degrees. The nurse tried unsuccessfully to reach the doctor and the baby died at 8:55 a.m. In a trial, the judgment for $150,000 was entered against Dr. Chi. Clearly telephone medicine is a problem of some proportions.

The part of the medical record identified as nurse's notes is important for legal purposes. In a malpractice suit, nurse's notes figure prominently. Sometimes the absence of noting routine care is viewed as negligence. The presumption in law is that if it was not documented, it was not done. Properly completed flow sheets with patient identification, date, activity, time, and identification of care giver can do much to solve this problem of routine and repeated activities at specified intervals.

In summary, all charting should be accurate and concise. It should be objective and completed promptly. No mention should be made of incident reports in the chart. Charting should be legible and include only standard abbreviations. Nurses and other health care givers should keep charting free of criticism or complaints. It is important not to destroy or obliterate documentation. No vacant lines should be left in charting and every entry should be signed. Do record date of return visit, cancelled or failed appointments, all telephone conversations, and all follow-up instructions. Charting timely, completely, and accurately can help the patient secure a better quality of care and it can protect nurses, physicians, and hospitals or agencies from litigation — or assist them to a favorable resolution of a dispute.

REFERENCES

1. Schaefer, M.S., "To Avoid a Lawsuit, Keep the Record Straight," *RN,* 44:81-84, Nov. 1981.

2. Ohio Nurses' Association, *Documenting Home Care,* Columbus, Ohio Nurses Assn., 1979.

3. Bailey-Allen, A.F., "Avoid Legal Pitfalls in Charting," *Orthopaedic Nursing,* 5:21-23, Jan-Feb, 1986.

4. "Proper Charting Protects You and the Patient," *Ohio Nurses Review,* 61:11, March 1986.

5. *Collins v. Westlake Community Hospital.* 312 N.E. 2nd 614 (Ill. 1974).

6. *Kenyon v. Hammer,* 688 P. 2d 961 (Ariz. 1985).

7. "RN Errs in Charting Rh Factor: Child Stillborn," *Regan Report on Nursing Law,* 25:1, Jan. 1985.

8. Murphy, E.K., "Documenting OR Nursing Care," *Today's OR Nurse,* 5:47-48, 54, May 1983.

9. *People v. Smithtown General Hospital,* 402 N.Y.S. 2d 318 (NY 1978).

10. *Hiatt v. Groce,* 523 P. 2d 320 (S. Ct. Kans. 1974).

11. *Wagner v. Kaiser Foundation Hospital*, 589 P. 2d 1106 (Ore. 1979).

12. *Thomas v. Corso*, 288 A. 2d 379 (Md. 1972).

13. *Goff v. Doctor's General Hospital of San Jose*, 333P. 2d 29 (Cal. 1958).

14. *Ramsey v. Physician's Memorial Hospital*, 373 A. 2d (Md. 1977).

15. *Norton v. Argnot Insurance*, 144 So. 2d 249 (Ct. App. LA 1962).

16. Calloway, S.D., *Nursing and the Law*, Eau Claire, WI, Prof. Ed. Systems, Inc., 1986, p. 65.

17. Bernzweig, E.P., *Legal Aspects of PHS Medical Care*, Washington, D.C., Dept. HEW, 1966, p. 63.

18. *Ahrens v. Katz*, 575 F. Supp. 1108 (Ga. 1984).

19. " 'Missing' Progress Notes: Nurses 'Whiteouts' X-rayed," *Regan Report on Nursing Law*, 25:1, March 1985.

20. *Carr v. St. Paul Fire and Marine Insurance Co.*, 384 F. Supp. 821 (1974).

21. *Pisel v. Stamford Hospital*, 430 A. 2d 1 (Conn. 1980).

22. *Thomas v. Corso*, 288 A. 2d 379 (Md. 1972).

23. *Cortez v. Chi*, 167 Cal. Rptr. 905 (Cal. 1980).

Nurse accountability program improves satisfaction, turnover

PHYLLIS ETHRIDGE, RN

This article describes one health care facility's project for restructuring nurses' organizational roles and improving their professional accountability. The project not only yielded increased job satisfaction and reduced turnover, but also produced several other unexpected positive results. Note: Summaries (shown in bracketed italics) condense extensive background material.

TODAY, 66 PERCENT of all registered nurses (RNs) are working within a hospital setting. A 1986 report by the Department of Health and Human Services predicted that the number of RNs working in hospitals will decrease to 47.3 percent by 1990 and to 40 percent by 2000.[1] Decentralization of hospital organizational structures and movement of nursing care delivery into the community can be facilitated when nursing administrators implement programs that emphasize high-quality, cost-effective care and promote networking and professional accountability.

A significant increase in the intensity of hospital care [that] patients require has had a tremendous impact on nurses' ability to provide continuity of care. The Medicare prospective payment system legislated in 1983 has shifted the use of complex technology to the home environment. Every year a larger percentage of outpatient procedures are performed on an outpatient basis. Hospital nursing administrators are seeking creative methods to maintain quality while increasing the hospital's market share to offset the decline of the inpatient census.

St. Mary's Hospital and Health Center, Tucson, AZ, responding to changes in health care reimbursement and society's need to maintain quality in health care, developed a comprehensive plan to strengthen nurses as professionals. Assessment of nursing's role and functions in the traditional health care system indicated a need for increased authority, responsibility, and autonomy to facilitate collaboration with other health care professionals.

The overall goal of St. Mary's comprehensive plan was to improve nurses' professional accountability. The objectives to be attained without increasing costs were increased efficiency, improved quality of care, increased job satisfaction, and decreased job stress. To accomplish these changes, a systematic program was phased in over a four-year period. A modified Shields[2] three-dimensional professional accountability model was used to depict the three major concepts of authority, responsibility, and autonomy....The project was based on the assumption that increased job satisfaction and decreased job stress for nurses in an acute care facility would improve retention and recruitment of nurses and facilitate decentralization of the hospital organizational structures through enhancement of professional accountability.

Before implementation of the plan, several programs were in place at St. Mary's that fostered RNs' accountability. These included a nursing practice organizational model similar to that of the medical staff, which promoted self-governance; and a joint practice committee co-chaired by the past president of the staff nurses' organization and an appointed staff physician, which promoted collegiality. Staff nurse bylaws were revised to allow development of the program. The components of the professional accountability program considered to be crucial to continued development of the plan were the following:

1. Identify and enhance qualifications of nurses through a credentialing mechanism
2. Restructure nurses' employment terms to professional salaried status
3. Implement a spiritual, holistic framework for nursing, thereby stressing the art of nursing
4. Identify programs to extend nursing's sphere of influence to activities that promote a continuum of care
5. Use the patient classification staffing tool as an acuity billing system
6. Decentralize the nursing organization and move it into the community, while maintaining quality and cost-effectiveness
7. Promote an environment conducive to two levels of nursing practice—professional nurse case managers and associate registered nurses.

[Implementation

St. Mary's took steps to implement the components of the professional accountability program. Staff nurses developed a credentialing program that evaluated and rewarded nursing competence in clinical practices, education, and leadership. After six months of nursing-management meetings, St. Mary's established professional salaried status for nurses. It held workshops in "traditional Indian medicine" to strengthen the nurses' holistic approach to health. Based on the results of an independent study, St. Mary's developed a system for variable billing by client acuity, which helped identify nursing as a revenue center. It started a pilot project in decentralized home care in which the nurse acted as the primary care provider and coordinated the client's care in the hospital and at home. (Because the project found that a lack of education in community health nursing hindered the provision of cost-effective care, the home care program now uses specially prepared nurse case managers.) Reliance on nurse case managers helped promote a continuity of care from acute care in the hospital to chronic care in the community. St. Mary's also established eight nursing centers that offered sessions on physicial activity, nutrition, medication control, stress management, and other topics to individuals, families, and groups in the community.

Evaluation

In 1983, several instruments were used to measure the nurses' job stress and job satisfaction before the accountability program was implemented. The same instruments were used again to assess these factors in 1985 and 1987. The instruments measured significantly lower job stress in several areas and significantly higher job satisfaction in four of six areas.

Other effects of the program include: decreased recruitment and orientation costs for nurses, reduced RN turnover rate from 15.2% in 1983 to 5.4% in 1986, decreased length of hospital stay for clients who receive care from nurse case managers, and financial savings of more than $500,000 over the past two fiscal years. Nurses, physicians, clients, and administrators have responded positively and benefited from the nurse accountability program.]

NOTES

1. U.S. Department of Health and Human Services Report on Nursing, *Fifth Report to the President and Congress on the Status of Health Personnel in the United States,* U.S. Superintendent of Documents, Washington, DC, March 1986.

2. Mary Shields, "An Evaluation Model for Service Programs," *Nursing Outlook,* 1974, pp. 418-451.

SECTION FOUR

Ethical aspects

BESIDES HAVING A legal responsibility, the nurse has an ethical responsibility to clients. Ethical responsibilities fall into two categories: personal for the nurse and professional for the nursing profession.

Sometimes, a nurse's personal ethics conflict with professional ones. For example, a nurse may believe that assisting in an abortion is ethically wrong. However, a nurse cannot refuse to care for a client because professional ethics require caring for any client who needs it.

At times, the nurse's professional responsibility (professional ethics) may be compromised by a client's ethical standards. For example, the nurse may not be able to provide adequate care to a client who declines life-supporting measures.

The nurse may encounter such ethical dilemmas in any type of practice. Other examples of possible ethical problems for a nurse include artificial insemination by a donor, *in vitro* fertilization, genetic counseling, child abuse, allowing a seriously ill or deformed neonate to die, behavior control, involuntary hospitalization, living will, euthanasia, confidentiality, informed consent, and substance abuse by a co-worker.

Some of these ethical issues relate to advanced health care technology. Others are created by the nursing shortage. Still others derive from conflicting ethical values. But all of them are ethical issues that will be faced with greater confidence by the nurse who has thought about and clarified personal and professional ethical values.

To help clarify personal ethical values, the nurse may consider these questions:

- Where do my personal values fit in with my professional decisions?
- What should my philosophy of nursing be?
- What do I think constitutes good nursing practice?
- Which qualities should I possess as a professional nurse?

To help understand professional ethical values, the nurse may turn to the American Nurses' Association "Code of Ethics" and the International Council of Nurses "Code for Nurses." These codes establish high standards of conduct to protect vulnerable, dependent members of society and to assure the public that individual nurses will not exploit their positions.

To help cope with ethical dilemmas, the nurse also may study ethics and discuss solutions to potential ethical problems. The articles in this section give the nurse an opportunity to do just that.

In "An Ethical Model for Decision-Making," Bunting and Webb begin with a brief overview of selected ethical theories and principles, including respect for persons, beneficence, and justice. Then they examine several decision-making models. After analyzing and synthesizing these models, the authors present a 10-question model to guide the nurse in ethical decision-making. Finally, they demonstrate how to apply this model to a clinical situation.

This article is particularly useful because its concepts and decision-making model are applicable to many different situations by nurses in various settings.

The second article, "Do Not Feed: Is Stopping Artificial Feedings Ethical?" by Collopy, et al., deals with halting artificial feedings to an elderly brain-damaged client. The ethical considerations in this case are discussed by an ethics committee including anethicist, a gerontology nurse, a physician-ethicist, and a nurse-ethicist. This article underscores that complex ethical dilemmas have no absolutely right or wrong solutions. It shows how different people apply personal and professional ethical values to the same situation to make different — but equally valid — ethical decisions. It also touches on the importance of discussing ethical problems with peers to help clarify one's values.

An ethical model for decision-making

SHEILA M. BUNTING, RN, MS; ADELE A. WEBB, RN, MS

...AS HEALTH CARE BECOMES more sophisticated and complex in its delivery, the ethical considerations become more complicated and difficult to untangle. It is not only the rapid growth of technology in diagnosis and treatment of illness, which brings its own particular dilemmas, but the perplexing social implications of diseases such as acquired immunodeficiency syndrome (AIDS) and genetic and congenital problems which pose new challenges to nursing judgment. These challenges arise in the realm of patient advocacy, confidentiality, protection of the community, and other duties and values vital to nursing. As the primary care providers, nurse practitioners (NPs) may find themselves in the middle of these types of controversies.

Because of their position of trust and their access to the deepest concerns of the clients, NPs may have information and be in situations separate from those experienced by physicians, social workers, and others. Problems are presented that cannot be adequately addressed by science alone, nor will the diagnostic manual or the policy and procedure book answer the difficult moral questions. NPs fulfill a unique role in the physical, psychological, spiritual, and social care of the client. They also command a specific body of knowledge in each of these areas. It is becoming clear that a basic knowledge of nursing ethics will need to be added to this list.

Normative ethics

The term "ethical" is often used interchangeably with the adjective "moral." It is used to describe the right or wrong aspects of human behavior in terms of good or evil.[1-2] Normative ethics is that area of ethics that is concerned with providing justification for moral obligations and with formulating basic moral principles through a process of reasoning.[3]

Characteristics of ethical decisions

Ethical decisions are made on the basis of ethical or moral principles rather than on the basis of medical, practical, financial, religious, or legal criteria, though these types of criteria may impact the ethical principles that guide the decision. The fact that ethical knowledge is required for ethical decisions means that physicians, who may have the expertise for making medical decisions to medicate or to intubate, may not necessarily have the best basis for making an ethical decision.

For example, in deciding to use or not to use chemotherapy in treatment of a malignancy, a physician might make a different medical decision, based strictly on scientific cytological studies, than would the patient himself based on his own knowledge of himself, his life expectations, and his own resources and values.

Ethical dilemmas

Ethical dilemmas are conflicts between two equally desirable or two equally undesirable choices. The knowledge needed to resolve an ethical dilemma does not fall within the sciences. It is philosophical in nature and is based on profoundly held systems of values. Individuals as well as diverse cultures and societies place dissimilar values on behaviors, so that two persons may reach very different conclusions about an act and both be "right" according to their own moral reasoning. Witness the conflicting ethical stances on abortion, heroic treatment of impaired newborns, and "do not resuscitate" orders.

Because of the influence of deeply and sincerely held personal values on ethical decision-making, nurses need to have an understanding of ethical theories and an ability to justify and to articulate their own methods of making moral choices. These choices, often made in very emotional situations, must be based on coherent ethical principles. Having this foundation for decisions will help the nurse to communicate the reasoning behind the decisions to other professionals and to feel more confident in [deciding] his or her own difficult dilemmas.

Ethical theories

Normative ethical theories are sometimes classified into consequential and non-consequential theories. In *consequential ethics,* an act is judged by whether it results in a good outcome. Utilitarianism is a form of consequential theroy that seeks the most happiness or the greatest good for the greatest number of people. The statement "the end justifies the means" is sometimes made regarding utilitarian theory.

Using this theory, nurses might, in their patient teaching, justify downplaying the side effects of a treatment in order to secure the outcome of a more relaxed, less anxious patient.

In *non-consequential ethical theory,* one considers whether the act itself is morally justified rather than basing the decision on the outcome alone. This type of justification for moral decisions (formalism) is sometimes called deontology or "rules ethics." In deontology, the principles or rules involved in the act are of primary consideration. Decisions are guided by precepts such as "never tell a lie" and "life is sacred and may never be sacrified for any reason."[4]

Benjamin and Curtis refer to deontological theories as duty-based or rights-based frameworks which "hold that there are certain basic duties that must be discharged no matter what."[5]

Codes of ethics such as the various codes of nursing (American Nurses' Association; the International Code of Nursing) are duty-based, while the Patient's Bill of Rights of the American Hospital Association derives from rights-based principles.[5] Complicating this distinction is the relationship between rights and duties. If a patient has a right, such as the right to information about his condition and treatment, then the caregiver has a corresponding duty to fulfill that right. The nurse practitioner would have the duty to provide information to the patient and, using rules ethics, would be prima regardless of the outcome.

It should be clear at this point that deontological (rules-based, formalism) and utilitarian (consequence-based) ethics are not mutually exclusive. The very idea of the greatest good for the greatest number is a principle in itself, and the rules of duty-based ethics originated because of the good for the majority of people that was expected to result from the application of these rules. Most persons, including philosophers and nurses, are not "pure" deontological- or utilitarian-based in their decision-making, but it is helpful to understand these two theories as they are used to justify moral action.

Ethical principles

Some broad ethical principles to which nurses appeal in making decisions are respect for persons, beneficence, and justice.

Respect for persons. The familiar notions of autonomy and self-determination, which guide so much of nursing practice, come from the principle of respect for persons. This ideal also dictates that nurses treat each person as an individual who has a right to privacy and a right to refuse treatment. The principles of confidentiality and truth-telling derive from respect for persons, as does the related concept of the

Case study and analysis

Case study

Barbara is an NP in a clinic that serves many clients who live in the high-rise apartments. She is familiar with Ms. D., 81, because she sees her on a regular basis in order to monitor Ms. D.'s hypertension and medications. Barbara finds Ms. D. to be a delightful, intelligent woman who continues to manage her own life and to enjoy her activities despite what she humorously refers to as "lapses." These are occasions that she describes to Barbara as times when she can't recall where she put away important papers or can't remember whether she did or did not take her dose of medicine.

In asking for help with her "lapses," Ms. D. has stressed confidentiality to Barbara. She fears she will be seen as incompetent or dangerous to herself by the management personnel of the high-rise, and she is even more concerned about the reaction of her daughter, Beth, who lives on the West Coast. "I think that Beth thinks she would rest much easier if I were in a nursing home," she confided to Barbara, "but I would hate that. I want to continue to control my life as long as possible even if I get mixed up and make a mistake once in a while."

Today Barbara meets Beth, who is in town for a visit. She is pleased to note Beth's obvious respect and affection for her mother before Ms. D. comes into the examining room. As her patient disrobes for her assessment, Barbara notices a huge bruise on Ms. D's buttocks. "I got dizzy and fell," Ms. D. admits. "I'm going to have to be more careful when I get up during the night. Please don't say anything to Beth. She can't do anything about it because she lives so far away, and I don't want her to start in again with that nursing-home talk."

Later, while Ms. D. is having her blood drawn, Beth draws Barbara aside. She expresses relief at finding that her mother is receiving good continuity of care from Barbara at the clinic, but says she is very concerned at what she perceives as deterioration in her mother since her last visit a year ago. "Can you tell me if my other has had any 'spells' lately?" she asks. "I'm so worried about her. Do you think something might happen to her living alone in that apartment?"

What do you think the NP should do? (See the analysis below.)

Analysis

1. Health issues.

Forgetfulness	Will this affect accurate self-medication? How much hazard exists for the patient and others (fire, electrical, chemical)?
Dizziness when getting up at night	What underlying pathology is indicated (neurological, hematological, metabolic, and so on)?
One incident of falling	Can the patient compensate for this problem through use of caution, assistive devices, and the like?

2. Ethical issues.

Principle of beneficence	Protecting the safety of Ms. D.: "One ought to prevent harm."
Principle of respect for persons: autonomy	Ms. D. has expressed her concern for self-determination and confidentiality.

continued

Case study and analysis *continued*

3. Further information required in order to make a judgment.	
Behavior	Is Ms. D. presently taking medication as prescribed? What hazardous situations has she realistically been in?
Physiological status	Questioning of routines, critical incidents, precipitating factors. Medical history, physical assessment, and lab studies. Common causes of vertigo are hypoxia, vestibular or cerebellar disease, side effects of medications, anemia, hypoglycemia, hemorrage, and toxic labyrinthitis.
Cognitive assessment	Plans Ms. D. has for dealing with her problems.
Resources available	Friends, neighbors, visiting nurse.
4. Persons who will be affected by the decision.	Ms. D. Beth, the daughter. Barbara, the NP. Possibly others: close friend, the physician, the manager of the high-rise.
5. Values of those involved.	
Ms. D.	Primarily values her independence and the confidentiality of her relationship with the NP.
Beth, the daughter	Values her mother's safety.
Barbara, the NP	Her value system will have been influenced by her life experience, her personal philosophy, her religious and ethnic background, her professional education, professional codes, and her professional experiences.
6. Conflicts between values or ethical principles.	Beneficence directs the prevention of harm; respect for persons directs the safeguarding of Ms. D.'s autonomy and confidentiality.
7. Must a decision be made and, if so, whose decison is it?	A decision must be made because not to decide would, in this case, be an ethical decision. It's the NP's decision because she has the information to give or to withhold from the daughter.
8. Available alternatives.	a) Tell Ms. D.'s daughter of the dizziness, the fall, and the forgetfulness. b) Tell someone else about the incidents (the high-rise manager, the physician). c) Keep the confidence of Ms. D. d) Attempt to persuade Ms. D. to tell her daughter herself (a variation on keeping the confidence of Ms. D.).

Case study and analysis *continued*

9. Ethical justifications for each alternative.	
Disclosure	It is justified by the principle of beneficence.
Keeping of confidence	It is justified by the principle of respect for persons, which embodies autonomy and confidentiality.
10. Probable outcomes of each alternative.	The NP should consider the possible outcomes of each alternative and assess the probability of each from her knowledge of the situation.
Outcomes of the action of disclosure	Harm to Ms. D. may be prevented. Harm to other residents of the high-rise may be prevented. Ms. D. may loose confidence in the NP because of the breach of confidentiality. Ms. D. may have her independence reduced or be persuaded to enter nursing home.
Outcomes of the keeping of confidence	Ms. D. may fail to take her medication and suffer deterioration in her medical condition. She may injure herself and others. She may change her behavior and manage her own care by calling on available helping resources.

responsibility of persons — the idea that individuals have obligations as members of the larger community. These rights as an individual and responsibilities as a member of society come into conflict in such cases as those in which a person's religious beliefs prohibit inoculation when the good of the community demands it.

Beneficence. Beneficence is the principle of doing good. Included under beneficence are the following rules: 1) one ought to inflict no harm; 2) one ought to prevent harm; 3) one ought to remove harm; and 4) one ought to do or promote good.[6]

Frankena states that, all things being equal, the first statement takes precedence over the others.[6] The astute NP will immediately realize that many treatments have harmful side effects and that balancing the four precepts is not so simple as it may first appear. Surgery to remove a harmful tumor may put the patient at risk, thereby doing harm, and many medications result in short- or long-term loss of function, though the long-range intent is to promote good or remove harm.

Justice. Justice is a basic principle for decision-making that enables a nurse to justify treating patients differently. In a world of scarce resources, such as the nurse's time, Medicaid funds, organs for transplant, etc., choices must be made. One criterion for selection is to distribute resources according to need. The patient needs the service the most is the one who will receive it. Another method is to appeal to fairness or equality.

Considered moral judgments

Considered moral judgments are determined by the nurse after appeal to the above moral principles and to the "categorical imperative" described by Immanuel Kant. This principle stated that one should "act only on that maxim which one can at the same time will to be a universal law."[5]

Using this principle as a universal, the nurse would ask himself or herself: "What if every nurse did what I am doing?"

The nurse may then ask, "What is the moral principle supporting the action I have chosen? Am I respecting this person as an individual and as a member of the comunity? What are the probable consequences of the action I have chosen?"

Decision-making models

Several nursing authors have outlined stepwise procedures for making ethical decisions. Bergman, in 1973, delineated a nursing-process type of procedure in which the nurse begins by identifying the major aspects of the problem, both ethical- and health-related, and then identifies and gathers what further information is required to formulate a decision.[7] Once the issues are clear, the nurse uses his or her own professional and personal philosophy to generate and select alternative courses of action. The next step is implementing decisions to the best of one's ability with ongoing review and flexibility. Flexibility is required because one's view of the ethical situation can change with more information — just as one's diagnosis of a health situation can be changed with added data and continued monitoring — and revising of the ethical decision is necessary.

The last steps, according to Bergman, are to evaluate the nursing decision and implementation in light of the results and to add these findings to the nurse's store of ethical knowledge to help her to make future decisions.

Murphy and Murphy[8] describe a similar procedure, and this is expanded further by Stanley.[9] These authors encourage nurses to look closely at the role of each person involved in the situation: family, other nurses, physicians, the patient, etc.

Authors of ethical decision-making models recommend considering as many alternative decisions as possible and, from a utilitarian point of view, considering the probable long- and short-range consequences of each alternative decision.

TABLE 1. A decision-making model for ethical assessment, planning, intervention, and evaluation

1. What are the health issues?
2. What are the ethical issues?
3. What further information do you require about either of the above in order to make a judgment?
4. Who are the persons who will be affected by the decision? (Include yourself and other persons involved in the care of the client if they will be emotionally or professionally affected.)
5. What are the values of the involved parties?
6. What are the conflicts between values or ethical principles?
7. Must a decision be made and, if so, whose decision is it?
8. What are the alternatives available?
9. What are the ethical justifications for each alternative?
10. What are the probable outcomes of each alternative?

Thompson and Thompson have devoted the second portion of their excellent book to the elaboration of a 10-step plan for bioethical decision-making.[1] A chapter is devoted to each step of the plan and includes discussion and examples, ending with evaluation of the results of the decision, and, finally, incorporation of the experience into one's own decision-making knowledge base.

There are no cookbook approaches that will simplify difficult moral questions, but these models will offer guidance to the nurse who is attempting to make a decision in an ethical dilemma. By combining and editing the points of these decision-making models, a list of questions has been compiled to guide the nurse practitioner through the process of ethical assessment, planning, intervention, and evaluation (see Table 1).

Once a decision has been made and implemented, the NP evaluates the results according to ethical principles (i.e., beneficence, justice, and respect for persons). The outcome that the nurse observes is compared with what "should be." This is done in all of practice for medical and health decisions, and can be done for ethical decisions as well. What a nurse learns from each case is incorporated into his or her knowledge base to be used in making decisions in the next case. How did the actual results compare with the intended outcome? What other actions are required? What would the NP have done differently had the outcome of the decision been known and what changes would he or she make in a future decision?

Conclusion

Ethical reasoning is an important skill for nurse practitioners because the nature of the practitioner role and of the nurse-client relationship is likely to bring about conflicts of values in today's technically and socially complex health care arena. This article has given a brief overview of some ethical principles and theories and reviewed several ethical decision-making models, From these, a 10-question model has been formulated to assist the practitioner in making a decision on ethical grounds.

REFERENCES

1. Thompson, J.E. and Thompson, H.O.: **Bioethical Decision Making for Nurses,** Norwalk, Conn., Appleton-Century-Crofts, 1985.

2. Krekeler, K.: "Critical Care Nursing and Moral Development," **Critical Care Nursing Quarterly,** 1987, 10:2 pp. 1-10.

3. Beachamp, T.: **Philosophical Ethics: An Introduction to Moral Philosophy,** New York, McGraw-Hill Book Co., 1982.

4. Aroskar, M.A.: "Anatomy of an Ethical Dilemma: The Theory," **American Journal of Nursing,** 1980, 80, pp. 658-60.

5. Benjamin, M. and Curtis, J.: **Ethics in Nursing,** New York, Oxford University Press, 1986.

6. Frankena, W.K.: **Ethics,** Englewood Cliffs, N.J., Prentice-Hall, 1973.

7. Bergman, R.: "Ethics Concepts and Practice," **International Nursing Review,** 20, September/October, 1973, pp. 140-2.

8. Murphy, M.A. and Murphy, J.: "Making Ethical Decisions Systematically," **Nursing '76,** May, pp. 13-14.

9. Stanley, T.: "Questions for Ethical Decision Making," handout for Ethics in Nursing Conference, St. Louis University School of Nursing, St. Louis, Mo., Oct 27-28, 1981.

10. Pearson, L.J. and Kotthoff, M.E.: **Geriatric Clinical Protocols,** Philadelphia, J.B. Lippincott Co., 1979.

11. American Nurses' Association: **ANA Code for Nurses with Interpretive Statements,** Kansas City, 1976.

12. The International Council of Nursing (ICN): **Code for Nurses,** Geneva, 1977.

Do not feed: Is stopping artificial feedings ethical?

ETHICS COMMITTEE

FEW ETHICAL ISSUES arouse more passionate debate than the question of whether to withhold food and fluid from a vegetative or terminally ill patient who can't feed himself. Feeding the helpless seems so central to compassionate care that many of us shrink from considering whether it's always appropriate.

But we can't keep ducking this issue. Now more than ever, artificial feedings seem to be preserving life for many patients who'll never again live in a meaningful way. Someday soon, one of those patients may be yours.

To illustrate this complex issue, we created a hypothetical case study and asked a panel of experts...to comment on it. We gave them these guidelines:

- Imagine that the patient, Mrs. Scott, is *your* patient and that you're participating in all treatment and care decisions.
- Assume that everyone in the situation is acting in good faith. For example, assume that Mrs. Scott's brother won't gain anything by her death.

Now, here's the case:

Ella Scott, age 81, worked most of her adult life as a music teacher. But several strokes have left her permanently unconscious and unable to communicate. Although she can breathe on her own and her eyes open occasionally, she's unaware of her surroundings. She now lives in a nursing home, where she's fed through a nasogastric tube. She tolerates most feedings well, although she does vomit some of them.

Mrs. Scott can never recover from the massive brain damage she's sustained — she'll only continue to deteriorate. But because her heart is strong and she has no underlying disease, she could languish in this condition indefinitely.

Mrs. Scott's only living relative, a younger brother, has asked the nursing home to stop the tube feedings. He says that his sister told him on several occasions that if she ever became incapacitated, she wouldn't want to be kept alive with extraordinary treatments. He believes that artificial feeding is an extraordinary treatment that's only prolonging his sister's death, not preserving her life.

However, Mrs. Scott's primary nurse, Marge Downing, strongly opposes stopping the feedings for these reasons:

- She doesn't consider tube feedings extraordinary; she considers them part of basic patient care.
- She believes that withdrawing the feedings would be the same as killing Mrs. Scott outright.
- The patient's wishes are unclear. Ms. Downing contends that no one knows what Mrs. Scott meant when she said she'd refuse "extraordinary treatments." Perhaps she meant only that she wouldn't want a ventilator to keep her alive if she had a terminal illness. Everyone agrees that she never specifically mentioned artificial feedings when she talked with her brother.

Mrs. Scott's doctor, Richard Morgan, has another viewpoint. Unlike Ms. Downing, he believes that artificial feedings are part of a patient's *treatment,* not her basic care. For support, he points to an American Medical Association position statement, issued in March 1986, that says doctors ethically can discontinue "life-prolonging medical treatment" —

including artificial feedings and hydration — for terminally ill or irreversibly comatose patients.

Dr. Morgan also believes that Mrs. Scott clearly expressed her wishes to her brother, and that she didn't want her life prolonged indefinitely with no hope of recovery. And although Mrs. Scott never specifically discussed artificial feedings with her brother, Dr. Morgan says that no one can reasonably anticipate every medical situation that might arise or every medical treatment that might be ordered. He favors stopping the tube feedings out of respect for Mrs. Scott's wishes.

What do you think? Should Mrs. Scott's artificial feedings be stopped? Here's what our four panelists said.

Bart Collopy, PhD, ethicist:

This is a difficult case. Personally, I agree with the brother and doctor that removing the feeding tube is justified.

I think Mrs. Scott expressed her wishes clearly when she talked with her brother. And I'm really not surprised that she spoke of "extraordinary treatments" without specifically mentioning artificial feedings. "Extraordinary treatments" is an ambiguous phrase, and perhaps health care professionals should avoid using it. A treatment that's extraordinary for one patient could be ordinary for another.

Instead of weighing an extraordinary treatment against an ordinary one, I would suggest weighing a particular treatment's *benefits* against its *burdens*. When a treatment becomes unduly burdensome for the patient, its continuation becomes morally optional. That doesn't mean we *must* discontinue the treatment. It only means that discontinuing it becomes a reasonable, moral choice. Viewed in this way, Mrs. Scott's tube feedings could be stopped.

But the doctor, and especially the nursing home administrators, have a responsibility to the nurse as well as to Mrs. Scott. After all, the nurse may be the one to remove Mrs. Scott's feeding tube, and she'll certainly have to continue caring for Mrs. Scott until she dies. In too many cases like this one, the nurse is left alone on a moral frontier, with no place to turn for advice or support.

So, to support nurses as well as patients, the nursing home should formulate a policy for similar situations: *What is our institution's position in cases like this? How should these decisions be made? And who should make them?* These policies shouldn't be fashioned "on high," either. The whole nursing staff should be involved.

Also, the nursing home administrators should decide whether to ask patients about their wishes as a matter of policy. Why not discuss some of these issues with each new patient when she's admitted and allow her to express her wishes and philosophy *before* she becomes incapacitated? Some of the agony of these dilemmas could be avoided if the patient's wishes were clarified before life-and-death decisions had to be made.

Theresa Mazullo, RN, gerontology nurse:

If I were Mrs. Scott's nurse, I'd feel morally obliged to continue the tube feedings. Otherwise, I'd feel responsible for her death by starvation.

I'm speaking from experience. I worked in nursing homes for nearly 10 years, and most nurses I discussed the issue with firmly believed — as I do — that providing nutrition is routine nursing care. It's not "prolonging" life; it's making the patient comfortable — the same thing as repositioning her, or bathing her, or giving her a drink of water. In my opinion, the fact that Mrs. Scott can't ask for these things makes no difference. In fact, if she couldn't tolerate tube feedings any longer, I'd favor inserting a gastric tube.

Recently I had a patient whose tube feedings were discontinued. The doctor wrote the order on the chart and a relative who had the legal authority to make medical decisions for the patient verified in writing that the family agreed with the order. But we nurses were the ones who cared for him while he died. Believe me, it was very difficult walking into that patient's room and seeing him lying there helplessly, starving to death.

Whenever relatives ask us to discontinue artificial feedings, I wonder how they'd feel if they were caring for the patient themselves. If his life were in *their* hands — could they let him die that way?

Kathleen Nolan, MD, physician-ethicist:
Mrs. Scott's situation prompts two questions:
1. Do we know what her wishes were before she became incapacitated?
2. Is artificial feeding a therapeutic intervention, or a part of basic patient care?

Regarding the first question: Mrs. Scott discussed the limits of treatment with her brother before she was hospitalized. Her brother has to interpret her statements in light of her current condition. In my opinion, he's the best person to do that. After all, who's more likely to know what the patient would have wanted — her brother, who discussed this issue with her, or the nurse, who may not even have known the patient before she entered the home? So I give greater weight to the brother's interpretation of Mrs. Scott's wishes.

As for the second question, I believe *oral* feedings are part of basic patient care, but *tube* feedings aren't. For example, I wouldn't be comfortable if Mrs. Scott's brother wanted to withhold food from her if she could still take it by mouth. But Mrs. Scott can't take food by mouth. Inserting a tube to deliver food is an invasive procedure — there's a big difference between invading a patient's body with a spoon and invading it with a tube.

If Mrs. Scott's brother doesn't think that she would have wanted this invasive treatment started in the first place, then it's been imposed without consent. Under such circumstances, discontinuing the treatment is justified.

Clearly, the decision to withdraw artificial feeding is going to have a tremendous emotional impact on Mrs. Scott's nurse. In fact, she may feel that by failing to provide artificial feedings, *she* is causing the patient's death. Of course, that's untrue; the disease is killing the patient by preventing her from taking nutrition.

But I think we can respect the nurse's feelings and her desire to care for the patient, without violating the patient's (or the family's) right to withdraw treatment. How? First, if the nurse objects to withdrawing the feeding tube herself, she should ask the doctor to do it. Second, she should ask the doctor to write an order permitting her to attempt mouth feedings after the tube is withdrawn. Some patients like Mrs. Scott do have enough brain stem activity to take small amounts of fluid by mouth; a few can even swallow enough nutrition to stay alive.

Of course, the nurse and doctor will have to discuss the risk of aspiration and so forth. But the nurse may find the patient's death easier to bear if she's permitted to continue providing some nourishment after the feeding tube is withdrawn.

Susan Salladay, RN, PhD, nurse-ethicist:
Whenever possible, this type of decision should be private, between the doctor and the patient or family. Nurses should write recommendations in their notes. But the patient or her family should be the primary decision makers.

But if the decision were mine to make, what would it be? I believe that the artificial feedings should be stopped. Mrs. Scott's brother says she wouldn't have wanted to be kept alive under these circumstances. To me, she was clearly against prolonging the dying process unnecessarily.

Of course, Mrs. Scott's prognosis is critically important. I'd describe her condition as "permanently vegetative." Medical science can't offer her a cure. But I don't consider this decision a precedent for other types of patients who have some degree of awareness, such as those with Alzheimer's disease.

Of course, after we withdraw Mrs. Scott's feeding tube, the nurse still has a moral obligation to continue all comfort measures, including medication, warmth, and touch. And if Mrs. Scott's level of consciousness changes, the decision to stop the feedings should be reconsidered immediately. No decision is final while she's still alive.

I don't think a nurse should violate a patient's wishes — we're patient advocates. And when recovery is impossible, that may mean being an advocate for death with dignity. That's *not* the same as abandoning the patient.

One point this case study doesn't address is the nursing home's position. If the home refuses to allow the tube to be withdrawn — and many homes would — the doctor and brother need to consider other options for carrying out the patient's wishes. For example, would the brother consider taking her home to die? If so, he's probably sure he's made the right decision. But if he's reluctant to take this step, I'd wonder if he's entirely comfortable with the decision. He may need more counseling — and more time.

No one should make a decision like this hastily. If Mrs. Scott were my relative, stopping the artificial feedings might not feel right to me at first. But in time, after weighing her wishes and prognosis, I think I'd come to accept it.

UNIT THREE

Study questions

1. According to "Therapy for Depression," the nurse should attend to a client's physiologic needs first, including food, fluid, shelter, warmth, air, rest, sleep, sex, and avoidance of pain. How might a nurse apply the five steps of the nursing process to meet the physiologic needs of a depressed elderly client?

2. Based on "The Impact of Nursing Diagnoses in a Long-term Care Setting," how do nursing diagnoses relate to the concept of nurse accountability?

3. In "Meaningful Dialogue," Burnard discusses the following elements of a therapeutic conversation:
• emphasis on the "here-and-now"
• focus on feelings
• development of empathic understanding
• nonprescriptive conversation
• maintenance of the client as the central focus of the conversation.
How do these elements facilitate a therapeutic conversation?

4. "No Longer a Silent Partner" explores the nurse's role on an interdisciplinary team. What kinds of skills can a nurse bring to such a team?

5. In "Legal Significance of Charting," Creighton suggests that the nurse follow these guidelines:
• Chart accurately and concisely
• Chart objectively
• Chart promptly
• Make no mention of an incident report in the chart.
• Write legibly and use only standard abbreviations.
• Keep charting free of criticism or complaints.
• Do not destroy or attempt to obliterate documentation.
• Do not leave vacant lines, and sign every entry.
• Record the date of each return visit, cancelled or missed appointment, and telephone conversation; specify all follow-up instructions.
How are these guidelines significant to nurses? Discuss the application of four of these guidelines to charting.

6. According to "Nurse Accountability Program Improves Satisfaction, Turnover," which three techniques can a hospital use to increase nurse accountability? What are the benefits of nurse accountability?

7. In "An Ethical Model for Decision Making," Bunting describes the ethical principles of respect for persons, beneficience, and justice. What are these principles? How can a nurse use them in making an ethical decision about a client?

8. If you were caring for the client described in "Do Not Feed: Is Stopping Artificial Feeding Unethical?", which issues would influence your decision to stop or continue artificial feedings? In what ways do these issues affect your decision?

UNIT FOUR

Life continuum in health and illness

THE BUSINESS OF NURSING is the improvement, promotion, and maintenance of health. But what is health? The word itself defies easy definition: It can mean different things to different people.

The World Health Organization (WHO) defines health as a "state of complete physical, mental, and social well-being, not merely the absence of disease or infirmity." (1974) This definition is not entirely adequate because it does not account for individuals from low socioeconomic groups or underdeveloped countries who may never be able to achieve this degree of health. Also, it does not specify at what point health ends and illness begins.

Individuals add to the complexity of health as a concept. They may have unique attitudes and beliefs about it. For example, a client may have diabetes. Yet if the disorder is controlled by diet and medication, the client may observe no change in how his body functions and may consider himself healthy. Therefore, any definition of health must account for personal views, which may differ from client to client.

In this unit, *health* refers to an individual's state of physical, emotional, intellectual, social, and spiritual well-being achieved by continual adaptation to internal and external environments. (For more information about environments, see Unit Two.) Because both environments change continually, the client must constantly adapt to maintain well-being. *Illness* is an abnormal process that diminishes or impairs a client's functioning.

Because many internal and external factors can influence a client's health, the nurse should further define health and illness in relation to a specific client. The nurse must consider the whole person, including the client's physical, emotional, and spiritual well-being, life-style, and health beliefs and values.

A nurse may view a client's health according to a model of health and illness. A model is a theoretical way to simplify and understand complex phenomena, such as health and illness. The health-illness continuum model looks at health and illness as relative states, rather than absolute ones as defined by WHO. One end of the continuum represents perfect health; the other represents illness that drastically impairs the individual's functioning. In between, the model describes a full range of health states. When using this model, the nurse compares a client's present position on the health-illness continuum with previous positions and establishes goals to move the client toward the perfect health end of the continuum.

Alternatively, the nurse may use Dunn's high-level wellness model (1961, 1977). This holistic model looks at all dimensions of the client's well-being as the basis for health. Dunn differentiates between good health, which is the absence of illness, and high-level wellness (achievement of the client's fullest potential within the limitations imposed by illness). This model emphasizes health promotion and illness prevention rather than just treatment of existing illness. It encourages the nurse to help the client maximize physical functioning and adapt emotionally, intellectually, socially, and spiritually to any limitations.

No matter how a nurse chooses to view health, the nurse's role is to improve, maintain, and promote health by providing care, teaching, administering health programs, reporting, investigating, and advocating on behalf of the client. To do this, the nurse needs a life-continuum perspective (a perspective for examining the changing needs of the client from the cradle to the grave).

This perspective requires an understanding of growth (quantitative measurable changes as an individual ages) and development (qualitative or behavioral changes as the individual adapts to the environment). For example, a pediatric nurse needs to know normal height and weight parameters to assess a child's physical growth. The nurse also needs to understand developmental milestones, such as a child's mastery of peekaboo. A geriatric nurse must be familiar with the changes that accompany aging, such as decreased temperature tolerance and the need for a slower pace. Each age has specific characteristics and requirements that affect the client's health and illness and the nurse's health promotion measures.

Health promotion and nursing

For many years, the health care system focused entirely on treating illness. Today, it emphasizes illness prevention and health promotion. Wilson (1988) explains this revolution in health care:

> The changing view of health strategies in America is, in part, the result of changing morbidity and mortality patterns. In 1900, the leading causes of death were influenza, pneumonia, tuberculosis, diphtheria, and gastrointestinal infections. Today, only 1% of the people in the United States who die before age 75 are killed by infectious diseases. In 1982, very different ailments predominated....Cardiovascular disease, including both heart disease and stroke, accounted for 46.3% of all deaths; cancer accounted for another 22%.... Accidents were also a major cause of death and disability. The primary cause of current diseases...is lifestyle choices....Examples of lifestyle choices influencing health include patterns of nutrition, exercise, substance abuse, occupation, and personal relationships.

In the 1970s, individuals began to realize that treating chronic disorders such as cardiovascular disease had limited success and that the cost of the treatment and related health care was astronomical.

These realizations led to a growing interest in preventing these disorders through fitness, self-care, and personal health. Individuals began to exercise more and change their eating habits. Industries and businesses established worksite wellness programs. Hospitals started health promotion programs to attract more clients. Changes such as these prompted a restructuring of the health care system and the nurse's role in that system (Wilson, 1988).

Since Florence Nightingale's time, the nurse has approached client care from a holistic perspective that includes health promotion as well as illness treatment and prevention. This perspective has prepared the nurse to adapt to the recent changes in the health care

Glossary

Development: qualitative or behavioral changes that occur as the individual adapts to the environment. Examples include the toddler's mastery of peekaboo or of responding with "Thank you" when a request is honored.

Growth: quantitative measurable changes, such as height and weight increases, dental growth, and sexual changes, that occur as the individual matures.

Health: state of physical, emotional, intellectual, social, and spiritual well-being achieved by an individual through continual adaptation to the internal and external environments.

Health-illness continuum: range of health states from perfect health to extreme illness; fundamental to the health-illness continuum model.

Health promotion: activities such as health education programs that focus on maintaining or enhancing the client's health.

High-level wellness: achievement of the client's fullest potential within the limitations imposed by illness; fundamental to Dunn's high-level wellness model.

Illness: abnormal process that diminishes or impairs an individual's functioning.

Life-continuum perspective: orderly approach to one's changing needs from infancy to old age.

system and to take the lead in defining the nurse's role as the system evolves.

Wilson (1988) identifies some aspects of nursing that complement the health care system's new focus on health promotion. These include the use of conceptual frameworks for holistic, humanistic nursing care that emphasizes the client's responsibility in moving toward health; and nursing research that defines health concerns and articulates effective nursing measures.

Health promotion across the life continuum

Unit Four examines the nurse's role as a promoter of health across the life continuum. Section One discusses basic concepts of growth and development; Section Two examines the nurse's role in health promotion for clients of all ages.

These issues build on the themes of earlier units. For example, health promotion is an extension of caring, which was discussed in Unit One. It demonstrates care that transcends the client's immediate needs and addresses the client's future well-being. The life-continuum perspective also reflects an aspect of caring by illustrating the extension of nursing care to clients of all ages. The internal and external environmental factors presented in Unit Two clearly influence health and illness. The interactive processes of nursing discussed in Unit Three are related to the nurse's ability to promote health and to assist clients throughout the life continuum.

REFERENCES

Dunn, H.L. (1972). *High Level Wellness.* (7th ed.). Arlington, VA: R.W. Beatty, Ltd.

Dunn, H. (1977). *High-Level Wellness.* Thoroughfare, N.J.: Charles B. Slack, Inc.

Wilson, L.M. (1988). The American revolution in health care. *AAOHN Journal, 36*(10), 402-407.

World Health Organization. (1974). *Chronicle of WHO.* Geneva: The Organization, Interim Commission.

SECTION ONE

Concepts of growth and development

To lay the foundation for health promotion and illness treatment and prevention across the life continuum, Section One presents two articles that illustrate some basic concepts of growth and development. Like most nursing literature, the first article approaches the continuum from a pediatric perspective that highlights psychosocial development. The second article departs from the norm by considering less investigated aspects of development — spiritual and religious development — from infancy to old age.

In "Chronic Childhood Illnesses: Developmental Issues," Yoos points out that a chronically ill child must cope not only with predictable developmental tasks, but also with a disease that may interfere with development and alter life experiences. To assist a child with these tasks, the nurse must assess the effect of the illness on the child's development and must identify obstacles to growth as well as resources in the child's environment.

Yoos presents a chart that helps the nurse do just that. First, the chart describes the developmental tasks for each stage of psychosocial development (according to Erikson) from the first days of life through adolescence. Then, it discusses the effects of chronic illness on task accomplishment. It concludes with specific nursing interventions that can help a child overcome the effects of chronic illness and reach normal developmental milestones.

Yoos reminds the nurse of the importance of understanding developmental issues when caring for a chronically ill child. Advances in technology, medical care, and health services have increased — and continue to increase — the number of children surviving with chronic illnesses. To meet the special needs of this growing group of clients and help them and their families cope with the impact of chronic illness, the nurse must be fully prepared to take a developmental approach to their care.

Hurley and Whelan (1988) support this approach. They studied children's responses to pain and analyzed them according to Piaget's four stages of cognitive development. They discovered major differences in pain perception at each developmental stage. For example, a preoperational stage child (age 2 to 7) responds to pain primarily as a physical experience and thinks that it will magically disappear. A concrete-operational stage child (age 7 to 11) understands that pain can be physical or psychological and has some idea of its cause and effect.

To provide appropriate care, Hurley and Whelan advise the nurse to adapt caregiving activities to the child's developmental stage. They conclude:

> As children grow cognitively, what they think about the nature and experience of pain changes. As a result, nurses must be aware of the developmental stages described by Piaget, and the behaviors expected from children at each level. Only then can children receive optimal care based on their cognitive as well as emotional needs.

Like the first article, Carson's "Spiritual Development Across the Life Span" relies on Erikson's theories. Unlike the first article, however, it does not limit its scope to childhood. Instead, this book excerpt describes how change occurs throughout life and illustrates the parallels between psychosocial and spiritual development. It also differentiates between religious and spiritual milestones and considers the nursing implications for clients from adolescence to late maturity.

Carson's excerpt presents nursing's holistic (body, mind, and spirit) approach to care and its life-continuum focus. It also expands the nurse's understanding of spirituality — a significant aspect of the client's internal environment, which was described in Unit Two.

REFERENCES

Hurley, A., & Whelan, E. (1988). Cognitive development and children's perception of pain. *Pediatric Nursing, 14*(1): 21-24.

Chronic childhood illnesses: Developmental issues

LORRIE YOOS, RN, MS, CPNP

DURING THE PAST 20 YEARS, the number of children with childhood chronic illness has increased substantially. Approximately 10% or 1 million of these children have such severe diseases that their daily life activities are severely affected. Because of advances in medical care and health services, more children with such illnesses are able to survive. These families face problems that must be handled according to the child's developmental status, the particular illness, and the family's emotional and financial resources.

What is chronic illness?

A chronic illness is a health condition that interferes with a child's usual activities on a daily basis for at least 3 months a year, leads to a hospital stay involving at least 1 month a year, or [can reasonably be] expected to meet one of these criteria (Pless & Pinkerton, 1975). Such illnesses usually last for a substantial time period and have sequelae that are debilitating for a long time period. Although we may encounter each individual chronic illness only rarely within a pediatric primary care setting, taken as a group, a moderate number of children will have chronic illnesses and handicapping conditions. Nevertheless, these children and their families have extensive and complex needs that require special attention from health care providers.

Common needs of families

Although biomedical research has provided tremendous advances in disease specific therapies, the value of the diagnostic label is less apparent when delivering basic primary health care and when dealing with the children's and their families' social and psychological needs. Stein and Jessop (1982) demonstrated that the psychosocial and developmental needs chronically ill children have are not disease specific. In fact, critical psychosocial concerns cut across diagnostic categories and are common to most children and families coping with chronic physical disease. When reviewing a large number of studies concerning children's adjustments to different chronic illnesses, Pless and Pinkerton (1975) found that all the children and their families faced similar problems. Despite specific health problems, the central issue for families seemed to be rooted in the very existence of the health problem.

This "noncategorical" approach to chronic childhood illness, in contrast with the high technological and subspecialization approaches, stressed an emphasis on the affected client as an individual and on the family unit, as opposed to the specific symptom or illness. For example, many chronic diseases are costly to treat and, obviously, many are accompanied by pain and discomfort. For the family, routine care may become burdensome. Access to highly specialized care as well as care with specialty coordination may be problematic. Chronic illness may impede the child's expected development and the family's developmental tasks (Perrin & Gerrity, 1984 [see Table 1]; Hobbs, Perrin & Ireys, 1985; Magrab, 1985).

Nurse practitioner responsibilities

Stein and Jessop (1984) and McInerny (1984) argue that the care for children with chronic illness should be the responsibility of the primary care provider working closely with appropriate subspecialists. Primary providers should assume greater responsibilities of coordinated care of the disease-specific and generic needs that chronically ill children and their families must face. The nurse practitioner can play an important role in support care, continuity service coordination, and advocacy.

Providing guidance. The American Academy of Pediatrics has stated that discussing and counseling are the most important elements of child health care. Similar to benefits from anticipatory guidance in well-child care, anticipatory guidance can help chronically ill children and their families with common questions and fears, what to expect from the health condition, treatment concerns, and reactions of friends and relatives. Moreover, normal growth and development issues, diet, behavior, and safety require reinterpretation for the child with a chronic disabling condition. Yet parents often report receiving insufficient guidance regarding the impact that the child's illness has on development and behavior (Stein, Jessop, & Reisman, 1983). For example, children need to be included in normal daily activities.

Assessing family dynamics. The nurse practitioner is in the best position to assess how the illness has affected family dynamics. Because the chronically ill child has a profound effect on the family system, the marital relationship and sibling reactions should be evaluated.

Easing transitions. The nurse practitioner can also help facilitate the child's transition from the family system to the school system. Teachers may feel uncertain about how to treat the child and tend to overprotect, which may produce secondary morbidity and handicap (Pless & Pinkerton, 1975). Although such secondary conditions are unrelated to the actual illness, they are caused by the way the illness has influenced or restricted the child's experiences. Having good reciprocal relationships and communication between personnel and health care providers within the community greatly benefits the child.

TABLE 1. Impact of chronic illness on children and families

- Cost of treatment is high.
- Treatment regimens are often complex, painful, and embarrassing.
- The daily burden of care falls on the family.
- The disease course may be unpredictable.
- Discomfort and pain may accompany illness.
- The child and family may experience social isolation.
- Access, coordination, and continuity of care may be difficult.
- Child's ability to engage in accustomed and expected activities may be impaired.

Developmental issues

Chronically ill children need to cope with the predictable tasks of child development as do their healthy peers. However, in addition, these handicapped children must cope with disease conditions that may modify development and life experiences. The nurse practitioner must assess how the illness interacts with the developemental process and identify impediments to growth as well as strength and opportunity sources within the child's social environment. An increasing number of researchers and clinicians have found a developmental approach to chronic illness to be a useful conceptual framework (Cerreto, 1986; Magrab, 1985; Perrin & Gerrity, 1984). Briefly, this model assumes that during various childhood stages, certain physical, emotional, cognitive, and educational tasks are required. Development, in the form of a series of devlopmental tasks, must be mastered before the child can function effectively in society. Factors that influence mastery need to be assessed and possibly manipulated to enhance growth and development (see Table 2).

TABLE 2. The effects of chronic illness on developmental tasks and intervention strategies

DEVELOPMENTAL TASK	EFFECTS OF CHRONIC ILLNESS	INTERVENTION STRATEGY
Neonate		
1. Achieving physiological stability	Chronic illness may decrease infant's access to environmental inputs if all his energy is needed to survive. Body rhythmicity may be disturbed. Physiological stability is essential [to develop] all other major areas.	Help caretaker become aware of and cope with the infant's patterns of sleep, feeding, and elimination. Infant's adjustment to extrauterine life needs to be assessed, and parents need to be taught important symptoms.
2. Developing bonding and attachment	Parental guilt, grief, or anger may interfere with attachment process as may the infant's inability to respond. Parents may withdraw. Attachment requires time to develop. Prolonged hospitalization may disrupt early relationship.	Encourage parents to express feelings...Give factual information about what is known about the...child's problem. Guide parents in establishing physical and emotional contact with the infant. Help parents develop a sense of competence.
Infant		
1. Continuing to develop attachment with the primary care giver	Major separations from parents when attachment is just being formed may interfere with process. Infant's social responsiveness may be decreased, thereby diminishing parents' attachment.	Help families to maintain a consistent presence in infant's life during hospitalization. Maximize opportunities for parents to participate in care. Help parents learn about their infant's characteristic responses. Teach when and how to stimulate infant and when to decrease the...interaction.
2. Acquiring a sense of trust	Developing trust is dependent on having needs met in a consistent manner, which is difficult to achieve in a hospital setting. Illness may violate expectancies of a nurturing, pain-free environment. Inconsistent care and separations from parents may lead to mistrust.	Meet expectancies about the environment whenever possible. Facilitate consistent care through communicating infant's characteristics with other care providers. Maximize parents' opportunities to provide their infant with care.
3. Developing an initial sense of individuality	May decrease the infant's sense of control and effect on his environment. Illness may lead to a sense of helplessness.	Encourage parents to give infant as much opportunity for exploration and mastery as possible.

TABLE 2. The effects of chronic illness on developmental tasks and intervention strategies *continued*

DEVELOPMENTAL TASK	EFFECTS OF CHRONIC ILLNESS	INTERVENTION STRATEGY
Infant *continued*		
4. Learning through sensorimotor exploration	Opportunities for exploration and manipulation of objects may be diminished.	Help parents use age-appropriate toys and activities adapted to child's needs. Help parents with creating useful play experiences. Parents may need help to think about what are usual, appropriate experiences and how to best approximate those experiences.
Toddler		
1. Developing autonomy	Autonomy is aided by opportunities for exploration and independence. Illness may hamper exploring and using motor skills. Parents may overprotect and be reluctant to set limits.	Help parents devise...methods so child can move [and play] independently...Give child simple choices...Help parents confront their guilt that may be preventing them from appropriate limit setting.
2. Mastering new skills in body control, hand use, and speech	May not have opportunity to engage in tasks requiring eye-hand coordination, assembling and categorizing objects. Some conditions affect ability to control bowel and bladder functions.	Help parents be creative in providing play experiences. Tasks involving successful toileting should be broken down into small specific behaviors.
Preschooler		
1. Mastering self-care skills	Parents may overprotect. Regression occurs in most children during illness.	Help parents verbalize concerns; suggest parents' strengths. Help parents to encourage independence and self-reliance.
2. Developing initiative and purpose	May lack exposure to new experiences. Parents may try to buffer interactions with the environment and peers and limit the child's opportunity to develop coping mechanisms. Initiative may be discouraged.	Explore possibilities for preschool experiences...May also need to work with school regarding the nature of child's illness, limitations, etc. Arrange for orientation or observation visit to preschool.
3. Using mental symbolization (although still has egocentric thought and focuses attention on only one part of an event)	Illness may be defined in terms of single external symptom. Illness cause may be attributed to punishment for bad behavior or something they did not do.	Encourage play to help child explore experiences and feelings about illness. Help child prepare for procedures by repeating facts ...and...playing out procedures.

continued

TABLE 2. **The effects of chronic illness on developmental tasks and intervention strategies** *continued*

DEVELOPMENTAL TASK	EFFECTS OF CHRONIC ILLNESS	INTERVENTION STRATEGY
School-age child		
1. Using concrete operations	Achieving this task is enriched by school, hobbies, and interactions with peers. May have diminished opportunities for learning and irregular school attendance.	Encourage and facilitate regular attendance. Nurse practitioner may need to act as liaison between school and family and advocate for the child. Educate teachers and healthy peers about chronic illness. Be creative when school is missed. Use computer break-up or home VCR.
2. Developing industry and initiative. 'I can do' (comes about primarily through mastering social interactional situations and concrete skills)	May have decreased interactions with peers. May feel different from peers. May miss out on experiences that lead to the normal development of self-esteem and a sense of mastery. May show a pattern of under achievement when compared to tested abilities (Pless & Pinkerton, 1975).	Encourage enhancing peer relationships through participating in clubs and sports. The importance of normalized school and life experiences cannot be over-emphasized. Health care providers need to collaborate with school personnel. (Magrab, 1985). School-age children should participate as much as possible in their own care and decisions affecting their treatment. Children need factual, honest information about their disabilities. Allow child to have control over diet or medications as child's ability to handle these situations develops.
Adolescent		
1. Establishing independence	Disease management may make independence difficult. Complying with medical regimen may become a problem. Relationships with parents and health care providers may become increasingly hostile. Job and career choice may be diminished.	Identify feelings of anger as normal and offer support. Encourage families to find areas in adolescents' lives where they can have independence. Assist parents in facing some of the complexities of possible living arrangements. Help develop skills for self-care. Referrals to vocational rehabilitation services may be appropriate.

TABLE 2. The effects of chronic illness on developmental tasks and intervention strategies *continued*

DEVELOPMENTAL TASK	EFFECTS OF CHRONIC ILLNESS	INTERVENTION STRATEGY
Adolescent *continued*		
2. Becoming comfortable with one's body	Preoccupation with bodily functions and changes is normal for all teens, accentuated for adolescents with chronic illness. Physical illness manifestations may make them feel markedly different from peers. Adolescents with visible physical defects experience sadness, grief, and anger.	Respect need for privacy. Assist in finding support groups. Acknowledge feelings; facilitate family sharing feelings. Teenagers need to understand the specifics about their physiologic condition and what treatment they are receiving. The ability to look at and care for one's own body, including those parts that are different, is necessary for the eventual acceptance of that body (Miezo, 1983).
3. Establishing sexual identity and building new and meaningful relationships	May have decreased opportunity to be part of a peer group. May have decreased access to peers with whom to discuss sexual questions.	Help parents understand that an adolescent with a disability is as much a sexual being as any other person. Encourage adolescents to participate in activities and initiate friendships. Provide information about birth control.
4. Developing formal operational thought	Deficit in previous stages may prevent this. Developing adolescent's cognitive abilities is aided by interaction and cooperation with others (Piaget, 1950). Ill adolescents may have fewer opportunities for confrontation with peers.	Encourage opportunities for adolescents to be faced with opinions, values, and beliefs that may differ from their own. Advocacy within school system.

REFERENCES

Cerreto, M. (1986). Developmental issues in chronic illness: Implications and applications. *Topics in Early Childhood Special Education. 5*(4), 23-25.

Hobbs, N., Perrin, J., & Ireys, H. (1985). *Chronically ill children and their families.* San Francisco: Joseey-Bass.

Magrab, P. (1985). Psychosocial development of chronically ill children. In N. Hobbs, & J. Perrin (Eds.), *Issues in the care of children with chronic illness* (pp. 698-715). San Francisco: Joseey-Bass.

McInerny, T. (1984). The role of the general pediatrician in coordinating the care of children with chronic illness. *Pediatric clinics of North America: Chronic disease in children* (pp. 199-209). Philadelphia: W.B. Saunders.

Miezo, P. (1983). *Parenting children with disabilities.* New York: Marcel Dekker, Inc.

Perrin, E.C., & Gerrity, P.S. (1984). Development of children with a chronic illness. *Pediatric clinics of North America: Chronic disease in children,* (pp. 19-31). Philadelphia: W.B. Saunders

Piaget, J. (1950). *The psychology of intelligence.* London: Routhlege and Kegan Paul Ltd.

Pless, I.B. & Pinkerton, P. (1975). *Chronic childhood disorder: Promoting patterns of adjustment.* Chicago: Yearbook Medical Publishers.

Stein, R.E. & Jessop, D.J. (1982). A non-categorical approach to chronic childhood illness. *Public Health Reports, 97,* 354-362.

Stein, R.E., Jessop, D.J., & Reissman, C.K. (1983). Health care services received by children with chronic illness. *American Journal of Diseases of Childhood, 137,* 225-230.

Spiritual development across the life span

VERNA BENNER CARSON, RN, MS

Drawing on Erikson's stages of psychosocial development, Carson examines spiritual development throughout the stages of life. Because Erikson's theories are based on a Judeo-Christian heritage, they may not be universally applicable. Nevertheless, this excerpt provides important information about spirituality and those nursing interventions that incorporate it into the care plan. Note: Summaries (shown in bracketed italics) and excerpts (marked by ellipses) condense extensive background material.

THE CONGREGATION WATCHES as the priest pours water over the infant's head. His parents and godparents join the priest in making the sign of the cross on the baby's forehead. As the ceremony ends, the child has been baptized and officially welcomed into the Christian community.

Similar rites of initiation take place in other faiths. Within 7 days after birth, the Orthodox Jewish couple present their baby girl at the temple to be named. At birth, the Islamic father whispers the prayer of Allah into the ear of his infant. The Buddhist mother brings her young infant to a monk for consecration. Each of these acts is a rite of passage established by a particular faith community. However, none of these ceremonies guarantees that children will practice their faith. For this to happen, children will need continual guidance, teaching, and support from family, friends, and faith community, as well as their own assent to the beliefs and practices presented.

Individuals may be born into a particular religion, but they are not born religious. Similarly, people are created with a spiritual as well as a physical and emotional nature. This does not guarantee that this spiritual nature will develop and flourish. Just as physical and emotional growth requires food for the body and the mind, a nurturant environment, and time, there are similar influences that contribute to spiritual and religious development....

Spiritual and religious development

Spiritual development. Growth in spirituality is a dynamic process in which an individual becomes increasingly aware of the meaning, purpose, and values in life. There is a two-directional process occurring in spiritual growth. The horizontal process increases the person's awareness of the transcendent values inherent in all relationships and activities of life. The vertical process moves the individual into closer relationship with a higher being, as conceived by the individual. It is quite possible to develop the horizontal and not the vertical process. Individuals may define their spirituality in terms of relationships, art, or music and never develop a relationship with a deity. Likewise, individuals who are drawn to a higher being in their spiritual growth may not develop other avenues of spiritual expression.

Religious development. Religious development refers to an individual's acceptance of a particular system of beliefs, values, rules for conduct, and rituals. Sometimes religious and spiritual development parallel each other and share common ground. This is not always true. An individual may strictly adhere to the tenets of a particular faith tradition yet never internalize the symbolic meaning behind religious activities. The individual gives the appearance of being religious but never examines the broader issues implied in spiritual growth. Religious development ideally leads to spiritual development; but just as people can get "hung up" in a particular stage of psychosocial development, so can their religious and spiritual growth be arrested.

Role of spiritual/religious milestones. Physical and emotional growth can be traced and studied according to predictable, sequential patterns. Infants crawl before they walk; they babble before they talk; they are dependent before they become independent. Parents are attuned to these developmental milestones — eagerly anticipating and rewarding each new step. A child's first smile, first tooth, and first tentative steps are reasons for parental joy. Likewise, most parents are cognizant of the child's increasing capacity to solve problems, to express self, to share, to control impulses, and to adjust to new situations.

Religious development is marked by the particular milestones established by a specific faith — such as infant or adult baptism, confirmation, Holy Communion, Bar or Bas Mitzvah, penance, or Buddhist infant initiation rites. These events are external and symbolic and may not correspond to either increased religiosity or spirituality for the individual.

The milestones of spiritual development are not as apparent as those marking physical and emotional maturity. Many of the influences that lead to physical and emotional health parallel the horizontal facet of spiritual development. It is therefore necessary to examine psychosocial milestones for their spiritual implications.

The vertical facet of spiritual development transcends earthly experiences because it occurs in response to a divine being. This call can be heard in the midst of a life filled with every material advantage or in a life devoid of all human pleasures. Sometimes in the most blessed lives individuals do not develop a relationship with a higher being. They may consider themselves quite spiritual in terms of creative endeavors and interpersonal relationships. There are many examples of individuals who are caught up in devastating life circumstances and who hear and respond to the voice of a supreme being or force. Because the vertical facet of spirituality develops in such different ways, it cannot be pigeonholed, staged, or sequenced as neatly as physical and emotional growth. It is possible, however, to examine potential milestones of spiritual growth.

[Spiritual development through the stages of life

Infancy. *According to Erikson (1963), the infant's developmental task is to balance trust with mistrust. The infant acquires the rudiments of trust through experience with caregivers who provide for the infant's needs. The infant also begins to hope by learning to anticipate that future needs will be met. By being involved in a totally dependent relationship with the mother, the infant develops faith in a greater being.*

By the end of this developmental stage, the infant has no clear spiritual or religious beliefs, but has the basics of trust and hope.

Early childhood. *From age 2 to 3, the child's developmental task is to master skills related to motor freedom. By successfully completing this task, the child acquires the virtue of willpower (Erikson, 1963). Through events such as toilet training, the child develops a sense of self-worth and power, which later allows the child to accept love, including the love of God.*

Preschool. *When the child reaches preschool age (age 4 to 5), the developmental task is to balance self-assertion with self-discipline. The virtue associated with this task is sense of purpose (Erikson, 1963). "Learning to balance what the child wants with what others demand is a crucial task — a task that has implications* *for both horizontal and vertical spiritual development."*

Spiritual and religious development begin in this stage as the preschooler develops a conscience, learns to obey parental rules, and comes to believe that God can reward good behaviors and punish bad ones.

School age. *From age 6 to 10, a child's task is to become proficient and knowledgeable in doing things. By mastering this task, the child gains a sense of industry and the virtue of competence (Erikson, 1963).*

"School age, with its emphasis on mastery, allows the child to begin to experience the transcendent dimension of creative activities as well as relationships. Children reared within a religious tradition feel a part of their religion. They may believe in God with their whole being, and they affirm the reality of the divine in their life."

Adolescence. *During adolescence, the child's developmental task is to develop a clear sense of identity. According to Erikson (1963), successful completion of this task yields the virtue of fidelity. "Adolescents must have a sense of self before they can be true to self, to another person, to a supreme being, or religious ideology."*

In this stage, adolescents may reject parental values and assume those of their peers. Some reject all organized religions to rebel against religious parents. Some embrace a religion that their parents reject. Others may join antispiritual groups that display antisocial and anti-God behaviors; still others join cults that prey on their need for identity, acceptance, and love.

Young adulthood. *The developmental task of a young adult is to commit to an intimate relationship — to balance intimacy with isolation. In completing this task successfully, the young adult gains the virtue of love, which adds to the horizontal and spiritual dimensions of spirituality.*

In the late teens or early twenties, a young adult may have a spiritual experience, which may be seen as a call from the Almighty or a self-actualizing event. The young adult who responds to this "awakening" makes a conscious choice to have a relationship with God.

Middle adulthood. *"Erikson (1963) describes the task of adulthood as achievement of a healthy balance between generativity and stagnation, with care being the resultant virtue."*

Spiritually, this developmental stage is characterized by nurturing of children (and teaching them spiritual and religious beliefs) and by increased turning inward. This stage may represent an adult's first spiritual awakening or a renaissance. An adult's faith "is very much alive and is experienced as unqualified love for the Almighty, self, and neighbor." This love is reflected in sacrifices and service to others.

Later maturity. *With age, the older adult faces the final developmental task — to balance ego integrity and despair (Erikson, 1963) — and achieves the virtue of wisdom. In this stage, the question arises, "Can I accept myself as I truly am?" To answer it positively, the older adult must review his or her accomplishments and failures and decide that "My life had meaning. It was the best I could do at the time, and I created a life like no other."*

During later maturity, religion may become more important. The older adult "may find comfort, solace, and affirmation in religious activities. Prayer and religious services facilitate the meditation that accompanies the life review process." The older adult's faith typically reflects unconditional acceptance and love of God.]

Nursing implications

Westerhoff (1976, p. 103) draws an analogy between faith development and the growth of a tree that is just as appropriately applied to spiritual development. The analogy is quite helpful to nurses in their attempts to incorporate a client's spiritual development into a plan of care.

> First, a tree with one ring is as much a tree as a tree with four rings. A tree in its first year is a complete and whole tree, and a tree with three rings is not a better tree but only an expanded tree. In a similar way, one style of faith is not a better or greater faith than another....Second, a tree grows if the proper environment is provided, and if such an environment is lacking, the tree becomes arrested in its expansion until the proper environment exists. Each tree, however, does its own "growing" and has its own characteristics.... Third, a tree acquires one ring at a time in a slow and gradual manner. We do not see that expansion, although we do see the results, and surely we are aware that you cannot skip rings, moving from a one ring to a three ring tree.... Fourth, as a tree grows, it does not eliminate rings but adds each ring to the one before, always maintaining all the previous rings as it expands.

...The nurse recognizes that spirituality is not something to be judged but rather to be assessed and accepted....The stress of illness can either cause the client to regress or to grow spiritually. The nurse's ministerial role cannot be minimized in assisting clients through their spiritual developmental crises....When nurses plan interventions geared to a client's psychosocial level, they are also meeting the spiritual needs of a secular or horizontal nature....A few examples illustrate the relationship between the client's spiritual development level and the appropriate nursing intervention.

> Mrs. Smith, a 66-year-old client crippled with rheumatoid arthritis, is hospitalized with a fractured left hip. The nurses responsible for Mrs. Smith's care notice her peaceful demeanor and her frequent periods of quiet contemplation. Mrs. Smith tells the nurses that she just wants to spend time with her God and that she does this best without words. The nurses recognize that Mrs. Smith's spiritual development is quite advanced. They make sure that she is provided quiet, uninterrupted time without being ignored.
>
> Gregory, 15 years old, is hospitalized with leukemia and is in protective isolation. His nurses are aware that his condition and his treatment are depriving him of the peer support so needed for his psychosocial as well as his spiritual development. The nurses encourage his friends to write and to call Gregory and to keep up communication from his church youth group.
>
> Jessica, 22 years old, is struggling with her spirituality. She questions all the beliefs that were so much a part of her upbringing. Her recent illness only increases her spiritual conflict and questioning. The nurses recognize that questioning about God, the meaning of life, and spiritual values is a vital and normal step toward spiritual maturity. The nurses recognize they are not a source of answers for Jessica, but rather they can act as a sounding board to allow her to find her own answers.
>
> Mr. Jennings, a client with terminal cardiac disease, prays for a complete healing of his heart muscle. His prayers are very much like a small child's. Mr. Jennings pleads and bargains with God, promising better behavior in return for healing. His nurses accept his prayer for what it is. He is reaching out to God in desperation, probably brought on by his fear of death. The nurses support Mr. Jennings's approach to God by telling him that they are praying that God will support and strengthen him in his struggle.

There are no pat answers or approaches for nurses to use when a client seems to be at a certain level of spiritual growth. However, the importance of the nurse's awareness that spirituality progresses over the life span and that the nurse has a role as a ministering person in this developmental process cannot be overemphasized....

REFERENCES

Erikson EH: Childhood and Society. New York: Norton, 1963.

Westerhoff J: Will Our Children Have Faith? New York: Seabury Press, 1976, pp. 79-103.

SECTION TWO

Nursing care throughout the life continuum

NURSING CARE IS associated with every age across the life continuum. At the moment of birth, a nurse is present to help the newborn adapt. When the child goes to school, a nurse offers health promotion and illness prevention. If the child is hospitalized, a nurse provides specialized care. As the child becomes an adult and wants to start a family, a nurse helps maintain a healthy pregnancy and teaches techniques of prepared childbirth, parenting, and breast feeding. Throughout the adult's working years, a nurse offers health care guidance from the job site or the inpatient unit. As the client grows older, a nurse attends to needs at home or in a nursing care facility. When the client faces death, a nurse stands ready to relieve pain, provide comfort, and offer support.

The articles in this section demonstrate the nurse's birth-to-death involvement with clients. They show some of the ways that a nurse may respond to needs that occur at different ages and stages of development.

In the first article, "Nurses' Responses to Changes in Maternity Care," Myers and Stolte investigate trends in maternity nursing, including family-centered care, shortened postpartum hospitalization, changes in client characteristics, increased probability of litigation, greater reliance on technology, and increased emphasis on health care cost containment. They examine the conflicts and rewards in these trends and their effects on maternity care and the nurse's role.

The next article, "Coping Skills for Children Undergoing Painful Medical Procedures" by Patterson and Ware, explores a part of the nurse's role in caring for children. It suggests several strategies to help the nurse reduce a child's pain during certain procedures. Although the child's psychological preparation may require additional time, money, and training, the authors believe that the effort and expense are justified because a child's initial experiences with health care providers and pain can dramatically affect future responses.

A child reaching adolescence develops special health care concerns that the nurse must address. In "Health Concerns of Adolescents," Smith et al. report, however, that the adolescent's concerns are not the ones that parents, the health care community, and the media expect. The typical adolescent is not overly worried about teenage pregnancy, drug use, alcohol abuse, anorexia, or smoking. Rather, the adolescent is concerned about getting along with family, handling emotions, and managing physical appearance. The authors remind the nurse to care for the adolescent as an individual, addressing his or her perceived health needs as well as the general health problems of the age group. By finding out what is most troublesome to the adolescent, the nurse can provide the most effective care.

The next article, Baldwin's "The Stress of Caring: Issues Confronting Mid-Life Caregivers," focuses on one aspect of care during middle adulthood. It begins with a profile of the typical mid-life caregiver. Then it examines the rewards — and stress — associated with caring for an elderly family member at home. Because stress can disrupt the caregiver's health, the article concludes with stress-management techniques the nurse can use to promote health and take care of the caregiver. Because increasing numbers of elderly clients receive care from family members at home, this article is particularly relevant for today's nurse.

In the next article, "Continence Through Nursing Care," Pearson and Droessler address an important aspect of geriatric care: continence. The importance of continence cannot be overstated because it is a hallmark of independence and adulthood and, as such, must be preserved. To help the nurse with this task, the article discusses risk factors for incontinence and specific nursing strategies to overcome each risk factor and help the elderly client regain continence. Another valuable facet of "Continence Through Nursing Care" is its demonstration of the importance of combining the clinical skills of a nurse clinician and the research and statistical skills of a nurse researcher to develop an effective clinical study.

The last two articles examine the nurse's role in assisting a dying client. The first one, "What Is It Like to Be Dying?" is a classic. In it, Elisabeth Kübler-Ross sensitively describes the stages that a client typically passes through when approaching death: denial, anger, bargaining, depression or grief, and acceptance. She cautions the nurse against using the stages as a strict measure of the client's success or failure in dealing with death. Rather, she presents the stages as a framework for understanding the complex and difficult task of dying. Throughout the article, Ross suggests ways for the nurse to help the client move through the stages of dying and reach the final stage, acceptance.

The last article, "Shalom, Melissa: Comforting the Terminally Ill Leukemia Patient" by Sherman et al., illustrates several of Ross's stages of dying in the true story of a dying client. It also depicts the efforts of nurses and other health care team members to meet the client's physical, emotional, and spiritual needs. It poignantly represents one of the nurse's greatest challenges and rewards: helping a client gain an acceptance of death.

Nurses' responses to changes in maternity care

SHEILA TAYLOR MYERS RN, MSN; KAREN STOLTE, RN, PhD

Originally published in two parts, this article presents the results of a descriptive study that identifies changes in maternity care and their effects on nurses. The study was based on semistructured interviews with 59 full-time registered nurses with at least three years of maternity experience from ten hospitals in Oklahoma and Kansas. The interviews, which used five open-ended questions, were taped, transcribed, coded, and cross-checked.

When analyzed, the interviews revealed changes in the following areas of maternity care (in descending order of frequency): "(1) family-centered maternity care; (2) technology [and] medical treatment; (3) characteristics of the consumer; (4) legal issues; (5) shorter patient stay; (6) economic pressures; and (7) care of the grieving perinatal patient."

This article is unique because, unlike other articles, it does not focus solely on new maternity care options,[1-4] maternity program implementation,[5-10] or economic or legal changes in maternity care.[12-15] Instead, it investigates the nurses' responses to these issues. Note: In this article, excerpts (marked by ellipses) condense methodologic and other background information.

Family-centered changes and short hospitalizations

...FIFTY-FIVE OF THE 59 NURSES mentioned some change that was classified as a part of family-centered maternity care, including prepared childbirth classes, sibling visitation programs, fathers in the delivery room, and open visiting hours.

Related to this service change, but mentioned frequently enough to be identified separately, were comments about changes that had been seen in the consumer of maternity care (n [number] = 41). Forty nurses described cognitive, attitudinal, or physiologic changes in client characteristics. Consumers were described as more educated and more assertive, knowing what to expect, having a better understanding of what is happening to them, and being more aware of their own rights. Yet, on a less positive note, patients were seen to expect the ideal, or perfection, in a situation in which no one has total control and the unexpected frequently occurs. Physiologically, clients were described as both younger and older than in the past. The nurses also noted that more patients, both mothers and infants, were sicker, or at least were at higher risk. This change was particularly striking in the postpartum units where increasing numbers of long-term antepartum patients are now admitted for care.

The shift to shorter postpartum hospitalization was mentioned by a large number of nurses (n = 35). Instead of the traditional 3 to 5 days, postpartum stays ranged from 6 to 48 hours for the woman with a normal vaginal delivery. Women who had had uncomplicated cesarean sections went home in three days from some hospitals.

Effects of maternity changes. Nurses consistently indicated satisfaction regarding changes toward family-centered care. Findings about effects on workload were contradictory; some nurses described increased workload and others thought it was decreased. Nevertheless, the nurses who said their workload was increased believed the advantages of family-centered care outweighed the extra work. One nurse noted that it was harder to work with the family than with an individual: however, once a relationship had been established, she thought the workload was less. The inclusion of other family members, particularly fathers, in the birth process was described as "fun." One nurse declared "the fathers always remember you." Nurses found working with families challenging and received a sense of satisfaction from doing so.

Increased patient contact and teaching were also described as outcomes of the change to family-centered care. A few nurses mentioned that they had become more knowledgeable since these changes had been initiated. In addition, in some hospitals, greater interdepartmental communication among the nurses was reported as well as an increased sense of responsibility for nursing care. Nurses from several hospitals that had replaced a traditional philosophy with family-centered care described a sense of accomplishment resulting from initiation and achievement of change.

Although the nurses were supportive of family-centered maternity services, they were also concerned about the effect of many visitors on the patients; some believed a large number of friends or relatives contributed to patient distraction during labor and to postpartum fatigue. Labor and delivery and postpartum nurses often felt like "traffic managers." One postpartum nurse said that the patients would not ask their friends to leave, but were visibly relieved when the nurse did so. At times, when visitors were present, the nurses felt that they were "intruding" if they entered the room to give care.

The nurses consistently reported that the changes in patient characteristics increased their workload because more time was spent in teaching or with patients who had complications. However, the nurses remarked that educated women were easier to teach. They described more involvement with patients than previously and noted that nurses were more "human." For instance, they could now express joy or sorrow to patients. The nurses liked this involvement, and showed pictures of themselves with mothers and infants to the interviewers. One nurse keeps a photo album of "my babies."

Feelings of stress, frustration, and increased responsibility were also described, most related to the increased complexity of care for patients with complications and the concomitant increase in workload.

The nurses were concerned about the trend toward short hospitalization for postpartum women. They did not believe that women had time to recuperate from labor or were ready to learn all that was needed about baby and self-care before discharge. The short time available for teaching also increased the nurses' workload since there was more to do in less time. Some units had initiated telephone follow-up to assess how the women were coping at home; however, these calls were not counted as part of the nurses' patient assignment, but merely added to her workload and created time management problems. Nevertheless, nurses who routinely did this follow-up saw it as a positive solution to their concern about the patients. Conversely, those who did not participate in this kind of program were discouraged about how to help prepare the women for discharge in the time allotted.

Some nurses described feelings of job insecurity because policies of early discharge had reduced patient census. They then had to work in other areas in the hospital or take days off without pay. Concern about staffing cuts were also evident.

Conflicts and rewards related to change. The nurses described philosophical, interdepartmental, and interdisciplinary conflicts that they attributed to recent changes in maternity care. One nurse stated that the biggest change for the experienced nursery nurse was the recognition that "the babies no longer belong to us, the nurses, but to the moms and dads." Although the nurses believed that family-centered care was best for both mothers and babies, some who chose the nursery as their area of employment because they liked to work with infants, not adults, were acutely aware of the limited time they now spend in direct care of babies compared to the past. Several contemplated moving to the neonatal intensive care unit to reestablish contact with infants. Other nursery nurses acknowledged the limited time spent in baby care, but felt compensated by their extended participation in helping the development of the mother-infant relationship.

In like manner, some postpartum nurses who did not enjoy taking care of infants but liked working with parents also felt a loss. Resolution of the conflict between a belief in family-centered care and the desire to give direct care to a particular group of patients has not been easy for some nurses.

Lack of experience in the care of either infants or postpartum women also contributed to nurses' discomfort in changing to a pattern of care that included both. When asked to identify what helped them adjust to the change, nurses repeatedly mentioned methods of inservice or continuing education such as workshops, professional journals, and autotutorial instruction.

The nurses described scheduling conflicts and lack of interdepartmental communication in some units. For example, because of the infants' presence on the postpartum unit, mothers were involved with their immediate needs for care and feeding and could no longer take sitz baths at a particular time. This reduced patient availability during doctors' rounds. In addition, babies often were left alone when the mothers took sitz baths, arousing concern among the nursery nurses. Because of the space required for family members, women were sometimes transferred to postpartum from labor and delivery before the time required for close observation ended. This occasionally caused conflict among nurses because postpartum units have fewer staff than do labor and delivery units.

Interdisciplinary conflict was also reported. In some cases, when the nursing staff attempted to implement family-centered care, the medical staff was not supportive of the nurses' independent judgments or incorporation of the family into care. Physicians sometimes withheld information from their patients that the nurse believed was needed by the clients to make informed decisions. At other times, physicians gave patients verbal prescriptions but left no written orders for them. The nurses often felt "in the middle" between the client and physician with simultaneous feelings of frustration, stress, and anger.

The nurses were able to identify only a few rewards related to the changes. Positive patient response was a major source of reward. Increased patient contact, in itself, was viewed as a reward by some nurses because of the trust and identity that they developed with the family. As a result of increased knowledge, skill, and responsibility, nurses recognized gains in self-confidence and feelings of importance. Several believed that maternity nursing is "coming into its own."

Discussion. Maternity nurses are dealing with a wide variety of changes, some directly related to the care of the childbearing woman and others evolving from the changing health care delivery system. In the attempt to adjust, nurses have experienced more conflicts than rewards. Yet, the authors were amazed at the nurses' commitment to family-centered care regardless of the personal and professional expense. Almost every change increased the workload of the nurse. In addition, the change in focus from the individual woman and infant to the family as the unit of care has forced the nurse to redefine her role. Much energy has been spent during this process. Some nurses had no difficulty with this role change since it was congruent with their own beliefs. Others are still involved in role transition with concomitant stress and frustration. Still others, who want to give care to babies exclusively, are considering an employment change from the newborn nursery to the neonatal intensive care unit.

The trend of short postpartum hospitalization evoked much concern among the nurses about lack of preparation of parents for discharge. Few solutions to this problem have been identified and the nurses expressed feelings of discouragement and powerlessness. However, one does not know if the patients are actually unprepared or if they are coping successfully at home.

The increased educational level of patients was noted as a positive change by the nurses; widespread availability of consumer education may account for this change. Two explanations for the larger proportion of sicker patients on the units are use of technology, which enables identification of high-risk patients, and improved medical care for those with chronic health problems.

Although effects of specific changes have been described in this article, interaction among them has also produced effects. Kroll [11] noted that the nurse of today "may have feelings of frustration...in coping with the expectations placed upon her." The nurses in this study were no exception. Increased workload, sicker patients, less time to give care, and lack of interdepartmental and interdisciplinary communication or cooperation have all contributed to feelings of stress and dissatisfaction. Hospital administrators, physicians, nursing administrators, and staff nurses all need to be involved in planning and implementing change. Communication and cooperation among these groups could help reduce stress, which, in turn, could result in better care for all — patients and nurses.

Technologic revolution, legal climate, and economic changes

...Changes in technology. Forty-eight of the 59 nurses interviewed identified technology as a continuing source of change, ranging from routine use of fetal and uterine monitors to arterial blood sampling. When discussing the technological impact upon their practice, nurses described less stress, improvements in professional identity, more interdisciplinary interaction, and both increases and decreases in workloads.

Generally, the nurses reported that their stress has been reduced by technology, particularly the use of monitors. For instance, they found comfort and confidence in the ability to predict patient difficulties. One labor nurse explained. "Before, we waited for something to happen, then acted. Now, with knowledge and assessment ability [we are] able to anticipate [impending complications]." Nursery nurses described increased ability to assess changes in babies due to the advent of arterial blood sampling and increased accuracy in treatment because they are able to titrate medications, formula, and oxygen flow.

The nurses also portrayed a strengthening of professional image and camaraderie. Increases in knowledge and skill were attributed to attendance at workshops and continuing education programs. This appreciation of one's own competence was typified by the nurse who said, "I feel more competent than I have in 21 years." Some nurses mentioned an increase in responsibility and self-reliance, while others talked about feelings of importance and being challenged. Repeatedly, nurses alluded to an elevated status that came with the advent of technology. Examples of these comments were, "With technology, obstetrics has come into its own," and "We have more to say about what goes on in treatment and care. A lot more is expected of me."

Workload distribution was a major topic when nurses discussed the technologic innovations in care. Although all agreed that the distribution of work has changed, the impact was interpreted in a variety of ways. Some nurses viewed technology as facilitating their work or actually decreasing their workload, recognizing the time saving associated with monitors and the capability of avoiding crises. Other nurses described an increase in workload and number of procedures. High-risk patients are being hospitalized who require frequent monitoring and high nurse-patient staffing ratios. Thus, nurses described their responsiblity for scheduling and monitoring antepartum diagnostic tests, and caring for long-term patients who remain hospitalized in order to maintain pregnancies or treat underlying chronic illnesses. Incorporation of these new roles into traditional nursing roles were seen as resulting in paradoxical patient care assignments, such as simultaneous care of regular and high-risk patients, those who are discharged quickly and those who remain for long periods of time, and antepartum and laboring patients. These assignments require the nurse to vacillate between normal and high-risk plans of care. Such shifts of thought increase workload and produce stress, fatigue, or frustration, and may reduce the quality of patient care.

The rise in technology has caused conflict among nurses, physicians, and administrators. For instance, nurses and physicians have learned about technology at differing rates, and occasionally are at odds in their interpretation of data, such as monitor strips. Implications for action and the professional scope of responsibility surrounding some technologies were reported as sources of conflict.

Standards guiding nurses in the use of technology and new medical treatments have been slow in developing or have been overridden by the pragmatism of physicians and administrators. At times, the nurses have been asked to do medical procedures such as amniotomies and administer prostaglandin suppositories. Although nurses have the technical skill to perform these procedures, some believe they are outside the scope of nursing. Because nurses on the same unit are often not consistent in these beliefs, conflict may ensue. Lack of clear hospital policies or appropriate definitions of nursing practice places nurses in the untenable position of either performing the procedures or facing reprimand from physicians or administrators.

Another conflict occurs because, although increased staff is required to give safe care to patients undergoing diagnostic testing and monitoring, at times it is not furnished. Nurses described their worries about limited space for machinery, fear of technology, overdependence on machinery, loss of observational skills, focus on the machine rather than the patient, and decreased time at the bedside.

Changes in the legal climate. Thirty-nine of the 59 nurses interviewed described changes related to the legal climate in maternity care. The possibility of litigation constantly guides these nurses' actions and thoughts, as reflected in such comments as, "Everything is malpractice-suit-conscious now...you feel like you are on a witness stand when charting or doing any type of care." "We must always be aware of legal repercussions for all (staff)." and "We think more about legal aspects than about nursing a lot of the time."

Many nurses knew of lawsuits and had attended workshops or seminars on legal aspects of practice. Litigation results in a defensive climate in which more laboratory tests and procedures are done than previously and doctors are quicker to intervene. Increased charting is needed to ensure that care is documented should litigation occur. The nurses repeatedly commented on the need for more frequent, complete notations than in the past, resulting in a vast increase in workload. A large proportion of time is spent in charting, sometimes to the detriment of patient care. Several nurses stated that conflict arises when they have to stay overtime to chart, because hospitals do not want to pay overtime. Those who wanted to be with patients resented the time they had to spend with paperwork. On the other hand, the nurses admitted that they were more aware of the reasons for records than in the past. One remarked, "The predominant factor in the amount of charting I do is to make sure I am covered (legally for my actions)."

Some nurses mentioned positive patient care outcomes resulting from increased legal awareness. For instance, they stated that nurses are more thorough and more aware of the care they give, make better observations, have more knowledge, and possess more skills than they did several years ago. They described more time spent with patients in order to verify information, ensure that monitors are working, or explain what is happening. The nurses believed in the importance of informed consent, and said that they give more detailed explanations of procedures, medications, and treatments than in the past. However, some expressed concern that such explanations might increase patient anxiety.

Recognition of legal responsibility has also had an effect on staffing: Although more positions have been created in some hospitals, particularly in labor and delivery, to provide adequate coverage so that more time is available for observation and documentation, other units have lost staff who could not adjust to the demands for detailed charting or who were so afraid of being sued that they moved to less threatening areas.

One nurse described in detail her struggle, which lasted several years, with the legal climate:

> The legal climate...made me inappropriately angry at the public in general....I would walk into a room and wonder if the person was going to try to get everything I worked for...and I hated feeling that way....I do have some ambivalent feelings....The public needs to be protected but it seems to me that...the lawsuits were brought against the most conscientious people....It is hard to accept that people have got around to making everything to do with medicine a legal thing....I considered doing something else...but it's so wonderful seeing somebody born...that would get me over my anger (for a while).

She stated that the climate seemed calmer now but, "I don't think you're ever really at ease because the statute of limitations is so long....You either let it cripple you and you quit or you go ahead and get the joy out of it." Nurses remarked that they were not as "at ease" in their work as previously. One nurse stated, "I've never been implicated but I always think, when is it going to happen to me?"

The nurses repeatedly mentioned increased stress as a result of the litigation pressures. They also noted that they are more cautious about what they say to patients. They were aware of a feeling of increased responsibility for good patient care.

Nurses reported that the nurse-doctor relationship has been markedly affected by the legal climate. Because of the threat of malpractice and the cost of insurance, some hospitals have fewer physicians practicing obstetrics. Those doctors who remain demand more from the nurses. For example, nurses must be present to verify the doctor's actions or to document that the patient was given an adequate explanation of events. At times, nurse-physician conflict has arisen when the nurse has been a patient advocate or when she recognized her own legal responsibility and did not unequivocally support the doctor. For instance, some nurses who gave detailed explantions to patients to reduce anxiety or to fulfill their own legal obligations have had to face anger from physicians who wanted to present the information, or wanted the patient to have less explicit detail. In these cases, the nurses often felt "caught between the patient and the doctor." Yet, on a more positive note, an increase in nurse-doctor collaboration was noted because the doctors now rely on the nurses' observations and recognize their competence.

Economic changes. Changes in the economy that have affected the delivery of services were noted by 27 nurses. At the time of the interviews, diagnostic related groups (DRGs) had been in effect in most of the hospitals for about a year, and a major economic downturn had occurred regionally with the demise of the oil industry. Hospital administrators were actively seeking ways to reduce costs. Nurses in almost all hospitals described some decrease in staff and vacant positions that had not been filled. Some maternity units have been staffed by a lone nurse who feels isolated because she must exercise professional judgment without peer consultation. In an attempt to compensate for this loss of staff, some hospitals were attempting to cross-train nurses so that they could function in more than one maternity area. In addition, nurses who had worked in maternity nursing for many years were asked to work in nonmaternity areas. Conversely, if the obstetric census was high, a nonmaternity nurse might be asked to work there. The nurses expressed concern about the quality of care in these instances.

Another trend was the competition among hospitals for patients. Unit planners have had to devise new or unique services to attract patients. Some of the changes related to family-centered care and shortened patient stay were initiated for this reason, but other, more general changes were also noted. Nurses stated that part of their responsibilities now included marketing of hospital services, and that telephone follow-up, home visits to high-risk antepartum patients, or teaching breast self-examination to all postpartum patients and women undergoing mammography had been added to their duties. In general, nurses believe they are having to "do more with less and less." On the other hand, more interdepartmental and interagency cooperation between nurses was reported. This cooperation has arisen from the outgrowth of economic pressure and the need to develop innovative services.

Frustration, anger, stress, low morale, and feelings of job insecurity plagued these nurses. One nurse pointed out, "It's hard to justify adding a person to a shift (because of increased requirements of technology) when the insurance companies are coming down on you (to reduce cost)." Some nurses voiced concern for their patients because of decreased availability of support services such as social workers, less patient contact, and reduced teaching time.

Conclusion

Technologic innovations, an increase in litigation, and economic changes in the health care delivery system are having a great impact on nurses and their practice in maternity care. These changes do not exist in isolation but are intertwined in such a way that nurses are experiencing the composite effect. Baker noted, "A medical care system which fosters the idea that more technology means better health care tends to breed a society that uses litigation as a solution to poor outcome"[16]. The maternity nurse is caught in this web of increased technology, increased litigation, and the pressure to reduce cost. The nurses' struggle to accomplish the role expansion necessary to incorporate these changes while providing quality care was clearly evident throughout the interviews.

In spite of increased stress, the nurses voiced consistent and abiding concern for patient welfare. As the intricacy of care of hospitalized patients is increasing, control over quality of care is elusive. The paradox in this situation is apparent. Even for nurses who know how to give quality care, it is more and more difficult to deliver that care within the constraints imposed. Most describe an increase in professional competence and satisfaction with their scope of practice, but question how to accomplish what is necessary with the time and resources available.

REFERENCES

1. Kelly M, ed. *Maternity Care in Ferment: Conflicting Issues*. New York: Maternity Center Association, 1980.

2. Young D, ed. *Obstetrical Intervention and Technology in the 1980s*. New York: Haworth Press, 1983.

3. Burst HV. The influence of consumers on the birthing movement. *Topics Clin Nurs* 1983;5:42-54.

4. Lubic RW. The effect of cost on patterns of maternity care. *Nurs Clin N Am* 1975;10:229-239.

5. Averitt SS. Adapting the birthing center concept to the traditional hospital setting. *JOGN Nurs* 1980;9:103-106.

6. Faison JG, Douglas, RG Cranch, GS, Lubic RW. The childbearing center: An alternative birth setting. *Obstet Gynecol* 1979; 54:527-532.

7. Notelovitch M. The single-unit delivery system—A safe alternative to home deliveries. *Am J Obstet Gynecol* 1978; 132:889-894.

8. Fraleigh DM. Combined mother-baby care: An experiment in patient assignment. *Can Nurs* 1984;80:25-28.

9. Daniels MG. The birth experience for the sibling: Description and evaluation of a program. *J Nurse-Midwif* 1983;28:15-22.

10. Avery MD, Fournier LC, Jones PL, Sipovic CF. An early postpartum hospital discharge program: Implementation and evaluation. *JOGN Nurs* 1982;11:233-235.

11. Kroll M. Handling stress in the marketplace. *Nursing Success Today*. 1985;2:5-10.

12. McCloskey JC, Grace HK. Economics in nursing. In: McCloskey MC, Grace HK, eds. *Current Issues in Nursing*, 2nd ed. Boston: Blackwell, 1985;741-743.

13. Young D, ed. *Proceedings of the Forum on Malpractice Issues in Childbirth: 1985*. Minneapolis: International Childbirth Education Association, 1985.

14. Cushing M. Fears of a float nurse. *Am J Nurs* 1983;83:297-298.

15. Dingwall R. Maternity care at a premium. *Nurs Times* 1986;82:38-39.

16. Baker SK. Statements from forum sponsors. In: Young D, ed. *Proceedings of the Forum on Malpractice Issues in Childbirth: 1985*. Minneapolis: International Childbirth Education Association, 1985.

Coping skills for children undergoing painful medical procedures

KATHERINE L. PATTERSON, RN, BSN; LEANNE LEWIS WARE, MEd, MA

A child with an acute or chronic illness may undergo many painful procedures, causing fear, anxiety, and stress in the child and the family. To help them cope with such procedures, the nurse can use psychological preparation and other strategies with the child as well as a handout for parents. Note: In this article, excerpts (marked by ellipses) condense an extensive literature review, summary, and additional guidelines for parents.

...WELL-CHILD CARE and the treatment of acute or chronic illness require that children experience painful and anxiety-provoking medical procedures. Children often develop negative responses to medical procedures or more generalized anxiety surrounding their health care.[1,2] To prevent these negative side effects, clinicians are studying methods to manage pain and reduce distress that children might experience during their medical treatment.

This paper reviews strategies currently used to manage procedure-related pain and distress in children. Considerations for using these strategies are discussed to assist the pediatric nurse in developing a plan of care for patients. Special considerations concerning parent preparation, the use of premedications, and indications for referral also are discussed. Finally, suggestions for intervention are presented based on current research findings as well as the authors' clinical experiences.

Psychological preparation procedures

The impetus for the development of interventions to help children cope with their medical experiences emerged from research demonstrating that many children experienced emotional upset both during and after hospitalization.[3,4] Since then, numerous techniques have been developed to assist children in coping with medical events such as hospitalization and medical procedures. These techniques, commonly referred to as psychological preparation procedures, have been shown to decrease emotional and behavioral distress in children undergoing various medical procedures.

Psychological preparation for medical procedures can be categorized by specific strategies. It is important to note that no single procedure is a panacea for children's pain or distress. Typically, several cognitive and behavioral strategies are used together to form a multicomponent intervention package. Future studies should seek to identify the active therapeutic ingredients of treatment packages, in order to reduce the personnel and time involved in preparing children for medical procedures.

The most basic approach involves giving the child information about the impending procedure. This can involve either sensory or procedural information, which is usually presented to the child through verbal dialogue, films, therapeutic play, rehearsal, or modeling.

Another type of strategy involves teaching the child skills to promote adaptive coping during a medical procedure. Coping skills such as emotive imagery, positive self-talk, relaxation training, breathing exercise, distraction techniques, and hypnosis have been used in intervention studies with varying degrees of success. Teaching a child to use coping skills

TABLE 1. Strategies for reducing children's pain and distress during medical procedures

STRATEGY	DESCRIPTION
Procedural information	Providing the child with specific information about the procedure (e.g., showing the child the instruments, examination room, describing how the procedure is done, how long the procedure will take, why the procedure is done, who will perform the procedure)
Sensory information	Providing the child with specific information about sensations that are likely to be experienced during the procedure (e.g., how it will feel, sound, smell, taste)
Relaxation training	Teaching the child to relax muscle groups of the body
Breathing exercises	Teaching the child to take slow deep breaths during the procedure
Distraction	Teaching the child to shift point of focus to things other than the procedure (e.g., counting ceiling tiles, reciting a nursery rhyme, talking about the day's activities, watching a cartoon)
Positive self-talk	Teaching the child statements to say to self while procedure is being performed (e.g., this will be over in a minute, I will be all right, this will help the doctor make me well)
Emotive imagery	Teaching the child to visualize positive and distracting images (e.g., going to the beach, riding a bicycle, being read to)
Hypnosis	Combining deep relaxation and shift of focus to produce trance state

usually requires verbal instruction, role rehearsal, or modeling the skill to the child. Contingency management procedures have been successfully used to reinforce children for attempting to use coping skills.

One final area of psychological preparation involves preparing the child's parent for the procedure. Parent preparation also employs information giving and coping skills training, but these interventions are directed toward reducing the parents' anxiety, as well as giving them tools to help their child through the procedure. Table 1 describes specific psychological preparation techniques, and Table 2 describes the methods commonly used to present these techniques to the child and/or parent....

General considerations for the use of any preparation strategy include the child's age and level of cognitive ability, the parent's and child's preference for a particular coping strategy, and the services available in the clinical setting. The following suggestions should be considered with each strategy.

Giving information. As a general rule, children younger than seven should be prepared as close to the time of the procedure as possible, probably no sooner than one hour prior to the procedure.[16] Children younger than seven are less likely to retain a great deal of information given too soon, and therefore may not fully benefit from early preparation. However, older children may benefit from and desire preparation in advance.[17]

It is important to ask about the previous experiences children have had with medical procedures before presenting information. Several studies suggest that if a child has had previous experience with a procedure, advance preparation may increase the child's anxiety.[16,18]

Verbal descriptions of stressful medical

procedures may not suffice for younger children. Pictures, films, peer modeling, or play techniques may enable the practitioner to provide information in a more concrete fashion. Consider the child's level of understanding when using verbal descriptions. Use simple words in short sentences for younger children. Older children can comprehend more detailed explanations, and generally will not appreciate being "talked down to." To establish and maintain children's trust, the descriptions must be accurate, particularly descriptions of the sensations they might experience.[5] It is important to assess the child's comprehension of the information after it has been presented, no matter what the child's age.

The child's individual coping style may have an impact on how he or she reacts to advance preparation. Parents' knowledge of how their children react to stressful situations will help the pediatric nurse determine the appropriate timing of preparation as well as which coping strategies will be most helpful. Researchers are beginning to investigate individual coping styles of children.[19,20] For example, children who exhibit a "repressive" or "blunting" coping style may try to actively ignore anxiety-provoking stimuli and those who are "sensitizors" or "monitors" cope by seeking information about the stressful event.[19,20] The practitioner can be sensitive to the child's individual coping style by attending to the child's initial responses to preparation. Practitioners must be flexible and alter their approach if a child shows signs of increased anxiety as information is presented.

Teaching coping skills. The child should be given an understandable rationale for learning and using each coping strategy. To simply suggest that a child should slow his or her breathing without explaining that this can help the child stay calm may reduce the likelihood that this technique will be effective. Also parents need a rationale for each coping skill. The parents must recognize the potential benefit of a coping skill if they are to encourage their child to learn and use the skill.

Relaxation and training can potentially reduce a child's anxiety as well as pain during procedures. Progressive muscle relaxation should be taught by a trained individual and must be practiced regularly to be most effective. The child could be told that "relaxed, soft muscles" will not feel as much pain as "tense, hard muscles." If the child must undergo repeated procedures, the importance of practicing this technique must be stressed. With practice, the child will be able to use this technique even more successfully with each subsequent procedure. The child can be provided with an audiotape of relaxation exercises to facilitate home practice. Parents can be enlisted to encourage home practice by providing praise and tangible reinforcers.

Breathing exercises are most beneficial when used as an adjunct to either relaxation training or distraction techniques. However, some children can use this technique successfully on its own. Modeling appropriate breathing patterns (slow deep breaths, with slow controlled exhalation) will prevent the child from hyperventilating. Imagination often facilitates proper breathing patterns with very young children (e.g., pretending to be a car tire that slowly fills with air, then develops a slow hissing leak). The parent can be encouraged to model the breathing pattern during the procedure which helps to refocus the attention of the parent as well as the child away from the procedure.

Distraction can be a very effective tool for children during painful procedures. In essence one helps the child focus attention away from the activity causing the pain. This method can be used easily by practitioners or parents because little preparation or training is required. Methods of distraction include watching a movie, counting, singing, listening to music, playing video games, and telling or reading a story.

Positive self-talk is a method of providing the child with coping statements that he or she can repeat during the procedure that reinterpret fears or negative assumptions about the procedure. Coping statements often center on such themes as benefits of the procedure, time limits of the procedure, the child's ability to get through the procedure, or positive experiences that might occur after the procedure (see Table 2). Parents can help by verbalizing these statements for the child. This method is especially useful for children undergoing repeated painful procedures. Thought stopping is a similar technique which focuses more on anticipatory anxiety.[21,22] Children are given a set of positive statements to repeat to themselves whenever they begin to feel anxious or frightened about an upcoming procedure.

Emotive imagery or guided imagery is a cognitive distraction technique that focuses the child's attention away from the procedure. The practitioner or parent helps the child imagine a pleasant visual image by describing sights, sounds, and physical sensations at the scene. In most cases the success of this technique requires that the child have an involved coach, helping the child to maintain a focus on the pleasant image. If the child is unable to completely ignore the sensations of the procedure, these sensations can be incorporated into the image. For instance, the child can pretend to be a Saturday-morning superhero who can endure this pain with the use of super powers in order to save friends.[6] Imagery is particularly successful for children who enjoy pretending and have vivid imaginations.

Hypnosis has been reported to reduce children's reports of pain and anxiety during repeated painful procedures.[7,8] Although it is reported that most children are easily hypnotized, hypnosis has been most effective with children older than eight years[7,8] when used as a pain-management technique for medical procedures. However, many clinical settings do not have personnel trained to offer this technique. The time constraints in most busy pediatric clinics discourage many nurses from using this technique in their practice. Even though the initial training in hypnosis may be costly and require a considerable time investment for the practitioner and the patient, this technique is effective for pain management and may be useful in other stressful situations.

Preparing the parents. Pediatric health care professionals and researchers have reported a positive correlation between parental anxiety and the distress their children exhibit during medical procedures.[1,23,24] Conversely, children whose mothers were given emotional support and information during their hospital stay were found to be less distressed and anxious.[9-11] In a series of stress point preparation studies[13-15] Wolfer and Visintainer prepared one group of children and their parents for hospitalization. They reported a reduction in distress for parents as well as children in the experimental group. These studies provide empirical support for including parents in the preparation process.

Parents may be reluctant to accompany their child during a medical procedure. Guilt, anxiety, or lack of exposure and knowledge of the procedure are possible reasons for parents' reluctance. The practitioner can allay some of these concerns by reassuring the parents that most children will actually do better if their parents are present.[15] Parents can be provided with specific roles designed to support their children during a procedure; however, parents should *not* be asked to help restrain their children. Involving the parent in supportive duties not only helps the child, but also distracts the parent from the actual procedure and reduces the feelings of helplessness that parents often describe.

Early in parent preparation, the practitioner should give parents opportunities to ask questions and discuss their concerns regarding the procedure. In addition, parents can be provided with both descriptions of psychological

TABLE 2. Methods used to introduce psychological preparation strategies to children

METHOD	DESCRIPTION
Play therapy	Using dolls to role play the procedure, letting the child observe the procedure or pretend to be the doctor. The child is allowed to "play through" his or her fears and concerns regarding a procedure. The practitioner can use this opportunity to correct the child's misconceptions about the procedure.
Modeling	The child is exposed to adaptive coping skills by observing a child model that is successfully using the coping skills while undergoing the medical procedure. It is important for the child model to exhibit realistic behaviors, that is, not an absence of pain and anxiety but rather coping with pain and anxiety.
Rehearsal	Allowing the child to "try out" new coping behaviors or role play a procedure, pretending to be both the patient and the person administering the procedure.
Contingency management	Providing the child with positive reinforcers (e.g., verbal praise, trophies, ribbons, small toys) for practicing or using coping skills.
Parent preparation	Addressing the parents' anxiety by providing information about the procedure and/or suggestions for helping their child.

preparation techniques and the rationales for these techniques.

Pharmacologic management. The use of premedications for children undergoing single painful procedures is commonplace in pediatric health care. The goals of premedication are to decrease apprehension and prevent attempts to resist treatment by the child. This intervention is usually reserved for procedures that cause considerable pain and anxiety, and require a cooperative patient; such as bone marrow aspirations, lumbar punctures, cast removal, fracture reduction, or suture placement. Below is a list of medications used in painful medical procedures:

Sedatives: Chloral hydrate
Barbiturates: Pentobarbital
Antianxiety agents: Diazepam, Lorazepam [not in young children]
Analgesics: Merperidine, Morphine, Codeine
Combination: Lytic cocktail (Merperidine, Promethazine, Chlorpromazine)

Little attention has been given to using medications for repeated painful procedures such as in the care of chronically ill children. The rationale for not using medications stems from concerns about repeated exposure to these agents as well as the potential interactions with other medications. In addition, many of these procedures are performed on an outpatient basis where time constraints limit the safe administration of these medications. The rationale for using or not using premedications should be discussed with the child's parent.

The use of pharmacologic interventions for painful medical procedures warrants further study. Comparisons with psychological techniques should be undertaken to try to identify how the child can be best helped during procedures.

General anesthesia for repeated painful procedures has not been widely used owing to the potential risks of anesthesia as well as cost and administrative factors. A recent report from the University of California at San Francisco describes a program in their Pediatric Oncology Clinic for the use of general anesthesia for repeated painful medical procedures.[25] While this program has met with wide acceptance from patients and their families, its usefulness in smaller centers might be limited by lack of hospital facilities and personnel.

The use of local anesthetics to less the pain of injections is commonplace for both children and adults. Traditionally, $^1/_2$% or 1% lidocaine is infiltrated subcutaneously to anesthetize the tissue prior to needle insertion. However, local anesthesia can also be achieved through the use of Frigiderm,[26] anesthetic patches,[27] or with the use of a jet infusion device (Syrijet-Mark II, Mizzy, Inc.).

Premedications should be considered as adjunctive treatment rather than a substitute for appropriate psychological techniques. Additional study is necessary to delineate the potential benefits of specific pharmacologic approaches as an adjunct to psychologic preparation techniques for children who undergo painful medical procedures.

Children requiring repeated medical procedures may develop significant distress surrounding these procedures. Even children who are initially very cooperative may become more distressed during subsequent procedures.[1,2,28] If a child's distress becomes severe enough to interfere with the safe performance of the procedure, a referral to a mental health practitioner skilled in psychological preparation is warranted. Often, this increase in distress is a conditioned response, and at other times the child's distress may increase if parents unintentionally reinforce distress rather than coping behavior. In either case, once maladaptive coping patterns have become established, considerable time and expertise in behavioral management are necessary to develop more adaptive coping during procedures. On occasion, the practitioner may observe a child to be so anxious initially that an immediate referral is necessary. Researchers are currently investigating ways to identify children who may be at risk for developing severe distress with medical procedures.[20]

Practical suggestions for the nurse

1. Before beginning a medical procedure, briefly assess both the child's and the parent's previous experience with the procedure. Parents are the best source for finding out how a child usually copes in stressful situations, which may help you select strategies best suited for the child.

2. If you sense anxiety in the parent, so will the child. Give parents concrete suggestions on how they can help their child during the procedure and let them know what kinds of reactions are typical in children of their child's age. If the parents still fail to cope well with repeated procedures, you may consider spending additional time exploring the cause of their anxiety, or refer them to a mental health practitioner. If a mental health referral is necessary, assure the parents that their feelings are normal, but that there are professionals who can help families cope with repeated medical procedures.

3. For long procedures, build in periods where the child (and you) can relax. Let the child know when this safe time is, and encourage him or her to relax as much as possible during this time. If relaxing during safe times is difficult for the child, try to distract the child with conversation. Let the child know when the procedure is completed. If the child is lying down, have him or her sit up as soon as possible or step down from the procedure table. Cues that indicate the procedure is over help relieve the child's distress more quickly.

4. When the child is doing something that helps to complete the procedure, or is otherwise adaptive, let the child know! Specific feedback and praise are helpful in producing adaptive coping skills. Give parents examples

of behaviors to look for during the procedure and encourage them to praise their child.

5. As much as possible, try to reduce the amount of time the child and parents spend waiting for the procedure to take place. Since this is not always possible, try to have interesting materials for all age groups in the waiting area.

6. Do not have the child and parents enter a procedure room that has not been set up. While you are preparing the room, they are watching you and their anxiety is increasing. Work as quickly as possible, and try to minimize interruptions.

7. Remember to give the child a rationale for using a coping technique as well as an explanation of why the procedure is necessary. Try to emphasize positive aspects of the procedure. ("This will tell us if your medicine is working," for diagnostic procedures. "This bleeding lets us know that your skin is healthy and will get well soon," with burn debridement.)

8. Especially with procedures that will be repeated, many children use several strategies to stall. Explain to parents that stalling behaviors may develop with repeated procedures and their help in discouraging them will actually help their child get through the procedure more quickly and with less distress. Remind parents to have the child go to the bathroom before the procedure.

9. Remember that each child will have different needs during procedures. Allow the child to watch the procedure if he or she so desires, and answer questions quickly and honestly. Children may become panicked if they feel that you are not listening to them.

10. Make sure that you talk to the child as well as to the parents, and have eye contact with the child as well as with the parents. The health practitioner's comments can be a source of verbal support, or possibly help the child focus his or her attention away from the procedure.

11. Some children's anxiety will be reduced if they are able to maintain sense of control. This can be done by giving the child choices during the procedure.

12. Encourage the child and parents to maintain physical contact, but do not have the parents restrain their child....

REFERENCES

1. Jay, S.M., Ozlins, M., Elliott, C.H., and Caldwell, S.: Assessment of children's distress during painful medical procedures. *Health Psychol.* 2:133, 1983.

2. Katz, E., Kellerman, J., and Siegel, E.: Behavioral distress in children with cancer undergoing medical procedures: Developmental considerations. *J. Consult. Clin. Psychol.* 48:356, 1980.

3. Vernon, D.T.A., Schulman, J.L., and Foley, J.M.: Changes in children's behavior after hospitalization. *Am. J. Dis. Child.* 111:581, 1986.

4. Prugh, D.M., et al.: A study of the emotional reactions of children and families to hospitalization and illness. *Amer. J. Orthopsychia* 23:70, 1953.

5. Johnson, J.E., Kirchoff, K.T., and Endress, M.P.: Altering children's distress behavior during orthopedic cast removal. *Nurs. Res.* 24:405, 1975.

6. Jay, S.M., Elliott, C.H., Ozlins, M., Olson, R.A., and Pruitt, S.D.: Behavioral management of children's distress during painful medical procedures. *Behav. Res. Ther.* 23:513, 1985.

7. Hilgard, J.R., and LeBaron, S.: Relief of anxiety and pain in children and adolescents with cancer: Quantitative measures and clinical observations. *Int. J. Clin. Exp. Hypn.* 30:417, 1982.

8. Zeltzer, L., and LeBaron, S.: Hypnosis and nonhypnotic techniques for reduction of pain and anxiety during painful procedures in children and adolescents with cancer. *J. Pediatr.* 101:1032, 1982.

9. Mahaffy, P.: The effects of hospitalization on children admitted for tonsillectomy and adenoidectomy. *Nurs Res.* 14:12, 1965.

10. Skipper, J.: Mother's distress over their children's hospitalization for tonsillectomy. *J. Marriage Fam.* 28:145, 1966.

11. Skipper, J., Leonard, R., and Rhymes, J.: Child hospitalization and social interaction: An experimental study of mother's stress, adaption and satisfaction. *Med. Care.* 6:496, 1968.

12. Roskies, E., Mongeon, M., and Gagnin-Lefebvre, B.: Increasing maternal participation in the hospitalization of young children. *Med. Care* 16:765, 1978.

13. Wolfer, J., and Visintainer, M.: Pediatric surgical patient's and parent's stress responses and adjustment as a function of psychological preparation and stress-point nursing care. *Nurs. Res.* 24:244, 1975.

14. Wolfer, J., and Visintainer, M.: Prehospital psychological preparation for tonsillectomy patients: Effects in children's and parent's stress responses and adjustment. *Pediatrics* 56:202, 1979.

15. Vistintainer, M.A., and Wolfer, J.A. Psychological preparation

for surgical pediatric patients: The effects on children's and parent's stress response and adjustment. *Pediatrics* 56:187, 1975.

16. Melamed, B., Dearborn, M., and Hermecz, D.: Necessary considerations for surgery preparation: Age and previous experience. *Psychom. Med.* 45:517, 1983.

17. Ross, S.: Impending hospitalization: Timing of preparation for the school-aged child. *Child Health Care* 12:187, 1984.

18. Melamed, B., Yurckeson, R., Fleece, E., Hutcherson, S., and Hawes, R.: Effects of filmed modeling on the reduction of anxiety-related behaviors in individuals varying in level of previous experience in stress situations. *J. Consult. Clin. Psychol.* 46:1357, 1978.

19. Goldstein, M.: Individual differences in response to stress. *Am. J. Community Psychol.* 1:113, 1973.

20. Schultheis, K., Peterson, L., and Selby, V.: Preparation for stressful medical procedures and person X treatment interactions. *Clin. Psychol. Review* 7:329, 1987.

21. Ross, D.: Thought-stopping: A coping strategy for impending feared events. *Iss. Comp. Pediatr. Nurs.* 7:83, 1984.

22. Ross, D., and Ross, S.: Stress reduction procedures for the school-age hospitalized leukemic child. *Pediatr. Nurs.* 10:393, 1984.

23. Johnson, R., and Baldwin, D.: Relationship of maternal anxiety to the behavior of young children undergoing dental extraction. *J. Dent. Res.* 74:801, 1968.

24. Vardaro, J.: Preadmission anxiety and mother child relationships. *J. Assoc. Care Children's Hosp.* 7:8, 1978.

25. Fisher, D., et al.: Comparison of Enflunane, Halothane, and Isoflurane for diagnostic and therapeutic procedures in children with malignancies. *Anesthesiology* 63:647, 1985.

26. Eland, J.: Minimizing pain associated with prekindergarten intramuscular injections. *Iss. Comp. Pediatr. Nurs.* 5:361, 1981.

27. Lubens, H. M., et al.: Anesthetic patch for painful procedures such as minor operation. *Am. J. Dis. Child.* 128:192, 1974.

28. Venham, L., Bengston, D., and Cipes, M.: Children's response to sequential dental visits. *J. Dent. Res.* 56:454, 1977.

Health concerns of adolescents

KATHERINE L. DUCHEN SMITH, RN, MS, CPNP; JOSEPH G. TURNER, PhD; R. BROOKE JACOBSEN, PhD

By presenting the results of a recent study, this article provides insight into the perceived health concerns of adolescents. The subjects of the study were 149 (75 male and 76 female) ninth graders ages 14 to 16. They each completed a 45-item questionnaire that asked them to check off their health concerns and then rank their top five.

After the questionnaires were tabulated and analyzed, they revealed that adolescents are more concerned about physical appearance, personal issues, and other concerns than about typical health problems. They also indicated that boys and girls differ greatly in the relative importance of their perceived health concerns (See Table 1). The following passage discusses the study's findings. Note: Excerpts (marked by ellipses) condense extensive background and methodologic information.

....GENERALLY SPEAKING, the 149 adolescents reported 2 predominant types of health concerns: (a) those of a social-personal nature (such as "worries about my future," "emotions and feelings," and "getting along with my family"), and (b) physical appearance types of concerns (such as weight, muscles, skin, and hair). This contrasts with more traditional "medical" concerns, including problems such as stomach and digestion, pregnancy, venereal disease, drug use, and others. Those issues were not significantly reported to be major health issues by the respondents in the study.

Testing certain assumptions. Much of the previous effort among pediatric nurses and other health clinicians has been directed at assumed beliefs about adolescent attitudes regarding their health and interpersonal concerns. Thus, the "helping professional" has frequently intervened based on a different frame of reference [from that of] the adolescent client. For example, the adolescent communicates on one level ("my weight's not right"), and the nurse anticipates a concern based on an adult response ("she must be worried she's ill"). By first assessing nursing research on what teenagers in general see as relevant health needs, nurses can increase their understanding to communicate more directly to youth and to support and implement appropriate health services.

Uniqueness of health concerns. These findings demonstrate that younger teens appear to have a unique set of health concerns influenced by both gender and family background. Pediatric nurses (a) need to identify the concerns of the individual or population with which they are working and (b) use these concerns when planning and directing educational, family, and health services.

Physique. Physical appearance and concerns are real to adolescents and it is important for the pediatric nurse to identify slow physical maturers, in particular within the clinical setting. Looking different in appearance from one's peers is often equated by a teenager to being inferior. The desire for peer acceptance and conformity grows in early adolescence. Any variation may have a negative influence on how that individual is related to by others as well as how the adolescent perceives herself/himself (Dwyer & Mayer, 1968-1969). The suggestions of Frazier and Lisonbee (1950), written over 30 years ago, apply to

TABLE 1. Most important rank-ordered health concern (boys vs girls: in descending order) (n = 149)

ORDER OF PREFERENCE	BOYS (n = 75)	GIRLS (n = 74)
1	My future	Weight
2	Weight	Hair
3	Vision	Getting along with family
4	Body build	Emotions and feelings, my future (tied)
5	Height, hair, acne, getting along at school (tied)	Skin, figure, acne (tied)

clinical nursing protocols and educational planning today. They reported significant concern among adolescents about physical appearance characteristics. By using adolescent growth charts, which described body stature by percentile of growth, the nurse can help the teenage client determine whether he or she compares to other teenagers of the same age and sex. Not only do the growth charts demonstrate percentile rank but also they can be used as a tool to initiate nursing teaching and counseling regarding body proportion, size, and nutritional requirements. Teenage girls, in particular, tend to see themselves as overweight and are frequently reassured about their weight by plotting out their body stature on a standard growth chart.

The adolescent's future. In terms of anticipatory guidance and the adolescent respondents' overriding concerns about their future, several nursing implications need to be discussed. For many teens around ages 15-16, a shift in cognitive development (Ausubel & Ausubel, 1966) occurs from concrete to more abstract thinking. It would be helpful for the nurse to assess the youth's cognitive understanding and to use this maturational ability, when appropriate, to assist the client in considering the long-term consequences when discussing health needs. For example, if counseling is to be effective for teenagers operating on an abstract cognitive level regarding alcohol and drug use, birth control and sexually transmitted diseases, pediatric nurses need to link these topics to factual discussion regarding their clients' futures. Examples of how to tie these concerns together include:

- "If you contract a herpes infection now, you will be a prime candidate for a Cesarean section someday when you want to have a baby."
- "By protecting yourself from teenage parenthood now, statistics show that you can have a firmer economic hold in the future."

Certainly, this type of discussion should not be used as a "scare tactic" but as a frank examination of health care facts as they pertain to future consequences.

Other suggestions for the nurse or educator who deals directly with adolescents include in-service workshops for effective application of these nursing research findings. An adolescent panel, at workshop sessions, discussing perceived health needs and optimal ways of meeting these needs can provide insight to nursing professionals involved in adolescent health care.

Conclusions

Pediatric nurses need to remember and reassure adolescents that their physical and emotional health concerns are normal and commonly expressed by others their age. Teenagers' self-image and esteem often will be bolstered by the knowledge that their worries are not unique. An adolescent's enhanced self-image may contribute to the diminished use of drugs, alcohol, and premature sexual experimentation, which is so frequently symptomatic of an adolescent's precarious feelings. Finally, this study demonstrates that although adolescence is often a medically healthy time of life for most young people, traditional medical issues are not necessarily important priorities for this age group. However, nurses need to be aware that it is a time, developmentally, when teenagers have significant perceptions about their health and well-being. Primary caregivers are in an ideal position to support adolescents' efforts to take on greater responsibility for their own health care, and to contribute to decisions that affect themselves and their bodies.

REFERENCES

Ausubel, D., & Ausubel, P. (1966). Cognitive development in adolescence. *Review of Education Research, 36*, 403-413.

Dwyer, J., & Mayer, J. (1968-1969). Psychological effects of variations in physical appearance during adolescence. *Adolescence, 3*(12), 353.

Frazier, A., & Lisonbee, R. (1950). Adolescent concerns with physique. *School Review, 58*, 397-405.

The stress of caring: Issues confronting mid-life caregivers

BEVERLY A. BALDWIN, RN, PhD

Five to eight million family members — mostly women — provide care for one or more adults. Many of these caregivers are 40 to 60 years old and must juggle several other roles, such as wife, mother, employee, and child caregiver. Because of this and because of the nature of caring for an older adult, mid-life caregivers are likely to suffer from stress and stress-related disorders.

Based on a study of mid-life caregivers, the following article takes a look at the caregiving experience and suggests ways that nurses can help relieve the stress of caregiving. Note: A summary (shown in bracketed italics) condenses background and methodologic information.

[An intervention study was conducted at the School of Nursing, University of Maryland, to assess the health consequences of caregiving and to compare stress-management programs for family caregivers. The study assigned 42 caregivers (daughters and daughters-in-law) to one of four groups: a treatment group using a classroom-didactic stress-management program, a treatment group using a support therapy stress-management program, a nonintervention control group, or a placebo control group. All caregivers underwent pre- and posttests that measured such factors as stress, psychobiological effects, and cardiovascular responses. They also kept stress-symptom diaries. Additionally, the caregivers in the treatment groups attended a two-hour session once a week for eight weeks.

The caregivers in this study are similar to those nationwide. The average caregiver was white, age 51, married, a mother of adolescent children, and a part-time or full-time employee. The average elderly adult under care was a frail woman, age 82, who is unmarried and must depend on others for activities of daily living. All of the elderly adults in this study attended an adult day care center for a portion of the day and lived with the caregiver.]

The caregiving experience

Family caregiving has inherent strains and conflicts, which, over time, may result in chronic stress for the caregiver. Caregiving does have a number of positive features both for the elder and for those providing the care, including reaffirmation of close parent-child ties, the perception of being needed, and an opportunity to repay parents for their caregiving in early development years. The fact remains, however, that caring for another adult, especially one who becomes more dependent and frail over time, can produce stress.

Family members providing ongoing care to the elderly state there are many reasons for the stress, such as the increased feelings of responsibility for another person; the burden of decisionmaking, often made alone; disruptions in one's life and lifestyle, especially at a time in one's life in which leisure time and retirement are anticipated; feelings of isolation or being apart from friends or other family members who are not involved directly or daily in the caregiving; feelings of alienation from friends, family, or co-workers; guilt; and the frustrations associated with not fulfilling one's or another's expectations.

Becoming a family caregiver may start in a crisis situation, such as the hospitalization of an elder for an emergency or acute event, a fall, other trauma, or recognition that the elder, due to physical and/or mental changes, can no longer function independently or without ongoing assistance. Many family caregivers are in the position of having to make decisions in haste with little preparation, thus leaving the caregiver with many questions, lack of information, and uncertainty. This uncertainty can continue for years beyond the initial crisis, and becomes amplified as the elder becomes increasingly frail and caregiving responsibilities increase.

When family caregivers in the intervention study were asked to describe their major concerns regarding their own well-being, they reported not having enough time for self, concerns over their own health, not having enough time for other family members, concerns about their marriage, not having enough time for fun and/or friends, the lack of privacy, interruptions in work and low work productivity, chronic stress and tension, fatigue and lower levels of energy, lack of freedom, and increasing impatience and temper.

The psychobiological consequences of caregiving vary among individuals. However, the daughters and daughters-in-law participating in the described study indicated five major areas of concern, related specifically to their health and health status. Generalized fatigue, even when not related to excess physical exertion, was highest on the list of problems. Coupled with fatigue and malaise were mood swings and moodiness, along with feelings of depression, often for the first time.

Sleep disruptions and bouts of insomnia were prominent among those caregivers having elders with sleep problems or nighttime incontinence. The lack of consistent, restful sleep seemed particularly evident with those caregivers experiencing chronic fatigue. Exacerbations of physical problems, such as high blood pressure, contributed to the sleep disturbances. Almost all caregivers indicated they experienced some form of gastrointestinal disturbances during the caregiving experience, which ranged from mild upset stomach to vomiting, diarrhea, and bouts of gastric ulcer episodes. Extremes in weight gain or loss were noted, especially during high stress times or when transitions occurred, such as moving the elder into a nursing home; or trauma, such as a fall or other related incident. Headaches, many experienced for the first time, were not relieved by non-prescribed analgesics. The relationship between headaches and blood pressure was not always clear, but presented an additional problem for these high-risk adults.

The caregiving experience, as reported by these women, presented responsibilities and concerns with varying impacts, depending on the circumstances of the caregivers and the degree of frailty of the elder. Surprisingly, even when adequate family and other social support was available to these caregivers, the sense of burden was not alleviated, since the assumption of responsibility for primary caregiving resulted in total commitment to the role by the caregivers.

Another unexpected response from these caregivers was the lack of recognition on their part of the connection between the stress (daily, ongoing, consistent) of caregiving and the psychosocial and psychobiological symptoms which were so prevalent in this group. Although they associated stress and health consequences generally, they did not make the same associations in their own individual situation.

Taking care of the caregiver

Although the two treatment methods utilized in the described study differed in structure and format, the focus of both was on identifying and reinforcing stress-management strategies that assist family caregivers to deal with the stress of the caregiving experience day by day.

The following techniques and rationale were used and reinforced throughout the intervention stage of the study. The caregivers were encouraged to practice the following techniques.

1. Identify the *stressors* in your life and in the caregiving role (a) making a stress list (i.e., what things, events, situations are most stressful), (b) starting a mood inventory (i.e., identifying what times of the day, week, month do mood changes, swings, or unexpected reactions occur), (c) establishing a stress profile (i.e., to chart the most and least stressful times and reactions), and (d) think through your reactions to stress — that is, mind reactions, body reaction, or both. By identifying stressors and spending time on outlining the antecedents and consequences, stress becomes real and therefore more manageable.

2. Learn and practice *stress management* techniques such as simple breathing exercises or other relaxation skills. Classes in stress and stress management may be taken through church groups, specialized support groups such as the Alzheimer's Disease and Related Disorders Asssociation local chapters, the YMCA, or other civic groups. Many of the basic stress-management techniques can be self-taught: books and audio and video tapes may be obtained through libraries or local book stores. It has been well-documented that stress-management techniques work, and the physical consequences for the caregiver are better health immediately and greater potential for dealing with stress over time.

3. Set *realistic goals* for yourself and for the elder family member by establishing short-term objectives that can be measured. Pick one small behavior that can be modified — for example, interrupting repetitive activities that annoy you — and measure the extent to which distractions or other interventions alter the behavior for a specific period of time. Take pride in accomplishments that are made, either by self or by the elder, no matter how small. Expecting unrealistic or impossible changes in yourself or in the elder in your care leads to self-fulfilling failure and to feelings of defeat. These feelings add to the stress of caregiving.

4. *Be good to yourself,* you deserve it! Don't wait for others to reward and praise you for patience, endurance, vigilance. Give yourself positive strokes, develop positive self-talk skills. As a positive attitude replaces feelings of defeat and failure, both the person and the body reaps the reward, with lower blood pressure, more relaxed breathing, and a muscular system free from tension and chronic stress.

5. Cultivate and maintain a *sense of humor!* Norman Cousins proved that laughter is the best medicine and laughter is contagious. The elder in your care will feel the tension ease if you inject humor into everyday events and if you don't take life and caregiving too seriously. Learning to laugh at yourself, your idiosyncracies and your biases, is the first step. With practice, a humorous outlook becomes second nature. You can then begin to defuse potentially stressful situations with a small dose of laughter.

6. *Place events in proper context* by not overreacting to each small crisis, situation, setback, or disappointment. Almost every situation has a "flip side" and the relative importance of any event must be considered in context. Your body will thank you for this attitude adjustment.

7. *Screen advice* and counsel from family, friends, and co-workers. Many caregivers report feeling overwhelmed and sensory overload when too much advice or too many alternatives are given for a specific problem. Although most people have good intentions and want to be helpful, some caregivers find unsolicited advice more stressful than helpful. Remember that most people want to show compassion; they don't always have the skill to do it effectively.

8. Realize that you *cannot erase the past history* of family relationships. Expecting the past to disappear when caregiving takes over is unrealistic. Actually, people tend to become more like themselves over time. Work on resolution and concentrate on "letting go" of old hurts, conflicts, disappointments, and unmet expectations. Focusing on the "here and now" is more manageable and more stress-reducing.

9. *Stay in touch* with friends, family, church and social groups, and community connections. Isolation from social support systems breeds loneliness and stress. Being with others keeps you in touch with life outside caregiving and gets you "out of yourself." It gives the body and the mind a "rest" from the burden of commitment perceived by some caregivers.

10. Actively *solicit and accept help/respite* from others. Respite from caregiving responsibilities may be a few minutes or hours, a day, or a weekend, a week or months. Don't expect friends and family to know automatically when you are in need. Martyrdom breeds stress. Respite and sharing of care is essential for refueling the body and the mind. Respite may be provided by others in your home, by placing the elder in foster or adult day care, or by sharing caregiving responsibilities with other family members on a day-by-day or task-by-task basis. Whatever form respite takes, it is essential for coping with stress over time.

11. *Take one day at a time* and try not to worry over what *might* happen. Practice distracting yourself or attending to something else when speculations, fantasy, or anticipation of worst outcomes for any situation dominate your thoughts. This stress-reduction takes practice and hard work — to refocus thoughts. But the alternative, that is, always preparing for the "worst scenario" requires that the body constantly get ready for fight or flight to combat stress, and, eventually, this constant readiness will cause wear and tear on the total system.

12. *Maintain positive health habits,* or, in other words, take good care of yourself! Adequate rest and sleep, regular exercise, strength-building diet, and regular physical health examinations are essential for confronting and coping with stress. Most caregivers ignore their own bodies until illness occurs. Illness poses another stressor and adds to the strain already being experienced as part of caregiving. It becomes important for caregivers to listen to their bodies, to learn more about how they deal with stress, both physically and emotionally, and to avoid the stresses of disease or other illnesses.

Caregivers as the invisible victims

For many family caregivers, the period of time spent in providing care for an elder parent is a positive and rewarding experience. For others, however, it may result in their becoming an invisible victim in a stressful and potentially overwhelming relationship. Based on the role of the family in caregiving today and the expectation by government that family members will continue to care for their elder member, the potential for being a victim is ever-present. Caregivers must become more visible and let their needs be acknowledged in order that their role is better understood and supported. Families need preparation for caregiving. Support networks must begin to focus on the caregiver and her needs, in addition to supporting the caregiver in meeting the needs of the elder. As more and more families continue to "take care," the problems and needs of caregivers must be examined and solutions found in order to prevent the caregiver from becoming the victim of her own willingness to provide care.

Continence through nursing care

Betty D. Pearson, RN, PhD; Sr. Dorothy Droessler, RN, MS

This is a clinical report of the results of the combined actions of a nurse certified in geriatric care and a nurse researcher. The nurse clinician reported that when noninvasive procedures were carried out elders had fewer catheters in place and fewer episodes of loss of urine control. In fact, some had gone from being incontinent to continent.

After listening to the clinicians tell about strategies that were used, the nurse researcher was impressed by the elegance of the care delivered but dismayed that only empirical knowledge could be reported because of the lack of a framework for collecting information. They decided to pool their talents and investigate the effectiveness of noninvasive strategies used to diagnose and treat actual and potential loss of urine control in elderly persons.[1,2]

The practitioner outlined her methods, concerns, and ideas. The researcher organized an extensive review of the literature (which they both studied), developed a framework for collecting and analyzing information, and wrote a proposal to obtain funds to conduct the study.

Classification

Data were collected from residents of a retirement facility that had 77 units for room and board and an attached 22-bed infirmary. The nurse practitioner collected urinary continence histories from 74 persons (average age 87 years) every month for 6 months. Of these, 60 were classified as at risk at the start and 14 as incontinent of urine. Six of those incontinent of urine were not previously known to be incontinent. Eight persons, classified as continent on the first history, were not followed for the remainder of the study.

The nursing classification of *urinary incontinence* was defined as the involuntary loss of urine more than once a month. This allows for a "key in the door" episode, that is, poor judgment by a person about how long they can delay urination after feeling the urge.[3] An example is walking in the park and stopping to talk, continuing the conversation long past noting the urge to urinate, and then not quite making it to the toilet.[3]

The classification of *at risk* for incontinence was defined for the purposes of the study to include persons able to control urination, but whose responses to *one or more* of the urinary continence diagnostic indicator questions were indicative of potential problems for urine control. The levels at which responses to these questions were deemed normal were drawn from the literature. *Continence* was defined to include persons able to control urination and free of any indications of potential problems of urine control.

Assessment

The continence history should be integrated into the nurse's physical assessment of the individual. The continence history used for this study was adapted from an incontinence history.[4] The pelvic and rectal examinations as presented by Cohen are excellent resources for the technique of examination to reveal atrophic vaginitis or urethritis, pelvic floor laxity, pelvic masses, fecal impactions, or prostate enlargements.[5] Cohen carefully directs the insertion of the examiner's fingers so as to protect the urethra while at the same time visualizing any exudate or urinary leakage.

Of course, assessments must be repeated at regular intervals, as well as when changes occur. Continence is not an isolated phenomenon; it is related to general well-being.

Treatment

The 74 persons classified as either incontinent or at risk started noninvasive treatment strategies during the first assessment. Monthly assessments afforded opportunities to reinforce or correct the manner in which treatments were carried out.

Prior to the study, the nurses of the facility had given meticulous attention to the appropriate management of medications. Diuretics, for example, were given early in the day. After consulting with the physicians, medications were discontinued as soon as it was feasible or they were reduced to the lowest effective dosage.

Environmental features also received attention. For example, the height of the beds and chairs allowed patients to place their feet flat on the floor; properly fitted walking aids were used appropriately; clearly labeled and well-lit toilets with requisite appliances such as grab rails were located no more than 50 feet from gathering places, as well as in the residents' rooms; and urinals and bedpans appropriate for hand and finger dexterity were provided.[6] In addition, clothing was modified to permit ease of toileting, such as eliminating girdles or belts from trousers and attaching suspenders to loose shorts and trousers and substituting footlets or regular hose for pantyhose.

A variety of liquids were readily available with cups and tumblers filled to only 1-½ in of the rim to reduce apprehension about spilling. These were refilled frequently to encourage fluid intake. Prunes and a variety of bran products were used to help residents maintain bowel regularity. Appropriate nursing assistance was provided at all times.

The treatments begun during the study were noninvasive strategies drawn from the literature and matched to specific risk indicators. These included a gradual increase of liquids with a goal of at least 2 qt (2,200 cc) daily, regular toileting, and pelvic floor muscle exercise.[7,8] Patients and staff regularly received praise from the nurse clinician for progress or effort expended on the treatments....

Regular toileting schedules have been proven effective in increasing urine control, especially when coupled with an adequate liquid intake.[9] An efficient means of accomplishing both for persons requiring assistance is to offer liquids following each voiding. Others should have a variety of liquids readily available.

Regular toileting was used for those individuals who voided fewer than 4 times a day or more than 8 times, and more than once a night. Individuals who void fewer than 4 times a day are at risk because the chronically overdistended bladder reduces blood supply and nerve enervation to the bladder, thus increasing the probability of overflow incontinence or infection.[10] Persons who void more than 8 times a day are at risk because either the bladder may be overdistended and not emptying completely, which increases the likelihood of infection, or the bladder is receiving only a little concentrated urine and is never stretched very much, which can lead to bladder muscle hyperactivity and, hence, incontinence.

Excessive frequency may also be indicative of psychosocial stress. The staff always looked for environmental or psychosocial factors aggravating urine difficulties; nursing interventions reduced or resolved many of these problems....

Other noninvasive means of promoting urine control included were prevention of urinary tract infection, especially common in women, and urinary tract irritation from use of shampoo for bathing or synthetic undergarments.[9,11,12] Urinary tract infections may be

Incontinence risk factors, normal criteria, and treatments

RISK	CRITERIA	TREATMENT
Flow	Awareness	Pelvic floor exercises (2)
Dribble	No dribbling	Pelvic floor exercises (10)
Stop then start	Able to	Pelvic floor exercises (17)
Atrophic vaginitis	Lubricated vagina	Pelvic floor exercises (19)
Full bladder	Recognition	Regular toileting (9)
Time to wait	10 minutes or more	Scheduled toileting (2, 15, 16)
Liquid intake	2 quarts daily	Gradually increase liquids (9)
Frequency	4 to 8 times per day, once per night	Increase liquids and regular toileting (7, 10)
Bowel constipation	No constipation	Prunes and bran and adequate liquids (18)
Burning	No burning	Proper perineal care and obtain urinalysis (18)
Loss of urine	Less than once a month	Treat appropriate risk factors (9)

eliminated if adequate liquid is coupled with emptying the bladder every 2 hours.

There are two reasons this works. The bladder is not overdistended and, hence, the mucosal lining receives an adequate blood supply, which in turn increases resistance to infection. If sufficient urine is received from the kidneys and released from the bladder about every 2 hours, bacteria are flushed out before they have multiplied sufficiently to cause infection.

Implementation

These techniques for assessment and treatment sound as if they are one nurse-one patient situations — not the real world of nursing. Although some authors advocate workshops, target dates, and involvement of all personnel to introduce change, here it is recommended to start by selecting one person and one nurse or nursing assistant. Give lots of verbal recognition for effort, progress, and success to both patients or residents *and* staff, even though some tasks remain or incontinence continues.

Continence maintained or regained may not require less nursing care, but does mean energy and time devoted to care are directed toward assisting persons maintain one definition of adulthood — continence. Belief in the importance of this problem to patients and excellence in nursing make a difference.

Evaluation

The noninvasive strategies used did result in 6 reversals of incontinence. Of the 14 persons incontinent at the beginning, 6 reverted to control of urine and were at risk for a lesser number of diagnostic indicators after 6 months. These reversals occurred after 2, 4, and 5 months of treatment. All 74 subjects significantly decreased the number of risk indicators experienced.

Statistical significance was computed using the *t* test. At the start, the range of combinations was 2 to 10 risks; in 6 months the range was 1 to 7. The 3 most frequently experienced risk factors were inability to wait 10 minutes or longer after experiencing the urge, liquid intake of less than 2,200 cc daily, and urinary frequency more than once a night.

The older adults increased their liquid intake by about 250 cc daily, which was statistically significant as an increase but did not reach the recommended level of intake. Liquid intake is important because concentrated urine serves as an irritant to the bladder and increases frequency of urination....

Further investigation is needed before the following questions can be answered. What is an appropriate amount of daily liquid intake for older adults? What is the best schedule for ingesting that amount? Are the risk factors identified necessary and sufficient to couple with noninvasive nursing strategies for promoting urine control? Are there groupings of these that can be identified as probable risk combinations so that when one of them is noted nurses would be alerted to investigating whether the others also exist?

How long do each of the strategies have to be practiced before a given risk is controlled? What is the fabric of meanings attached by elders to continence?

Excellence in nursing includes the assessment, treatment, and evaluation of actual and potential urinary incontinence. Continence of urine is a hallmark of adulthood and must be protected.

REFERENCES

1. American Nurses' Association. *Nursing: A Social Policy Statement.* (Publ. No. NP-63) Kansas City, MO, The Association, 1980.

2. Pearson, B.D., and Droessler, D. *Urinary Incontinence Diagnosed and Managed by Nurses.* (Research Report to American Nurses' Foundation) Milwaukee, WI, 1985.

3. Freed, S.Z. Urinary incontinence in the elderly. *Hosp.Pract.* 17:81-94, Mar. 1982.

4. Brink, C. Assessing the problem. *Geriatr.Nurs.* 1:241-247, Nov.-Dec. 1980.

5. Cohen, S. Patient assessment: examination of the female pelvis: part I; part II, Examination of the male genitalia (Programmed Instruction) *Am.J.Nurs.* 78:1717-1747, 1912-1945, Oct. 1978; 79:689-712, Apr. 1979.

6. Wells, T., and Brink, C. Helpful equipment. *Geriatr.Nurse* 1:264-269, 276, Nov.-Dec. 1980.

7. Clay, E. Habit retraining: a tested method to regain urinary control. *Geriatr.Nurs.* 1:252-254, Nov.-Dec. 1980.

8. Mendelstrom, D. Special techniques: strengthening pelvic floor muscles. *Geriatr.Nurs.* 1:251-275, Nov.-Dec. 1980.

9. Demmerle, B., and Bartol, M.A. Nursing care for the incontinent person. *Geriatr.Nurs.* 1:246-250, 275, Nov.-Dec. 1980.

10. Brocklehurst, J.C., ed. *Urology in the Elderly.* New York, Churchill Livingstone, 1984.

11. McConnell, J. Preventing urinary tract infections: nursing measures alone dramatically reduced UTI in a nursing home. *Geriatr. Nurs.* 5:361-362. Nov.-Dec. 1984

12. Urinary tract infection from shampoo (Nurses' Drug Alert) *Am.J.Nurs.* 86:66-67, Jan. 1986.

What is it like to be dying?

ELISABETH KÜBLER-ROSS, MD

...SOME FIVE YEARS AGO, four theology students asked me if I couldn't help them in a project. They had to write a paper on crisis in human life, and they had chosen dying. That's the biggest crisis people have to face, they said, and they asked, "How do you go about it? How do you do research on dying? You can't experience it. You can't experiment with it, you can't verify it, you can't do all the things that one ought to do with a good research project."

So I suggested to them that it would be very simple to ask dying patients, "What is it like? How does it feel? What fears, needs, fantasies do you have? What kind of things are we doing that are helpful? What kind of things do we do that are detrimental?" The students agreed, and I volunteered to work with them and to find a seriously ill patient for our first interview.

How naive I was: I discovered that there was not a single dying patient in a 600-bed hospital! I went from ward to ward and told the nurses and the doctors that I would like to talk to a terminally ill patient.

"What about?"

"About dying."

"Oh, we have nobody dying."

If I pushed, they said, "He's too weak" or "too sick" or "too tired" or "he doesn't feel like talking." A lot of not only denial and rationalization but also hostility and some very aggressive behavior emerged. One nurse asked me, "Do you enjoy playing God?" and another: "Do you get a kick out of telling a 20-year-old that he has one week to live?" And, of course, there was much well-meant protectiveness for the patients.

I had had the same experience a few years earlier in another hospital. There, the only way I was able to find a dying patient was to go through the wards and look at the patients and guess that somebody was very sick. That way I saw an old man who looked very sick and who was reading a paper with a headline, "Old Soldiers Never Die." I asked him if he wasn't afraid to read that, and he said, "Are you one of those doctors who can't talk about it when you can't help us no more?" So I gave him a pat on the back and said, "You're the right kind of man and I want to talk with you."

Eventually, though, we started to receive an ever-increasing number of referrals. Our first patient was perhaps the most troubling one — to me, anyway. I went to see this old man the day before I was to see him with the students. He put his arms out and with pleading eyes said, "Please, sit down *now*." With the emphasis on *now*. But I did what we always do. I could only hear my own needs, I was frustrated and tired of running around, and tomorrow was the day I was supposed to see him with the students. So I told him "No, I can't stay now, I'll be back tomorrow," and I left.

When I came back with the students the next day, it was too late. He was in oxygen, he could hardly breathe, and the only thing he was able to say was, "Thank you for trying, anyway." And he died a short time later. He helped us a lot, however, although not in any verbal way. What he told us was that when a terminally ill patient says, "Sit down *now*," you have to sit down *now*. Because somehow these patients sense that *now* is the time that they can talk about it. There may not be such a time again, so even if you can sit down only two or three minutes, you will feel better, and so will the patient. The students and I had so many feelings when we left that man's room that we did something that we have continued to do for almost five years now: we went to my office and shared our gut reactions. Not nice things. Not the kinds of things that one ought to say and feel: those come from your head. But how does it feel in the gut? That's what we talk about. We try to get to know each other's feelings — to understand them, not to judge them. We try to help each other express them so that we can learn to listen to our gut reactions and to differentiate between the patient's needs and our own.

So far, we have interviewed over 400 terminally ill patients. By "terminally ill," I mean patients with a serious illness which may end fatally. They don't necessarily die the next day or the next week. Many of them have gone home or have had a remission. Some have lived only 12 hours, and others have lived for a year or two.

What have we learned from them? We have learned that our patients all know when they are dying, and I think that's consoling for us to know. Half of them have never been told that they have a serious illness. We are often asked what or whether a patient should be told. Actually, I don't think any patient should be told that he is dying. He will tell *you* that when you dare to listen, when you are able to hear it.

But patients should, I think, with very few exceptions, be told when they have a serious illness. Our patients say that they would like to be told this under two conditions: one is that the person telling them allows for some hope, and the second is that "you are going to stick it out with me — not desert me — not leave me alone." If we can, indeed, "stick it out" with them, then I think that we can help them the most.

We have learned, too, that dying patients generally go through a series of stages. The stages don't always follow one another; they overlap sometimes and sometimes they go back and forth.

Most patients, when told they have a serious illness, react with shock and denial. "No, it can't be me. It's not possible." Only three of our 400, however, maintained this denial to the very end, although many have maintained denial in the presence of other people — usually family or staff members — who need denial themselves. If a family needs denial, the patient will not talk to them about the seriousness of his illness or how he feels. But if they, or we, can tell him that we are ready to talk about it, that we are willing to listen, he will drop the denial quite quickly and will talk about his situation.

Our patients usually drop part of their denial when they have to take care of unfinished business or financial matters, especially when they begin to worry about their children. But they also drop their denial if they know that the person with them will help them to express the multitude of feelings that emerge when they face the given reality.

Perhaps the second most important and common response is anger. When a person can no longer say, "No, not me," the next question is usually "Why me?" The patient should be allowed to express this, and you don't have to have an answer because none of us will ever have an answer to that question. Just listen.

At this stage these patients will be very difficult: not only with the family (they visit too early or too late or with too many people or not enough people), but also with the nurses. You come in and shake a pillow and the patient complains, "Why are you bothering me now? I just want to take a nap." When you leave him alone, he protests that you don't straighten out his bed. The physician doesn't have the right prescriptions or the right diet or the right tests. In short, these are extremely "difficult and ungrateful" patients.

What do you do when you have a patient like that? What is your gut reaction? Remember, the harder you try, the harder the time he gives you. What do you do? You withdraw, you get angry at him, maybe you wait twice as long until you answer his light.

In one study, they measured the time it took nurses to answer patients' lights. And they discovered that patients who were beyond medical help — terminally ill patients — had to wait twice as long as the others.

That, too, you have to try to understand and not judge. It is very hard to be around patients like this for very long, especially if you try to do your best and all you get is criticism and abuse. What we have found to be most helpful to the patients and ourselves is not to get angry back at them or take their abuse personally (which we normally do) but to try to find out what they are so angry about.

We asked our patients about this. What came out was that the peppier, the more energetic, the more functioning you are when you come into that room, the more anger you often provoke. And the patient says angrily to you, "*You* can walk out of here again, you know. *You* can go home again at five and see your kids. *You* can go to work." They're not angry at you as a person, but at what you represent — life, functioning, pep, energy, all the things they are in the process of losing or have already partially lost.

We tried to see if it would help if we poured fuel on the fire, if we let them ventilate, let them express their anger. If we can say to them, "You know, I would be angry, too. Get it off your chest. Scream if you feel like screaming," then they will express their rage and anger, but it never comes out as loud and frightening as you might think.

The best example is the mother of a small child who died. She looked very numb, so I said to her, "You look as though you need to scream." And she said, "Do you have a screaming room in the hospital?" She was serious. I said, "No, but we have a chapel," which was a silly answer because she immediately replied, "I need just the opposite. I need to scream and rage and curse. I've just been sitting in the parking lot and cursing and screaming at God. 'God, why do you let this happen to my child? Why do you let this happen to me?'" And I said, "Do it here. It's better to do it *with* somebody than out in a parking lot all alone."

And that's what I mean by the stage of anger, of rage, of a sense of impotence, of helplessness. You can help not only the patient to express this rage and anger, but the family, too, because they go through the same stages. And, from a practical point of view, the nursing staff will be saved many, many steps. The nurse will be called less, the patient will be more comfortable.

Sometimes the patient gets to this point — loses his anger — without any external help, and you wonder what happened. Very often it is because he has entered the state of bargaining. Most bargaining is done with God. "If you give me one more year to live, I will be a good Christian or I will donate my kidney or this or that." Most of the time it is a promise, in exchange for some prolongation of life.

We had one patient who depended on injections around the clock to control her terrible pain. She was one of our most difficult patients, and it became very hard to keep on visiting her. Then one day she was very friendly and she said, "You know, if you help me get out of this hospital for one single day, I will be a good patient." She wanted that one day to get up and get dressed and attend her son's wedding. This was finally possible, and she left, looking like a million dollars.

And we began to wonder, "What is it like? How must it feel to ask only for one single day? It must be terribly difficult to come back to the hospital."

When she returned, she wasn't happy to see me. Before I could ask a single question she said, "Dr. Ross, don't forget I have another son." That's the briefest, quickest example of the bargaining stage I know.

In the denial stage it's "No, not me!" In the anger, "Why me?" In the bargaining, "Yes, me, but..." When the patient finally drops the "but," then it's "Yes, me." And "Yes, me" means that he has the courage to acknowledge that it has indeed "come nigh" to him, and he is naturally very depressed.

After a while these patients become silent. It's a kind of grief which is difficult for us to accept — where they don't talk much any more, where they don't want any more visitors. How do we react to them when we come into their rooms and find them crying or silently mourning? What do we do? Can we tolerate this?

This is sometimes even more difficult to bear than the angry patients. As long as they complain about all the things they have lost, it's something we can grasp. But when they become quiet and the tears are running down — and especially if it's a man — then it's very hard. We have a tendency to say, "What a beautiful day outside. Look at those lovely flowers. Cheer up. It's not so bad."

It *is* bad. If I were to lose one beloved person, everybody would allow — even expect — me to grieve. It would be perfectly normal because I would have lost one person I loved. But the dying patient is about to lose not just one beloved person but everyone he has ever loved and everything that has been meaningful to him. That is a thousand times sadder. If the patient has the courage to face this, then he should be allowed to grieve, he has a right to it.

We call this the preparatory grief. If he can prepare himself slowly, if he is allowed to grieve and, if necessary, to cry, then he becomes able to decathect, to separate himself. He will have the courage to ask for no more relatives to come after a while, no more children. And at the very end he will want perhaps only one loved person — someone who can sit silently and comfortably by his side, without words, but just touching his hand or perhaps stroking his hair or just being there.

That's when a patient has reached the stage of acceptance. And acceptance is not resignation! Resignation is a bitter kind of giving up ("What's the use?"), almost a defeat. But acceptance is a good feeling. "I have now finished all of my unfinished business. I have said all of the words that have to be said. I am ready to go."

These patients are not happy, but they are not terribly sad. They usually have very little physical pain and discomfort, and they slip into a stage which very often reminds us of the beginning of life: when a person has physical needs and needs only one person to give him some tender, loving care and compassion — who can be with him but doesn't have to talk all the time. It's the comfort of being together that counts.

"Do you have to be a psychiatrist to work with these people?" I am often asked. Many of our patients are angry when a psychiatric consultation is called because they have dared to become depressed. What I have talked about so far is the normal behavior of a dying patient, and it doesn't take a psychiatrist to help him. It doesn't take much time, either — only a very few minutes.

Last fall, we saw a young man who was the father of three small children. He had never been sick, never been in the hospital before, and now he was admitted with acute leukemia. Every day when I saw him, he was on the verge of talking. He wanted to talk but he couldn't. So he would say, "Come back tommorrow." And I would come back the next day, but he would say again, "Come back tommorrow."

Finally, I said to him, "If you don't want to talk about it, that's all right." He quickly responded, "No, if I don't do it now, I'll never be able to do it. Why don't you come back tomorrow morning very early, before rounds, before anybody else comes? I have to get it out." (We never talked, by the way, about what "it" meant, but both of us knew.)

The next day I came very early and the nurses told me that this patient had been dying during the night, that he had put up a physical fight for about three and a half hours, that he was really not in a condition to talk. But when I promise a patient I will see him, I keep that promise even if he is comatose or not in a position to communicate. So I went to his room and, to my surprise, he almost sat up in his bed. "Come on in," he said; "close the door and sit down." And he talked as he had never talked before.

He said, "I have to tell you what happened last night, you will never believe it." (I'm using his own words because I want to show you what we mean by talking about dying. Patients do not always use the word "dying" but you can talk about dying in many languages.)

"Last night," he continued, "I put up a fight for several hours. There was a big train going rapidly down the hill toward the end, and I had a big fight with the train master. I argued and fought with him. And I ordered him to stop this train one tenth of an inch short.''

Then he paused and asked me, "Do you know what I am talking about?" I said, "I guess the train that goes rapidly down toward the end is your life. And you had a big fight with the train master — for just a little bit more time." Then I smiled and added, "You made it." (That's bargaining. He bargained for one tenth of an inch.)

At that moment his mother came in and I said, "How can I help you with the tenth of an inch?" using his language since I didn't know on what level this mother and son communicated. And he said, "Try to help me convince my mother that she should go home now and bake a loaf of bread and make my favorite vegetable soup; I want to eat that once more." And the mother did go home and he did get his bread and soup — his last solid food. He died about three days later.

I think this man went through all the stages of dying in this overnight struggle. He tried to maintain his denial as long as possible — and then he dropped it in that one night. The anger, the bargaining, and the depression preceded the final stage of acceptance.

My last example is a woman whose story illustrates what hope means and how the nature of hope changes from the healthy to the sick to the dying. If we can elicit the patient's hope and support *his* hope, then we can help him the most.

This woman came to our hospital feeling very sick and weak, and her doctor said that she should go to a specialist in another hospital. So she hoped at that time that it was nothing serious, that it could be treated, that she would get well. After a while she was told that she had a serious kidney disease; then she hoped for treatment that would cure it. Next, she was told that her life could be prolonged if she were accepted on a dialysis program for indigent people. This, too, was something for her to hope for — but she was rejected.

The social worker and the nurses, who were really fond of this woman, could not accept this. It was hard for them to visit her after dialysis had been denied, so they asked us to see her in our death and dying seminar.

The patient was very relieved when we were frank and told her why we wanted to see her. Many little but unfortunate things had happened to her at the hospital to which she was sent — hurriedly and unprepared — to be considered for dialysis. Confusion and misunderstanding grew until finally, when all the doctors stopped at her bedside on rounds, she realized that this was the moment of truth.

"A big cloud came over me," she said, "and I had the idea that I had a kidney operation and didn't need those doctors. When I woke up they were gone." In other words, she had a fantasy that she didn't need the doctors to save her life. Considered to be psychotic and hallucinating, she was rejected for dialysis.

We explored a lot of feelings about that, and then we discussed with her what kinds of things we could do now to make whatever time she had left more meaningful or more bearable.

She said, "Don't be so upset. When I die, it will be just like going from this garden to God's garden." But something was really bothering her, she added. She didn't quite know what it was and it was hard to talk about it.

Two days later, I said to her, "You know, there was something that bothered you, and that's what we call unfinished business. What is it?" And she kept saying, "I'm bad, I'm bad, I'm bad." And we tried to find out together why she was bad. Because what she was really saying was that she had to confess something that she felt guilty about, but she didn't know the origin of this guilt. And we searched like two children who are looking in the dark for something they have lost.

Finally, I gave up and I said, "God only knows why you should be bad," which was a genuine gut reaction on my part. And she looked up and said, "That's it: God. I called on God for help for the last few days. 'God help me, God help me.' And I heard Him say in the back of my mind, 'Why are you calling me now, why didn't you call me when things were all right?' What do you say to that, Dr. Ross?" And my gut reaction was to take off. Why couldn't a priest be here? Or a minister? Or somebody? But not me.

But you can't give a patient like this a phony answer. You have to be you and you have to be honest. So I struggled, and finally I said, "Just imagine that the children are playing outside and the mother is in the house and the little boy falls and hurts his knee. What happens?" And she said,"The mother goes out and helps him back on his feet and consoles him." I said, "OK, and he is all right now. What happens next?" And she said, "The boy goes back to his play and the mother goes back in the house." "He has no use for her now?" I asked, and she said, "No," and I said, "Does the mother resent this terribly?" She looked at me almost angrily and said, "A mother? A mother wouldn't resent that." And I said, "If a mother wouldn't resent that, do you think that our Father would?"

Then the happiest, most beautiful smile came over her face, and she asked me something I'll never forget: "What is your concept of death?" (I felt like saying, "How dare you ask me!" It shall not "come nigh" to me, even after seeing so many dying patients.) So I said something about liking her idea about the garden, but she just shook her head and asked again, "What is your concept of death?" Then I looked at her face and said, "Peace." That was a genuine answer. And she said, "I'm going very peacefully, now, from this garden into the next one."

This patient taught us how hope can change: from hoping it's nothing serious, then hoping for treatment, then hoping for a prolongation of life. And finally hoping that "If I'm not accepted in this garden, I hope I'll be accepted in the next garden."

It is the patient's hope that we should support. I had known this woman less than an hour, yet I learned from her. And I think I helped her.

It didn't take much time. But what it did take, and will always take, is a sense of comfort in the face of death as part of life. When we have learned this, then maybe we can help our patients learn it, too.

Shalom, Melissa: Comforting the terminally ill leukemia patient

DEBORAH WITT SHERMAN, RN, MSN; DONNA MULLIGAN MACDONOUGH, RN, MSN; MARK TUCKFELT, MD; DIANE DURANT, RN, BSN; RABBI RONALD GERSON

Deborah Witt Sherman, RN, MSN: The familiar name on the report sheet caught my eye. *Melissa Cohen.* Could this be the same Melissa Cohen I knew from the synagogue? She and her husband were very active at Temple Beth Shalom, though it had been some time since I'd seen them at services.

I read the diagnosis next to the name — *acute myelogenous leukemia.* With a sinking feeling in the pit of my stomach, I headed for Room 331 on the continuation care unit.

Tentatively, I knocked on the door and entered the room. One look at the woman in the bed confirmed my worst fear. It was Melissa.

She recognized me as I approached the bed. Taking her outstretched hand, I looked into her sunken, frightened eyes. We had never been close friends, but we'd chatted on occasion at the synagogue. The change in her appearance since the last time I saw her was startling. I noted her pallor, the sparse red hair, the bruises on her arms.

Headaches and no energy

In a tired voice, Melissa told me what had happened during the last 6 months. I'd been on an educational leave of absence and didn't realize that this was her third hospitalization.

Her illness started last December, Melissa said. She started getting headaches and complained to her family about a lack of energy. Hoping it was just the stress of her job as a bank teller, her husband, Harry, took her on a Florida vacation. Melissa returned feeling a bit more rested, but still not herself. She began running a low-grade temperature.

One day, she was surprised to find several large bruises on her thighs. She also noticed that when she brushed her teeth, her gums bled. Her menstrual flow also became unusually heavy.

Knowing that something was wrong, Melissa made an appointment with her family doctor. He examined her and found marked splenomegaly, minimal lymphadenopathy, and sternal tenderness. Suspecting leukemia, the doctor ordered a battery of blood tests.

The results weren't good. Melissa's white blood cell (WBC) count was very high, with a pronounced shift to the left showing 92% myeloblasts. Her platelet count had fallen. Her hemoglobin and hematocrit were both below normal, reflecting the severe anemia commonly seen in leukemia patients.

Following an oncology consultation and a bone marrow tap, Melissa's condition was diagnosed as acute myelogenous leukemia (AML). Her only chance of survival was to undergo intensive chemotherapy, which might bring a remission.

Melissa was hospitalized immediately and started on chemotherapy. She went into remission, but it only lasted about a month. Another round of chemotherapy induced a second remission, but now her WBC count was rising once more, her platelet count was falling, and the latest bone marrow tap showed roughly 50% myeloblasts.

"I thought God had given me a second chance," Melissa said, crying. "All I want is to see my kids grow up and to enjoy my life with Harry."

My eyes filled with tears. What could I

say? I knew the reality of her condition. Getting up from my chair, I sat on the bed and held Melissa in my arms. As we cried together, I sensed the beginning of a deep bond of trust.

Before leaving the room, I promised Melissa that I would be there for her when she needed me.

Reassuring words

Later that evening I met Harry Cohen in the hallway. Like Melissa, he was happy to see a familiar face. I asked how he was managing at home with the children — Cindy, who was 13, and Brian, 11. He told me that some of the women from the synagogue were bringing over meals and that the children had been spending a lot of time with friends.

Harry knew that I was a nursing supervisor. I could tell by his questions that he needed to be reassured by someone in authority that we were doing everything possible for Melissa. I told him I couldn't control Melissa's disease, but I could control the quality of care she received. By coordinating the efforts of the health care team, I could see to it that Melissa's physical, emotional, and spiritual needs were met.

Harry also needed to know that someone understood that he was suffering, too. Although he never came right out and said it, I knew he was well aware that his wife was dying.

Poor prognosis with AML

Mark Tuckfelt, MD, oncologist: Acute myelogenous leukemia is a malignant disease that affects people of all ages and carries a very poor prognosis, even with aggressive medical treatment. The hallmark of acute leukemia appears to be the unregulated proliferation of early precursor cells. In AML, the proliferating cells — namely, myeloblasts — replace normal bone marrow. The myeloblasts then migrate and invade other tissues. The most common complications of AML are infection, anemia, and hemorrhage, all of which result from the diminished production of granulocytes, red blood cells (RBCs), and platelets.

Like other leukemia patients, Melissa underwent intensive chemotherapy in an attempt to kill tumor cells in various stages of development. After two cycles of this so-called consolidation therapy, using high doses of chemotherapeutic drugs, we were about to start Melissa on maintenance therapy. That's when she relapsed again and had to be readmitted for a third time.

Our goal now was to induce another remission with chemotherapy so we could try a bone marrow transplant. During this third cycle of chemotherapy, we tried to keep Melissa hemodynamically stable. With the fall in her hemoglobin and hematocrit levels and her platelet count, she needed transfusions of packed RBCs and platelets.

We also had to protect Melissa against infection. That was a concern because, in leukemia, immature WBCs can't defend against infectious organisms. The use of chemotherapeutic drugs, which may cause immunosuppression, compounds the problem.

Several cultures were taken, but they revealed no pathogens. Finally, we diagnosed bilateral interstitial lung infiltrates and started aggressive antibiotic therapy. But Melissa's temperature continued to rise. This led us to suspect that she might have an occult fungal infection, which often develops in patients with impaired immunity caused by chemotherapy. We administered amphotericin B to combat this potentially life-threatening infection. The other possibility was that the chemotherapy itself was causing her high temperature.

Realistically, though, we knew that if we couldn't induce another remission, Melissa's death was inevitable. Our only recourse then would be to try to alleviate her physical and emotional pain with supportive care.

Realistic care plan

Donna Mulligan MacDonough, RN, MSN: The care plan we drew up for Melissa was based on the realization that she probably wouldn't go into remission again. The best we could hope to do was minimize complications from the AML and chemotherapy and keep her as comfortable as possible.

We structured the care plan around these four goals: (1) controlling infection, (2) maintaining the treatment regimen, (3) preventing complications from hematopoietic imbalance, and (4) providing physical and psychological comfort.

To reduce the risk of infection, Melissa was put in reverse isolation. Her nurses followed strict sterile technique during all procedures. They tried not to disturb her any more than necessary so she could rest and conserve her energy. And they started administering total parenteral nutrition through a subclavian intravenous (I.V.) line to build up her strength.

Melissa's vital signs were taken every 4 hours. Her nurses assessed all potential sites of infection (such as the lungs, urinary tract, mucous membranes, and the subclavian I.V. site) routinely. Melissa was receiving trimethoprim and sulfamethoxazole (Bactrim DS [one tablet, b.i.d.]) for her suspected pulmonary infection. To improve her respiratory status, she was also receiving oxygen by nasal cannula.

Problems with amphotericin B

One treatment-related problem that came up involved the amphotericin B that was ordered for the suspected fungal infection. Melissa's nurses administered this drug once a day, the dosage being 0.25 mg/kg, given in 100 ml of D_5W over 1 hour. Unfortunately, Melissa experienced some unpleasant adverse reactions to the medication — namely, increased fever, chills, headache, and nausea.

To reduce Melissa's febrile reaction, she received 50 mg of oral diphenhydramine (Benadryl) an hour before the amphotericin B, along with 50 mg of I.V. meperidine (pethidine, Demerol) 30 minutes beforehand. Hydrocortisone (50 mg) was also added to each infusion bottle. This combination of drugs finally did bring Melissa some relief from the effects of the amphotericin B.

Because amphotericin B is nephrotoxic, Melissa's nurses monitored her renal function daily. This included a review of her electrolyte, blood urea nitrogen, and creatinine levels and a close check on intake and output. Also, because hypokalemia may develop with amphotericin B, they watched her potassium level carefully. As a precaution, they added potassium supplements to her I.V. infusion of D_5W and normal saline solution.

Bleeding episodes

To prevent complications from hematopoietic imbalance, Melissa's nurses assessed her skin frequently for further ecchymosis and petechiae — both signs of her reduced platelet count. To minimize tissue trauma and keep her as comfortable as possible, they placed an eggcrate-like mattress on her bed.

Melissa did have two episodes of epistaxis, but in both cases the bleeding was stopped with gentle pressure. Her nurses were very much aware of the risk of bleeding from all puncture sites. After performing venipunctures, they were careful to maintain gentle pressure on the site for 5 minutes, apply cool compresses, and elevate the extremity.

The nurses avoided rectal temperatures and intramuscular (I.M.) injections when possible because of the potential for serious bleeding. As a further safeguard, Melissa's urine, stools, and emesis were tested routinely for the presence of blood.

Comfort measures

Despite everything that was being done for her, Melissa became increasingly uncomfortable. Her fear of dying made her very tense and nervous and acutely aware of her generalized aches and pain. Acetaminophen (Tylenol [650 mg]) was given every 4 hours p.r.n. to alleviate her discomfort and to treat a temperature above 101° F. (38° C.). Promethazine (Phenergan [50 mg I.M.]) was also given p.r.n. for nausea. And Dr. Tuckfelt ordered 50 mg of I.V. Demerol given as necessary to make her more comfortable. After Demerol was administered, Melissa's vital signs, especially her respiratory rate, were closely monitored.

But the most effective comfort measures were the reassuring words from her nurses and the touch of their hands. A cool washcloth to wipe the perspiration from her brow, a soothing, gentle backrub — these interventions did as much, if not more, than all the drugs in the world could have done.

Often, in the middle of the night, Melissa would cry out, tormented by the fear of dying. Keeping her close to the nurses' station allowed the staff to respond promptly and provide the contact with another human being that she so desperately needed.

Mental health consultation

Diane Durant, RN, BSN: I became involved in this case when nursing supervision requested a mental health consultation to help meet Melissa's emotional needs. The initial challenge I faced was getting Melissa to talk about how she felt.

My first inclination was to let Melissa direct the conversation. But I soon realized that her fear of dying was so strong that it prevented her from opening up. By not talking, she was withdrawing more deeply into herself, which made it that much harder to help her through this period of grief.

Changing my approach, I found that being direct at times, even innocently blunt in my questions, helped open up the lines of communication. I came right out and asked her how she felt about dying, what she thought it would be like. At first it was difficult for her to begin, but together we did finally explore her feelings and put them into perspective.

Melissa's predominant fear was losing her family. She was very possessive in her feelings toward Harry and the two children. She seemed obsessed by thoughts of never seeing them again, of their lives going on without her, of another woman possibly taking her place someday as wife and mother.

The point I wish to make here is that sometimes a dying patient will become so immobilized with grief that she can't find the strength to confront her situation realistically. But even in the face of imminent death, there is room to grow, to learn, and to share.

To help Melissa cope with her depression and loneliness, I introduced music therapy and relaxation techniques into her care plan. The gentle tones of Melissa's favorite classical music seemed to ease her physical and emotional pain. The relaxation techniques — guided imagery and deep breathing — helped give her a sense of peace.

Accepting death

Deborah Witt Sherman, RN, MSN: It had been only 3 weeks since I first saw Melissa on the continuation care unit. I had spent a lot of time with her since then, as a nursing supervisor and as a friend. She shared her innermost thoughts about her marriage, her children, and her relationship with God. (See *Melissa, you have made a difference....*)

Melissa had begun to accept the reality of her impending death. There were still times, however, when she would cry and say, "I don't want to die."

Doctor Tuckfelt had already informed her that she had only a few weeks to live. The chemotherapy had failed to induce another remission. We all realized that Melissa's battle was nearing an end.

Transfer to ICU

Melissa's condition soon became critical. She complained of severe chest pain. A chest X-

"Melissa, you have made a difference..."

Rabbi Ronald Gerson: As Melissa's rabbi, I visited her regularly throughout her hospitalization. I tried to give her hope and encouragement—not a false optimism, but rather a genuine spiritual strength that would enable her to accept the reality of her situation.

I brought to her the love, support, and prayers of the congregation at the synagogue where she worshiped. But Melissa still felt very alone and isolated by her fear of dying and the anger she felt toward God.

Melissa was a devoted religious woman. She wondered how a God she worshiped so fervently could inflict such heartache and pain.

"What have I done to deserve this?" she asked me.

"Melissa," I said, taking her hand, "I can't answer that question. I don't know why things like this happen to good people like yourself. There are many things that we don't understand about God. But I truly believe that we are here on earth at this time and place for a reason."

As a humble and at times self-critical person, Melissa needed help in realizing that it wasn't the length of her life but the quality of her life that mattered most.

"Melissa," I said, "reflect back on your life. It was through your love and careful nurturing that your children have grown so beautifully. Your husband has many wonderful memories to cherish. And you have touched the lives and hearts of many other people through your active involvement in your faith. Melissa, you have made a difference in this world."

Again Melissa asked: "But why has God shortchanged me? I will do anything He wants—if He'll just let me live."

"I understand your anger," I said, "but let's think back on all the wonderful things in your life that you have thanked God for."

As we openly discussed her life's blessings, Melissa's anger gradually subsided. Her love of God re-emerged, and she turned to Him for strength rather than interpreting her illness as His wrath. Though it was difficult and painful for her, Melissa finally reached the point where she could openly express her fear of death and the loss of her family without anger.

Together we hoped. Together we prayed. Together we grieved.

ray and lung scan revealed severe bilateral lower lobe pneumonia. Bilateral gurgles could be heard in her lungs. Her respiratory rate rose to between 40 and 50 breaths per minute; her pulse rate was 150.

Intravenous aminophylline was administered every 6 hours to dilate her airways. Unfortunately, Melissa's rapid respiratory rate caused her to blow off too much carbon dioxide, producing respiratory alkalosis.

With the consent of the family, Dr. Tuckfelt ordered Melissa transferred to the intensive care unit (ICU) for closer observation. The nurses on the continuation care unit understood why that was necessary, but the separation from Melissa was difficult. It was hard on Melissa, too. Being separated from the nurses she had known and trusted for so long only added to her fear and insecurity. Eventually, we worked out an arrangement with the ICU staff, whereby one nurse from the continuation care unit would visit Melissa during each shift.

Within 2 days of her transfer to the ICU, Melissa's temperature rose to 103° F. (39.4° C.). She was given Tylenol suppositories and cool sponge baths and placed on a hypothermia blanket.

To help ease her respiratory difficulty, Melissa was given 40% oxygen through a venturi mask. A left radial arterial line was inserted to monitor her arterial blood pressure; the line was also used to obtain samples for arterial blood gas analysis. Melissa's respiratory status did improve slightly, but her hemodynamic status remained critical.

A family's grief

Harry stayed close by his wife's side. At times, I would meet him in the hallway and we would walk together. Harry talked about the pain he felt, knowing he would soon be losing Melissa. Putting an arm around his shoulders, I comforted him and shared his grief.

Melissa's son Brian was a frequent visitor. He didn't seem to realize just how sick his mother was. His smile and hugs broke and mended his mother's heart at the same time. Cindy, Melissa's daughter, on the other hand, found it very hard to see her mother so close to death. When Cindy did visit, a nurse would accompany her to the bedside and encourage physical contact with her mother. Melissa would stroke her daughter's hair and say, "Cindy, I love you." Cindy, crying, would reply, "I love you too, Mom."

Final days

Four days after her admission to the ICU, Melissa began having periods of confusion. Her abdomen became markedly distended, with diminished bowel sounds, suggesting an ileus. A nasogastric tube was inserted. The tube drained moderate amounts of black fluid, and Melissa started vomiting coffee-ground-like material — both signs of gastrointestinal bleeding. Her hemoglobin count dropped to 7.5; her heart rate increased to 188, with frequent premature atrial contractions, and her blood pressure dropped to 100/60. Two units of packed RBCs were ordered, and a Foley catheter was inserted to monitor her intake and output.

I stopped in to see Melissa on my evening rounds. By now, she was covered with petechiae, the result of an extremely low platelet count of 7,000. I noted that she was also cyanotic, and her arterial blood gas measurements reflected carbon dioxide retention. When I called her name, she opened her eyes briefly to acknowledge my presence. As I stroked her thinning hair, I knew this would be the last time I would see Melissa.

At 10 the next morning, my telephone rang at home. It was Donna MacDonough. She told me that Melissa had gone into respiratory arrest during the night. Cardiopulmonary resuscitation was started, but it was unsuccessful.

Enriching experience

Dr. Tuckfelt and the nurses who cared for Melissa attended the memorial service. Together we grieved for this woman who had fought so valiantly against the ravages of AML. We took comfort in knowing that we had done everything we could to make her as comfortable as possible during the last months of her life, and that we had helped her come to terms with death.

For all the pain and sorrow, caring for Melissa ultimately enriched our lives. She taught us to not take life for granted, to live each moment to the fullest, to cherish our families and friends. In loving memory of our dear friend, the sisterhood at the synagogue dedicated a tree of life in Melissa Cohen's name. This was fitting because when we think of her, we think of life, not death.

Shalom, Melissa.

SELECTED REFERENCES

Jaffe, H., et al: *Why Me? Why Anyone?* New York, St. Martin's Press, 1986.

Long, B., and Phipps, W.: *Essentials of Medical-Surgical Nursing:* A Nursing Process Approach. *St. Louis, C.V. Mosby Co., 1985.*

Moeller, K., and Swartzendruber, E.: "Suppressing the Risk of Bone Marrow Suppression," *Nursing87*. 17:52, March 1987.

Wyngaarden, J., and Smith, L.: *Cecil Textbook of Medicine*. Philadelphia, W.B. Saunders Co., 1985.

UNIT FOUR

Study questions

1. Based on "Chronic Childhood Illnesses: Developmental Issues," how should nursing care for a chronically ill toddler differ from care for a chronically ill adolescent?

2. Because she has leukemia, Lisa Bowman, age 16, is placed in protective isolation. According to "Spiritual Development Across the Life Span," what effects may isolation have on her spiritual and psychosocial development? How can the nurse intervene to promote Lisa's development?

3. "Nurses' Responses to Changes in Maternity Care" identifies changes in the following areas of maternity care: family-centered maternity care; technology and medical treatment; consumer characteristics; legal issues; shorter client stay; economic pressures; and care of the grieving perinatal client. How have these changes affected the maternity nurse? (Pick any two.)

4. "Coping Skills for Children Undergoing Painful Medical Procedures" describes nursing strategies in the following categories to reduce a child's distress: procedural information, sensory information, relaxation teaching, breathing exercises, distraction, positive self-talk, emotive imagery, and hypnosis. How might a nurse apply these strategies to a six-year-old who must undergo a painful medical procedure?

5. As described in "Health Concerns of Adolescents," an adolescent boy's concerns typically include his future, weight, vision, body build, height, hair, acne, and getting along at school. How might a nurse address these concerns when counseling an adolescent boy about alcohol use, drug use, birth control, or sexually transmitted diseases? (Pick any two.)

6. As "The Stress of Caring: Issues Confronting Mid-Life Caregivers" points out, a mid-life caregiver faces stresses that can cause such problems as fatigue, malaise, moodiness, depression, and sleep disruptions. What stress-management strategies can a nurse suggest to a mid-life caregiver to prevent or relieve stress?

7. According to "Continence Through Nursing Care," noninvasive techniques for correcting incontinence in an elderly client include pelvic floor exercises, regular toileting, increased fluid intake, increased fiber intake, and proper perineal care. How do these techniques reduce the risk of incontinence? (Pick any two.)

8. In "What Is It Like to Be Dying?" Ross identifies five stages of dying: denial, anger, bargaining, depression or grief, and acceptance. Give two examples of typical client behaviors in each stage.

9. As demonstrated in "Shalom, Melissa," which physical, emotional, and spiritual interventions might a nurse use when caring for a terminally ill client with cancer?

UNIT FIVE

Diversity in health care settings

UNIT FOUR INVESTIGATED the diversity of nursing in meeting people's needs from birth to death. Unit Five examines nursing practice in various settings.

In response to increased emphasis on health promotion (described in Unit Four), consumer demand, and federal legislation and funding (particularly Medicare and Medicaid), the health care delivery system has expanded in size and complexity. Today, health care services are available to clients of all ages in all states of health and in various settings.

Health care services

Basically, today's health care system offers four basic types of services: health promotion, illness prevention, illness diagnosis and treatment, and rehabilitation.

Health promotion services help the client reduce the risk of illness, maintain optimal functioning, or develop positive health habits. Offered in various settings, these services include, for example, childbirth education classes and nutrition counseling for pregnant women and their families, stress reduction, smoking cessation, and aerobic exercise classes. In such programs, the nurse may act as a teacher and role model of healthful behaviors.

Illness prevention services usually are directed to a specific client and family. They consist of regular physical examinations, identification of familial or environmental risks for illness, and nursing care that teaches positive health practices to prevent illness. Examples of these services include cholesterol- and blood pressure-screening programs, community mental health programs, and occupational health programs such as the ones that promote respirator use by coal miners to minimize coal dust inhalation and reduce the risk of lung disease. Illness prevention activities sometimes receive legislative support. For example, many states have laws that require the use of seat belts and infant car seats to reduce the risk of injury.

Traditionally, the diagnosis and treatment of illness were the most common health care services because, in the past, an individual sought health care only after illness. This pattern is changing as health promotion activities become more popular. (For more information, see Unit Four.) Diagnostic techniques and treatment methods also are changing, primarily as a result of new technologies and scientific knowledge. Many diagnostic methods now are noninvasive and painless; some treatments are simple enough to perform at home.

In schools, clinics, and other community settings, the nurse is involved in diagnosis by teaching techniques for early detection of illness, such as breast self-examination, and by educating the client about forthcoming diagnostic procedures. The nurse is involved in treatment by managing therapeutic care in all settings and by teaching the client and family how to perform treatment at home.

Finally, the health care system offers rehabilitation services that restore an individual to the fullest possible functioning after a physical or mental illness, injury, or chemical dependency. At one time, the health care system offered rehabilitation services primarily to clients with central nervous system illnesses or injuries. Today, it offers them to many types of clients, those who need cardiac rehabilitation after a myocardial infarction or who need to learn independent living skills before moving back into the community after mental illness. To design a rehabilitation plan tailored to the client's needs, the entire health care team — the nurse, physician, social worker, physical therapist, occupational therapist, dietitian, psychiatrist, and speech therapist — works with the client and family. Each health care team member supplies expertise and emotional support for the client's rehabilitation.

Health care organizations

At one time, hospitals were the only organizations that offered health care services. Today, many organizations provide health care services, including outpatient, community-based, volunteer, and institutional organizations; hospices; and health maintenance organizations (HMOs).

Outpatient organizations. A client who does not require hospitalization may need outpatient services, which may be provided in a physician's office, clinic, or other ambulatory care facility. Diagnosis and treatment of acute and chronic illnesses is performed in such settings, where the nurse assumes various roles. For instance, in a physician's office, the nurse's role may range from registering the client, taking vital signs, and preparing the client for examination to collaborating with the physician as a nurse practitioner in providing primary care to a client in stable health.

In a clinic, the nurse assumes similar roles. In an ambulatory care facility, however, the nurse usually functions as a nurse practitioner with a specific client caseload and is responsible for providing follow-up care for all her or his clients.

Community-based organizations. A community health care agency typically provides care to clients in a particular neighborhood. Such agencies include day care centers that provide health care to specific client populations during the day, crisis intervention centers that offer emergency psychiatric care to clients experiencing extreme stress, home health agencies that bring health care to the client's home, drug rehabilitation centers that provide long-term care to the chemically dependent client, and agencies such as Alcoholics Anonymous, which can help a client stop drinking and remain sober.

Volunteer organizations. A volunteer agency is designed to meet a specific health need, usually related to prevention and detection of a specific illness. It also may provide financial support for research, medical training for physicians and nurses, and education and support for clients and families dealing with a specific illness. Because this type of organization is not run for profit, it must rely on professional and lay volunteers. Volunteer organizations include the American Heart Association, the American Cancer Society, and Ronald McDonald House (a nationwide network of resources used to keep the family intact during hospitalization of a chronically ill child).

Institutional organizations. This category includes hospitals, extended care facilities, rehabilitation centers, and psychiatric hospitals.

Once the major source of health care, hospitals are still a major provider of inpatient services. They also provide other health services as well. Depending on a hospital's size, its services can range from only inpatient care of acute illness to a full range of inpatient, outpatient, and support group services to meet the community's needs. Because a hospital may offer so many different services, a nurse who works there may assume various roles, including, for example, specialization in critical care or obstetrics.

Extended care facilities provide long-term medical, nursing, or custodial care to chronically ill or disabled clients. They usually offer round-the-clock nursing care and require the nurse to possess special skills. Examples of these institutional organizations include intermediate-care facilities, skilled nursing facilities, nursing homes, convalescent homes, and some residential institutions.

A rehabilitation center is a residential center where a client receives therapy and training to promote greater independence. The center may focus on physical rehabilitation such as that required after a cerebrovascular accident (stroke); psychosocial rehabilitation and detoxification related to chemical dependency; or psychosocial measures to return a mentally ill client to the community. The nurse who works in a rehabilitation center needs skills that are specific to the type of center. For example, a nurse who is employed by a physical rehabilitation center requires knowledge about normal physical function and skills that promote maximal functioning; a nurse who works in a detoxification center needs an in-depth understanding of drugs and excellent counseling skills.

Psychiatric hospitals provide inpatient and outpatient care to clients with emotional illnesses. The treatment goals include cure or, if cure is not possible, assistance with behavior control and adaptation to the illness. A nurse who works in a psychiatric hospital needs strong communication skills to develop a meaningful relationship with each client. This relationship allows the client to feel accepted, test reality, experience appropriate limits to behavior, and explore the meaning of the illness and alternative ways of responding. The psychiatric hospital nurse actively participates in group, occupational, recreational, and family therapies.

Hospice organizations. Hospices, family-centered institutions for terminally ill clients, grew out of consumers' dissatisfaction with traditional hospital care offered to dying clients. Hospices provide care to clients who have reached the terminal phase of any illness, including cancer, AIDS, cardiac disease, renal disease, or respiratory failure. Because hospices aim to maintain the quality of the client's life, their care includes pain relief and comfort measures, but not emergency procedures such as cardiopulmonary resuscitation. Hospices maintain open visiting for families in a home-like environment.

A hospice may be an independent agency in the community, a unit in a hospital, or a complement of services offered by a home health care agency. A nurse who works in a hospice functions with relative independence, providing care and support to the client and family and, after the client's death, offering emotional support to the grieving family.

Health maintenance organizations. HMOs provide health maintenance and treatment services to voluntary enrollees who pay a predetermined, fixed group rate. They differ from hospitals and other health care agencies primarily in their financing methods and organization. A client with private insurance typically is not limited to a particular agency or health care provider for health care services. An HMO member, however, must use the organization's facilities and health care providers. In HMOs, the nurse usually functions as a nurse practitioner.

Glossary

Community-based organization: health care agency that provides care to clients in a particular neighborhood. Examples include day care centers, crisis intervention centers, home health agencies, and drug rehabilitation centers.

Health maintenance organization (HMO): group health care agency that provides health maintenance and treatment services to voluntary enrollees who pay a predetermined fixed rate.

Hospice organization: health care agency that provides family-centered care for terminally ill clients.

Institutional organization: established health care agency, such as a hospital, extended care facility, rehabilitation center, or psychiatric hospital.

Outpatient organization: health care agency that provides services to clients who do not require hospitalization. Examples include physician's offices, clinics, and other ambulatory care facilities.

Rehabilitation: restoration of an individual to the fullest possible functioning after a physical or mental illness, injury, or chemical dependency.

Volunteer organization: nonprofit health care agency that meets a specific health care need,

The importance of understanding diversity

The selections in this unit present a sampling of the diversity in health care settings. The nursing student should be aware of this diversity for several reasons. First, the student may receive a clinical placement in any of these settings. Knowledge about it may facilitate the student's orientation.

Second, in each setting, the nurse must know which skills to use, including the nursing process and interactive skills (see Unit Three), knowledge of client systems (see Unit Two), growth and development information (see Unit Four), knowledge of environmental factors (see Unit Two), and caring principles (see Unit One) as well as specialized skills for the specific setting. This reinforces the importance of learning the basics well. Finally, exposure to the diversity in nursing opens up vast possibilities for the student about to begin an active career.

S E C T I O N   O N E

Nursing care in institutional settings

THIS SECTION DISCUSSES nursing care in two of the most common settings where nurses work: hospitals and nursing homes.

With the advent of shorter hospital stays, outpatient diagnostic services, home care treatments, and increased health care options, in-hospital nursing care has been affected greatly. Today's hospital nurse confronts increased client acuity and must possess astute assessment skills and technical expertise.

The first article, "Critical Care for the Multiple Injured Patient" by Fought, investigates aspects of hospital nursing that also may apply to multiple injured clients in a prehospital care setting or emergency care facility. After providing an overview of the mechanisms of life-threatening injury and the predictors of survival and mortality, the article examines the effects of pulmonary, cardiovascular, neurologic, musculoskeletal, and genitourinary trauma. Then it examines the nurse's role in critical care of trauma victims, highlighting appropriate assessment tools, nursing diagnoses, and nursing interventions.

This article is particularly relevant to the hospital nurse because injuries account for one of every eight hospitalized clients. Also, injuries cause more than 140,000 deaths in the United States each year, making them the number one killer of Americans up to age 44 (Committee on Trauma Research, 1985) and the number four killer overall (Wilson, 1988). The nurse with sharp assessment and critical care nursing skills can help decrease fatalities from trauma and injury. The second article, "Harvest Moon: Portrait of a Nursing Home" by Tisdale, provides a glimpse at nursing in a long-term care facility. Through a series of vignettes, it describes the differences between nursing home care and other types of nursing care, the frustrations related to Medicare regulations, the demands on the health care team, and the challenges and rewards for the nurse who works in this setting.

An enlarging older population demands nursing home care and related nursing skills. According to Patterson (1987), "All nursing home care should be directly supervised and planned by a professional nurse." In an experiment at a teaching nursing home, Patterson divided the residents into "districts" of 15 each. One registered nurse was named leader for each district and "assumed 24-hour-a-day, 7-day-a-week accountability for the clinical management of all residents within [that] district."

As a result of this "district nursing," Patterson reported greater autonomy for the nurses who provide comprehensive care for a controlled number of residents, rather than providing limited, specialized care for all residents. Under district nursing, the nursing students began to "see the nursing home setting as an arena for autonomous, challenging, and satisfying practice." Furthermore, the residents experienced small improvements in their health.

REFERENCES

Committee on Trauma Research. (1985). *Injury in America*. Washington, DC: National Academy Press.

Patterson, J. (1987). Maximizing RN potential in a long-term-care setting. *Geriatric Nursing, 8*(3), 142-144.

Wilson, L.M. (1988). The American revolution in health care. *AAOHN Journal, 36*(10), 402-407.

Critical care for the multiple injured patient

SHARON GAVIN FOUGHT, RN, PhD

The nurse may assess and care for a critically ill trauma victim in a prehospital care setting, emergency department, operating room, critical care unit, or in transport to any of these locations. Typically, nursing care is based on the setting where the traumatically injured client is treated rather than the severity of the client's condition. Fought challenges the nurse to reconceptualize critical care to reflect the client's condition rather than the setting. Note: Summaries (shown in bracketed italics) and excerpts (marked by ellipses) condense extensive background information.

[Mechanisms of life-threatening injury

Penetrating injuries, caused by one or more penetrating missiles, can cause death directly by disrupting one or more organs or structures or indirectly by leading to organ or system failure. Blunt injuries may cause death through direct trauma to the organs or structures or through fractures that cause trauma to adjacent organs.

Although an initial injury may not seem life-threatening, it can lead to organ system failure and death, especially in a high-risk client who is elderly or debilitated, depends on drugs or alcohol, has a chronic disease or osteoporosis, or is receiving radiation or chemotherapy.

Predictors of survival and mortality

The nurse may use one of the following tools to assess a trauma victim and predict the chance of survival: MIEMSS Trauma Score (MTS), Trauma Score (TS), Injury Severity Scale (ISS), and Abbreviated Injury Scale (AIS).[1-6]

The nurse should perform ongoing assessments, set priorities, and implement care in the same way, whether the client is in an ambulance or a critical care unit.]

Mechanisms of organ system failure

Whether the first hours after life-threatening injury are in the emergency care facility or critical care unit, the factors primarily responsible for organ or organ system failure should be understood in order to deliver effective care. Although complications of injury may be a cause of death, often the priorities for care in the first several hours do not address the identification and therapies or interventions to prevent such complications. Selected examples follow.

Pulmonary trauma. Trauma to the pulmonary system is most likely to result in death through respiratory failure. This is particularly true if the patient was involved in a high-speed, motor vehicle accident, suffered major blunt trauma, experienced a mean arterial pressure of less than 60 mm Hg for any period of time, had 20% or more of blood volume replaced, or experienced a decrease in level of consciousness.[7] Other injuries likely to produce severe, life-threatening situations include injuries to the trachea, larynx, subclavian vessels, and lung (resulting in hemothorax, pneumothorax, or tension pneumothorax) and inhalation injuries.[8]

Preservation of airway and breathing is the first step in resuscitation of the trauma victim. Restoring ventilation and blood flow to supply oxygen to tissue are also interventions to prevent death initially from consequences of pulmonary trauma. Interventions to restore the integrity of the pleural space and airways are essential in maintaining the effectiveness and function of the pulmonary system.

The secondary level of involvement, or sequela likely to be a factor resulting in death, is decreasing compliance concurrent with increased minute ventilation — resulting in adult respiratory distress syndrome (ARDS). Interventions should be instituted to prevent the development of respiratory distress and atelectasis. As soon as the patient is physiologically stable and a cervical or spinal-cord injury is ruled out, the patient should be turned and taught to take deep breaths to prevent atelectasis. Monitoring should include surveillance for signs and symptoms of fat emboli, which occur in the first 24 to 48 hours. Of significance are increases in circulating fat levels and decreases in arterial oxygen tension....All organs and organ systems suffer irreversible damage when inadequately oxygenated. Myocardial infarction secondary to hypoxemia is but one example of a secondary effect of pulmonary trauma that can result in a life-threatening situation.

Cardiovascular trauma. Direct trauma to the cardiovascular system may cause inadequate circulating volume and, if not corrected in a timely fashion, death. Myocardial contusion, trauma to the great vessels, and massive loss of volume secondary to severe burns or blood loss are usual injuries associated with cardiovascular trauma. In addition to identifying the source of and intervening to halt the loss [of blood] and replac[ing] volume, the use of inotropes is an effective method to preserve cardiovascular function.

Sequelae of cardiovascular trauma often develop as a result of severe hypotension. The consequences of inadequate tissue perfusion of the brain, heart, and kidneys are well known and frequently result in death. The presence of a palpable blood pressure is not an adequate clinical indicator of systemic circulation and perfusion.

Effective fluid resuscitation, rapid preparation for and transport to an environment for surgical intervention, and maintenance of renal function are essential to prevent delayed onset of or continuing hypotension as a result of cardiovascular trauma.

Neurologic trauma. Neurologic trauma that threatens life generally involves brain trauma or high cervical-cord lesions. Specifically, these injuries are likely to be cervical-spine lacerations with concurrent fractures, basilar skull fractures with air or cerebrospinal fluid leaks, brain lacerations or hematoma development, and Le Fort's III fractures.[8]

Another predictor of life-threatening crisis is the brain-trauma patient who is unconscious for 15 to 59 minutes. When direct destruction of vital brain or high cervical- cord tissue is the mechanism responsible for life-threatening injury, effective oxygenation and immobilization of the cervical cord are essential interventions.

The development of secondary problems of cerebral ischemia or edema results in life-threatening situations. The use of aggressive respiratory therapy, anti-inflammatory agents, and analgesics is frequently effective in preventing the progression of these situations. Bladder and gastrointestinal-tract decompression, through the insertion of urinary catheters and nasogastric tubes, facilitates effective monitoring of fluid balance and kidney perfusion and prevention of aspiration.

Musculoskeletal trauma. Musculoskeletal trauma causing life-threatening illness is most likely to involve thoracic trauma, resulting in flail chest, above-the-knee amputations, or pelvic crush injuries. These become life-threatening when unstable bone structures damage underlying vital organs or reduce circulating volume. Stabilizing fractures, restoring function of underlying structures (such as

TABLE 1. **Proposed nursing therapies for critically ill trauma patients**

NURSING THERAPY	EVALUATE EFFECTIVENESS
Positioning	To treat dyspnea, pain To prevent increased intracranial pressure, atelectasis, instability of fractures, edema, aspiration
Suction-drainage	To treat hemothorax, pneumothorax, occluded airway To prevent hypoxemia, problems resulting from dysfunctional gastrointestinal (paralytic ileus) and genitourinary systems (distended bladder)
Activity prescription (bed rest)	To treat unstable fractures, pain To prevent continuing damage to soft tissue, tendons, nerves, vessels
Crisis intervention	To treat ineffective coping by patient or family To prevent inadequate coping, increasing anxiety, inaccurate perception of events

the heart in flail chests), and replacing circulating volume are essential interventions.

Following the initial injury, frequent and usual complications that can result in life- (or limb-) threatening injuries include infection, sepsis, acute pulmonary emboli, and compartmental syndrome. Appropriate interventions to prevent infection include early debridement, cleansing, tetanus toxoid administration, and use of antibiotics. The use of heparin, urokinase, and vena cava umbrellas should be considered in the prevention and treatment of pulmonary emboli.

Genitourinary trauma. Crush injuries can result in acute tubular necrosis (ATN), with a mortality rate of up to 60% from ischemic change and circulating nephrotoxins.[9] Appropriate fluid resuscitation and oxygenation at the cellular level are essential prerequisites for maintaining renalfunction. Direct injury to or perforation of the kidney, bladder, or penis can also cause life-threatening crises.

Potentially life-threatening sequelae that can occur in hours or days include renal failure, excess circulating fluid volume, and increased susceptibility to infection.

Critical care of trauma victims

Surveillance instruments. Based on preliminary data, MTS explains variability in mortality of critically injured traum patients more accurately than other trauma scores, systems, or instruments. For example, MTS explains variability in mortality for 45% of cases more accurately than either TS (explaining 31% of variability in mortality) or ISS (explaining only 22% of variability in mortality).[4]

There are two instruments more widely used in the critical care environment than in the emergency care environment that warrant consideration by the nurse caring for critically ill trauma patients. The Acute Physiologic and Chronic Health Evaluation (APACHE) instrument is widely used in the critical care unit and perhaps should be considered for pre-hospital care or emergency care facilities as well. The APACHE is based on 34 physiologic factors and the patient's most abnormal state in the first 32 hours of care.[9,10] The Therapeutic Intervention Scoring System (TISS) takes a comparable approach and assigns scores to therapeutic interventions, providing for the critically injured patient a measure of acuity of illness.[11]

Suggested nursing therapies. In addition to

TABLE 2. Nursing diagnoses for selected traumatic injuries resulting in threats to life

INJURED SYSTEM	POSSIBLE NURSING DIAGNOSES
Pulmonary system	Impaired gas exchange Ineffective airway clearance Ineffective breathing patterns
Cardiovascular system	Inadequate cardiac output Inadequate gas exchange at the cellular level Inadequate tissue perfusion Fluid volume deficit
Neurologic system	Alterations in mobility Alteration in consciousness Alteration in comfort Decreased adaptive capacity
Musculoskeletal system	Impaired mobility Impaired skin integrity Potential for infection Alteration in comfort Potential for inadequate tissue perfusion

the functions associated with ongoing surveillance and monitoring, implementation of medical therapies, and institution of pharmacologic and nutritional therapies, there is a need to create a date base and develop protocols for nursing thrapies. The proposed use of selected nursing therapies to prevent and treat life-threatening problems in critically ill trauma victims is outlined in Table 1. For life-threatening trauma to to selected systems, nursing diagnoses associated with each injury and proposed use of therapies are delineated in Table 2.

The effectiveness of implementing selected nursing therapies, in conjunction with medical and pharmacologic therapies, must be evaluated. Although these therapies have been used traditionally with critically ill patients in the critical care environment, the time between the initial injury and admission to a critical care unit would indicate that these therapies not only might be instituted in the emergency care setting, but also may be effective in preventing and treating actual or potential life-threatening situations. Consequently, nursing protocols involving the therapies should be implemented and evaluated for their effectiveness....The use of the APACHE and TISS may also be of value in evaluating effectiveness of these approaches.

REFERENCES

1. Champion HR, Sacco WJ, Hunt TK: Trauma severity scoring to predict mortality. *World J Surg* 1983;7:4-11.

2. Greenspan, L., McLellan BA, Gerig H: Abbreviated injury scale and injury severity score: A scoring chart. *J Trauma* 1985;25: 60-64.

3. Sacco WJ, Champion, HR, Gainer PS, et al: The trauma score as applied to penetrating trauma. *Ann Emerg Med* 1984;13:415-418.

4. Dunham CM, Gens DR: The evolution of trauma indices. *Trauma Q* 1986;3(1):25-31.

5. Wilson RF: Trauma, in Shoemaker WC, Thompson WL, Holbrook PR (eds): *The Textbook of Critical Care*. Philadelphia, WB Saunders, 1983.

6. Ayres SM, Schlichtig R, Sterling, MJ: *Care of the Critically Ill*, ed 3. Chicago, Year Book, 1988.

7. Thompson J, Dains J: Indices of injury: Development and status. *Nurs Clin North Am* 1986;12:655-672.

8. Swearingen PL (ed): *Manual of Nursing Therapeutics Applying Nursing Diagnoses to Medical Disorders*. Reading, Mass, Addison-Wesley, 1986.

9. Knaus, WA, Zimmerman JE, Wagner DP: APACHE—acute physiology and chronic health evaluation: A physiologically based classification system. *Crit Care Med* 1981;9:591-597.

10. Knaus WA, Draper EA, Wagner DP: APACHE II: A severity of disease classification system. *Crit Care Med* 1985;13:818-829.

11. Cullen DJ, Keene R, Waternaux C, et al: Objective, quantitative measurements of severity of illness in critically ill patients. *Crit Care Med* 1984;12:155-160.

Harvest Moon: Portrait of a nursing home

SALLIE TISDALE, RN, BSN

FLORENCE TAUGHT ME TO SING, not well, and we would sing and skip and laugh out loud. I knew her years ago, in my first job in a nursing home. I was a nurse's aide, I was 17, and she was in her seventies. Florence was confused, happily so, unsure from moment to moment of her age, her history, her condition and status in life.

She was not inclined to wonder, happy to accept whatever explanations I and others would offer for the apparent inconsistencies in her life. She sang a few songs many times —"I ain't had no loving since January, February, June, or July" — and skip a step on her walk to the dining room.

One afternoon she beckoned me to her room. She leaned over close to me to whisper in my ear, pointing surreptitiously to her roommate, an obese and balding woman sleeping in a chair by the window. "That woman," Florence told me, enunciating carefully, "She told me her family put her in a *nursing home*." She widened her eyes in proper shock at such a thing. "Can you imagine? Isn't that *awful*?"

Oh, yes, Florence, I wanted to say. Oh, it is awful. Age is the last place and time most of us will inhabit, and the fact that age seems so foreign to most of us, as though cleft from the known world, is one of life's sly tricks. It is outside the compass points, outside the native land we dwell in till we reach it. The time comes, for most of us, when we have to consider — for ourselves or someone we love — those awful places, those terrible, necessary institutions, those nursing homes.

This terribleness is not always obvious. Ordinary, even familial things happen here, though often unwitnessed. Wounds are healed, muscles strengthened, faces washed, and hands held. Each small movement is tiny in its fruition, huge in its absence. But in spite of these gestures, to most people the nursing home remains a cockeyed slanting world, without common reference, begging despair. Finding no one to blame for old age, why not blame those who house it?

Harvest Moon Care Center is a nursing home for 100 people, located in a residential neighborhood in a medium-sized West Coast city. The architecture is undistinguished, the landscaping ordinary and not quite finished. The walls inside are painted in cheap, dull colors, decorated with amateurish oil paintings of fruit bowls and flower vases. In these characteristics, Harvest Moon is like most nursing homes.

In some respects, though, Harvest Moon is different, even unique. It is owned by a large fraternal organization with a long-standing interest in caring for the elderly, and it has a good reputation in the community. People sometimes wait months for a vacancy here. In a market turning toward for-profit corporate control at an almost frantic pace, Harvest Moon remains decidedly nonprofit, surviving partly on donations and second-hand equipment, and run by a board of directors determined not to sink in an increasingly cut-throat market.

Village life

Nursing homes are terrible places, people murmur to me. Terrible places. I know what they mean — this going on, this repetition, this sense of *consignment*. It explains some of the surge in home health nursing. The advertisements for home health often play on the guilt that is the particular burden of families who find themselves played out, unable to continue caring for an elderly and ill family member; families who reluctantly begin searching for a nursing home. What kind of person puts her mother in a nursing home? How can a family condemn Grandpa to an institution?

The choice to keep a frail or ill relative at home is sometimes the right one — but sometimes it is not, and it is this failure to admit the proper place of the nursing home that bothers me. We don't live in extended families; the home hearth is often empty. Round-the-clock home nursing is often more expensive than a nursing home, depending on the patient's needs. But there are other factors, too.

The most obvious is exhaustion. Nursing is hard work, and it goes on all day and all night long. Grown men are not babies, no matter what illness they suffer from, and months of lifting, bathing, and turning take their toll.

Months of broken sleep and interrupted meals add up, too. And at home, there is no relief. The son and daughter cannot go home, take a day off, freshen up, and come back lively. After a few weeks or months the bell is answered less quickly, the many small needs attended to more perfunctorily. Proximity has its rewards, and its price.

One side to the terribleness of the nursing home is the fear that the patients are not well cared for, their needs not met. It is not always obvious how well a nursing home cares for its residents, because so much of what can be seen — so much of what appears terrible, smells and sounds and looks terrible — is not the fact of the nursing home, but of age and illness.

A visitor may see only a restraint, and a small woman pressing pitifully against it; the nurse nearby sees the woman's confusion and weakness, the broken hip lying in wait past her next step. The visitor hears the cries for help and the ringing of bells, and senses neglect, laziness; the nurse finishes one task and moves to another and another, making mental notes, and knowing all along that the cries for help often don't cease when help is given — the cries for help have an almost metaphorical place in the work being done. They are the work-songs in the field.

Little mercies

Mary Ann Bigler has worked at Harvest Moon for 13 years, longer than any other employee. She is 33 years old. Her plump face is heavily made up with bright eye shadow, thick black eyeliner, red lipstick that somehow fails to age her looks past those of a world-worn 15-year-old. She wears her fine, curly hair short and pulled back with bright barettes, each bearing a sprig of plastic poinsettia leaves and holly berries.

She fills her white stretch pants and the pink smock worn by female aides tightly; the pocket of the smock is decorated with medallions and pins; employee of the year for 1979, the nurse's aide certification pin, small metal clips given in honor of one year's, five years', and ten years' steady employment. In mild defiance of policy, she wears a BORN AGAIN button tacked to her lapel. Her eyes are dull and sleepy in her fleshy face and she tells her own kind of war stories.

"You wouldn't believe the stories I've heard. There was this one woman, Mrs. Jepsen, us girls, we could sit and listen to her for hours on end because of the things she and her husband did at the turn of the century.

"And this other, Edna Crane, she was 101 years old. She had a lot to say — back in the turn of the century, the kinds of cars, you know, the changes in the clothing styles, horse and buggy days, you know, are really interesting.

"I think the one I kind of miss the most — what was her name now? Mary something, it's been a few years. But she worked 30 years in the trainyard, *in the yard* with the men, pushing 300-pound greasecarts around. That woman was strong as an ox and ornery as all get-out.

"You can listen to some of them people and get just as good a history lesson as reading it. I know some people put down the geriatrics because they're senile or this or that, but you stop and think: everything from the past is *still there!* You ask them, and they'll just ramble on. It's amazing."

After 13 years of service, Mary Ann Bigler makes $5.05 an hour. Odd, that caring for our fellows' most intimate needs is considered unskilled labor....

Attention isn't cheap

A woman slowly wheels into the physical therapy area and turns her chair around in a corner, where she silently watches the proceedings with a mournful face.

No one pays her any attention. She has lived in B Wing for years, with no medical orders for physical therapy. She has no medical diagnosis to justify the expense to the family, and neither insurance nor Medicare will pay for such vague gifts as increased flexibility, a parcel more of strength or endurance, the warmth of a small portion of individual attention.

Individual attention isn't cheap. Like most patients who live in an intermediate-care facility (ICF), her doctor — whom she sees three or four times a year — has ordered "activity as tolerated," an open-ended and almost meaningless statement that gives the nurses and aides permission, but no mandate, to help the woman walk and exercise. They often haven't time; always the days are full of tasks that *have* been mandated.

So several times a day she comes to the therapy room and waits, hoping one of the assistants can find a few extra minutes to walk with her. They try to accommodate her. But today Martin (the physical therapist) is scurrying the aides through the most vital treatments, hoping to send them home as soon as possible, worried about a coming ice storm. After half an hour of silent observation, the woman leaves.

Medicare criteria

People with broken hips — either pinned for repair or replaced with steel — are the second biggest group at Harvest Moon, behind strokes. Some hips shatter as though made of glass, splinter like smashed wood; some have so little fabric left that the rags cannot be sewn together.

Paula Schulz, the nurse practitioner at Harvest Moon, suspects that Margaret Bond faces this in her innocent optimism: "Her bones are full of holes," she says in her bluntness. So Margaret waits in her room, paying out dearly saved hundreds of dollars a week, waiting, probably in vain, for her hips to tolerate a fraction of her weight.

Because Medicare regulations reflect a world where every fractured hip is the same, there is no room for such a hiatus, no money, no time. Margaret has only so long to recover, and so she saves her days, her precious Medicare days, for the possibility of renewal — and more expensive treatment — in the future. In a sense she is on vacation from her own rehabilitation, which Medicare claims should be a straightforward and predictable journey. She waits on a side road until she is well enough to travel further.

One part of Medicare pays the cost of nursing care, drugs, equipment, and rehabilitation therapy — but not doctor's services — for the first 20 days of a stay in a skilled facility. For the twenty-first through the hundredth day, it pays all but $50 a day. After 100 days, it pays nothing. There are no extensions. To qualify for a new 100-day benefit period, the patient must leave the facility and be gone for 60 days, and not receive any hospital or skilled nursing home care in that time. Because Margaret can't leave for home, and can't go forward with her therapy, "saving days" is her only choice.

Although the HCFA system manages Medicare, the actual distribution of money and assortment of claims is done by "third-party payers," or administrators. These are large insurance companies that bid for the right to handle Medicare claims in their area. The choices are limited; in Harvest Moon's metropolitan area of over a million in population, there are only two Medicare payers. Harvest Moon has chosen to use Blue Cross.

"I never get to talk to Medicare," groans Paula. "Who's Medicare?" She imitates the voice on the phone when she calls the Medicare offices; it is a weird and shrill monotone, the voice of an irritated robot: "Well, you know what the three criteria are, do they meet the three criteria, if they meet the three criteria then they are skilled, if they do not then they are not, why are you bothering us?"

She returns to her normal voice. "That's how they are. It's like there's this Medicare monster. Then there's this Blue Cross monster, too, who blames Medicare for everything, when indeed it is them and their doctors. If you ask Blue Cross who denies you, they say it's Medicare. But if you call Medicare, they deny *that.* You say, 'Who is Medicare, who denied this?' 'Well, our doctor, it's our doctor.' Who's the doctor?" Paula shakes her head.

"There's no humanitarianism in the rules," she continued. "If you stick a tube down someone's nose, they're skilled. If you feed him and plead with him and coax him to eat and watch his nutrition and watch his hydration, which takes ten times as long as dumping formula down a tube, then he's not skilled." Since without Medicare many people must turn to welfare, it is in the interest of a facility to keep a person on a tube as long as possible, to actually *discourage* the progress Medicare demands until it threatens to stop payment for lack of it.

But not every worse-than-average patient can be sent home from the hospital. This has proved to be a boon of a kind to the skilled facilities like Harvest Moon. The number and variety of patients being admitted is growing rapidly, and their stays are shorter. Rapid turnover, as it were, was unheard of five years ago, and so were the complexities required for their care. The skilled wing of Harvest Moon now boasts medical problems and treatments even more varied than an average hospital ward. In extended care there are no specialties but perseverance.

Decline and fall

"In 12 years I've done a lot of it,'' says Mary Ann Bigler, referring to the hours at the bedside of a person dying. "It takes a lot of guts to take care of the terminals. It's hard on the feelings 'cause you get close to them. We've had some that we just bawl like babies after they go, you know.''

In a sense all of long-term nursing is a death watch, which bothers me not at all, because I think all of life is a death watch. But certain deaths I remember, because of how they surrounded me, of how I was enveloped for a time in their colossal, world-shaking motion.

I remember one death, and a death watch, from one of my first shifts as a supervisor, alone on a weekend, tentatively in charge of the aides, the patients, the other nurses. I walked carefully and tensely through the halls. One of my many charges that day was Pearl, who had been declining for months. She was an obese and silent woman, fed by a tube and the slow spoonfuls of puree offered by the aides. She watched the proceedings around her with what appeared to be a jaded and critical eye.

She never spoke, nor cooperated, but neither did she fight. She simply allowed, without protest, the care we gave. She had a mild case of pneumonia, which we treated, by the family's wish, without great effort, and sooner or later she was bound to die from it.

Pearl's aide that morning was a young, frizzy-haired girl named Liz, new to the nursing home, as tentative as I. She watched Pearl's stertorous breathing with rapt and fearful attention. Several times in the morning Liz asked me to come look at Pearl, listen with what she assumed were more experienced ears. Finally I called the priest listed on Pearl's chart, and tried, without success, to call a relative. The priest came, jovial and kind, and pulled up a chair to Pearl's bed to read his Bible. About 20 minutes after he left, Liz found me, tearful. "I don't think Pearl's breathing," she whispered.

I realize now, though it didn't occur to me then, that Liz somehow thought she was responsible for Pearl's death. "I was feeding her and she just — stopped."

And Pearl was dead, and dead she was different — what was still and distant before was a complete absence now. She was sitting up in bed, propped with pillows to be fed, her head lolling on her neck. Her skin was already waxen, and I imagined I could feel it begin to cool under my hand. It was as though the hairs on her arms themselves had died.

In my own tense inexperience I began the rote tasks, the list of protocols to follow. I'm still sorry I didn't take a few moments to explain them to Liz, to take *her* by the hand. I sent her for wet warm washcloths and towels, lowered the bed so that Pearl lay flat. I pulled out the feeding tube and threw it away, cut off and removed the catheter that had drained her urine. Liz returned and together we gave Pearl a bath, dressed her in a clean gown, and pulled the sheet up to her chest.

And then I called the funeral home, and finally reached one of her daughters, and explained. The men in dark suits with the long black bag came and rolled Pearl away. I went back to my medicines. Two weeks later Liz quit.

My friend who runs a nursing home that has many problems just told me a story, with a story inside it. An elderly man admitted his wife to the facility. She was in a deep coma from a stroke that had destroyed all but the most primitive parts of her brain. She was fed by a tube, and a few days after her admission the family and physician decided to remove the tube.

The tube came out on a Sunday, when my friend was off work. She had a little difficulty with that, because of the problem with thirst — and sure enough, when she went to the woman's husband with her concerns, he admitted that he was taken aback, that he hadn't realized she would get no water.

They agreed to have the tube put back in to allow a small amount of water every day. It spared, before he knew of it, the old grieving man another difficulty, perhaps a sadder one. Without the feeding tube the woman would have had to be moved to another wing, because she would lose her Medicare coverage and no longer qualify for skilled care. The nursing home's tight budget had no room for a few charity weeks in that lucrative section.

The woman would have gone to the intermediate-care wing, to a new room, to new nurses and aides, lower staffing ratios, and more distractions. The woman died a short time later, apparently in peace, and my friend just shuffles her pile of Medicare reports and fee schedules and shakes her head.

SECTION TWO

Nursing care in noninstitutional settings

As the client's options in health care settings have expanded beyond the hospital, so have the nurse's choices in specialized care and employment. This section investigates two important noninstitutional settings for care: clients' homes and hospices.

Since diagnosis related groups (DRGs) have prompted shorter hospital stays, clients typically have been discharged from hospitals in need of complex, professional nursing assistance. (For more information, see Unit Nine.) In response to this need, home care nursing has grown. Although this rapidly expanding, changing field of practice has not yet become standardized, it promises to have a dramatic effect on the health care system.

The first article, "The Home as a Setting for Care: Clarifying the Boundaries of Practice" by Humphrey, takes a look at the various definitions of home health care. Then Humphrey clearly delineates the differences between home care nursing and house calls (a technical service provided by an agency that may supply medical equipment and products, but not professional health care). Although both types of services are necessary, Humphrey feels that clear distinctions between their roles and functions are needed to avoid confusion for consumers and payers and to ensure the best possible care for the client. To help all home care providers make this distinction, she provides a "litmus test" for home care.

In many homes, a family member provides most or all of the care for a chronically ill or dying loved one. Because the family member may be totally responsible for providing care 24 hours a day, he or she may suffer from physical, emotional, and spiritual stress. (For more information, see "The Stress of Caring: Issues Confronting Mid-Life Caregivers" in Unit Four.) Fortunately, a respite care nurse can relieve some of this stress by providing care and giving the family member a chance to rejuvenate.

In the second article, "Rx for Care Givers: Respite Care," Zelewsky and Dietrick suggest nursing strategies that address the home care needs of the client and the caregiver. They provide an assessment tool that helps the nurse analyze the needs of both client and caregiver, which the authors call "the caregiving dyad," within the home environment. Then they explain how to use this information in the nursing process.

Both home health articles benefit the nursing student by providing an understanding of nursing care in the home. As the elderly population increases and the cost of institutional health care continues to rise, the home will become an increasingly common setting for care; and nursing knowledge about home care will increase in value.

Another health care setting, the hospice, is gaining in popularity. In 1988, the National Hospice Organization reported that more than 1,650 hospices existed in the United States and that the number of hospice clients had increased more than 40% in the previous three years.

The growing interest in hospices may be because the hospice offers a humanitarian alternative to acute care in a hospital for a client who faces death. The hospice provides physical, emotional, and spiritual support to ease the dying client's suffering and the survivors' grief.

To help prepare the student for nursing in this setting, Martin depicts the special qualities of the hospice nurse in "How Nursing Takes Over When Medicine Gives Up." She tells how the hospice nurse achieves two main goals: keeping the client comfortable and helping the client's family deal with their grief. By describing the care for several different hospice clients, Martin illustrates the challenges and rewards of hospice nursing. (For additional readings on death and dying, see Unit One, Section Two.)

The home as a setting for care: Clarifying the boundaries of practice

CAROLYN JOY HUMPHREY, RN, MS

As home care nursing grows in popularity, so does the need to define its boundaries. In this article, Humphrey lays the foundation for this definition and helps distinguish home care nursing from other forms of home care assistance. Note: Summaries (shown in bracketed italics) and excerpts (marked by ellipses) condense extensive background information.

IN THE PAST FEW YEARS home care nursing practice has changed and expanded greatly. Hospitals and for-profit organizations have entered the home care field, providing services that had historically been given exclusively by nonprofit community agencies. Of the 5923 home health agencies in the United States as of February 1987, only 500 were visiting nurse associations and 1172 official agencies. The number of hospital-based and proprietary agencies providing home care at that same time was 3064.[7]

The aging population in the United States is increasing, with record numbers being projected by the year 2000.[4] This increase in the number of elderly, their increased life expectancy, and advances in medical technology for all age groups have resulted in the need for the current and future health care systems to treat more patients with complex medical and nursing needs.

With the advent of the diagnostic related groupings (DRGs), patients are being discharged from the hospital "sicker and quicker," requiring home care services to be more diverse and available. Often a patient is not admitted to a hospital at all but is required to have needed care provided in the home with the support of the family. This can be a large problem when there are no willing or able caregivers to assist with the person's care on a 24-hour basis.

Along with this need for increased quantity of care come additional demands from reimbursement sources to cut health care expenditures while maintaining quality. This shift in emphasis and reimbursement from acute institutionalized care to the provision of care in the home has meant that home care nursing is a growing, constantly changing field of practice. Although more nurses work in home care today than at any other time, confusion exists about what exactly home care nursing is and how it differs from other services and products provided in the home....

[The foundation and structure of home care practice

Public health nursing began in 1877 when the first trained nurses began to visit the sick in their homes. By 1893, this type of nursing included some preventive care, too. For many decades, its emphasis on comprehensive care for sick and well clients continued relatively unchanged.

In the 1970s, the advent of Medicare and the growing interest in health promotion and disease prevention prompted nursing leaders to examine the scope of public health nursing, which was becoming known as community health nursing. The American Nurses' Association (ANA) called community health nursing "...a synthesis of nursing practice and public health practice applied to promoting and preserving the health of populations."[1] The

ANA pointed out that community health nursing is more than nursing practice that takes place outside a hospital.

In 1980, the American Public Health Association (APHA) offered this definition of community health nursing:

> The specialty of public health nursing is professional nursing directed toward a total community or population group. Consideration is given to environmental, social, and personal health factors affecting health status....Emphasis is on planning for the community as a whole rather than on individual health care.[2]

Home care nursing is based on community health nursing, but with a difference. It focuses primarily on illness care for individuals and families, whereas community health nursing emphasizes disease prevention and health promotion for population groups. Both types of nursing share an emphasis on family-centered care and on environmental, social, and personal factors that affect health.

To date, a universally endorsed definition of home care nursing does not exist. However, various professional organizations have developed their definitions of home care, which eventually may aid in defining nursing in this field.]

Definitions of home care

As home care has been given more attention in the press, business circles, and reimbursement arenas, it seems to be a term everyone talks about, yet if questioned, various individuals and organizations would yield definitions that conflict in many areas. Some professional and trade organizations have issued formal definitions of home care which are presented below.

American Medical Association definition of home care. The American Medical Association has defined home health care as "The provision of nursing care, social work, therapies, vocational and social services, and homemaker-health aid services may be included as basic components of home health care. The provision of these needed services to the patient at home constitutes a logical extension of the physician's therapeutic responsibility. At the physician's request and under his medical direction, personnel who provide these home health care services operate as a team in assessing and developing the home health care plan."[3]

American College of Physicians definition of home care. In a recent position paper developed by the Health and Public Policy Committee of the American College of Physicians, home health care is broadly defined as "the provision of health care services in the patient's home rather than an institutional setting or a provider's office."[4]

American Hospital Association definition of home care. Rather than a definition, the American Hospital Association provides a listing of what constitutes home health care as shown in Table 1.[3]

National Association for Home Care definition of home care. The National Association for Home Care, which represents the nation's home health agencies, hospital home care programs, homemaker-home health aide organizations, and hospices, defines home care as "service to the recovering, disabled, or chronically ill person providing for treatment and/or effective functioning in the home environment. Home care can also assist in the provision of services to adults and children in danger of abuse or neglect. Generally, home care is appropriate whenever a person needs assistance that cannot be easily or effectively provided only by family members or friends on an ongoing basis for a short or long period of time."[6]

Friedman's definition of home care. In her book designed for the consumers of home care, Friedman defines home health care as "the provision of care at home for a person

TABLE 1. American Hospital Association home care constituents

Medical care and supervision	Speech therapy
Nursing care and supervision	Inhalation therapy
Social work services	Medical technician services
Physical therapy	Appliance, equipment, and sterile supply services
Occupational therapy	Pharmaceutical services
Availability of hospital inpatient services	Transportation for patient and equipment
Nutritional guidance	Homemaker and health aide services
Laboratory and radiology services	

who is sick or disabled to the extent that he or she is unable to function in the same manner as a 'normally healthy' person in our society."[3]

Development of home care

These broad definitions emphasize the extension of institutional medical care into the home to the individual and say almost nothing about the other factors in the home that impinge upon a patient's health, recovery from illness, attaining maximum level of functioning, or dying in a home environment. These components are the foundation of the practice of community health nursing and should be the basis for the professional practice of home care....

Present practice of home care nursing as contrasted with past history

Community health nursing, as defined previously, can be practiced today in an organization that focuses primarily on disease prevention and health promotion. This practice setting allows the nurse to work with population groups rather than individuals. As Williams points out, these patients are selected by the organizations as "an aggregate of individuals who have in common one or more personal or environmental characteristics that contribute to their risk for a certain disease."[8]

This focus on primary and tertiary prevention allows the nurse to apply concepts of public health and nursing to these groups and effect change that can decrease the impact or occurrence of diseases and disabilities. It also allows the practitioner to study the relationship of environmental, social, and economic factors on this subgroup of patients at risk.

Home care nursing, on the other hand, is practiced in organizations that stress the clinical management of personal health service programs for the treatment of disease or disability. In this setting, patients are referred to the agency based on their diagnosis of disease, need for treatment of a condition, or assistance in working through the end stages of a terminal disease. The focus with these patients is on secondary prevention, assistance to families, and direct treatment in the home.

Currently, in most home care settings the environmental, social, psychological, and economic impact on the patient is assessed and included in the treatment plan. The emphasis on reducing costs by payers, however, is causing many home care agencies to decrease this emphasis or cut them out entirely. Some home health agencies send nurses in on "dressing visits" or "catheter visits" in which the nurse only does the treatment or procedure. This omission of total patient care should not be accepted as professional home care nursing practice.

Need for boundaries. In professional practice, there is a need to set boundaries so that practice roles and expectations become clear. Additionally, in the regulated health care industry, these boundaries must be present to ensure adequate reimbursement and interpretation of regulations and to assure the payers they are receiving appropriate services. The rationale for providing care to individuals and groups should be based on the boundaries set for practice by professionals, not by reimbursement sources. These boundaries must be clear and simple so consumers of the care can also understand the scope and content of practice.

Nursing's internal boundaries. Community health nursing has long been in conflict with other specialties in nursing since it has been known as a field of generalists, not specialists. The emergence of clinical specialists, nurse practitioners, and various professional specialty associations within nursing served to make the community health nurse's expertise even more confusing to members of the profession as well as to consumers and other practitioners.

Nursing has repeatedly set boundaries for professional practice by identifying its specialist groups with specialties in medicine, using disease categories or body systems as foundations. This is evident in the practice of psychiatric nursing, obstetric nursing, medical-surgical nursing, oncology nursing, and so on. These specialties base a great deal of their practice on the medical diagnosis and treatment of the patient integrated with the basis of nursing practice. Additionally, some specialties in nursing are defined by population groups and settings such as gerontology nursing and intensive care nursing.

Since the patient groups and individuals seen by community health and home care nurses have various disease conditions and needs as well as consideration of environmental factors that have an impact on their health or illness, nurses in these practice settings are required to be generalists. This often results in questions about the validity of their specialty as compared to that of others.

Although home care nursing is not defined by disease category or population group, there are still concepts and principles specific to community health nursing that make it a specialty area of nursing. These principles should not be ignored in the practice of home care. Community health nursing has included expertise in nursing care relative to diseases but has additionally considered personal, environmental, and social factors as well as provided care with a family-centered focus. Now, with the advent of home care as a new specialty area of practice, nursing must determine boundaries so that home care nursing becomes a specialty area of its own, still retaining these important concepts.

As Williams stated, practice cannot be defined purely by the setting in which it takes place. Home care is not just medical-surgical or oncology nursing provided in the home rather than the institution. To develop a comprehensive definition of home care nursing is not within the scope of this article. However, professional nurses involved in the field should rise to the challenge and ensure that home care nursing is defined as a specialty and that home care practice boundaries are set within the professional domain of nursing, remembering the important roots of community health nursing practice. These internal boundaries must be developed before external boundaries within the field of professional home care can be effectively set.

External boundaries. Now that the home has become a popular site for the delivery of health care services, numerous problems, external to nursing and the other professional providers,...have arisen that call for the need to set clear boundaries to differentiate who is providing home care and who is providing housecalls. I contend that professional services constitute home care, and technical services provided in the home rather than in an institution constitute housecalls.

Organizations that supply durable medical equipment (DME), such as oxygen, wheelchairs, hospital beds, walkers, and disposable supplies, or assist patients with transportation or home-delivered meals are product driven. That is to say they are motivated by the selling of a specific product and the bottom line of profits, not necessarily what product may best fit the specific needs of a patient. Most businesses that are involved in these sales are reputable; however, they are neither governed by professional standards nor regulated by criteria that ensure sound patient management and quality patient care. This lack of standared and criteria is how technical services provided in the home significantly differ from...professional home care....

The boundaries governing technical-housecall types of products must be differentiated from professional-home care services if patients are going to fully benefit from the provision of services in the home. To those professionals who have worked in the field of community health prior to the home care boom of the past few years, the history of community health practice that prides itself on standards and management of patient care is seriously jeopardized by technical providers who label themselves home care experts.

The litmus test of home care. With the various definitions of home care presented previously in this article, it becomes clear that home care is used by many as a generic term to cover a wide variety of technical and professional services provided to patients in the home. In its position statement on home care, the American College of Physicians stated that the primary factor in the successful delivery of home care was that the medical needs of patients and the ability of patients and families to manage an individually designed treatment plan at home should only be done with assistance from a team of home health professionals.[4]

Today the home care professional team is made up of doctors, dentists, nurses, homemakers, home health aides, and physical, speech, occupational, and respiratory therapists as well as clinical dietitians. High-technology health care equipment is now available in the home, including renal dialysis machines, equipment for intravenoud infusion therapies, respirators, and many other sophisticated medical devices. Since there are currently no formal reviews of new technologies for their safety and effectiveness in the home setting, it is imperative that home care be delivered by professionals who are trained to handle this equipment and manage patient care in this independent environment.

The growing number of patients being cared for at home plus the increased reimbursement for supplies and equipment used in the home have spawned numerous new ventures to provide these needed and often lucrative services. DME companies have proliferated, publicizing that they deliver home care. Other companies provide oxygen in the home, IV therapy infusion, transportation, housekeeping, shopping, meals on wheels, and other assistive services provided in the home. These organizations also advertise that they provide home care. How is a consumer, payer, and provider of services to define and differentiate these services from professional home care unless clearer boundaries are set?

The home care professionals discussed previously utilize the concepts and standards of care specified by their various professional organizations in their daily practice. All are licensed and/or certified by professional boards on state and national levels. Many of these professional organizations are reviewing or are in the process of examining the practice of their professions in the home environment.... The role of physicians in home care, for example, should be strengthened to work together with the home care team in implementing the care plan in the home. First, physicians must become more educated about home care and the various team member roles as well as their own roles as advocates in the policy-making arena relative to home care. [4,5]

It is this factor — the utilization of standards of practice — that becomes the litmus test of home care. If the standards of professional practice are not applied and the patient's care is not provided and managed by a professional team, then the service is purely a housecall and should be seen as such. If these delineations could be made clearer by providers and by payers, the provision of home care services could be more easily assessed and justified for planning as well as reimbursement. It is far easier to determine payment methodologies relative to products such as DME, oxygen supplies, medical supplies, and meals-on-wheels. The multiple variables inherent in professional home care practice must be defined more clearly by the professions. To begin this process, nursing can take the lead in defining home care nursing's role and the scope of practice of the professional team....

REFERENCES

1. American Nurses Association: Standards for Community Health Nursing Practice. Kansas City, ANA, 1974 2. Clark MJD: Community Nursing—Health Care for Today and Tomorrow. Reston, Virginia, Reston Publishing Co, 1984

3. Friedman J: Home Health Care: A Complete Guide for Patients and Their Families. New York, WW Norton & Co, 1986

4. Health and Public Policy Committee, American College of Physicians: Home health care position paper. Ann Intern Med 105:454-460, 1986

5. Koren MJ: Home care—who cares? N Engl J Med 314:917-920, 1986

6. National Association for Home Care: How To Choose a Home Care Agency. Washington, DC, 1987

7. National Association for Home Care: NAHC Report No. 227, August 21, 1987, Washington, DC, p 5

8. Williams, CA: Community health nursing—what is it? Nursing Outlook 25 (4):250-254, 1977

Rx for caregivers: Respite care

MARIANNE G. ZELEWSKY, RN, MSN AND EMILY P. DEITRICK, RN, MSN

Increasingly, the community health nurse needs to assist those who care for a dependent elderly family member. Zelewsky and Deitrick prepare the nurse for this respite care by describing how to assess and meet the needs of the caregiver and care receiver through the nursing process. Note: Excerpts (marked by ellipses) condense extensive background information.

"I WANT TO KEEP HER AT HOME, but I'm getting so tired." The words echoed in my ears as I drove away from the Grover home. Mr. Grover had just celebrated his 85th birthday. He enjoyed excellent health and was totally committed to continuing to care for Grace, his wife of more than a half century.

Six months earlier, Mrs. Grover had been discharged from the hospital following a 2-week stay for the treatment of a recurrent depression. In addition to the depression, she had problems with urinary incontinence, anorexia, an idiopathic cardiac arrhythmia, and newly diagnosed pernicious anemia. She could manage most activities independently with some verbal cuing. In fact, she was likely to become angry if it was suggested that she required help. She needed the sensitive supervision provided by her husband.

During these 6 months in my role as the Grover family's community health nurse, I had watched the insidious decline of her health status. Initially, my monthly visits to administer vitamin B_{12} shots had revealed a pleasant and generally cooperative elderly woman. Now she was becoming increasingly agitated, often hostile, and occasionally nonresponsive. Meal times had become a battleground for Mr. and Mrs. Grover. Her worsening anorexia was causing significant changes in her nutritional status. She needed more help with her personal hygiene, but was more and more resistant to assistance. Mr. Grover's role as care giver became overwhelming. The situation demanded intervention before his fatigue and mounting stress affected his ability to continue in his care-giving role.

The Grover case is typical of those encountered by the community health nurse. There is perhaps no more arduous task than providing care around the clock, 7 days a week, for an increasingly dependent, frail, elderly person. The challenges accompanying this task of care giving include significant financial, social, and physical costs for a family. The drain on family resources must be both understood and addressed by the community health nurse. Furthermore, the nurse must develop a plan of care that meets the needs of the client and the primary care giver....

The community health nurse and respite care

For most of this century, the number of people aged 65 and over has been increasing at a rate much faster than that for the remainder of the U.S. population. People 85 and older are the fastest growing segment of this group. This very old population will grow from 2.2 million in 1980 to 16 million in 2050 (Chicago Hospital Council, 1985). The needs of this population will create new demands for health-care programs and services.

Community health nurses, who will be serving growing numbers of elderly clients and their families, can respond positively to this major demographic trend. Understanding the impact of the increasing age of their service populations is essential. Community health nurses must also assess community needs and develop appropriate services for elderly clients and their families. To address the needs of the care-giving dyad, the nurse must use the four steps of the nursing process: (a) assessment, (b) planning, (c) implementation, and (d) evaluation.

Assessment. Accurate needs assessment is the first step in assisting families to cope successfully in the care-giving role. Home-care nurses must include both the client and the care giver in the initial assessment. Failure to identify care giver needs may lead to a crisis situation, resulting in institutionalization of the dependent client and heightened stress and frustration for the care giver. The nurse must assess three areas of potential need: (a) the dependency needs of the client, (b) the home environment, and (c) the care giver's capacity to meet the needs of the client as patient. Observations can provide insight into the quality of life for both the care giver and the care receiver. For example, where does the care recipient spend most of his or her time in the home? A hospital bed in the middle of the living room is a good indicator that the patient may be very much an integral part of the family. If the patient spends his time isolated from family activities, the potential for sensory deprivation is greater.

The assessment tool presented as a checklist in Table 1 is designed to aid the community health nurse in focusing on the needs of the care receiver and care giver and on the efficiency of the home environment. This assessment tool is based on the clinical experiences of the nursing staff in a medium size (35,000 visits per year) home health agency, serving a predominantly elderly population.

Assessment of the care giver's needs should include the relationship within the caregiving dyad. Several key behaviors are mentioned in the guidelines including touching behaviors, communication patterns, and rewards for being a care giver. The nurse must realize that even in the healthiest of relationships, there is still the potential for escalating care giver stress, especially as the patient's needs intensify. The nurse must be alert to symptoms of care giver burnout including chronic fatigue, declining health, role conflict, insomnia, depression, excessive irritability, and guilt.

Planning and implementation. A comprehensive nursing care plan includes interventions for providing respite, a service intended to improve the care giver's effectiveness. Respite care may range from a volunteer visit once a week to around-the-clock, 7-day-a-week support. Initially, the care giver may dismiss the need for help with a casual "I can do it myself." This does not eliminate the need for respite, but alerts the nurse to another care giver need, the ability to occasionally let go of care-giving responsibilities and accept some help. Indeed, the only way the care giver can continue to function in this demanding role is to seek occasional relief from the burdens of providing care.

In some situations, the family willingly accepts the opportunity to escape from caregiving tasks immediately. In other situations, several weeks or even months may elapse before the family agrees to respite care. Often a referral to a social worker may speed the process, but only if the family agrees to this option. Respite care must always reflect the family's needs and wishes, for no one is more knowledgeable about the needs of those providing the care than the care givers themselves.

Evaluation. Evaluation, realized by goal achievement, could incorporate the following outcomes. The care giver may demonstrate a renewed capacity for coping and use the extra time provided by respite in the most personally effective way possible. The care re-

TABLE 1. Guidelines for assessing the care-giving dyad and home environment

Care receiver

1. Where and how does the patient spend most of his or her time?
2. Can the patient be left alone? For how long?
3. Does the patient express concerns about being a burden?
4. What can the patient do for himself or herself?
5. Has the patient's dependency increased significantly in the past month?

Care giver

1. How old is the care giver?
2. How healthy is the care giver?
3. What is his or her relationship to the care receiver?
4. How long has he or she been providing care?
5. Where does the care giver live? If in the same house, where does the care giver sleep?
6. How much time does the care giver spend every day meeting the needs of the care receiver?
7. Are there certain patient-care tasks that the care giver feels uncomfortable performing?
8. Does the care giver receive any outside help in the management of the patient's care?
9. Would the care giver be willing to accept some help to ease the care-giving burden?
10. Is the extended family a part of the care-giving dyad's support system?
11. Does the care giver have other responsibilities (e.g., child care, home management, job, etc.)?
12. Does the care giver know about and use community resources?
13. How do the care giver and care receiver communicate with each other?
14. What are the touching behaviors between the care giver and the care receiver?
15. Is the care giver's nightly sleep routinely interrupted by the needs of the care receiver?
16. Is there a plan in place in case the care giver becomes sick or has an accident?
17. What rewards does the care giver receive from the care-giving role?

Home environment

1. Is the room where the care receiver spends most of his or her time conveniently arranged so that the patient can do things independently when possible?
2. If bedbound, is the patient in a bed that facilitates providing hands-on care?
3. Is the home environment safe?
   Appropriate modifications in the bathroom?
   Commode available, if needed?
   Cleared pathway in traffic areas?
4. Can the home environment be conveniently modified to conserve energy for both the care giver and the care receiver?
5. Is meal preparation difficult for the care giver?
6. Is the home well-equipped to do extra laundry, or other extra needs?
7. Is the temperature of the home safe?
   Neither too hot nor too cold?

ceiver's social isolation may be decreased with the initiation of respite care. This outcome, of course, is predicated on a well-trained respite worker, sensitized to the needs of the care-giving dyad. Finally, the ultimate goal of the successful care plan, which implements respite strategies, is to prevent rather than to treat care giver burnout....

Conclusions

Community health nurses can be actively involved in assessing the need for respite care and in implementing appropriate adult respite-care programs. Families and the staff of community agencies should be able to describe and plan a variety of programs to meet the increasing demand for respite-care services. Offered to vulnerable families on a preventive basis, respite care may help prevent family burnout, extend caregiving abilities, conserve family and community economic reserves, prevent institutionalization, and enable the dependent elderly to remain in the community.

And how was the Grover dilemma resolved? Eventually Mrs. Grover was rehospitalized, more diagnostic tests were performed, and a nasogastric tube was inserted for tube feedings. At this time she was transferred to a nursing home. Mr. Grover tolerated this arrangement for 3 months but then made plans to bring Grace home. The family (six children ages 45 to 60) were all supportive of Mr. Grover's decision although understandably concerned about Mr. Grover's stamina and his continued ability to care for their mother. Fortunately, the Grovers could afford 24-hour help. Arrangements were completed to place a home health aide, and Mrs. Grover returned home. Her health improved slightly in the more therapeutic home environment, and the Grover family was both relieved and committed to keeping the parents in their own home as long as possible.

REFERENCES

Cantor, M.H. (1983). Strain among caregivers: A study of experience in the United States. *The Gerontologist, 23*, 597-604.

Cantor, M.H. (1985). Families: A basic sourde of long-term care for the elderly. *Aging*, 349, 8-13.

Chicago Hospital Council. (1985). Older adults in metropolitan Chicago. Chicago: Chicago Hospital Council and the University of Illinois School of Public Health.

Collins, G. (1986, January 6). Many in work force care for elderly kin. *The New York Times*, p. 14.

Dobrok, R., & Litwak, E. (1981). *Maintenance of family ties of long-term care patients: Theory and guide to practice*. Rockville, MD: National Institute of Mental Health.

Fengler, A., & Goodrich, N. (1979). Wives of elderly disabled men: The hidden patients. *The Gerontologist, 19*, 175-182.

Goldstein, V., Regnery, G., & Wellin, E. (1981). Caretaker role fatigue. *Nursing Outlook, 29*, 24-30.

Johnson, C. (1983). Dyadic family relations and social support. *The Gerontologist*, 23, 377-383.

Jones, D.A., & Vetter, N.J. (1984). A survey of those who care for the elderly at home: Their problems and needs. *Social Science Medicine, 19*, 511-514.

Macken, C.L. (1986). A profile of functionally impaired elderly persons living in the community. *Health Care Financing Review, 7*(4), 33-49.

Metropolitan Chicago Coalition on Aging. (1985). *Respite care policy recommendations*. Unpublished document.

Montgomery, R. (1984). Services for families of the aged: Which one will work best? *Aging, 347*, 17-21.

Reece, D., Waltz, T., & Hageboeck, H. (1983). Intergenerational care providers of noninstitutionalized frail elderly: Characteristics and consequences. *Journal of Gerontological Social Work, 5*(3), 21-33.

Scharlach, A., & Frenzel, C. (1986). An evaluation of institution-based respite care. *The Gerontologist, 26*, 77-82.

Upshur, C. (1983). Developing respite care: A support service for families with disabled members. *Family Relations, 32*, 13-20.

Zarit, S., Reever, K., & Peterson, J. (1980) Relative of the impaired elderly: Correlates of feelings of burden. *The Gerontologist, 20, 649-654*.

How nursing takes over when medicine gives up

NORMA F. MARTIN, RN, BSN, MS

TED RUSK WAS ONLY 42 YEARS OLD when he learned that he had terminal cancer. A devoted family man, he shrank from the idea of a very long and costly hospital stay. "I want to die at home," he told his physician.

The doctor referred Mr. Rusk to our hospice. When he finally passed away some five months later, he was right where he wanted to be — at home with his family around him.

Mr. Rusk's experience captures the essence of hospice, which enables a terminally ill patient and his family to make the most of the time he has left. Hospice nursing lets the patient live at home, keeps him as comfortable as possible, and prepares him for a peaceful, natural death.

A hospice nurse also gives psychological support to the patient's family, teaches them how to properly care for the patient, and helps them to work through their grief.

The concept dates back to the Middle Ages, when a hospice was a place where pilgrims could find food, shelter, and comfort. The first modern hospice — a residence for dying patients — was founded in London in 1967, and the first hospice in this country opened in Connecticut seven years later.

Today, most hospices are home care programs. Our own was started three years ago, when two of the local hospital-based hospice programs merged with a visiting nurse service.

Who's eligible for hospice?

Whenever a patient at one of our hospitals has less than six months to live, a hospice nurse visits him to see if he may be interested in our program.

To be eligible, the patient must want to go home, and his family must be willing and able to care for him there. Perhaps most important, the patient must understand that his entry into our program marks the end of aggressive efforts to cure him and the beginning of palliative care.

A nurse coordinates the hospice team

Taking care of terminally ill patients and their families is too big a job for one nurse to handle. That's why hospice programs rely on teamwork.

Generally, a team includes a nurse, a doctor, a social worker, a home health aide, and a chaplain. There can be other participants — pharmacists, physical therapists, dietitians — as well as volunteers who provide respite care and emotional support for the family.

A team meets regularly, usually once a week, to discuss the physical, psychological, and spiritual aspects of a patient's care. In most cases, it's the nurse who coordinates the team, referring other members to the patient or his family as needed.

The nurse herself visits the patient at least once a week and as often as once a day. What's more, she or another nurse is on call around the clock, seven days a week.

If a hospice patient must temporarily return to the hospital, his team cares for him there, then follows him back home. After he dies, the social worker, chaplain, or a trained volunteer provides bereavement counseling for his family.

An emphasis on comfort

While the patient is alive, his hospice nurse tries to keep him comfortable, both physically and psychologically. Whenever possible, she teaches him relaxation techniques and makes sure he gets as much pain medication as he needs.

If a patient is on morphine, for instance, she urges the doctor to order a large enough dose and the least painful method of administration. She tells the family to give medication at regular intervals, instead of waiting until he's in pain. Her goal is to find the optimum level of the drug—one that relieves his suffering yet leaves him alert.

The nurse also gives the patient as much control over his life as possible. She explains the effects of a particular drug or procedure, for example, and encourages him to make decisions about his care.

In Ted Rusk's case, the nurse told him he could decide to stop his blood transfusions whenever he was ready. He chose to discontinue the treatment after he celebrated his 15th wedding anniversary and his daughter's 11th birthday.

Helping families work through grief

Grieving begins many months before death, usually when the patient and his family first hear the fatal prognosis.

Helping them deal with their feelings is one of the most demanding jobs a hospice nurse faces. At our hospice, we give each patient and his family a 10-page pamphlet on grief, recommending that they read it and talk about it as soon as they're ready. It includes a detailed description of the stages of grieving—denial, bargaining for time, depression, anger, and acceptance.

If a nurse discovers that any member of the family is having a particularly difficult time emotionally—problems often arise, for instance, because a patient and his family experience grief at different times and in different ways—she'll ask that the team's social worker visit the family more often.

One such instance involved a man named Arthur Gardner. His wife had accepted the prognosis that she had only few months to live, but Mr. Gardner insisted that "Bonnie's not dying."

With extra counseling from the social worker and the nurse, Mr. Gardner was able to accept the fact that his wife was close to death. Indeed, he finally told her she had his "permission" to die. Once she heard that, Bonnie Gardner seemed at peace, and she died two days later.

Recently, I spoke about grief and healing to a support group for bereaved spouses. I reminded them of a line in our pamphlet: "We are helped by working on our feelings, and not suppressing them."

Only by allowing themselves to experience the sadness and despair, I said, can bereaved families regain the feeling that life is worth living. Hospice care not only helps patients die in peace and comfort, it helps their families face life again.

BIBLIOGRAPHY

Hope for Bereaved. Hope for Bereaved. Syracuse, N.Y.

Hospice Volunteer Handbook. Visiting Nurse Service and Hospice, Fort Wayne, Ind. 1985.

Spencer, R. and Nichols, L. *Clinical Pharmacology and Nursing Management.* Philadelphia: J.B. Lippincott Co., 1983.

UNIT FIVE

Study questions

1. In "Critical Care for the Multiple Injured Patient," Fought describes nursing care for trauma victims. Based on her suggestions, which nursing diagnoses may be used for a critically ill client with pulmonary trauma?

2. According to "Harvest Moon: Portrait of a Nursing Home," how might Medicare payments affect the care of an elderly client with a fractured hip?

3. In "The Home as a Setting for Care: Clarifying the Boundaries of Practice," Humphrey contrasts home health care with house calls. What is her "litmus test" for distinguishing between these services?

4. "Rx for Care Givers: Respite Care" proposes that the nurse identify the need for respite care through a special assessment. Name at least two factors that the nurse should assess for the care receiver, caregiver, and home environment. Why are the two factors significant?

5. When caring for a dying client, a hospice nurse tries to achieve two main goals: to keep the client comfortable and to provide emotional support to the client's family. According to "How Nursing Takes Over When Medicine Gives Up," which specific steps can a hospice nurse take to achieve these goals?

UNIT SIX

Psychosocial concepts in nursing

PSYCHOSOCIAL CONCEPTS reflect a client's mental and social functioning. They include the client's understanding of self and relationships with others. Psychosocial concepts are integral to the client's holistic nature, which includes body, mind, and spirit.

The client's body, mind, and spirit are not separate, distinct forces, but dynamic, interactive ones. When their interaction is balanced, the client is in a state of healthy equilibrium. An internal or external stressor can upset this balance and disrupt the client's equilibrium. For example, a myocardial infarction (heart attack) that affects the client's physical health also can influence the client's mental and spiritual health, causing fear and distress.

Unlike other health care professions, nursing emphasizes holistic care — addressing all aspects of the client. The nurse realizes that physical disorders can cause psychosocial problems and that psychosocial problems can lead to physical symptoms. The nurse also understands that psychosocial problems do not conflict with the client's physical symptoms, but present a fuller picture of the client with an illness or injury.

When health care is needed, the client typically reevaluates the meaning of the world and the nature of the self. This psychological reevaluation can upset the client's normal way of thinking and responding to the external environment. Whether the outcome is positive or negative may depend on the nurse's understanding of the client's psychosocial concerns.

By paying attention to psychosocial concerns, the nurse can uncover the client's subjective world — a world as extensive and as real to the client as the objective one. She or he also can help the client make the best of perplexing or adverse life experiences that may seem to contradict the meaning of self and help him accept unexpected circumstances that may seem beyond the client's comprehension.

Through psychosocial concerns, the nurse also can understand the client's subjective experience of illness. The client's perception of the meaning of a health problem or its treatment will directly affect the client's psychological well-being and compliance with the treatment.

The self-concept

The self-concept explains a client's ideas, feelings, and attitudes and their interrelationships. Self-concept includes body image, moral and

Glossary

Crisis: emergency of the mind and body that typically occurs when circumstances overwhelm the client's abilities to cope with them.

Crisis intervention: therapeutic actions that help resolve an immediate problem and restore the client to pre-crisis functioning.

Denial: defense mechanism in which a client refuses to accept facts, thoughts, or feelings that are consciously intolerable.

Drug dependence: physical or emotional addiction to drugs, including alcohol.

Ego boundaries: psychological lines that separate a client's "internal" (body, mind, spirit) and external environments.

Fear: dread of an imagined or real occurrence; behavioral manifestations are characterized by a shutting down of perceptual awareness to avoid unacceptable problems and stress.

Grief: pattern of physical, emotional, and other responses to bereavement, separation, or loss.

Hostile behaviors: conflict or emotions expressed through defensive, destructive, or other neurotic actions.

Loneliness: awareness of being apart from others.

Psychosocial concepts: self-reflections on a client's mental and social functioning.

Self-concept: a client's ideas, feelings, and attitudes and their interrelationships — including body image, moral and ethical views, emotional awareness, and intellectual and spiritual insights.

Self-esteem: feelings of personal worth.

Suicide: intentional taking of one's life.

ethical views, emotional awareness, and intellectual and spiritual insights. Through the self-concept, a client can evaluate the total effects of a health problem.

A client's self-concept and psychosocial nature can help the nurse understand the client's behaviors and interact positively with the client. However, the nurse must remember that various health problems can alter the self-concept, leading to nursing diagnoses such as *disturbance in self-concept, body image; disturbance in self-concept, self-esteem; altered role performance; and disturbance in self-concept, personal identity*. Therefore, the nurse's continuing assessment of the client's self-concept is essential to effective nursing practice.

Common psychosocial concerns

A stressed client may develop a common psychosocial concern, such as denial (the unconscious refusal to accept painful facts), loneliness (awareness of being apart from others), fear (dread of an imagined or real occurrence), and grief (physical, emotional, and other responses to bereavement, separation, or loss). These concerns can affect any client at any time, cutting across specific diagnostic categories, client classifications, age groups, and ethnic considerations.

The nurse may encounter these psychosocial responses in various health care settings. For example, the nurse may see denial as a defense mechanism in a client with newly diagnosed cancer. The nurse may find grief in a client in the terminal stages of an illness or with a radical alteration in body image. The nurse may find loneliness in a frail elderly client in a nursing home. And she or he may encounter fear in any client who faces the unknown, such as surgery, a new diagnosis, or a difficult or painful treatment. In each case, the client's physical comfort and psychological security can alter self-concept, and the nurse must be aware of the client's changes.

Severe psychosocial syndromes

Common psychosocial concerns occur regularly as exaggerated, but *normal*, behaviors. However, when these concerns are unresolved and when they are overwhelmed by other problems, they can lead to *abnormal* behaviors. These behaviors may take the form of a severe psychosocial syndrome, such as drug dependence (physical or emotional addition to drugs, including alcohol), acting-out behaviors (actions that express painful emotions through defensive or destructive behaviors), internalized anxiety through neurotic behavior, or attempted suicide.

Circumstances that exceed the client's coping abilities can disrupt the holistic balance and place the client in crisis (an emergency for mind and body). An acute, unexpected psychosocial condition, a crisis is characterized by a life-or-death sense of immediacy and, usually, by serious psychosocial or physiologic problems. Crisis has three basic phases: stress, response, and resolution or disintegration. To help a client resolve a psychosocial or physiologic crisis, the nurse must use crisis intervention techniques that help therapeutically resolve an immediate problem and restore the client to a pre-crisis level of functioning. (For more about crisis resolution, see Unit Seven.)

Psychosocial concepts in caring

Although psychosocial concepts are just one aspect of the whole person, they are vitally important. By applying them, the nurse can better assess a client's psychosocial response to a health care problem and its effects, more accurately evaluate the physical responses to a psychosocial or physical problem, intervene appropriately to prevent more severe problems, and help heal the whole person — body, mind, and spirit.

For these reasons, the psychosocial concepts in this unit are fundamental to the study of nursing and of special relevance to the student who soon will become a nurse.

SECTION ONE

The self-concept

Because the self-concept is a subjective and psychological judgment, it does not lend itself to an easy or precise definition. However, Hamachek (1985) offers this description of the self-concept and other aspects of the self:

> ...each person has (a) a *self* (a sense of personal existence), (b) a *self-concept* (an idea of personal identity), (c) a certain level of *self-esteem* (feelings of personal worth), (d) an *ego* (a barometer of psychological and emotional strength), and (e) *ego boundaries* (gauges of psychological and emotional resiliency).

Because illness and tragedy can reactivate a client's earlier developmental stages, the nurse must be able to assess a client's current developmental stage — and related self-concept — to provide optimum care. Erikson's theory of personality development (1963) is the most common framework for this assessment. (For more information, see Unit Four.)

Erikson identifies eight developmental stages throughout life. Each stage presents a psychosocial task that can help the self-concept develop from undifferentiated in infancy to sharply defined in old age. Self-concept development parallels the client's physical, moral, and ethical development and is influenced by culture and by various experiences.

To develop normally and function effectively, the client must successfully complete each psychosocial task. Incomplete development can hinder the client in interpersonal relationships — and in life. A mentally ill client may be handicapped in all stages of development or fixated with one stage.

An understanding of the client's developmental status helps the nurse select interventions that are most likely to be successful. "Self-Concepts in the Nurse-Client Relationship" by Arnold and Boggs addresses this understanding. It examines development — especially of the self-concept — in each of Erickson's stages. Then it describes the assessment guidelines, stressors, and core pathology associated with each stage. Finally, it shows how to order psychosocial nursing interventions using Maslow's hierarchy of needs. (For more information, see "Therapy for Depression" in Unit Three.)

According to Hamachek (1985):

> One cannot see another person's self-concept — that is private — but one can see expressions of that self-concept in behavior, which can be interpreted as reflections of an individual's ego boundaries. For example, a person might say, "Mary has a strong ego, she can handle the criticism" or "John has a fragile ego, he cracks easily under pressure." That person would probably not say, "Mary has a strong self" or "John has a fragile self." The self is something the other person already has; the ego is something added to it, usually by way of assessment of strength or weakness. Thus, when people talk about someone having a weak or strong ego, they are implicitly saying something about the sort of boundaries that help to keep that individual's sense of self intact. Hence, the term *ego boundaries*.

The nurse can obtain important information about the client's self-concept and determine the most effective interventions by assessing individual behavior.

In "Human Interaction and Personal Boundaries," Scott defines a client's boundaries holistically as a separation between a client's "internal" (body, mind, spirit) and external environments that varies in its degree of openness and flexibility. The author tells how boundaries function and why they are needed. She describes how to assess a client's boundaries, which may range from closed (the client may be withdrawn and rigid) to open (the client may be social and willing to take risks). A flexible client functions between those extremes — that is, quiet and withdrawn at times (as when the environment seems unsafe) and outgoing and social at other times. She also discusses ways to help a client maintain flexible boundaries, such as assisting the client to become aware of needs, to develop support, to communicate effectively, and to perceive reality more accurately.

A client's boundaries can hinder care or facilitate it. Through this article, the student can learn to modify detrimental boundaries and promote more effective care.

Note: Some nonessential details have been deleted from both selections (marked by ellipses).

REFERENCES

Erikson, E. (1963). *Childhood and society*. New York: Norton.

Hamachek, D. (1985). The self's development and ego growth: Conceptual analysis and implications for counselors. *Journal of Counseling and Development*. *64*:136-142.

Self-concepts in the nurse-client relationship

ELIZABETH ARNOLD, PhD; KATHLEEN BOGGS, RN, PhD

Erikson's approach

SELF-CONCEPTS DEVELOP and change over time. Erik Erikson's theory of personality development (1963) is used in the nurse-client relationship as a way of organizing psychosocial data about a client. It gives the nurse direction in looking at the critical life issues the client may be facing concurrently with the health-related problem. It can be used to assess an individual's psychosocial progress through the life span, and it provides an initial, global analysis of the person's behavioral performance designated as healthy and growth-producing by society. The nurse should have an awareness of the clinical behaviors associated with Erikson's stage theory of ego development.

Trust versus mistrust

Erikson's first stage of personality development is labeled Trust versus Mistrust. Trust is the feeling that someone important to one's well-being will be there emotionally and physically when needed. Consistency and reliability are two very important constituents of trust building.

Babies from the moment of birth are considered active, not passive creatures, capable of giving behavioral cues and eliciting responses from their caregivers. The quality of the mother-infant relationship is more important than the particular words spoken or particular type of care given. Babies who regularly have their needs met are most likely to successfully resolve the first task of psychosocial development. Since this relational experience is so important, hospitalization represents a major disruption in the resolution of the first psychosocial task. While the nurse cannot totally bridge the gap, paying as much attention to responding to the infant's psychosocial need to trust as one does to the physical care of the infant is an important facet of comprehensive nursing care.

The first indicators of social trust in the infant are the ease with which it feeds, the absence of excessive irritability, and the regularity of sleep. Around the age of three months, the infant begins to show differential responses to relationship by smiling, responding with eyes and body movement to the caregiver's attention. The infant recognizes at a sensory level that it is dependent for its very existence on the mothering figure and around eight months begins to protest whenever the primary caregiver leaves the room. The anguish of abandonment is felt with the baby's whole being, expressed through inconsolable crying and stretching of the whole torso in the direction of the retreating figure. For this reason, allowing the primary caregiver as much access to the infant and teaching the mother about this very normal behavior that is likely to intensify in the hospital are valuable adjuncts to the physical and emotional care the nurse extends more directly to the infant in the hospital. Assigning the same personnel to the infant is another nursing strategy likely to promote trust.

The baby's beginning perceptual differentiation from the mother is evidenced by its willingness to let the mother out of sight for short periods. The mother has been found trustworthy and the infant has confidence that she will reappear. The object of trust has become somewhat internalized, and the baby has beginning trust in its own perception that she will reappear, as well as enough confidence (trust) in itself and the interpersonal environment to survive until her return. Babies who do not experience trust with one primary caregiver will go to anyone without discrimination, or they are likely to withdraw from physical contact.

Later, in new and unfamiliar situations, the threads of this developmental task reappear. The older child or adult may react with hesitancy or avoidance when confronted with new experiences. For example, the child may cry on the first day of school, or in the hospital. The anticipatory apprehension most people experience before a job interview or in a new job situation is reflective of the interpersonal dilemma of needing to develop trust.

In the adult client, lack of trust is seen in guarded verbal expressions, a childlike acceptance of all treatments without question, or the opposite: passive noncompliance. Strong prejudices, overconcern about whether the individual is "liked" or is "doing it right," hopelessness, and helplessness suggest a lack of trust in self and others in the environment or in life itself. Interpersonal control is experienced as external to the self. The institutional analogue for the development of trust is found in many organized religions....

Autonomy versus shame and doubt

Once a baby becomes physically mobile and begins to experience its social environment as supportive and trustworthy, the child needs to develop coping strategies to handle the emerging physical and emotional autonomy. This developmental stage assumes ascendancy as the child focuses on developing motor autonomy and learns the magic of the word "no" in choosing between alternatives. Behavioral control in its most rudimentary form is experienced as internal as well as externally applied. If denied an opportunity to practice beginning autonomous behavior or the family support to express legitimate feelings freely without fear of reprisal, the child instead develops a sense of vulnerability, shame, and self-doubt when confronted with situations calling for autonomous action. Denial of legitimate free choices and interpersonal experimentation, labeled as wrong or unacceptable by significant others, leads to a lack of discrimination and loss of desire of acquisition and analysis of new information. The child learns that it is unsafe to choose any action unless it is sanctioned by someone in authority.

The opposite of too much rigidity is lack of limits. The toddler is not equipped physically or emotionally to be completely autonomous in its choices or decisions. [Because it lacks] discrimination, many of its choices can lead to shame and self-doubt without parental direction. Provision of safeguards for maintaining the legitimate dignity and rightful independence of self and others helps the child learn the limits of freedom and develop an expectation of free expression without getting hurt in the process. The child learns to express the self so that legitimate personal needs are met without significantly antagonizing others. Developing a sense of autonomy includes behaviors related to self-control, order, and predictability. The human strength associated with this stage is will — not the reasoned will of the adult, but the inception of fundamental knowledge that it is possible to influence the reactions of others, and that one's personal action can affect the outcome of an interpersonal situation. The institutional analogue of autonomy in society is the concept of law and order.

In the adult client, behaviors reflecting an inability to make uncomplicated decisions, marked lack of assertiveness, disregard of doctor's orders, a defeatist attitude, overconcern with duty, self-doubt, feelings of inferiority, stubbornness, hoarding, compulsiveness, or obsessional thinking suggest a continuing struggle with the developmental task of autonomy versus shame and doubt. Children and adults in danger of "losing face" in any interpersonal situation are likely to reexperience conflictual elements of this task. Encouraging client participation in all aspects of health-related decision making, providing privacy, and respecting the dignity of all clients at all times, regardless of condition or age, acknowledges the importance of this developmental task....

Initiative versus guilt

Initiative broadens the development of autonomy to include the skills involved in deliberately planning and undertaking activities. Autonomous actions become more purposeful and goal-directed. As the child discovers pleasure in manipulating tools and experimenting with different roles in play activities, enterprise is reflected in the increasing number of questions asked and the eagerness with which the child seeks goal-directed activities. Playing games such as "house," "doctor," and "store" allows the child to experience different life roles, preparatory for the larger task of developing a career identity in adolescence. Beginning collaborative skills are activated. The initial movements of this stage are the foundation on which the later sense of identity will build.

Failure to develop the skills associated with the development of initiative leads to a sense of guilt and lowered self-esteem over what might have been if the individual had acted on the patterns of action readily accessible to every human being. In adulthood, passivity, some forms of noncompliance, psychosomatic illness, denial of accomplishments, unwillingness to compete when necessary, perfectionism, excessive or inadequate planning, and implementation of needed activities suggest a conflict with initiative versus guilt. The social institution supportive of initiative can be found in the heroes of fairy tales, myths, legends, and action-filled books, as well as the idealization of real-life heroes....

Industry versus inferiority

From the beginning strivings for cooperation and team play emerges the need for skills to finish projects. In this stage, the child begins to experience the pleasures associated with task completion. There is a pride in producing something. The child begins to see itself as a worker and to experience the self in relation to others, both competitively and cooperatively in mastering skills and tools. Group play becomes team play. Industry is a forerunner of the more integrated task of forming an ego identity based on career and ideological commitment. It includes the specific strategies needed to complete work-related tasks and establish collaborative relationships with peers. The desire to learn, to know facts, and to understand how things operate is unparalleled in this stage.

The ego strength associated with this stage is competence. Developing competence as one adjusts to inevitable changes is a lifelong process. Schools, extracurricular activities, and sports support the activities needed to achieve a sense of proficiency. In the hospital setting, by using the child's natural need for knowledge, the nurse can provide activities and information that lead to a personal commitment of meeting the continuing shifts and demands of life.

Inferiority refers to the sense of helplessness or lack of control individuals feel when they sense their skills and abilities are not equal to the challenge at hand. To successfully resolve the task of developing competence, individuals must feel that they either possess the capabilities or have the potential to develop the interpersonal and technological skills necessary for successful interaction with the larger environment. Without the family support that fosters activities to help the child experience the inner self as capable and independent, the child is likely to develop feelings of insecurity and inferiority in competitive situations. In the hospital, the nurse can enable clients to feel more competent by helping only to the point where the client's self-help capacity can take over the process.

Adult clients struggling with feelings of inadequacy about unfinished tasks, and vagrants, workaholics, and burnout victims may have conflicts related to industry versus inferiority. Once physical mastery over the environment is achieved, the emerging self begins to tackle the more arduous task of emotional mastery. Prior to adolescence, primary patterns of life experience integrations occur through relationship with the parental unit. In preadolescence, there is a shift in emotional energy from parents to peers....

Identity versus identity diffusion

Establishing a clear, firm sense of identity that can be assaulted but not destroyed by unfavorable life circumstances is considered by Erikson to be a pivotal life task. Identity is characterized by a continuity of self. Through the reflected images of self revealed in relationships, personal identity becomes clearer. All of the truths about self learned from others, the inner strivings of self developed through competencies and values, and the unspoken expectations of significant persons in our lives contribute to a composite sense of self.

In the natural progression of ego maturation, adolescence marks the transition from child to adult. The separation of self from parental figures, which began at birth, reaches a period of ascendancy as the adolescent begins to establish physical and financial independence and finally emotional independence from parental figures through the preparation and acceptance of a distinct career as well as ideological commitment. Peers, first of the same sex and later of the opposite sex, become the people who make life meaningful and to whom the adolescent looks for continuity of relatedness. These experiences contribute to the development of ideological commitments and then later to seeking or rejecting intimate connections with others. A certain amount of identity diffusion or emotional upheaval in the process is considered healthy and normal. There is clearly a loss associated with giving up dependence, and the process of learning the skills necessary to consolidate a workable sense of personal and professional identity is disconcerting.

Much of the teenager's emotional turmoil and ambivalence relates to a search for identity — an identity separate from yet very much built upon what has come before. The childhood form of self represents the core of adolescent identity. Yet the sense of identity defined in late adolescence or early adulthood is more than simply the total of earlier developed self-images. The integration of all previous developmental stages including threads of negative self-images is present. In successful achievement of the task, the positive self-images dominate and allow for an optimistic reevaluation of past self-images in present self-assessment. Erikson believes the psychosocial sense of identity goes beyond personal identity, serving to link the past with the future in the context of the present.

Three components define a sense of identity. Erikson speaks of an ideological commitment, career identity, and sex role identity as bench-marks of identity. No one achieves a totally balanced sense of identity. Some cultures emphasize formation of an individualized, enterprising identity, whereas other cultures favor a more collective approach and deliberately sabotage such solo efforts. Generally, people who choose a commitment that corresponds with their talents, skills, and interests are more satisfied in their self-definitions.

From a process perspective, important features include the quality of consistency and the existence of a functional unity amoung all parts of the personality. Consistency represents the characteristic stable way in which an individual operates interpersonally with life so that others can relate to their knowledge of it and trust it to be valid in most situations.

The ego strength associated with identity versus identity diffusion is fidelity. Expressed through an ideological, religious, occupational, or emotional commitment, fidelity includes faith in self as well as in others. Cults, causes, religious experiences, and many organizations provide important social agencies for the development of commitment. The teenager affirms the chosen sense of self by pledging loyalty to the group. In turn, the group confirms the individual as affiliated with a certain community. Whether the commitment chosen is capable of providing the needed confirmation is not easily discerned by the adolescent initially, but there is a growing discrimination in choice of commitment, more in line with personal values and attributes as the adolescent grows and matures. Internal rather than external standards are used increasingly to measure appropriateness of behavior.

Not all identity crises are age-related. Events that call into question real or perceived changes in relationships, parenting, responsibilities, work, lifestyle, and economic status can precipitate a temporary identity crisis. Colleges, career training, and the armed services...offer institutional support for the development of identity. Identity diffusion is seen in delinquency, psychosis, gender confusion, adult irresponsibility, and fanatical behaviors....

Intimacy versus isolation

Once a person has chosen a vocation, the next life task represents an extension of self in a shared relationship with another human being. Intimacy is the ability to join with another human being, to connect emotionally as well as physically in mutually satisfying ways. The ability to trust another's goodwill, a good sense of individual identity, and enough confidence in one's ability to relate effectively in the world build on previously learned interpersonal skills; they are necessary prerequisites to intimacy.

The ego strength associated with intimacy is love, described not simply as warm feeling, but rather as a complete commitment to merge with another person without fear of ego loss. In the development of intimacy, each partner brings a strong personal identity and chooses to share it for the mutual enrichment of both partners. If a clear sense of personal identity is not well established prior to choosing partnership, [intimacy will be difficult]. Others can enrich, complement, and offer feedback about the self; they should never be allowed to define it.

Intimacy can be physical, expressed through touching, hugging, sex; it can be intellectual, expressed through sharing of one's ideas; or it can be emotional,...finding expression in the nonpossessive sharing of the hopes, fears, and vulnerabilities that are in each of us. In its highest form, true emotional intimacy is made up of loyalties, interdependencies, shared experiences, memories of emotional meetings, conflicts, triumphs, disappointments, and a strong appreciation of...differences [and] similarities. Reduced to its simplest meaning, it is a respect for and a cherishing of the other person, just as he or she is, with no reservations. Intimacy acts to strengthen a sense of personal identity because it provides a powerful additional resource for expression and exploration of self within a safe relationship.

Isolation, the feeling of emptiness that often accompanies the sense that nobody cares, that there isn't anyone to share with, is the polar opposite of intimacy. Failure to risk being vulnerable in significant relationships or full emotional expression leads to insensitive responding and further feelings of loneliness. Friedman (1984) suggests that prolonged grieving may represent the unresolved part of the relationship, the things one wished one had expressed during the course of the relationship, but failed to share with the significant other....

Generativity versus stagnation and self-absorption

Generativity is the developmental stage associated with midlife. It "encompasses procreativity, productivity, and creativity" (Erikson, 1982). Having established a sense of intimacy with one other human being, the individual becomes eager to extend the sense of community. Once again, the individual reaffirms the sense of identity by investing the self in the interest of the larger society. The self-concept continues to evolve as honoring commitments and sharing one's talents with others reaches ascendancy. The benchmarks associated with this stage of ego maturation are not necessarily related to the number of family or community obligations, but rather to the quality of investment made to one another. It is quite possible to fill one's life with activity without being generative or to make many commitments without satisfying any of them. Generativity is expressed through work, community service, and creative endeavors as well as by procreation. The ego strength associated with generativity is caring, expressed through commitment.

A sense of self-absorption or stagnation evolves when an individual makes choices that sever personal commitments to one's fellow human beings. Unfinished tasks, unfulfilled obligations, and unrealized promises suggest an unsatisfactory resolution of this important life task. In times of stress, it is not unusual for energetic, dedicated individuals to lose the sense of generativity that characterized their previous dedication to the betterment of self and others....

Integrity versus despair

Erikson's final stage of ego development, Integrity versus Despair, focuses on the meaning and worth of one's life. Generally, if on balance a person has done all that is possible, given the information and situation known to the person at that time, life feels well lived. There is a basic integrity to one's life, the feeling "my job is done, I have done the best I could, and I am willing to go, knowing that other generations will carry on with what I have started. My life has mattered!" All other ego strengths are incorporated into this final stage of human development "so that a wise Indian, a true gentleman, and a mature peasant share and recognize in one another the final stage of integrity" (Erikson, 1968a). In old age, the self-concept turns inward for understanding, partly because of the need to understand the meaning of one's life and partly because some external reflections of human experience — work, family, spouse — are not as readily available. For this reason, life review is an important nursing strategy with elderly clients. A sense of despair develops when an individual realizes that life is almost over and that the opportunity to do things differently no longer exists. The nurse performs an important service in helping a client maximize the time left by making changes in attitude that permit fuller acceptance of the positive elements present in every situation.

The virtue of wisdom is associated with integrity. Wisdom comes from having lived life to the best of one's ability, from having few regrets about choices made, and from the person's willingness to share this experience with others. Because wisdom stirs from within, there is a growing sense of detachment from the things of the world, with the realization that the true treasure lies within....

Within each of us, the developmental remnants of earlier experiences persist and are reworked and interwoven into every individual's life (Erikson and Erikson, 1981).

Certain ritualizations, ceremonial acts, or culturally natural ways of doing things provide continuity between self and community by outlining guidelines for the social processes one must engage in for successful human adaptation in the community....

Prioritizing self-care needs

Abraham Maslow's theory of self- needs...is used by many nurses to classify health needs in the nurse-client relationship. Behaviors related to level of self-care needs are presented in Table 1.

Need deprivation in early childhood can lead to an almost insatiable hope for need satisfaction in adulthood. Illness, trauma, environmental changes, and developmental stages during the lifespan are naturally occurring variables that affect need satisfaction in some immediate and strange ways. Deprivation can arise from unmet needs or it can evolve as a consequence of overindulgence. Adults who give excessive need satisfaction — childhood overfeeding, overprotection, and permissive child-rearing — can cause children to expect similar treatment from others. When this behavior is not forthcoming, the individual feels insecure and sometimes bitterly deprived.

Although Maslow's theoretical hierarchical-need model is portrayed as linear and progressive, each stage of development is only partially independent of the others. Assessment of needs can be revised at any time in the life cycle when the situation dictates it. In the course of a hospitalization, need priorities may need to be updated, as circumstances can interfere with the client's need satisfaction. Applying this idea to the implementation of the nursing process, consider the following example:

> Mr. Rodgers has been admitted to the cardiac ICU with an acute myocardial infarction. He is a middle-aged businessman, internationally known, a corporate vice-president of a major company, and very well liked by his employees. His blood pressure for the past two years has never gone below a diastolic reading of 95, and he is being treated with a mild diuretic. His wife is always telling him to "slow down," and his two sons complain that their father is rarely home. Before this hospitalization, he had never seen the inside of a hospital.
>
> After his condition stablizes, Mr. Rodgers is discharged to the cardiac step-down unit and gradually begins the rehabilitative process that will necessitate some changes in his lifestyle.

Prior to admission, Mr. Rodgers could be seen as trying to meet love and belonging needs through his work, and perhaps also his self-esteem needs. His...heart attack changes the picture dramatically. If the nurse were to analyze client changes in need priority, upon admission, Mr. Rodgers' basic physiological needs would assume precedence. The nurse must see that he is continuously monitored by an EKG, provide the necessary medications, and measure intake and output; these aspects of care are required to maintain the balance of life processes. All other client needs recede in importance until the client's basic dynamic equilibrium [is restored].

Once Mr. Rodgers' condition has stabilized enough so it is no longer life threatening, the nurse might turn her attention to safety and security needs. Mr. Rodgers needs to briefly understand the implications of having a heart attack and should be oriented to the ICU and what he can expect from the ICU staff. Most people feel much more secure when they know what to expect. At this stage in his hospitalization, the nurse might designate safety and security needs as...priority, with the knowledge that, should Mr. Rodgers fail to maintain his current physiological equilibrium, the more basic physiological needs would again assume the highest priority.

As Mr. Rodgers improves and is transferred to the cardiac step-down unit, providing safety and security through a full orientation to the unit and staff remains a priority. Educative support regarding needed modifications in diet and lifestyle allow the client to begin regain-

TABLE 1. Psychosocial behaviors related to self-care needs

LEVELS OF NEED DEPRIVATION	PSYCHOSOCIAL BEHAVIORS
Physiological needs	Overfocusing on physiological need; difficulty sharing; compulsive eating; real or potential difficulty with body functions (respiration, elimination, digestion).
Safety needs	Separation anxiety, phobias; fear [of] new experiences; overdependence or noncompliance, helplessness; excessive worry about finances and future; rigidity; free-floating anxiety.
Love and belonging needs	Feeling of loneliness, alienation; demandingness; frequent illness; joining cults, gangs; some forms of juvenile delinquency; preoccupation with finding a friend or partner; teenage or out-of-wedlock pregnancy; affairs; difficulty trusting others; jealousy.
Self-esteem needs	Competitiveness; expressed feelings of low self-worth; controlling relationship behaviors; overachievement, underachievement; workaholism, narcissism; inability to complete commitments; midlife crisis; daydreams; seeking recognition and power; threatened by success of others; critical of and insensitive to needs of others.
Self-actualization	Dissatisfaction with life; boredom; inability to choose or reach realistic goals; self-absorption; expressed feelings of failure.
Self-transcendence	Egocentricity, selfishness; expressed feelings of emptiness [or dissatisfaction]; thrill-seeking; inability to forgive others.

ing physical and emotional control over his changed circumstances. But, once nursing actions related to security needs are accomplished to the satisfaction of nurse and client, secondary questions regarding sexuality and fitting back into the family and community begin to emerge. Since a heart attack is a warning sign of needed changes in lifestyle, the support of family is crucial to task accomplishment....

Maslow's hierachy of needs offers a useful framework for assessing the immediacy of need fulfillment for a given client. The behaviors suggested above can be used as an indication of inner needs. Paying attention to the client's need priorities gives the nurse some direction in planning nursing interventions that maximize client motivation and need satisfaction....

REFERENCES

Erikson E, Erikson J. On generativity and identity: From a conversation with Erik and Joan Erikson. Harvard Educational Rev 51:249, 1981.

Erikson E. Childhood and Society. New York, W.W. Norton, 1963.

Erikson E. Eight Ages of Man. *In* Gorlow L, Katkovsky W (eds.). Readings in the Psychology of Adjustment. New York, McGraw-Hill, 1968a.

Erikson E. The Life Cycle Completed: A Review. New York, W.W. Norton, 1982.

Friedman E. From a speech to a group of family therapists. Bethesda, MD, 1984.

Human interaction and personal boundaries

ANNE L. SCOTT, RN, MSN

Upon walking into Sarah's room you feel as if you have run into a cement wall. You have been her primary nurse for two days and thought you had a good relationship. Now you feel as if you are separated from her by an invisible wall.

While giving Mrs. J. some medication, you see her roommate get out of bed and pull her curtain closed between the two beds.

Sixteen-year-old Joe is going home in the evening and needs to be taught about his medication. You know his girlfriend is visiting, but doubt that he would object to your brief interruption. However, when you enter the room you strongly sense that your presence is not wanted.

THESE SITUATIONS ILLUSTRATE the concept of boundary. What is a boundary, how does it function, and why is it needed? What qualities should nurses look for in assessing their clients' boundaries, and how can nurses intervene in assisting clients in boundary regulation?

Clarification of boundaries

...From the literature and the characteristics of the various uses of the concept, the following attributes of boundary may be derived: A boundary separates a system from its external environment, defines the system's borders or limits, delineates the space and qualities belonging to the system, varies on a permeability continuum from closed to open, and is dynamic or flexible in an attempt to adapt to the environment.

An important step is to separate nursing's definition and use of boundaries from psychology and other disciplines. Nursing views man as a whole person consisting of body, mind, and spirit. The whole is greater than the sum of the parts. Thus, rather than looking just at ego boundaries or body boundaries, nursing defines the boundaries of a person in terms of the *whole* person. Boundary will be defined in this article as a dynamic line of demarcation separating an individual's internal (body, mind, and spirit) and external environments, and varying in permeability and flexibility. In the first example, when the nurse felt the wall between herself and her client, Sarah, she could sense that Sarah did not want to be touched (physical), talked to (mental), or even have anyone close to her (spiritual).

How boundaries function

The major characteristics of boundaries are permeability and flexibility. Permeability is defined as the degree to which a boundary is opened or closed, and varies on a continuum from closed to open. If the boundary is closed, then there is very little exchange between a person's internal environment and his external environment. If the boundary is open, the person may be talkative, social, and enjoy taking risks.

Flexibility is the ability of a person to move along the permeability continuum. If an individual is sometimes closed and sometimes opened (thus using the entire permeability continuum), then he is flexible. If, however, he is always toward the closed end of the continuum, having a low degree of flexibility, he could be described as "rigid closed." If a person is always open and never closed, he could be described as "rigid opened." The rigid closed person would be quiet and withdrawn most of the time. He would seldom, if ever, share his intimate secrets, dreams, and thoughts with even his best friend or spouse. A person who is rigid opened would nearly always be outgoing, talkative, ready to listen to others, and sharing intimate secrets with those he hardly knows. The flexible person is one who is quiet and withdrawn sometimes, usually when he senses an unsafe environment, and outgoing and willing to share himself with others at different times. The process of obtaining and maintaining a boundary begins with a person's need to individuate and adapt to the environment, and results in either a rigid closed boundary, a rigid opened boundary, or a flexible boundary. The individual with the flexible boundary is the only one who can successfully achieve individuation and adaptation (Landis, 1970; Reich, 1949). The ability to have a flexible boundary begins in the second half of an infant's first year and is attained prior to age three (Piaget, 1954; Mahler, 1975). However, even if one has the *ability* to be flexible, five other components are needed to maintain flexible boundaries: awareness of needs, communication, mental and spiritual strength, support, and an accurate perception of reality. One then needs to negotiate one's boundaries with others. For example, a person may feel threatened and fearful prior to surgery. To respect this person's boundaries would be to eliminate the pre-op medication and cancel the surgery. However, since this is unrealistic, the nurse and client may negotiate the boundaries. The nurse could acknowledge the client's fear and express empathy. She could then ask if she could help in any way (thus increasing safety in the external environment). Then she could say she had to give the pre-op medication now, but would close the curtains and leave the client alone for the next ten minutes (thus allowing for closed boundaries).

Why boundaries are needed

The purpose of a boundary is to facilitate individuation or separation from the environment. Developmentally, this begins at approximately six months of age. Mahler (1975) describes an infant's first attempts at separation-individuation as consisting of behaviors such as pulling at the mother's hair, ears, or nose, and straining the body away from the mother to have a better look at her. At seven to eight months, the infant begins to differentiate from the mother. The child closely examines the mother's glasses and jewelry and exhibits anxiety towards strangers. These crucial developmental steps are indicative of the child's beginning formation of his boundary. The process of boundary formation continues through the toddler stage. In the third year of life a fairly stable sense of identity (self-boundaries) is attained.

The second purpose of a boundary is to assist the individual in adapting to a continually changing environment. If a person is viewed as an open system, one can imagine the stimuli or energy entering and leaving the system in an attempt to regulate the internal environment to adapt to the external environment. The cell wall is an excellent example of this process as it varies in permeability in response to external environmental conditions in order to permit fluids and positive and negative ions to cross the cell wall (boundary). The result of this dynamic process is adaptation. The cell wall or boundary is what permits or possibly controls this function.

Assessment of boundaries

Landis (1970) conceptualized boundaries on a permeability continuum ranging from open to closed. However, he classified people into two categories: permeable-dominant (primarily opened) or impermeable-dominant (primarily closed). There is value in assessing the degree of flexibility in a person's boundary, since there are positive consequences [at] both ends of the continuum. The greater the flexibility in a person, the greater will be the ability to adapt. The studies done by Landis and Gruenthal (Landis, 1970) provide highly useful assessment criteria for the nurse (see Table 1). If a client has behaviors only in the permeable-dominant (opened) category and never (or rarely) in the closed category, the client would be considered to have "rigid opened" boundaries. If, however, the client exhibits some of the behaviors in both categories he would have "flexible" boundaries.

The flexible person is able to *choose* to be closed when perceiving an unsafe environment, but can also *choose* to be opened when perceiving a safe environment. The rigid person is either unable to choose to be closed or opened, or else his perception of the safety (or lack of safety) in his environment is inaccurate. Therefore, the flexible person is the healthiest and most adaptable.

Nursing interventions

Two major variables appear to have a direct effect on a person's ability to regulate his boundary: choice and perception of environmental safety. In order to choose, one needs to be aware of personal needs, have the mental and spiritual strength to communicate those needs and/or alter one's environment, have support, and communicate [with] others. In order to perceive the safety or lack of safety in the environment, one has to accurately perceive reality. Nurses can assist an individual in maintaining flexible boundaries by assisting them in these five areas: awareness of needs, mental and spiritual strength, support, communication, and accurate perception of reality. However, the client must have the ability to separate and individuate. If he does not have this ability, which is the case with many schizophrenics (Tausk, 1967), then although the nurse can help the client using these principles, the process will be less effective.

The nurse needs to first assess whether the client has rigid closed, rigid opened, or flexible boundaries. If the client has flexible boundaries, no interventions are required. If the client has rigid closed or rigid opened boundaries, the nurse should assess which of the five components of facilitation of flexible boundaries are lacking.

For example, Mr. R., the president of a large, successful firm, expresses continual anger at the nurses. He refuses medications and other forms of treatment. He has not formed any relationships with anyone since he was admitted two days ago, and has had no visitors. He emphatically demands that his set schedule of routines be adhered to by the health care staff.

The nurse's assessment indicated a "rigid closed" boundary. Of the five components, Mr. R. had mental and spiritual strength, and was able to communicate his need for control. However, he was unaware of his need for explanations of the medications and treatments he was receiving, lacked support, and perceived the environment as more threatening that it actually was.

To assist Mr. R. in attaining the three components he was lacking, the nurse first validated his need to understand his medications and treatments and then thoroughly explained them to him. She also explained the times he would be getting each medication and that the nurse would be in to give him the medication anytime from one-half hour before to one-half hour after the scheduled time. She offered to answer any questions he might have (which were many), and then continued to check on him closely throughout the evening. Because of this simple exchange, Mr. R. became aware of his need to know what was happening to him (medications

TABLE. Behaviors found in people with opened and closed boundaries

Open behaviors (permeable-dominant)
- Risk taking*
- Move rapidly into relationships*
- Little control over impulses*
- Overresponsive*
- Easily attracted to objects and people*
- Easily distracted*
- Perceive other people and objects in constant motion*
- Feel they are being drawn into action or acted upon*
- Spontaneity often accompanied by helplessness and infantile dependence*
- Aggressive impulses expressed but denied (conflict)*
- Ambivalence and hypersensitivity in relation to environment*
- Rush into relationships, then retreat, then rush in again (strong dependence accompanied by fear of being overwhelmed)*
- Cognitively try to grasp the totality of a situation before exploring different aspects, then show great flexibility*
- Enjoy being around people
- Talkative
- Share selves with others
- Admit errors easily
- Like to touch and be touched
- Readily show emotion
- Seek close relationships
- Democratic
- Short attention span

Closed behaviors (impermeable-dominant)
- Fear of closeness in interpersonal relationships*
- Cautious about relationships*
- Maintain emotional detachment*
- Protective mechanism*
- Dependency needs under conscious control*
- Expend greater effort maintaining impenetrable facade and firm controls (compulsive)*
- Have fear of not being able to maintain facade*
- Passive-aggressive conflict takes place on more conscious level—feelings of guilt and fear of punishment lead to conscious efforts to control these unacceptable hostile impulses*
- Fear of disclosure, of exposing themselves to the scrutiny of the environment*
- Consciously strive for internal and external control*
- Overemphasize structure—fear of weakness, softness, impotence*
- Tend toward manipulative control of environment*
- Initially tend to survey the overall situation; however, examine one part at a time with great scrutiny—as a detective or diagnostician tends to become absorbed by minor and sometimes insignificant details*
- Prefer being alone
- Quiet
- Do not share selves with others
- Hold grudges
- Do not like to touch or be touched
- Highly [organized]
- Protect secrets and territory
- Do not take risks
- Avoid close relationships
- Autocratic
- Long attention span
- Stoic

*Behaviors found in studies by Landis (1970).

and treatments), and gained the support of his nurse. Thus he began to perceive the hospital environment as safer than before. His boundaries began to open gradually as evidenced by his decreased hostility and increased friendly relationships with the health care staff.

Conclusion

Boundaries surround every individual and affect how that individual interacts with his environment. The nurse who understands how and why boundaries function, how to assess boundaries, and how to intervene can assist clients in individuating and adapting to their environment.

REFERENCES

Landis, B. Ego boundaries. *Psychological Issues* (Monograph No. 24). New York: International Universities Press, Inc., 1970.

Mahler, M., Pine, F., Bergman, A. *The Psychological Birth of the Human Infant.* New York: Basic Books, 1975.

Piaget, J. *The Construction of Reality in the Child.* New York: Basic Books, 1954.

Reich, W. *Character Analysis* (3rd ed.). New York: Orgone Institute Press, 1949.

Tausk, V. On the origin of the 'influencing machine' in schizophrenia. *The Psychoanalytic Reader* (rev. ed., Vol 1). New York: International University Press. 1967.

SECTION TWO

Common psychosocial concerns

COMMON PSYCHOSOCIAL PHENOMENA that a client may experience include denial, loneliness, fear, and grief. These can occur in diverse clinical settings, and can have devastating effects on the client.

By considering these psychosocial concepts, the nurse can help redefine the client's self-concept in the face of illness or tragedy. Through caring, the nurse can help the client discover new meanings about the self and others, and, through interpersonal relationships, find personal reward and career satisfaction.

Denial, the refusal to accept unpleasant facts, is a common psychosocial concern in clients who face painful or anxiety-producing situations. For example, a client may deny the death of a child or minimize the need for treatment. To help such a client, the nurse must know how to deal with the client's denial.

In "Denial," Forchuk and Westwell show the nurse how. They begin by defining denial and explaining how it can be a defense mechanism or a cognitive process. Then the authors describe how denial can be normal, as when it is part of the normal grieving process (see Unit Four), or abnormal, as when it forces a client to live in a fantasy world. Finally, the authors discuss nursing interventions for a client who uses denial and present methods of coping with the frustrations in caring for such a client.

Loneliness is an emotional state in which a client feels separated from others and experiences a need to be with people. It can cause feelings of sadness, despair, meaninglessness, and emptiness and can lead to mental illness. Although loneliness is common in elderly clients (as discussed in Unit Two in "Social Risk Factors: Impact of Elders' Perceived Health Status"), it can affect clients of any age.

Copel's "Loneliness: A Conceptual Model" provides an understanding of the factors that can lead to loneliness and offers a concrete way to visualize its effects. This valuable article describes how to help the client identify and cope with specific stressors that exacerbate loneliness. By mastering the techniques discussed by Copel, the nurse can help prevent the potentially devastating effects of loneliness.

Another common psychosocial concern, fear represents dread of an imagined or real occurrence—an automatic shutdown of perceptual awareness to protect the client from unacceptable problems and stress. In most health care settings, the client fears the unknown. For example, lack of knowledge can cause fear in a client who is undergoing a new diagnostic procedure or receiving an unfamiliar treatment. But fear is especially common in a client with a devastating disease, such as acquired immunodeficiency syndrome (AIDS).

Kennedy's "AIDS: Coping with the Fear" focuses on one of the most debilitating consequences of AIDS: fear. Kennedy investigates the nature of this psychosocial concern and discusses nursing strategies that can be used to reduce fear in the client, his or her family and friends, other clients, and even other health care professionals. This article is particularly relevent because the number of clients with AIDS is growing and because the nurse must know how to release the client from the paralyzing effects of fear before healing can begin.

According to the North American Nursing Diagnosis Association (NANDA, 1987), hopelessness is a "subjective state in which an individual sees limited or no alternatives or personal choices available and is unable to mobilize energy on one's own behalf." Other sources supply different definitions, but all agree that hopelessness can be far more devastating than a disease. Without hope, a client is compromised spiritually, psychologically, and possibly even physically.

The last article in this section, "Sorrow Has Many Faces: Helping Families Cope with Grief" by Archer and Smith, addresses the psychosocial concern of grief — a pattern of physical, emotional, and other responses to bereavement, separation, or loss. The authors assert that no single approach exists for grieving: Grief is different for each person. They advise the nurse to let each client experience grief in a personal and individual way rather than to expect the client to experience it precisely according to the five stages of grief (described in Unit Four in "What Is It Like to be Dying?").

Unusually sensitive in its approach, this article gives attention to concerns not normally discussed in the literature about grieving. It provides examples of discussions with family members and friends who have just suffered a sudden loss and points out physical, emotional, mental, social, familial, and spiritual dimensions of their grief. It reminds the nurse to assess a grieving client like any other client — that is holistically — to individualize interventions to meet the client's special needs.

REFERENCES

North American Nursing Diagnosis Association. (1987). *Classifications of Nursing Diagnosis: Proceedings from the Seventh National Conference*. St. Louis: C.V. Mosby Co.

Denial

Cheryl Forchuk, RN, BScN, BA, MScN; Jane Westwell, RN, BScN, MScN

This article provides an understanding of the theories of denial and then translates these theories into practice. It offers guidelines for assessing denial and for subtle interventions that avoid direct confrontation and aid resolution. Note: Some (marked by ellipses) background material has been deleted.

...Denial is a very broad concept that at times may seem to overlap with other terms such as avoidance, negation, allusion, self- deception, minimization, or even positive thinking (Lazarus & Folkman, 1984). Agreement is reflected in the definition of denial as consisting "of an attempt to disown the existence of unpleasant reality" (Campbell, 1981). The looseness with which the word is used in general conversation may interfere with its clarity in the clinical setting. At times, any "no" will be labeled as denial and the underlying dynamics are obscured. In this article an attempt will be made to clarify the process of denial and discuss appropriate nursing interventions.

Frameworks in which to view denial

Denial can be viewed from within several frameworks. Denial will be examined as both a defense mechanism and a cognitive process. The model the nurse uses has direct implications for nursing practice.

Denial as a defense mechanism. Defense mechanisms alter a person's perception of reality (Vaillant, 1971). This function is in direct conflict with another ego function — to determine reality. The process of how the defense mechanism denial operates, although simplified, is based on the four phases described by Dorpat (1983)....

The first phase of the process of denial is the "preconscious appraising of danger or trauma."...Dorpat believes that the appraisal of danger or trauma is usually carried out at a preconscious level, but states that conscious appraisals may also occur.

The second phase is called "painful affects and defensive actions." The individual has already determined that danger or trauma may be present; therefore, defensive action is initiated to avoid the unpleasant affects. At each stage of cognition there is an affective component that will determine whether a given stage of thinking will become conscious. Certain stimuli may register at the unconscious level, but will be blocked from conscious awareness.

During the third phase, "cognitive arrest," threatening information is actively excluded from conscious awareness. Attention is refocused elsewhere. Dorpat likens this process to what Sullivan (1953) called "selective inattention."

Dorpat views the process of excluding this material from conscious awareness as occurring in primary process thought. He states that the individual who is using denial unconsciously fantasizes about actively destroying that which is causing the unpleasant affect. These attacks prevent conscious awareness of the painful object; therefore, conscious cognition is prevented....

The cognitive arrest phase is usually followed by the fourth phase, screen behavior. "Screen behavior refers to the ideas, fantasies, affects, and overt behaviors activated by the...(individual's) need to fill the gaps formed in the cognitive arrest phase and to support its defensive aims" (Dorpat). In other words, screen behavior provides a cover story, which will make the information credible and internally consistent....

Denial as a cognitive process. Denial can also be conceptualized as a cognitive process. The works of Lazarus and Festinger will be discussed.

The appraisal process. Lazarus views denial as a cognitive process that may be used as a valuable first step in coping with stress (Goleman, 1979; Lazarus, 1981; Lazarus & Folkman). Within Lazarus' framework, stress is viewed as occurring in the transaction between the environment and the person. The individual's appraisal of an event and perception of her or his ability to cope determines how stressful the event will be for the individual. For example, Westwell (1983) found that women perceive a wide variation in the degrees of stress encountered in the early postpartum period. While some women experience great stress interpreting and responding to their infant's needs and behaviors, other women experience little stress and felt they responded intuitively and with ease.

Two ways of coping with stress are problem-focused and emotion-focused strategies (Lazarus & Folkman). Denial is an example of an emotion-focused way of coping. Emotion-focused strategies do not...change the situation but act to change how a person feels about the situation. Lazarus and Folkman state that there are many stresses where the individual cannot alter the situation. Therefore the effective strategies, which include denial, may be helpful, providing they do not prevent adaptive action.

Cognitive dissonance. Denial can be viewed within a framework of cognitive dissonance (Festinger, 1957). Cognitions are described as "any knowledge, opinion, or belief about the environment, about oneself, or about one's behavior." Dissonance occurs when there are inconsistencies or conflicts among an individual's cognitions. Festinger hypothesizes that the existence of dissonance is psychologically uncomfortable....This discomfort will motivate the person to reduce the dissonance between cognitions. Festinger states that the individual who experiences dissonance will also avoid situations and information that might be likely to increase the dissonance. Dissonance can be reduced by rejecting or altering an inconsistent cognition or adding a new cognition. This rejection of a cognition may be observed as "denial." For example, according to Forchuk (1984), a person who has alcoholism may experience dissonance if attempting to accept all three cognitions:

- "You are alcoholic";
- "You are worthwhile";
- "Alcoholics are not worthwhile."

The individual may reduce the dissonance by denying their alcoholism....An example of steps to be used within this framework is illustrated in Figure 1.

Is denial normal?

Denial has been described as both a pathological and normal ego defense mechanism. Anna Freud (1980) viewed denial as a normal, accepted mechanism for children, except when the child was unable to make the transformation from fantasy to reality readily or tried to shape...actual behavior according to the fantasy. Denial seems less likely to be perceived as a normal process as the person matures. Historically, denial "is usually ranked toward the bottom of ego hierarchies as indicating disorganization, primitivation, or distortion of reality and is considered inherently maladaptive" (Lazarus & Folkman). Kübler-Ross (1969) viewed denial as one of the normal stages of coping with a terminal illness. "Denial functions as a buffer after unexpected shocking news, allows the patient to collect himself and, with time, mobilize other, less radical defenses." Denial was seen as a tempo-

FIGURE 1. Assessing denial within a cognitive framework

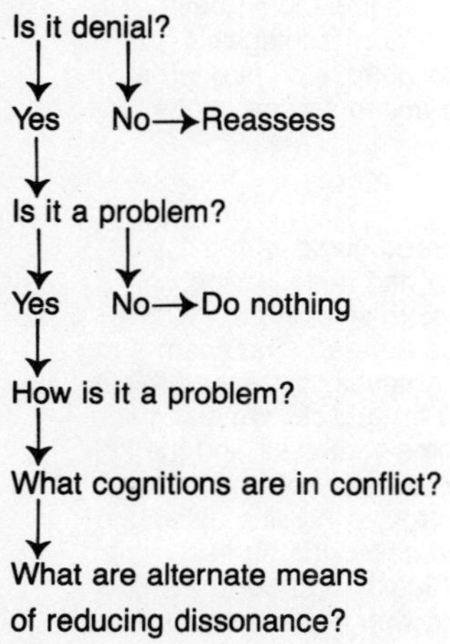

rary defense usually replaced by partial acceptance. Lazarus and Folkman view denial as a potentially helpful coping strategy.

Integrating theory and practice

The nurse may have difficulty translating theories related to denial into nursing interventions. For example, the nurse may have difficulty determining if what is being observed is actually denial. Confusing denial with lying or refusing to acknowledge the nurse's truth or reality are common pitfalls. However, when the nurse focuses on whether or not what she is seeing is "true" denial (as opposed to lying) the nurse's focus is on collecting the "proof" rather than enhancing an understanding of the patient's experience. Labeling every "no" as denial is as untherapeutic as forcing the patient to "prove" denial. For example, a person refusing to discuss an issue may not be using denial, but may consciously be deciding not to discuss the issue.

Part of comprehending the patient's experience involves understanding how the denial maintains the patient's sense of well-being. The nurse needs to keep in mind that denial protects the ego from having to acknowledge unpleasant realities.

Anxiety is implicitly or explicitly an important component of all the models described. Anxiety is an indication or symptom of perceived anger, threat, challenge, or conflict. It is not always readily apparent, however, what it is that the patient perceives as the danger, threat, challenge, or conflict. Peplau (1971) described the unpleasant experience of anxiety and how individuals may use specific behaviors in order to reduce their anxiety. Denial may be viewed as an example of an anxiety-reducing behavior. The nurse needs to listen to what the patient is saying about his or her experience and perceptions. The patient's behavioral and situational factors also require consideration. In Case Report 1, this understanding was very important for the nurses caring for Ms. A, who had delivered a stillborn baby. Ms. A was diagnosed as having a postpartum psychosis with her major defensive style being denial. Staff recognized the symbolism of her actions, but did not verbalize these with her or confront her. Instead they discussed her feelings around wanting the baby.

Understanding that denial serves a protective function makes it clear why confronting denial directly can be viewed as ineffective and untherapeutic. Not only would direct confrontation serve to increase the individual's anxiety, causing the need for denial to increase, it may undermine the nurse-patient relationship....

Because a direct confrontive approach is not generally indicated with the models described, the nurse needs an alternative approach. Denial serves a protective function and sometimes the alternative is to do nothing or at least to delay action. The patient's interpretation of the nurse's actions and the nurse's

Denial as a defense mechanism

Case 1
Ms. A was seven months pregnant when she was admitted via the Emergency Department in premature labor. She delivered a stillborn baby, but seemed to be coping well. "I'm fine...everything will be all right." On the day of planned discharge she was observed stuffing tissue paper into her ears, nose, and later into her vagina and rectum. When questioned about this behavior, she responded by asking staff to feel the baby kick and asked to have the fetal heart rate monitored.

Case 2
Mr. B was a self-employed businessman who had always prided himself on his good health despite smoking two packages of cigarettes daily. When informed he had terminal lung cancer he stated simply, "I know there has been a mistake...I'm just tired. There's nothing wrong with me." He proceeded to "tidy up" his business and personal affairs so he could take a "long vacation."

Mr. B's wife called the public health unit to ask a nurse to visit her dying husband and help him talk about his impending death. On the day of the visit Mrs. B apologized profusely for her husband, who had left saying he saw no need to talk to a nurse as he had no problems.

Case 3
Ms. C was a registered nurse with three young children. She had been having increasing difficulties in sleeping at night. A physician friend had ordered lorazepam 2 mg b.i.d., but she had gradually increased this to 8 mg b.i.d. "I'm not an addict...I'm just going through a difficult time with work and the kids and need some extra help, but I have the situation under control." A nursing colleague was concerned and called the nurses' "addiction hotline." Ms. C agreed to a confidential meeting with a nurse counselor to "get them off my back."

understanding of the patient's situation will vary according to the stage of the relationship. Another facet in considering what, if any, action should take place is how fixed or how temporary the denial may be. Because denial may be temporary, time may be all that is needed. This is illustrated in the nursing interventions planned for Mr. B, the businessman denying his illness. The nurse helped Mrs. B ventilate her feelings of concern and frustration and did health teaching around normal stages of grief and dying. Neither Mrs. B nor the public health nurse confronted Mr. B with his illness or his denial.

Another possible intervention is to find a "back door" approach. The "back door" approach enables the patient to work on a less anxiety-producing part of the issue rather than dealing with the more anxiety-producing parts. An example is the situation described earlier where the cognition "Alcoholics are not worthwhile" was dealt with rather than directly confronting the denial reflected in "I am not alchoholic." A similar cognitive approach was used with Ms. C, the nurse who abused lorazepam. The nurse counselor discussed with Ms. C her interpretations of "addict" and gave some brief nonjudgmental health teaching related to addiction. The "label" issue was put aside and nonpharmacological strategies to help her cope were explored over several outpatient visits.

Nurses frequently describe feelings of frustration and fear that they are being manipulated when caring for patients who are using denial. It is difficult for the nurse to experience these feelings and not assume a judgmental attitude and project blame onto the patient. Awareness of one's own defensive structure, which includes denial, may help the nurse in avoiding this common pitfall. Recognizing the interpersonal and intrapersonal dynamics may help the nurse to have an intellectual and affective understanding. This understanding allows the nurse to remain emotionally available to the patient.

Nurses may be concerned that they will be reinforcing the patient's denial unless they confront the patient with "reality." A helpful technique (drawn from the assertiveness literature) is "fogging" or "agreeing with truth" (Smith, 1975). The nurse can agree with the part of the denial that is based in reality. For example, a statement such as "It sounds like you believe you are not abusing your medication" could be used with Ms. C without direct confrontation ("It sure sounds to me like you've been abusing your medication") or reinforcement of denial ("You're not abusing your medication").

The myriad of emotions generated within both patient and nurse make denial a very complex and difficult issue. There is no easy solution to assist patients with denial, but understanding the theoretical process of denial gives the nurse a framework within which alternatives can be found.

REFERENCES

Campbell, R.J. *Psychiatric Dictionary,* ed. 5. New York: Oxford University Press, 1981.

Dorpat, T.L. The cognitive arrest hypothesis of denial. *Int J Psychoanal* 1983; 64:47-58.

Festinger, L. *A Theory of Cognitive Dissonance.* Evanston, Illinois: Row, Peterson and Company, 1957.

Forchuk, C. Cognitive Dissonance: Denial, self-concepts and the alcoholic stereotype. *Nursing Papers* 1984; 16:57-69.

Freud, A. *The Ego and the Mechanisms of Defense,* rev. ed. New York: International Universities Press, Inc., 1966.

Goleman, D. Positive denial: The case for not facing reality. *Psychology Today* 1979; 13: 44-60.

Kübler-Ross, E. *On Death and Dying.* New York: Macmillan Publishing Company, Inc., 1969.

Lazarus, R.S. The costs and benefits of denial, in Dohrenwend, B.S., Dohrenwend, B.P. (eds.): *Stressful Life Events and Their Contexts.* New York: Prodist Publications, 1981.

Lazarus, R.S., Folkman, S. *Stress Appraisal and Coping.* New York: Springer Publishing Company, 1984.

Peplau, H. A working definition of anxiety, in Burd, S.F., Marshall, M.A. (eds.): *Some Clinical Approaches to Psychiatric Nursing.* London: The Macmillan Company, 1971.

Smith, M. *When I Say No, I Feel Guilty.* New York: Dial Press, 1975.

Sullivan, H.S. *The Interpersonal Theory of Psychiatry.* New York: W.W. Norton & Company, 1953.

Vaillant, G.E. Theoretical hierarchy of adaptive ego mechanisms. *Arch Gen Psychiatry* 1971; 24:107-108.

Westwell, J.M. *Coping Processes and Resources Used by Primiparous Women in the Postpartum Period,* thesis. Toronto: University of Toronto, 1983.

Loneliness: A conceptual model

LINDA CARMAN COPEL, RN, PhD

According to many health care professionals, loneliness is a precursor of mental illness. Fortunately, the nurse is in a strategic position to identify loneliness and help the client deal with it. By studying the model presented in this article and learning to use a framework for loneliness assessment, intervention, and evaluation, the student can prepare for this vital role. Note: Extensive background and theoretical material has been deleted (marked by ellipses).

...LONELINESS IS A UNIVERSAL experience which can threaten feelings of personal worth, undermine confidence in interpersonal relationships, and disrupt decision-making abilities and thought processes. Any or all of these factors may inhibit therapeutic treatment of the client. The phenomenon of loneliness in the client can be perceived and dealt with by the nurse. Since nurses assist patients to cope with both physical and psychosocial experiences of illness, it is essential that nurses strive to recognize the manifestations and effets of the phenomenon of loneliness.

Sullivan (1953) discussed loneliness and proposed that humans are social animals with a need for contact and interaction with others. When this need is not fulfilled, it is expressed in loneliness. When people take action to avoid or to relieve the tension impeding their desire for interpersonal intimacy, there is enhancement of self-esteem and decreased potential for the development of loneliness....

There is in every person an innate longing or desire for interpersonal intimacy. This inherent drive stays with the human being from infancy through adult life. During the life cycle a person constantly strives to fulfill this need by connecting to another person or persons. As one matures, the need for a satisfying social network extends beyond family members. In the process of living, a person realizes the need to develop and maintain relationships. Human contact prevents one from feeling isolated or estranged, and thus separated from human caring. The feelings of acceptance, support, and love enable one to experience a sense of wholeness and fulfillment.

Confronting the individual's movement towards establishing a connection with others is internally and externally caused tension. During the course of life, all individuals experience physical, social, and emotional tensions which influence whether or not they encounter loneliness. Tension arises primarily from feelings of lack of trust, shame, grief, alienation, social obstacles, cultural patterns, and pain.

The ability to trust is basic to all human interactions. Trust is believed to begin with the dependent relationship that the infant has with the primary caretaker. Basic survival of the infant revolves around the creation of this bond of trust. Being able to rely on others positively affects one's maturational process. As one ages, a multitude of living experiences shapes one's ability to trust and to discriminate [among] interpersonal expectations (Beard, 1982).

The caretaker's failure to satisfy basic needs results in a lack of trust. If the ability to trust is not cultivated and nurtured as part of the individual's developmental process, a decrease in positive interactions will be noted.

Not being able to trust heightens the person's sensitivity to feelings of being unaccepted, devalued, and misunderstood by others. Lack of trust generates increasing tension as the person struggles to establish and sustain interpersonal relationships.

The concept of shame reflects feelings of inadequacy and insecurity. When a person feels shame, there is a tendency to withdraw from others and avoid interpersonal relationships. Like the ostrich, the person experiencing shame hides from others and continually lives with the fear of having unacceptable aspects of self-exposure to others. A person feels threatened by the presence of social disapproval (Shane, 1980). Severe tension is generated from feelings of being scrutinized by others.

The process of responding to a loss is grief. Loss, whether observable or perceived, occurs whenever the person is faced with either lifestyle adaptation or changes. The ability to experience grief is learned. How well an individual cultivates and maintains relationships will influence that person's expression of grief. Grief is a social process and it needs to be shared and supported by others. The focus during stressful times is directed towards proceeding through the grieving process. Tension generated by the loss and accompanying grief work is overwhelming.

The experience of alienation is one in which a person feels detached from self and society. There is avoidance of emotional connectedness and general feelings of estrangement. Often alienation results when an event precipitating physical separation or isolation occurs. May (1953) believed that whenever a person acknowledges feelings of being on the outside of life or being out of touch with the self, alienation exists. The stress of alienation further deteriorates relationships and self-investing opportunities (Yoder, 1977).

Social obstacles represent anything that impairs social connectedness between people. Among the examples of social barriers is anything that facilitates isolation, boredom, or despair. Common examples include poverty, family dysfunctions, friendship changes, financial difficulties, deteriorating neighborhoods, altered living accommodations, and physical or mental limitations. Underlying each of the examples cited is the feeling of decreased worth as a human being. Social obstacles impede opportunities for social contact and are major sources of tension for the individual.

Within each person there are cultural patterns which provide the roles and directions which provide the roles and directions for daily living. All beliefs, values, and behaviors are rooted in one's culture. The roles one takes on, the norms for a group, and how communication is processed are influenced by culture. The layers of culture consist of religion, politics, economics, health, social class, and geographic environment. These layers impact to some degree on each individual. Changes in any of the layers foster anxiety within the cultural system. Conflict among beliefs, values, and behaviors disrupt the individual's world. Tension can be mild or severe depending upon how deviant the behavior is viewed.

The last factor, pain, is viewed as a perception of some degree of discomfort based on the influences of physiological, psychological, and social phenomena. Pain is a personal and complex multifaceted experience which defies simple definition. Numerous factors may cause the person to have pain or modulate the pain experience. A person's response to pain reflects the struggle of the cycle of pain. Pain begets tension which begets more pain which begets more tension.

The identified sources of tension can independently or collectively influence the individual's risk for loneliness. Individuals attempt to use their resources and opportunities to overcome these various tensions. The ability to cope effectively with tension moves the person away from a loneliness experience. If the person lacks the abilities to conquer or defend against these stressors, loneliness results.

Every person who successfully deals with stressful life situations demonstrates adequate decision making. The ability to make positive decisions regarding one's behavior facilitates human interaction. A person makes decisions with a direct or indirect goal in mind. Either the direct or indirect approach is an acceptable way to attain goals. Individuals may consistently select one approach over another or use the approach that best produces the desired outcome. The direct goal approach constitutes the person's desire or attraction toward a group, another person, God, or tradition (Reisman, 1979). With an indirect approach, a person chooses to be removed from activities with others and seeks aloneness or solitude.

The experience of aloneness is the physical separation of self from others. Removing the self from others allows the person to pause, reenergize, and focus on a particular aspect of the self. This activity is at least neutral and at best an opportunity to maintain or revitalize the self. Solitude is the emotional state where the person withdraws into an activity or fantasy of that person's own creation. The state of solitude is actively sought out, and one's conscious awareness focuses on maintaining that state. Moustakas (1961) postulated that true solitude facilitates the opportunity to become introspective, to concentrate, and to focus one's energy on particular work or dilemmas. The process of achieving these goals culminates in a person's growth, increased self-esteem, creative expression, productiveness and self-actualization (Reisman, 1979).

Use of model in clinical practice

A nurse in any setting may use this model to assess a client for loneliness. During a formal interview or in any nurse-client interaction, the nurse discusses or observes stressors and how these stressors impact on the client. The quantity and intensity of tension places a person at risk for loneliness. Appropriate coping mechanisms enable the client to deal with tension. Examining the client's capacity to make decisions directly influences movement away from loneliness. People who make decisions can become involved in human interaction and distance themselves from loneliness. The nurse can use this model to assist in focusing the assessment process on stressors which generate tension and promote loneliness. Identifying behaviors such as sadness, resignation, despair, emptiness, and meaninglessness provides the nurse with the awareness that these behaviors are the consequences of loneliness.

Nursing interventions are based on assisting the client to identify and deal with specific tensions that exacerbate loneliness. To build adequate coping mechanisms effectively, the nurse encourages [the] client to use or refine...abilities to make decisions. Often [a] client [is] not aware of the options. [The nurse can assist] the client to problem solve, determine goals, make decisions, and become familiar with how to promote human interactions....

The nature of loneliness is such that the nurse may expect repeated episodes of loneliness to occur as the client faces additional stressors. The client may move through the [various stages of loneliness] multiple times.

Nursing care evaluation reflects the client's ability to overcome tension, make decisions, establish goals, and demonstrate positive outcomes. The model outcomes can be demonstrated in a variety of ways. Positive outcome will be the completion of a goal that in some ways demonstrates fulfillment of self-esteem needs.

A clinical example

The following example illustrates the practical applicability of the model for the nurse clinician. A six-year-old child experiences the disruption of the family as her parents divorce and she moves with mother and other siblings into a small apartment. Mother now works two jobs, and several new neighbors in the apartment complex babysit the children. The child experiences difficulty in first grade. Teachers suggest that the child undergo evaluation for learning disabilities and other related health screenings. The school nurse meets with the child and observes an underweight, sad, relatively non-communicative child in need of improvement with hygiene practices. A subsequent meeting with mother and child reveals the stressors of divorce, relocation, financial difficulties, and loneliness. Nursing diagnoses for the family include:

1) Loneliness related to changes in interpersonal relationships, family and environmental losses, grief, and feelings of inadequacy and insecurity.

2) Ineffective family coping related to disruption of lifestyle from divorce, relocation, and financial difficulties.

3) Disturbance in self-concept related to decreased self-esteem, change in role performance, emotional pain, and feelings of sadness and despair.

Interventions are directed at mother and child. Mother is referred to a community mental health woman's support group run by a psychiatric facility. The nurse group leader verifies the impressions and assessment of the school nurse and formulates interventions to assess the need for human interaction, development of coping strategies, and future goal determination. At the school the nurse meets with the child. Together they work on development of trust, promoting the child's adequacy, and facilitating nurturing and social approval.

Brief frequent conferences with the teachers yield strategies to facilitate interpersonal relationships with peers, and feelings of acceptance and value. Arrangements for an evaluation of learning disabilities with the school psychologist, as well as a physical exam with the school district's pediatric nurse practitioner or physician, are made. Six months later, a follow-up [report shows the child's] improved academic performance after [she was transferred] into the guided learning classroom setting, increased self-initiated interaction with peers, and beginning ability to talk about life at home. A weight increase of five pounds now reflects the appropriate height-weight growth and development parameters for a six-year old female. A follow-up report on the mother states that she continues to participate in the woman's group, has acquired a female friend, and verbalizes more positive feelings about her ability to provide for the children....

REFERENCES

Beard, M. Trust life events and risk factors among adults. *Advances in Nursing Science* 1982; 4(4):26-43.

May, R. *Man's Search for Meaning*. New York: W.W. Norton, 1953.

Moustakas, C. *Loneliness*. Englewood Cliffs, NJ: Prentice-Hall, 1961.

Peplau, H. Loneliness. *American Journal of Nursing* 1955; 55:1476-1481.

Peplau, L.A., Pearlman, E. Perspectives on loneliness. In Peplau, L.A. & Pearlman, D. (eds). *Loneliness: A Sourcebook of Current Theory, Research, and Therapy*. New York: John Wiley, 1982.

Reisman, J. *Anatomy of Friendship*. New York: Irvington, 1979.

Shane, P. Shame and learning. *American Journal of Orthopsychiatry* 1980; 50:348-354.

Sullivan, H.S. *The Interpersonal Theory of Psychiatry*. New York: W.W. Norton, 1953.

Yoder, S. Alienation as a way of life. *Perspectives in Psychiatric Care* 1977; 15:66-71.

AIDS: Coping with the fear

MARGARET KENNEDY, RN

CARING FOR PATIENTS with acquired immunodeficiency syndrome (AIDS) means grappling with its most contagious, debilitating effect: fear. But our experience has taught us that nursing interventions can help keep fear from overwhelming the patient, his family and friends, other patients, and even staff members.

Our patients, our teachers

Two years ago, when we learned that our medical/surgical unit would be accepting AIDS patients, many of us began to read everything we could find about the disease. That certainly made the clinical picture clearer.

Little information was available, however, about the AIDS patient's emotional status. That meant our patients would become our teachers. Meeting Richard, my first AIDS patient, gave me an insight I would draw on again and again. I'd returned from a day off to find the nurses on my unit buzzing about the AIDS patient with Kaposi's sarcoma who'd been admitted the night before. Seems he'd made his presence felt — strongly — with incessant, irritable demands. I assigned myself to him for that evening.

When I went into his room, my "challenge" was lying in bed, covers pulled up to his chin. He interrupted my "Hello, I'm Margaret" with a testy recitation of what he would and would not do, and what he would permit *me* to do and not do.

"Stop!" he commanded, as I approached his bed. "Stay right where you are. Don't come near my I.V. — I was bruised enough last night when the nurse inserted this needle, and I don't need you to dislodge it.

"What you *can* do is call whoever's in charge. I want to register a formal complaint about the maid service here. Look at that sticky gunk on the floor and the dust on my nightstand. If I don't get prompt action, I'm calling my attorney."

"Well, that sounds fair enough," I said calmly.

I promised to look at — but not touch — his intravenous line. While I wiped up the orange juice on his floor and dusted off his nightstand, I chatted about using him as a reference to apply at the local Hilton. That small joke eased the tension, and he seemed to relax somewhat.

I started to leave the room, replaying the whole scene in my mind. "Unbelievable," I thought. "What's *really* happening here?" Suddenly it came to me: Richard was in crisis. Overwhelmed by his situation, he was sending out distress signals to everyone.

Turning back, I met Richard's eyes: I'll never forget the helpless, desperate look in them.

I touched his shoulder and said, "I have a feeling you and I are going to become very good friends." For the first time, I saw the little smile that would later become so familiar. All he said, though, was, "You know, you may be right."

In charting my assessment, I used a single word to describe Richard's number one problem — fear. Helping him cope with that fear would be my number one goal.

"I'm a dying man"

As I would discover during the next 2 years, AIDS patients may respond to their disease differently — with denial, anger, depression, or withdrawal. But the underlying emotion is fear. That's hardly surprising, given the disease's devastating effects and the fact that there is no cure.

One night while I was in Richard's room, a newscaster reported the latest mortality figures for AIDS. "Just a friendly reminder from the media that I'm a dying man," Richard said. Then he started to cry.

I tried to reassure Richard that his diagnosis didn't mean he'd die immediately: Infectious disease episodes are treatable; he could possibly live for a number of years. The point was to focus on living, not dying.

Other threats *are* more immediate, such as loss of income. Richard ran a very profitable real estate firm, which of course involved a great deal of public contact. A handsome man, he considered his attractiveness a business asset. But as his Kaposi's sarcoma worsened, he liked what he saw in the mirror less and less. Once he said to me, "Who would want someone with these ugly sores on his face showing people their home? How am I going to make a living?" Another fear weighing on the patient is that AIDS may also strike those he cares about (and needs so much now). I remember Gary, a patient who had Kaposi's sarcoma, confiding to me, "I shudder whenever the phone rings — I've lost over 20 friends to AIDS in the past year. And I'm really worried about my roommate Tom. He has some sores on his legs, but he won't see a doctor." Gary's sense of guilt about having possibly passed the disease along to Tom was nearly as overwhelming as his concern for his friend's health.

When Tom came to visit, I asked if I could speak to him alone. We talked for over an hour; mostly, I listened as he tried to sort out his feelings. He finally agreed to see a doctor.

Fear among friends and family

As Tom's denial of his symptoms demonstrates, those close to the patient have fears of their own. Like Tom, many partners of AIDS patients remain loyal, spending a lot of time at the bedside. But they're dealing with a double-edged fear — anxiety about their partner's welfare and their own health ("Am I next?"). Information about safe sex practices and human immunodeficiency virus (HIV) screening can help allay some of that fear.

If an AIDS patient is married, the spouse may carry the added burden of worrying about their children's health. One patient's wife didn't know of his bisexuality until he became ill. After she and their infant daughter tested positive for the HIV virus, she rarely visited, despite pleading phone calls from him. Shortly before he died, she called only to tell him she'd given away his dog. Fear and anger here had turned into retaliation.

Because most AIDS patients are young, their parents are usually still living. The death of a child, regardless of his age, is a special grief, complicated by the stigma associated with AIDS. Besides worrying about losing their son, parents may dread public disclosure of his sexual preference. A mother of a young heterosexual male with AIDS told friends that her son had an immunodeficiency disease, but not AIDS. Unfortunately, some parents learn about their son's homosexuality or bisexuality only when they learn his diagnosis. Richard once joked, "The hardest part of having AIDS is...how do I tell my mother I'm Haitian?" Not a very funny dilemma, though, for the patient, nor for parents dealing with two disturbing revelations.

Even friends of the patient may find their fears keep them from giving him the support he needs. Some of Richard's friends, for instance, asked if inviting him to their homes for dinner after his discharge would be "safe." I reassured them that transmission of AIDS occurs through direct contact of body secretions, primarily blood or semen. There is no evidence that the disease can be transmitted through casual contact.

Other patients' concerns

Although infection-control procedures can protect other patients physically, they may need *emotional* protection as well. They're afraid, too: AIDS may be the most talked about but least understood disease of our time.

While walking in the hall with her husband, a patient paused at a door that had an isolation sign. She gasped as if it read "Live Explosives." I heard her say, "I wonder if that patient has AIDS, because if he does, I'm getting out of here fast."

What should we say when patients ask, "Do you ever get AIDS patients on this unit?" As nurses, we can convey the *facts* about AIDS to patients and visitors. Usually, once they understand the means of transmission, their fear lessens.

Here's an example of how facts can reduce fear. A postsurgical patient refused to have a blood transfusion unless I would "guarantee" that she wouldn't get AIDS. After I reassured her about the blood bank's HIV virus screening and testing, she felt less threatened and agreed to the transfusion.

Confronting your own fears

Of course, before they can offer anyone else information and support, health care workers caring for AIDS patients must confront their own fears — fears that may be heightened by their families' concerns for their safety. My husband, for example, used to worry that I'd stick myself with a needle when starting an intravenous line for an AIDS patient. As time passed without any incidents, that fear faded.

The staff did have legitimate concerns. What if an AIDS patient needs cardiopulmonary resuscitation? Our unit's answer is to have a disposable Ambu bag and oral airway available.

Should nurses assigned to AIDS patients also care for other immunosuppressed patients? Could we spread the disease to these patients through some error in technique? Again, because time has shown us that careful technique is the best safeguard against infection, the nurses on our unit care for *all* patients.

Research suggests that some health care professionals display signs of homophobia — fear of homosexuals. (Some may even see AIDS as God's punishment for the "sin" of being homosexual.) To determine if such attitudes exist at our hospital, we're circulating a questionnaire to identify the feelings and concerns of those caring for AIDS patients. Based on the results, we'll plan interventions to ensure quality care.

Generally, though, our experience with AIDS has already taught us that the more staff members know about this disease — and the more AIDS patients they've cared for — the more comfortable they are.

Something else happens, too: Just as panic is contagious, patients and visitors seem to take on the staff's confidence.

Important thing is to try

We can do much to help the AIDS patient and those around him deal with their fears. But we also must recognize that we won't always succeed.

Despite constant and conscientious efforts, we were never able to help Richard cope with his fears. After many long hospitalizations, he had an emotional breakdown. When his friends withdrew, he depended on us more and more. We did our best for him, but when Richard died he was still a frightened man.

The important thing is we *tried* to help him. Had we done nothing, we would have failed in a far worse way. When working with AIDS patients, we have an obligation to use our skills and knowledge not just to prevent transmission of the disease itself but also to control the fear it creates, a fear to which no one is immune.

Sorrow has many faces: Helping families cope with grief

DAREN N. ARCHER, RN, MSN; ANNE CLARKE SMITH, MS

WHO HASN'T FELT inadequate when talking to family members after a loved one has died? What can you say to lessen their pain? Surprisingly, what you've read or learned about the stages of grief in your nursing education may be as much of a hindrance as a help.

The main weakness of the typical stages-of-grief model is its narrow focus on psychological responses — denial, anger, bargaining, depression, and acceptance. This emphasis overlooks other grief reactions, including social, spiritual, familial, and physical responses.

Moreover, because the stages-of-grief model is easy to remember, understand, and teach, some practitioners have altered it into a how-to model, implying that a mourner need only progress through the stages to recover from grief. As your real-life experience with grieving families has probably taught you — and as we've learned from our own painful experience with personal loss — that's not necessarily so.

To overcome those shortcomings, we've developed a holistic model of grief, one that recognizes that each person relates to his world in many different ways. Incorporating the findings of various disciplines, this model can help explain some of the responses you've seen that don't fit the traditional stages of grief.

Reactions to sudden loss

Perhaps the best way to explain the holistic model is through an example. Imagine yourself in this scenario: You're an emergency department nurse. Early one Saturday night, the ambulance crew brings in a 2-month-old baby named David. When his 14-year-old baby-sitter checked on him in his crib, she discovered he'd stopped breathing. The emergency team responding to her call was unable to resuscitate him.

The baby-sitter lived next door to the baby's family; her mother, Mrs. Avery, rode with the baby in the ambulance. The baby's parents, Bob and Ellen Carr, were attending a wedding reception with his maternal grandparents, the Stoners. They are all waiting in a private lounge to talk to you.

After you introduce yourself, you say, slowly and deliberately, "I understand Dr. Young told you that your son, David, is dead. He also explained that because David was a healthy baby, the cause of death might have been sudden infant death syndrome. To be sure, an autopsy must be performed. But before David's body is removed for the autopsy, you could see him to say good-bye. Would you like me to arrange that?"

Knowing the stages-of-grief model, you expect to encounter denial, shock, or numbness in the bereaved family. But these are the responses you do encounter:

Mr. Carr: "I don't want my son to suffer any more than he already has. I don't want an autopsy. I just want them to give David to us. We can take care of him ourselves."

Mrs. Carr: No response at all. She looks past you into the hall and seems to be listening to something outside the room.

Mrs. Stoner: "I've never heard of anyone wanting to see a dead baby. I don't think it's right for us to see him. My goodness, people don't really do that, do they?"

Mr. Stoner: "We all need to stay calm. I don't think the children should be upset any further. Let's not have any more talk about seeing the baby."

Mrs. Avery (addressing Mrs. Carr): "Honey, I know David's passing has upset you, but remember that God will take care of your little angel now. We can thank God that David will never suffer again."

No one response

Obviously, denial isn't the only response found here. Each person reacted to the loss differently. The holistic model recognizes such individual responses because it assumes that a person relates to his world from many interconnected dimensions. The death of a loved one is a wound to the inner self: Emanating from within, pain is felt in all dimensions of a person's life — physical, emotional, mental, social, familial, and spiritual.

The following list doesn't include all the possibilities, but it does suggest the variety of grief responses that the holistic model recognizes:

• ***physical.*** Short-term responses include: crying, insomnia, fatigue, decreased or increased appetite, headaches, heart palpitations, dizziness, nausea, vomiting, diarrhea, constipation, heaviness or crushing feeling in the chest, lump in the throat, and emptiness. (Although these symptoms generally don't last long, they may recur on anniversary dates of the death for years to come.)

Long-term responses include: rheumatoid arthritis, peptic ulcer, irritable bowel syndrome, ulcerative colitis, substance abuse, heart disease, angina, eating disorders such as anorexia and bulimia, menstrual irregularity, migraines, and other chronic conditions.

• ***emotional.*** A range of negative emotions is possible: from moderate irritation to anger to irrational rage; from mild anxiety to fear to paralyzing terror; from slight wistfulness to sadness to suicidal despair; from vague doubts to regrets to immobilizing guilt.

• ***mental.*** Transient responses include shock, denial, forgetfulness, disorganization, inability to concentrate, and absentmindedness. Chronic responses may include intellectualization. This factual awareness without emotional response might be seen in someone who repeats expressionlessly, "I know my baby's dead." Another response is determined optimism, which leads to an unrealistic expectation of rapid resolution of grief: "Don't worry about us, we'll be fine." Rationalization is also possible — premature acceptance and avoidance of "why me?" The mourner may say, "This happens to other families all the time" or "I know he'll be better off now."

• ***social.*** Because our culture doesn't prescribe set mourning rituals, those who want to console the bereaved are left largely to their own devices. "Comforting" remarks or gestures usually fall into two categories.

Appropriate consolation is usually offered by those who recognize the deep, enduring pain caused by the loss. They don't try to minimize the loss or cheer up the bereaved prematurely. On the other hand, people who are blinded by their own ignorance, discomfort, insensitivity, or malice are more likely to offer inappropriate consolation. They'll try to rationalize, deny, or minimize the grieving person's pain.

• ***familial.*** At one end of the spectrum is the optimally functioning family, in which each member tolerates and supports the grieving of every other member. At the opposite end is the dysfunctional family, in which one of these four coping mechanisms is used almost exclusively:

1. One family member grieves too much, virtually to the point of being immobilized; other members don't grieve enough, but busy themselves with day-to-day responsibilities.

2. To minimize their sense of loss, one or both members of a grieving couple may become involved with another person. A husband or wife may have an affair after the death of a child. Or they may become obsessed with

the thought of having another baby. Or they may become unduly concerned about another child's problems.

3. Emotional distancing occurs. Each family member mourns alone, unable to share his grief with other family members.

4. Marital conflict can develop around a variety of issues. Sometimes one member of a couple feels guilt or blames the other for the death. The conflict may center on a recurring problem that is exacerbated by the loss. Or it may be a misunderstanding about the depth of the spouse's grief in relation to one's own.

• ***spiritual.*** A grieving person usually seeks answers to philosophical questions, which may include: Is there a God or higher power? Did He allow this death or cause it to happen? Is death part of God's plan for our lives or just a random event? Does God have the power to perform miracles? If so, why didn't He perform one for my loved one? What did I do to deserve this suffering? Why me?

The answers to these questions will form the person's world view for years after the loss — often until another deeply felt crisis occurs to renew the questions.

Back to the scenario

With these various dimensions of the holistic model of grief in mind, let's reconsider the responses described in the above scenario. How should *you* respond to each person?

Mr. Carr's concern about his son's body suggests a physical response. He may be feeling very real physical pain himself because of the shock he's received. So don't challenge Mr. Carr's statements outright, even though, of course, his son will feel no pain during the autopsy. Instead, reassure him that his son's body will be handled with great care. Mr. Carr also needs physical validation of his son's death — he'll need to see the body. Be sure to stress that his son's death, though sudden, was most likely painless.

Mrs. Carr's blank response is characteristic of emotional shock. As you speak to her, stand physically close to her, touch her, and use a calm, gentle voice. You should also encourage Mrs. Carr to see her baby, but the choice must be hers. She's retreated from the pain of the moment; don't force her to accept its reality.

Mrs. Stoner's concern about what others do in this situation — her desire to know what is "correct" — is an inappropriate social response. You should reassure her that many people choose to see their dead child to say good-bye; it's a healthy and acceptable thing to do.

Mr. Stoner's take-charge attitude indicates that he's overfunctioning for the members of his family. He wants to minimize their pain by making decisions for them. Explain to him that couples who've lost a child appreciate being allowed to consider their options and to make their own choices. Suggest that he give the Carrs some privacy so they can talk.

Mrs. Avery's attempt to console Mrs. Carr shows that she has called upon her own spiritual beliefs to cope with this death. She doesn't understand that her faith can't help her friends — only *their* faith can do that. You might remind her that the Carrs haven't had time to absorb what has happened to their son: It's too soon to expect them to be happy that he's in heaven. Suggest that Mrs. Avery go to the chapel to pray and to allow the family some time alone.

Finally, what about *your* response to the situation? It's rooted in the mental dimension: You've remained calm and objective, relaying information and helping the family make some very difficult decisions. This is an entirely appropriate response, but be careful: If carried to an extreme, it could make you seem unfeeling.

Don't be afraid to respond in other ways. Many families appreciate the physical and emotional responses shared by nurses who touch them, hug them, cry with them, handle their loved one's body gently, or simply remain physically close to them.

Families are also extremely sensitive to inappropriate social comments made by health care providers. Never do anything that seems to minimize the family's tragedy. Comments such as, "It's for the best," are difficult for families to accept — even if they occasionally make similar comments themselves.

Not a manual

The holistic model is not meant to be a how-to manual. Because its various dimensions overlap to some extent, you may find it hard to determine just how a person is responding. For instance, Mr. Carr was clearly upset and irritable about the autopsy request (an emotional response), although the content of his words focused on the physical — his concern about his son's body. Also, as a person grieves, his response will shift from one dimension to another. Only tactful questions and careful listening on your part can help you find the right approach.

Remember, too, that your interaction with the bereaved person typically ends early in the grieving process. He won't complete his active grieving until he has explored the impact of the loss on all dimensions of his life. Even then, the adjustments he's made in his inner world will go with him throughout his life.

Some final thoughts

You won't find any new information in the holistic model of grief presented here. But it is a new *synthesis* of the work of thinkers, writers, and researchers going back thousands of years. People have struggled with grief since the first loved one died and are still far from understanding it. But perhaps this model can help you at least recognize the enormously complex and individual nature of grief and respond to it in a caring and humane way.

SELECTED REFERENCES

Bowen, M.: *Family Therapy in Clinical Practice.* New York, Jason Aronson, 1985.

Gyulay, J.: *The Dying Child.* New York, McGraw-Hill Book Co., 1977.

Kübler-Ross, E.: *On Death and Dying.* New York, Macmillan Publishing Co., 1969.

SECTION THREE

Severe psychosocial syndromes

THIS SECTION BEGINS by examining three of the most serious responses to overwhelming stress: drug dependence (a physical or emotional addiction to drugs, including alcohol), acting-out behaviors (conflict or emotions expressed through defensive, destructive, or other neurotic actions) and suicide (intentional taking of one's life). It concludes by discussing crisis intervention for these and other severe psychosocial problems. Throughout, it provides helpful guidelines for the nurse who encounters these behaviors in clinical practice.

The first article, "Drug Dependency in Hospital Patients" by Adams, helps the nurse provide appropriate care for a drug-dependent client. It investigates the multifaceted nature of drug dependence and provides a chart of controlled substances and their effects to help the nurse identify a drug user. It also discusses manipulative strategies a drug-dependent client may use, such as buying a roommate's narcotics or causing staff divisiveness by playing off one person against another. Finally, the article presents special nursing interventions to help the drug-dependent client, including development of realistic goals and health care teamwork.

The nurse also should be aware of the effects of another form of drug dependence: alcoholism. An alcoholic client may be admitted to the hospital for treatment of cirrhosis, organic brain damage, or other alcohol-related disorders. During the hospital stay, however, the client may suffer from withdrawal symptoms, such as tremors, anxiety, insomnia, nausea, vomiting, confusion, hallucinations, sweating, and convulsions. If withdrawal symptoms occur, the nurse must take a similar approach to that used with other drug-dependent clients: Try to prevent withdrawal complications and, when the crisis has passed, develop a relationship with the client that fosters open discussion of alcoholism, its effect on the client's life, and possible treatment options.

A client with an undiagnosed borderline personality disorder can wreak havoc in any health care setting, especially the hospital. Such a client displays a wide range of hostile behaviors, being divisive, becoming violent, and creating major management difficulties. The article, "The Borderline Patient on the Med-Surg Unit" by Runyon, Allen, and Ilnicki, helps the nurse cope with such a client. It describes the defense mechanisms most frequently used by a client with borderline personality disorder and the nursing problems related to caring for such a client. Then it presents a standard care plan that includes expected outcomes and nursing interventions for a client with these nursing diagnoses — ineffective individual coping; anxiety; altered comfort: pain; or potential for violence. Because this care plan has been successful in various med-surg areas, it should be especially useful to the student who plans to work in a hospital or similar setting.

Suicide is the ultimate response to an overwhelming situation. In this severe psychosocial syndrome, the client sees no other options. When a client feels this way, the nurse must provide support until the client is out of danger. In "At Risk for Suicide," Bydlon-Brown and Billman advise the nurse to identify suicidal tendencies by watching for specific behaviors: suicidal ideation (thoughts about ending one's life), lack of rapport, poor compliance with the treatment plan, limited socialization, hyperactivity or abrupt changes in activity, and frequent mood changes or constant feelings of anger or frustration. Then they present an assessment tool for the nurse to rate these behaviors and determine the client's suicide risk — and the amount of nursing supervision needed. This particularly useful article gives the nurse a concrete way to assess a client's suicide risk based on subjective *and* objective data and allows the nurse to provide proactive care that can save a client's life.

The nurse also can use the suicide prevention contract. Mentioned briefly in the previous article, this contract is "a bilateral commitment and contribution toward the avoidance of the client's self-destruction." (Assey, 1985) It has three major components:

- *balance* between trusting the client with some freedom and protecting the client from self-inflicted harm.
- *open expression of caring* to reduce the sense of aloneness by letting the client know that someone cares.
- *reinforcement of the contract* by facilitating and witnessing the client's pledge to uphold the contract's terms (Assey, 1985).

The nurse and the client negotiate the contract's terms together, which may be a simple declaration such as "I will not kill myself without talking to you first" or "I will not kill myself accidentally or on purpose, no matter what" or it may be a more detailed statement tailored to the specific situation.

For a client in crisis — that is, for a client emergency in which circumstances exceed the client's mental or physical ability to cope with them — the nurse must be prepared to use crisis intervention.

According to Wolterman and Miller (1985), crisis intervention is "...a series of activities designed to influence the course of a crisis so as to produce a more adaptive outcome; one that also will strengthen the ability to cope with future crises" (Jacobsen et at., 1968). Zund (1974, p. 9) identifies the ingredients of a crisis as: (1) a problem that cannot be solved in usual ways; (2) a situation in which a normally self-sufficient person (or family) must depend on others to act; (3) a client's feelings of uncertainty, fear, loss, and anxiety; (4) a situation where the client has few, if any, situational supports; (5) a client who has distorted perceptions of events; and (6) a client who feels extremely helpless, which may lead to despair.

In "Crisis Intervention and Suicide," Hradek explains the six essential steps to use with the client at risk for suicide to resolve the problem that precipitated the crisis. Hradek also presents the case study of a young alcoholic in crisis, highlighting the nurse's use of crisis intervention techniques within the nursing process.

The last article, "Helping the Family Through a Crisis" by Baird, explores crisis intervention from the perspective of the family rather than the individual. A crisis can affect a family in different ways and typically strains a family's support systems and established coping methods. The nurse must assess the causes and effects of a crisis in the family's context. Baird explains how to intervene by helping the family explore their options and test different coping methods. Then she discusses how and when to evaluate the family's progress and reinforce their coping methods. This article provides specific questions to ask in various types of crises, preparing the student to manage diverse situations.

REFERENCES

Assey, J.L. (1985). The suicide prevention contract. *Perspectives in Psychiatric Care, 23*(3): 99-103.

Jacobsen, G., Strickler, M., & Morley, W.E. (1968). Generic and individual approaches to crisis intervention. *American Journal of Public Health, 58*:339-342.

Wolterman, M.C., & Miller, M. (1985). Caring for parents in crisis. *Nursing Forum, 22*(1):34-37.

Zund, R. (1974). Deterrents to crisis intervention in the hospital unit. *Nursing Clinics of North America, 9*(1):27-36.

Drug dependency in hospital patients

FRANCES E. ADAMS, RN, MSN

THE PATIENT MAY be a heroin addict or a crack user; or she may be a housewife who uses Valium, an adolescent on amphetamines, or someone in chronic pain taking an analgesic prescription. When the drug-dependent person is admitted to a general hospital, the profile and the problem can vary widely.

The reasons for admission are diverse. They may be related to the patient's drug problem — or not. It could be acute appendicitis that brings someone in, or a heroin addict's need for intravenous antibiotics to treat the cellulitis caused by "skin popping" — intradermal heroin injections. The problem may be AIDS, hepatitis, or subacute bacterial endocarditis from contaminated needles. Some addicts feign illness, such as renal colic, because its severe pain is treated with narcotics. Or there may be traumatic injuries — fractures or knife wounds.

Regardless of the immediate reasons for... admission, however, the basic illness they share — drug dependence — creates unique problems both for hospital staff and for the addicts themselves.

Admission is likely to cause drug-dependent patients great anxiety; they may be afraid of their pain and of losing their accustomed means of relief. Compounding this is the drug-dependent person's already weakened self-esteem that may have led him into conflict with groups and people in authority. Such a person is likely to struggle with staff about decisions; most frequently, about drug decisions.

These personality traits can lead to difficulties all around and create situations ranging from the mildly disruptive to near havoc on the unit. Nurses and physicians are caught between the fear that they are "feeding into the patient's problem" (when they medicate as the patient wishes) and the fear they are causing unnecessary suffering (when they withhold drugs and hear the patient complain of pain and poor care). Planning and careful teamwork can largely defuse the tensions.

ER tactics — his and yours

Not all drug-dependent persons disturb hospital routine. The health team's first task, therefore, is to identify accurately those who may. Beginning in the emergency room or clinic, [the nurse's] familiarity with the signs of drug intoxication is crucial (see chart).

Identifying a drug user isn't, however, always easy. If an I.V. drug abuser isn't "high," he may try to avoid detection of his tracks by rolling up the sleeve of his trackless arm before his blood pressure is taken. An easy way to counter this is to tell him you want to check the BP in the other arm.

Then there are those whom Chappel describes as patient hustlers, skillfully manipulating ER physicians to get drugs.[1] One such "hustler" may *feign illness,* reporting only vague symptoms, but on being asked which drug has helped in the past he names the drug and sometimes specifies a dose. Another may be *deceptive* by stealing prescription forms or returning to the ER or clinic before the prescribed dose has run out, claiming the drug was lost or stolen. (One man said his cat had pushed the open bottle of pills into the toilet.) A third "hustler" tactic is *pressuring,* which consists of playing on sympathy, overt bribery, or even making physical threats.

Controlled substances and effects

DRUGS	TRADE OR OTHER NAMES	DURATION (HOURS)	MEDICAL USES
Narcotics			
Opium	Dover's Powder, Paregoric, Parepectolin	3-6	Analgesic, antidiarrheal
Morphine	Morphine	3-6	Analgesic, antitussive
Codeine	Empirin Compound with Codeine, Robitussin A-C, Tylenol with Codeine	3-6	Analgesic, antitussive
Heroin	Diacetylmorphine, Horse, Smack	3-6	Under investigation
Hydromorphone	Dilaudid	3-6	Analgesic
Meperidine (Pethidine)	Demerol, Mepergan	3-6	Analgesic
Methadone	Dolophine, Methadone	12-24	Analgesic
Other narcotics	Darvon, Fentanyl, LAAM, Lomotil, Numorphan, Percodan, Talwin*, Tussionex	Variable	Analgesic, antidiarrheal, antitussive
Depressants			
Chloral hydrate	Chloral hydrate	5-8	Hypnotic
Barbiturates	Amytal, Lotusate, Nembutal, Phenobarbital, Seconal, Tuinal	1-16	Anesthetic, anticonvulsant, sedative, hypnotic
Benzodiazepines	Ativan, Dalmane, Diazepam, Halcion, Klonopin, Librium, Paxipam, Restoril, Serax, Tranxene, Valium, Xanax	4-8	Antianxiety, anticonvulsant, sedative, hypnotic
Methaqualone	Quaalude	4-8	Sedative, hypnotic
Glutethimide	Doriden	4-8	Sedative, hypnotic

**Not designated a narcotic under the Controlled Substances Act*
***Designated a narcotic under the Controlled Substances Act*

Controlled substances and effects *continued*

DRUGS	TRADE OR OTHER NAMES	DURATION (HOURS)	MEDICAL USES
Depressants *continued*			
Other depressants	Equanil, Miltown, Noludar, Placidyl, Valmid	4-8	Antianxiety, sedative, hypnotic
Stimulants			
Cocaine**	Coke, Flake, Snow	1-2	Local anesthetic
Amphetamines	Biphetamine, Desoxyn, Mediatric	2-4	Hyperkinesis, narcolepsy, weight control
Phenmetrazine	Preludin	2-4	Hyperkinesis, narcolepsy, weight control
Methylphenidate	Ritalin	2-4	Hyperkinesis, narcolepsy, weight control
Other stimulants	Adipex-P, Cylert, Didrex, Lonamin, Plegine, Sanorex, Tenuate, Tepanil	2-4	Hyperkinesis, narcolepsy, weight control
Hallucinogens			
LSD	Acid, Microdot	8-12	None
Mescaline and peyote	Buttons, Cactus, Mesc	8-12	None
Amphetamine variants	2,5-DMA, DOB, DOM, MDA, MDMA, PMA, STP, TMA	Variable	None
Phencyclidine	Angel Dust, Hog, PCP	Day	Veterinary anesthetic
Phencyclidine analogs	PCE, PCPy, TCP	Days	None
Other hallucinogens	Bufotenin, DET, DMT, Ibogaine, Psilocin, Psilocybin	Variable	None

continued

**Not designated a narcotic under the Controlled Substances Act*
***Designated a narcotic under the Controlled Substances Act*

Controlled substances and effects *continued*

DRUGS	TRADE OR OTHER NAMES	DURATION (HOURS)	MEDICAL USES
Cannabis			
Marijuana	Acapulco Gold, Grass, Pot, Reefer, Sinsemilla, Thai Sticks	2-4	Under investigation
Tetrahydrocannabinol	THC	2-4	Under investigation
Hashish	Hash	2-4	None
Hashish oil	Hash oil	2-4	None

**Not designated a narcotic under the Controlled Substances Act*
***Designated a narcotic under the Controlled Substances Act*

A medication history may provide other clues. Begin by asking nonthreatening questions about coffee, cigarettes, prescription drugs, and alcohol. Then ask about nonprescription drugs. Patients tend to give more accurate responses when the question is worded in a way that implies drug use is expected. For example, you might ask, "When was the last time you used a narcotic?".[2]

If a patient admits to illicit drug use, note its onset, frequency, amount, and type. Keep in mind that reported amounts may be exaggerated in the hope of proving a high tolerance and thus the need for large doses of pain medication. The reverse is true about alcohol. A rule of thumb is that drug abusers will claim they use twice as much of a drug as they actually use, while alcoholics will claim only about half of what they actually drink.

If an ER patient says he or she is in a methadone maintenance program, call the program to confirm this. Ask about the onset of treatment (as it indicates cooperation with the program) and dosage schedule. Chart these data and the program representative's name.

Clock-watchers, buyers, splitters, and visitors

Drug dependency may not be apparent until the patient has been admitted. Again, unit staff need to be aware of physiological and behavioral indicators of dependence or drug seeking, as well as the signs and symptoms of acute intoxication or withdrawl within the various classifications of drugs. Post this information where it is easily accessible (see chart).

The behavioral clues to dependence soon show up. Patients may complain of inadequate pain relief but may not appear to be in pain. Because pain is subjective, it is difficult to evaluate. However, if staff or roommates *consistently* observe that a patient behaves as if he is in pain when others are nearby but in their absence appears comfortable, it can indicate drug seeking or dependence.

You may also encounter a patient who watches the clock for the next medication dose and, each time, asks what and how much he is getting. By making a direct but nonaggressive statement such as, "It seems you have some concern about your pain medication," you can encourage the patient to express any worries he may have. A very defensive or angry response to your comment may suggest a drug abuse problem.

It is not uncommon for a drug-dependent patient to buy narcotics from his roommate. Be alert to the patient who shows unusual interest in a roommate's medication schedule, or to any increases without apparent cause in the roommate's requests for medication. (This is another good reason to make sure that a patient takes his medicine when it is offered.)

Staff splitting — playing off one staff member against another — is a divisive tactic drug abusers employ to manipulate people. It may involve complimenting team member A while comparing her to B and criticizing B's performance. Subsequently, the process may be reversed so that B feels praised and "one up" compared to A. Or the split may start with an apparently innocuous patient request that a different nurse bring the pain medication because "my nurse can't seem to find the time."

When a split occurs, problems can multiply. Team members become competitive or think that their peers are treating the patient improperly. Staff may argue about approaches or, worse, say nothing to one another and provide inconsistent care.

If the patient's mood or consciousness level changes markedly during or after visiting hours, and other questionable behaviors are also observed, consider various approaches. You may decide to ask the patient if he has taken any nonprescribed drugs, or you may decide to obtain a urine toxic screen. If you suspect that the patient brought drugs into the hospital with him, notify your supervisor or the person who is designated by your hospital's policy to authorize having a hospital security guard help you check the patient's belongings in the patient's presence.

Staff noted a change in one patient's behavior following every visit by one specific person. The security guard, called during the next visit, found a variety of pills in the visitor's purse. In another instance, staff observed a change in a patient's behavior and holes in the I.V. tubing following a visit. Visitors were then prohibited. Another option, undesirable but sometimes necessary, is to discharge the patient, but in the two cases cited both patients were too ill to leave the hospital.

Let's agree on (realistic) goals

To help drug-dependent patients, the first step is to hold a patient care conference to gather complete data and decide on goals and approaches. Include the patient's primary and associate nurses, physicians, and ancillary personnel who have worked with the patient, a psychiatric liaison nurse, and a social worker.

Health care goals will depend on the nature of the patient's drug problem. If the patient has a long history of street-drug abuse or of shopping from doctor to doctor for pain relief, it is probably not realistic to set the goal of ending the drug dependency. More feasible goals would be to prevent withdrawal complications and to develop a rapport with the patient that permits open discussion of the abuse, its effect on the patient's life, and treatment options.

Often it's best that a small group of nurses provide care, rather than rotating care among many different nurses, to avoid staff splitting. Whatever the plan, consistency is imperative.

Immediately after the conference, the patient's primary nurse and physician discuss with the patient the staff's observations and plans, and answer any of his questions or concerns.

Never challenge the patient's pain by saying, "We don't think your pain is real" or "It's not normal to have this much pain at this point." Either remark could set up a power struggle over trust issues between the patient and staff. Instead, tell the patient, "We know you are in a lot of pain, but we're concerned about how much medicine you've been receiving, so we're gradually going to reduce the amount." This approach places the responsibility squarely on the team, not on the patient. Hearing it from the physician and nurse simultaneously will forestall any splitting tactics.

Teamwork works

At change of shift, the nurse going off duty and the oncoming nurse can tell the patient, together, that the plan has been discussed and will be continued. This concretely demonstrates the team's cohesiveness. In the case of some very manipulative patients, it is decided that only one physician, usually the attending one, will prescribe narcotics.

This strategy is particularly important in teaching hospitals, where interns and residents write prescriptions and patients may persuade exhausted house officers to increase narcotic doses late at night. Each time new drug prescriptions are written, the patient's primary or assigned nurse and the designated physician together see the patient and explain any changes and the reasons for them.

This type of management is not accepted by all experts. John Fultz and others, for instance, suggest that when a street narcotic addict is hospitalized and methadone is being started or titrated, the patient should not be told the dose.[3] If the patient questions the dose, these authors advise asking why he doesn't trust the staff.

I believe, however, that because addicted persons usually have great difficulty with trust issues, engaging in a superficial discussion of trust is probably futile. All patients have the right to know the drugs and doses they are taking; denying this right is punitive. It is better to answer patients' questions and respond to complaints directly, in a matter-of-fact way, at the time they are raised. One reason for this approach is its honesty; another is that it discourages patients from splitting staff over the issue of drug administration and eliminates nurse-patient conflicts about which physician to call for more medicine. Over time, such honesty should increase the patient's trust of staff because nothing is hidden. Even with accurate information about their drug regimens, however, patients may continue to act out their frustration at losing control by attempting to split the staff. Several responses are possible. The best is to recognize the process and direct the patient back to the team member against whom the criticism was leveled. "It would be best if you spoke to B about your concern" is a simple statement that may avert a struggle. If the patient later repeats the criticism, ask if he spoke to B as you suggested. If not, offer to ask B to speak with the patient.

When a woman whose pain regimen had been described to her in detail continued complaining about her physician and his "lack of explanation about my pain pills," the nurse paged the physician and the two of them confronted the patient. Her complaints stopped.

Undermedicating pain

In my practice, I often encounter nurses who worry that giving patients narcotics will lead to life-long addiction. Consequently, some patients are undermedicated for postoperative pain and their recoveries are prolonged. Nurses and physicians need to realize that most hospitalized patients will not become drug dependent and, even if they do, they can be tapered off the narcotic before discharge.

For example, a patient with a traumatic crush injury required an amputation after weeks of effort to save his leg. He needed a great deal of medication for his pain and became dependent. As discharge approached, however, his narcotics were gradually tapered off and he went home in no danger of continued drug dependence.

The incidence of addictive behavior is small compared to the number of persons exposed to drugs. This was abundantly evident among Vietnam War veterans: fewer than 1 percent of those who had taken heroin while in Vietnam continued daily use after returning to the United States.[4]

Discharge

If a heroin abuser is started and maintained on methadone during hospitalization, offer *early* assistance in gaining placement in a methadone maintenance program. Most programs have long waiting lists, but if the patient is genuinely interested and you offer him names, addresses, and telephone numbers, and he phones for an appointment, there is hope that he will persevere and stop abusing drugs.

On the other hand, when a patient who has been maintained on methadone does not seek help, staff often express futility because they believe they have merely reinforced the habit or prevented withdrawal symptoms. A staff meeting often helps air lingering frustrations or unrealistic hopes. It *is* discouraging to treat someone for a life-threatening illness such as subacute bacterial endocarditis only to have him return to street drugs immediately after discharge. But staff can focus on the therapeutic care they *did* provide.

For drug abuse, as with many chronic problems, the nursing goal is not cure but care. If we assist drug-dependent persons in seeking further treatment, we are doing what is reasonable and realistic.

REFERENCES

1. Chappel, J. N. Patient manipulation of the physician. In *Drug Abuse: A Guide for the Primary Physician.* ed. by Bonnie Baird Wilford. Chicago, IL., American Medical Association, 1981.

2. Lake, C. R. The acute psychiatric diagnostic interview. *Psychiatr.Clin.North Am.* 7:657-669, Dec. 1984.

3. Fultz, J. M. When a narcotic addict is hospitalized. *AJN* 80:478-481, Mar. 1980.

4. Dole, V. P. A clinician's view of addictions. In *The Basis of Addiction: A Report.* ed. by Jack Fishman, Berlin, Dahlen Konferencen by Abkon Verlag Sgesell Schaft, 1978, p. 42.

The borderline patient on the med-surg unit

NELL RUNYON, RN, MS; CATHERINE LA MATTINA ALLEN, RN, BSN; SUSAN HESTER ILNICKI, RN, BS

DISTINCTLY DIFFERENT from other patients in their patterns of interaction, people who have borderline personality disorders frequently are labeled "hateful," "hostile," "difficult," "unmanageable," "impossible," or "dangerous." They stir up trouble between everyone, creating anger and turmoil around them — and make it difficult for you to give warm and genuine care. They are demanding and manipulative, and no matter what you do for them, nothing is ever good enough. They frequently disrupt treatment, refuse care, can become violent, and may ultimately leave against medical advice.

People with an undiagnosed borderline personality disorder can wind up on your med-surg unit for any number of reasons — surgery, trauma, illness, or problems related to alcohol or drug abuse. Typically, the patient's hostile and manipulative behavior manages to erode the unit's morale; only then do the staff recognize the need for psychiatric consultation.

What makes a borderline tick?

Considering himself a victim, the borderline expects to be mistreated and misunderstood. He envisions himself alone, pitted against a cold, unfeeling world. When he becomes a patient, the uncertainties of his illness stress his already tenuous grasp on reality. His defense mechanism — the source of his interpersonal conflicts with the staff — are his only armor.

Projection. When a person disowns a feeling — that is, decides it comes from outside himself — he is projecting. For example, "*I'm* not angry, *you* are"' is the projector's response to his own anger. Projection distorts the person's perception of others' intentions. People are no longer real to him, but mere reflections of his *own* feelings.

The borderline personality retains images of his parents as both cruel and loving, weak and omnipotent, hated and idealized.[1] Because he sees other adults as parental figures, he assigns parental "traits" to them. His expectations and beliefs are that all adults will behave toward him as he perceives his parents did. In effect, therefore, he "writes the script" for his own behavior. He reacts to people as he *expects* they will behave toward him — namely, mistreating and misunderstanding him. He reacts angrily to anything he perceives as the slightest hint of rejection. The more he looks for mistreatment, the more he creates it, all the while unaware of what he's doing.

Since the borderline has no idea *why* he acts as he does, he will not accept responsibility for his actions. If someone says, "You're making me angry," he is likely to reply, "Who, me? I didn't do anything. You're the one who's causing the problem here, not me." Such negative interactions become a way of life for the borderline. It comes as no surprise to others that he often goes through life a victim of assault and abuse.

Identification. To the borderline, all adults are parents and he is a powerless child. Identifying with that role, the patient has little trust that his needs will be met, so he *demands* that they be met. Staff who genuinely want to help often find themselves trapped into acting out the patient's parental projections. Yet if they confront him directly by counterattack, without thought to the impact, they are in effect accepting his challenge and perpetuating the whole negative cycle.

Behaviorally, projection and identification take forms more likely to cause the staff to sit up and take notice — **entitlement** and **splitting**.[1] The borderline feels that he did not get all the love he deserved as a child; thus he is entitled, now, to demand it from others. It is not these feelings per se but the *intensity* of these feelings that characterize the borderline personality. He views the world as "owing" him, and he intends to make it "pay up." This may explain why he characteristically demands help — although he is unlikely to accept it.

Just as the borderline sees parental figures as all good or all bad, he categorizes each staff member the same way. He splits the staff — idealizing some, yet finding the others incompetent, cold, or indifferent. The "split" staff react to him just as he perceives them, but eventually the idealized staff (or shift) fail to meet the borderline's grandiose expectations of them. Typically, the patient then makes angry calls to administrators to decry everyone's level of competence. The staff feel angry, threatened, and helpless.

We've designed a goal-oriented approach to the borderline patient. Our standard care plan is written in language approved for clinical testing by the North American Nursing Diagnosis Association (NANDA), and follows Carpenito's model.[2] Its success in a wide variety of med-surg areas has made it a valuable management tool at our hospital.

As we set our standard plan in motion, we intend to:

• reduce the patient's anxiety to a level tolerable for him, thus lessening his impulsivity

• defuse the power struggle between patient and staff so that staff are able to deliver optimal care

• manage the patient's behavior purposefully — that is, by *acting* and not *reacting*

• collaborate with other disciplines to obviate disruptions and follow the plan.

The plan addresses the following problems:

Ineffective individual coping. We know how difficult it can be to deal with a patient whose actions are prompted by his feelings of entitlement. The anger flows freely — and inappropriately — between patient and nurse. Using the plan, though, you *expect* anger from the patient. Alerted to it, you save your own angry feelings for the patient care conference, where you can acknowledge them with colleagues instead of counterattacking the patient.

In conference, you can get past your own anger to an understanding of how the patient's projected anger works. Then you can proceed to recognize the valid stressors the patient has and work with him to structure his activities accordingly. Nothing defuses a potential crisis quite like maintaining professional composure.

Team conference, in fact, is your best weapon against staff splitting. Once everyone understands what the patient is doing, everyone can agree on one consistent approach, delivering the message that the staff works together and will not tolerate splitting.

The unit's manager can also ensure that the same nurses are always assigned to the patient. The fewer staff the patient interacts with, the less opportunity he'll have for splitting.

Anxiety. The borderline patient feels disabled without frequent interaction with staff and fears that he will be abandoned. As he demands more attention, though, staff tend to avoid him, which only makes him even more anxious.

Using the plan, you *routinely* give the patient attention. He feels cared for and less afraid that his caretakers will not come back. You tell him exactly when you will return and you return at that time. You invite him to participate in the plan.

Establishing a contract with the patient makes a care plan explicit. Tell the patient beforehand that the staff will be preparing a con-

Our standard approach to a borderline personality

PROBLEM	EXPECTED OUTCOME	INTERVENTION
Ineffective individual coping (the inability to manage stressors well enough to control anger and fear) related to inadequate psychological resources *Manifested by:* • entitlement behaviors —makes demands —has angry affect —is easily rejected —rejects care that is offered —is never satisfied with care —provokes angry confrontations and power struggles • splitting behaviors —criticizes and complains about staff —attempts to set staff against each other —makes angry calls to administration and others in authority	• will comply with the treatment plan and manage activities of daily living (ADL) without excessive anger and disruption • will show acceptance of caregivers • will direct complaints to the appropriate management	• recognize patient's feelings of anger early • maintain professional composure • avoid confronting patient about unrealistic demands • acknowledge valid stressors in patient's situation (trauma, surgery, pain) • allow patient to structure activities whenever possible (bath, dressing) • recognize and deal with splitting behavior early —acknowledge complaints; reassure patient he will get excellent care —call a team conference —discuss plan with other shifts —designate manager for complaints —collaborate with other disciplines on treatment plan —document plan to assure consistent approach • assign nurses consistently when possible —three nurses, one each shift, as primary nurses —three associate nurses to relieve the primaries
Anxiety (feelings of uneasiness or apprehension in response to a vague, nonspecific threat) related to an actual or perceived threat to self-concept *Manifested by:* • frequent demands for attention • excessive ringing of call bell • vague, unfocused somatic complaints • expressed feelings of apprehension	• will tolerate solitude and will ring the call bell less often • will express fewer vague complaints	• at shift change, greet patient briefly, explain new procedures, and again describe routine treatments • be direct in setting time limits of treatments and return visits • give options whenever possible. Establish a contract with patient when appropriate • give unsolicited attention—for example, when patient has not rung the bell

Our standard approach to a borderline personality *continued*

PROBLEM	EXPECTED OUTCOME	INTERVENTION
Alteration in comfort: pain related to trauma, surgery, or illness *Manifested by:* • an intense, excessive experience of pain	• will feel enough relief of pain to comply with pain management and manage ADL	• administer analgesic as prescribed • coordinate pain management with other disciplines • educate patient regarding analgesic • discuss any anticipated change in analgesic with patient • anticipate intense pain. Give analgesic around the clock, especially the first 24 hours postop
Potential for violence (aggressive behavior directed at self or others) related to antisocial character, new stressors, frustration, perceived threat to self-esteem, and/or drug or alcohol abuse *Manifested by:* • hostile words • self-destructive threats • self-abuse • assaultive behavior • rage	• will control violent behavior • will not harm self or others	• set limits with kind firmness —be direct, clear, and confident —do not confront or challenge patient —visit patient often to help him stay in control • assess immediacy of threat —encourage patient to talk about his feelings of anxiety or loss of control • help patient to gain control —assure him that his safety and well-being is a priority —remove potentially harmful objects from his room —bring a colleague with you when necessary —determine his need for psychiatric consultation —determine his need for physical or chemical restraint —determine whether security officers are needed

tract for his care. Find out what he wants regarding at least one major issue. Design the contract to begin with the goals that allow the patient the fewest options and end with those offering him the widest choices. Write the contract care-plan style and then present it to the patient.

After you and the patient go over the contract (with the head nurse and/or physician, if appropriate) and adjust it to fit, he'll know exactly what you expect of him and what he can expect of you. When both of you sign it, the power struggle lessens considerably. Be sure the appropriate manager reviews the contract for compliance at least once a week.

Altered comfort: pain. A borderline patient in pain feels extremely anxious when he thinks he has to convince the team that he does, indeed, have pain. And because many borderlines are substance abusers, managing their pain takes a great deal of expertise and collaboration.

Around-the-clock (rather than PRN) dosing is the best practice for many patients, but it is essential for postop pain control in borderline patients. Anticipate that the patient will have pain and tell him what to expect, as well. Inform him of any changes in analgesic routine *before* they begin, not after the fact.

Potential for violence. Frustration, anger, and anxiety are volatile emotions. Borderline patients typically threaten or enact violence. We recommend setting limits with "kind firmness." With this technique, you avoid challenging the patient and contributing to potentially aggressive behavior.[3]

Tell the patient clearly and confidently what you expect, but keep alert to the possibility that he may need chemical or physical restraints until he regains control. To use this technique effectively, you need to release any feelings of anger you may still have. Avoid an authoritarian or hostile stance. Take advantage of any support systems the patient may have to help him regain and maintain a sense of control.

REFERENCES

1. Stoudemire, A., and Thompson, T. L., 2d. The borderline personality in the medical setting. *Ann. Intern. Med.* 96:76-79, Jan. 1982.

2. Carpenito, L. J. *Nursing Diagnosis: Application to Clinical Practice.* Philadelphia, J. B. Lippincott Co., 2d ed., 1987.

3. Groves, J. E. Management of the borderline patient on a medical or surgical ward: the psychiatric consultant's role. *Int. J. Psychiatry Med.* 6(3):337-348, 1975.

At risk for suicide

BARBARA BYDLON-BROWN, RN; ROBERT R. BILLMAN, RN

"WILL YOU HELP ME? I'm going to kill myself!" This frequent chant of 65-year-old Ms. C, a patient on our closed, acute-care psychiatric unit, was familiar to staff. Diagnosed as a chronic, agitated depressive person, Ms. C was being treated with electroconvulsvie therapy and a PRN antianxiety agent.

Besides her constant refrain, Ms. C has a pattern of inappropriate behavior. She rarely communicated with staff, which made us anxious. She sometimes lay on the floor in the middle of the hall. Mood swings from cheerfulness to anger, sometimes accompanied by aggressive behavior, were becoming frequent.

One night her chants were louder than usual. Then Ms. C went to bed and appeared to sleep. The night shift reported that when she awoke she was calm and in good spirits. But things were not as they appeared. Shortly thereafter, the nurse caring for Ms. C found a cloth restraint hidden in her room. Ms. C confided to the nurse, "I'm going to kill myself."

Nurses on units similar to our 29-bed psychiatric unit frequently face such situations.[1] We use primary nursing to provide continuity of care, and we use routine suicide supervision levels [frequent, regular checks on a suicidal client]. Every shift we also check rooms for sharp items such as nail files and razors.[2] But what, we asked ourselves, are *appropriate* levels of supervision for the suicidal patient?

Are 5- to 10-minute checks adequate? Is one-on-one observation enough? Is there a correlation between patient behaviors and the intensity of nursing supervision?

To explore these issues, we formed a suicide assessment committee and observed nursing care given to suicidal patients. We found that many factors can interfere with suicide assessment, among them patient and staff transference [unconscious redirection of feelings by the client from an important figure (usually from childhood) to a therapist or other caregiver]; biased attitudes toward the diagnosis; reliance on intuition; and inconsistency because of differences in experience, expertise, education, and patient contact.[3]

To begin to enhance our assessment technique, we realized we needed to standardize the way we took psychosocial histories on suicidal patients. Our subjective (gut-level) responses to patients were *based* on objective data. However, we were not integrating our subjective feelings with our objective observations.

We also recognized that countertransference [conscious or unconscious emotional response of a therapist or caregiver to a client] with specific patients had a major impact on which suicide supervison levels were used. In turn, these supervision levels affected patients' self-esteem. Observing a patient more closely to assure optimum safety may be perceived by the patient as mistrust. Consequently, he may become angry, feel he has lost control, and believe his condition is deteriorating.[2]

However, to be less restrictive while attempting to maintain optimum patient safety places nurses in a difficult position. We realized we needed to balance risk factors and supervision levels with patients' rights and all the other factors influencing nurses' judgments. One way to achieve our goal was to develop a framework to assure assessment consistency.

The suicide assessment tool (on page 267)

is based on subjective and objective data. When used in conjunction with nursing judgment, it helps determine the supervision level needed for suicidal or impulsive patients. The tool relies on the nurse's judgment of the way a patient is behaving.

What to watch for

Suicidal ideation is the thought of wanting to end one's life. When discussing such ideation with a patient it is important for the nurse to establish the patient's intent.[4] If the intent (often called a suicide threat) is there, the patient is at greater risk of attempting the act. The act of planning a way to commit suicide (even if it is not a lethal plan) indicates the patient is prone to act on the thought.

Once the assessment is made, the nurse may make a contract with the patient.[5] The patient agrees *not* to act on his suicidal thoughts until he first contacts the nurse, or he agrees to delay carrying out his threat for a specific time. If the patient cannot or will not agree to such a contract, the risk of his attempting suicide is greater.

Rapport, the ability of the patient to speak about his feelings to the nurse, eventually results in mutual trust. The less rapport there is, the freer the patient is to act on his thoughts.[2]

How closely does the patient follow a *treatment plan?* Does he take medicines as prescribed? Does he attend assigned group therapy? If he does these things, he probably feels more hopeful about his ability to change and less helpless about his illness. The patient who does not, or cannot, comply with treatment is at greater risk of attempting suicide.

Socialization is another key issue. The patient who isolates himself may act on suicidal thoughts.[1] Some minimally withdrawn patients will respond when spoken to but have little desire to make social contact. They will participate in social interaction if urged by the nurse. The highly withdrawn patient, even with constant encouragement, will not or cannot interact with staff and others. Thus, he should be considered at more risk of acting on suicidal thoughts, since he is not communicating his need for support. There is also less information on which to assess him.

What is the patient's *activity level?* The more anxious and hyperactive the patient, the higher the risk of attempting suicide.

Be alert to sudden changes in activity level: Note the highly withdrawn patient who becomes very agitated or the highly agitated pa-

A case in point

Our unit's nurses were well acquainted with Mr. W, a manipulative and attention-seeking 30-year-old. He had been admitted to our unit several times over the last five years. Diagnosed with a bipolar illness, he was treated with an ECT series because his symptoms worsened after medication had failed. We checked him every 30 minutes.

One day, Julie, a staff nurse, approached the charge nurse with a concerned look on her face. "What's wrong?" asked the charge nurse. "Well, it's Mr. W," replied Julie. "I have him sitting in the lounge where I can observe him, but I don't know what to do. He says he has a plan to kill himself, and he is willing to come and get me before he acts on his plan. He's been withdrawn, anxious, and his thoughts are disorganized. I have a strange feeling about it. I don't want to overreact to his behavior by paying too much attention to his threats. At the same time, I'm afraid he might actually do something."

"Let's use the assessment checklist and see what it tells us," suggested the charge nurse.

After reviewing Mr. W's history and Julie's interactions with him that day, together they filled out the suicide assessment tool (at right) and were struck by the number of behaviors circled at the bottom of the third column.

"Even though manipulative, he is at risk and needs more observation," said the charge nurse.

"Yes, you're right," replied Julie. "Now that I see all the parts together, it's obvious that Mr. W needs to be checked every 5 to 10 minutes."

Guidelines for assessing suicide risk

Current checks Q 30 min

Any gestures in past 24 hours No

Number of days of hospitalization 35 days

Medications available No

OFF CHECKS	OBSERVATION EVERY 30 MINUTES	OBSERVATION EVERY 15 MINUTES	CLOSE-OBSERVATION EVERY 5-10 MINUTES	1:1 RESTRICTION	RESTRAINT OR SECLUSION
Verbalizes no suicidal ideation Congruence shown in verbal and behavioral information 100% compliance with treatment plan Has perception of support in community Verbalizes concerns on a feeling level to present nurse	Verbalizes suicidal ideation Verbalizes no plan Verbalizes no intention Cooperative with treatment plan Withdrawn low Multiple previous attempts Verbalizes superficially to present nurse	Verbalizes suicidal ideation with plan and/or intent No perception of support Little compliance with treatment plan Subjective or objective frustration Anger Labile affect or mood Mute or decreased amount of verbalization Avoidance of staff and others Withdrawn high Intoxicated Impaired reality testing Hyperactive Demonstrates limited problem-solving ability	Sudden change in activity level ...not chronic anxiety Unable to agree not to [attempt] suicide Makes suicidal gesture currently	Concealing equipment that could be used to harm self with available specific plan Attempt made while hospitalized to kill self	Attempt made to kill self in front of staff; i.e., even 1:1 cannot resist impulse to kill self

Guidelines for assessing suicide risk *continued*

Significant contributing data

Lives with parents.

Mother & father unable to visit—exhausted by pt's. illness.

Previous attempt 3 yr. ago by carbon monoxide.

Paternal grandfather schizophrenic; suicide 10 yr. ago by carbon monoxide.

Tenth-grade education.

Oriented to person, place and time.

Slight short-term memory loss.

tient who suddenly becomes calm.[4] Either change may herald a patient's decision to kill himself. Close observation is needed.

What is the patient's *mood?* Does it change often, or is he constantly angry or frustrated? If the latter, he is at greater risk.[6]

Supervision stages

Once the nursing judgments are made, the behaviors are circled on the assessment form. The team leader or charge nurse will validate the data with the primary nurse. Then both nurses decide the supervision level for the patient.

For example, if many behaviors are marked in one column of the form, the patient may need to be supervised at the higher level of frequency. If the patient's behaviors range over several columns, the nurse considers how the lower-risk behaviors affect the higher-risk behaviors. (Higher-risk items appear at the bottom of the supervision columns.)

New confidence

We were pleased with the results of using the assessment tool on our unit. Staff members exhibited increased confidence in making assessments. They also became more aware of the complex issues surrounding suicide intervention, leading to a heightened professionalism.

As a result of this new understanding, recently employed staff benefited from the close collaboration with experienced staff. At the same time, experienced staff were relieved that their judgments were no longer considered primarily subjective in nature but were based on a structured, systematic assessment.

REFERENCES

1. Webster, M. Assessing suicide potential. In *American Handbook of Psychiatric Nursing*, ed. by Suzanne Lego. Philadelphia, J. B. Lippincott Co., 1984, p. 29.

2. Barile, L. The client who is suicidal. In *American Handbook of Psychiatric Nursing*, ed. by Suzanne Lego. Philadelphia, J. B. Lippincott Co., 1984, p. 40, 400-402.

3. Clunn, P. A., and Payne, D. B. *Psychiatric Mental Health Nursing*. 3d ed. New Hyde Park, NY, Medical Examination Publishing Co., 1982.

4. Carmack, B. J. Suspect a suicide? Don't be afraid to act. *RN* 46:43-45, 90, Apr. 1983.

5. Reubin, R. Spotting and stopping the suicide patient. *Nursing* 9:82-85, Apr. 1979.

6. Hatton, C., and others. *Suicide: Assessment and Intervention.* 2d ed. Norwalk, CT, Appleton & Lange, 1983, p. 76.

Crisis intervention and suicide

ELIZABETH A. HRADEK, RN, BSN

Suicide precautions such as close nursing supervision and removal of dangerous objects from the client's room may prevent self-destructive behavior in the hospital, but they do not correct the client's underlying problem or decrease the risk of suicide after discharge. On the other hand, crisis intervention, which also can be used in the hospital, offers more lasting suicide prevention.

Whenever a suicidal client who is basically healthy cannot resolve a stressful situation with his or her usual problem-solving skills, the nurse can use the crisis intervention model of problem solving described below. Note: Summaries (shown in bracketed italics) and excerpts (marked by ellipses) condense extensive background material.

...KUS (1985) DESCRIBES six essential crisis intervention steps that the nurse assists the client through. First, the nurse must help the client identify and describe the precipitating problem. This step may be very difficult due to the person's anxiety level. The nurse must assist the client in focusing only on the immediate problem and convey a firm belief that resolution is possible. Writing out the problem as identified will assist in problem clarification.

Second, the nurse must assist the client to generate possible solutions and list these in writing under the identified problem. It is important to find out what the person usually does when confronted with problem situations. Any adaptive coping skills that are present can be positively reinforced. It is also important to find out what, if any, situational supports are available to the client. If the nurse is familiar with alternatives that have helped others in similar situations, suggestions may be made.

Third, the nurse assists the client in evaluating the possible consequences of the proposed solutions. This will be facilitated by having the client write down each possible alternative and list the pros and cons.

Fourth, the client decides which alternative will be chosen. It must be the client who makes this decision. The nurse must support the client's decision (although not necessarily agree with it) as well as support the client's right to change his or her mind if the alternative chosen does not achieve desired results.

Fifth, the client implements the chosen plan. Sixth, the nurse helps the client evaluate the implementation. There are two basic questions to be answered. Did the solution solve the problem and resolve the crisis? Does the person feel at least as comfortable psychologically as before the crisis occurred?

[Using the crisis intervention model, the nurse assesses the immediate problem. The assessment must evaluate risk factors related to suicide, such as suicidal ideation, a history of psychiatric illness or previous suicide attempts, alcoholism, loss of pleasure, and feelings of hopelessness.

Nursing interventions should be active, focusing on specific problems. The nurse must remain flexible and act as a resource person, teacher, and family liaison. She or he also should implement safety measures, guide the client through the problem-solving steps, and help evaluate the effectiveness of the solution.]

...The following case study demonstrates application of crisis intervention techniques to a client with suicidal ideation.

Case study

Sam, a 20-year-old college junior, was brought by ambulance to the emergency room of a large midwestern teaching hospital with a self-inflicted stab wound in the abdomen and a lacerated left wrist. Sam refused treatment in the emergency room, stating "I need to die. Why don't you let me die?" A court order for involuntary hospitalization and treatment was obtained by the emergency room staff and Sam was taken to surgery for repair of his abdominal and wrist wounds. He was admitted postoperatively to a general surgery floor. The nursing staff instituted "suicide precautions" and requested a consultation with a psychiatric clinical nurse specialist.

Assessment. The first contact with the psychiatric clinical nurse specialist occurred about five hours after surgery. Sam had a flat affect and poor eye contact. He repeatedly verbalized embarrassment and shame regarding his suicide attempt. He denied current suicidal ideation but said he wished he had died. He was able to sign a written contract with the clinical nurse specialist stating that he would not harm himself while in the hospital and that he would notify staff if he needed help keeping this contract. The clinical nurse specialist also contracted to meet daily with Sam to assist him in looking at his current problems and consider possible actions he could take. Sam agreed to this arrangement, adding that he did not really think it would help and was probably a waste of time. From the very beginning, ambivalence was apparent.

Nursing assessment focused on identification of specific and immediate problems. Sam was able to rapidly identify the following changes in his life [that] he felt to be sources of stress. He was living away from home for the first time...and missed his family a great deal. He was fearful about their reactions to his suicide attempt. He had enjoyed school and had achieved good grades prior to this semester, but was currently having difficulty getting his school work done. Finances were a source of concern for Sam. His family was experiencing financial hardship related to the farm economy and he felt guilty accepting what financial assistance they could give him. A brief, but important, relationship with a female friend was terminated by mutual agreement two months earlier.

By the third one-hour session with the clinical nurse specialist, Sam was able to identify three specific problems. These included: loneliness related to missing his family and his old girlfriend and not forming new friendships at school, financial concerns, and fear of school failure.

Nursing assessment included factors known to be frequently associated with suicidal behaviors. Specific questions [were asked about] alcohol use, frequency, and impact on social role....This assessment indicated that Sam also had a significant drinking problem. He reported frequent fighting and one arrest resulting from intoxication. School failure and financial problems were also related to daily drinking until intoxicated. Sam felt his frequent drinking had contributed to his not making friends at school. He was irritable when drinking and had experienced blackouts. Sam was intoxicated the night of his suicide attempt. Together, Sam and the clinical nurse specialist prioritized his problems as alcohol abuse, loneliness, financial difficulties, and fear of school failure.

Intervention. After discussion,...Sam, the clinical nurse specialist, the surgeon, and the consulting psychiatrist,...decided that treatment for the alcohol abuse was a primary need. The clinical nurse specialist provided Sam with information on three different alcohol treatment programs and arranged for him to visit with counselors from two of the programs he found most attractive.

Sam selected a program and made an appointment for his intake interview the afternoon of discharge from the hospital. Sam was encouraged to initiate more frequent contacts with his family while in the hospital. He found them to be anxious to help and non-critical of his suicide attempt. Immediate financial concerns regarding payment for hospitalization were referred to a social worker

Sam's primary reason for refusing treatment had been his inability to pay for hospitalization. After various options for payment were explained to Sam, he voluntarily consented to admission and the involuntary hospitalization order was dismissed. Sam dropped his current classes because of poor grades and a three-week absence due to his abdominal wound. This decision allowed him to work full-time, which helped diminish his financial concerns. He planned to re-enter classes at a later date.

Evaluation. Sam's hospitalization lasted...11 days. During that time his affect went from flat to full and spontaneous. His speech became fluent, goal-directed, and laced with some humor, rather than halting and monosyllabic. Problems [that he felt were] hopeless and overwhelming were now manageable. Relationships with family were renewed and strengthened. Sam reported confidence in his plans for alcohol treatment and gratitude that he was not allowed to give up on himself 11 days earlier. Sam was seen six weeks after discharge. At that time, he was engaged in outpatient alcohol treatment and was also active in Alcoholics Anonymous. His full-time job and his contacts with Alcoholics Anonymous had both fostered new friendships. His family ties remained strong. Sam was certainly functioning at a level at least as good as his pre-crisis level and probably considerably higher because of his control of his alcoholism.

REFERENCES

Augilera, D.C., Messick, J.M. *Crisis intervention: Theory and methodology*. St. Louis: C.V. Mosby, 1978.

Benter, S.E. Crisis therapy. In G.W. Stuart and S.J. Sundeen (Eds.). *Principles and practice of psychiatric nursing*. St. Louis: C.V. Mosby, 1983.

Kus, R.J. Crises intevention. In G.M. Bulechek and J.C. McCloskey (Eds.). *Nursing interventions: Treatments for nursing diagnoses*. Philadelphia: W.B. Saunders, 1985.

Roy, A. Suicide in depressives. *Comprehensive Psychiatry* 1983; 24:487-491.

Helping the family through a crisis

SALLY FELGENHAUER BAIRD, RN, MSN, PhC

PREMATURE BIRTH, sudden infant death syndrome, leukemia — many things can put a family in crisis. When that happens, your goal is to help them start functioning normally again. The strategies you'll use range from assessing the crisis to planning for the future. Let's start with assessment.

Assessment: Cover all bases

First, you'll want to see if the family is actually in crisis. There are many potential crisis-producing events, but not all families will go into a crisis over them.

What should you look for? Signs of rising tension and disorganization because of their inability to cope with an event that's happened in the last 6 weeks. Family members may cry, look exhausted or depressed, complain of insomnia, or not want to eat. Some show their stress by asking the same questions time and again.

Look at their general appearance and note their behavior. Are they upset? Nervous? Are they neat? Disheveled? Is their speech nervous? How do they describe their feelings? Is their behavior inappropriate?

Watch for family members who don't show physical symptoms but have changed their usual living pattern. For example, parents who recently learned their oldest child has leukemia may completely ignore the needs of their other children. Remember, what may be a crisis to one family may not be to another. Some families experience a crisis when faced with a seemingly small problem; others have enough coping mechanisms to withstand most stressful events.

What caused the crisis?

Once you've determined that the family is indeed in crisis, look for the cause. It may be something obvious, such as a death or a premature birth. Or it may be the "last straw" in a series of problems; in this case, your assessment is more difficult because the family might not recognize what precipitated the crisis. To get to the root of the problem, ask questions such as:

- Why did you come to the emergency department *today?*
- When did you begin to feel tense?
- What occurred at that time?
- Did you receive any unexpected news?
- Did you receive any visitors then?
- Do you have a new baby in the home?
- Have your lost your job?
- Is there an illness or death in the family?

Listen for anything that might have triggered the crisis: a mother-in-law visiting an already upset home, the news of a job relocation, the discovery of alcoholism in the family, a poor prognosis for a family member, and so on.

When did the crisis start?

Timing can be important, so find out when the crisis started. If a handicapped child was born 5 weeks earlier, family members might be less open to intervention than they would have been when the child was first born. This isn't to say that they won't benefit from later intervention, but your efforts could be less effective as time passes.

How does the family perceive the problem?

The next strategy is to determine the family's perception of the problem. This gives you an idea of why the event provoked a crisis. For example, a mother who's just resumed her career after raising her children may perceive another pregnancy as a threat to her career. You might ask these questions to learn how the family views the event:

- What does this event mean to you?
- How has it changed things?
- How do you think it will affect your future?

To clarify the problem for the family, discuss the relationship between the crisis and the precipitating event. This is especially important if the family doesn't see the relationship between a previous situation and their current stress.

What support systems are available?

Next, assess the family's support system. People in crisis know who can help better than anyone, so be sure to ask them. They might be able to call on neighbors or relatives to assist with household chores during the crisis. Some families, however, won't ask for help and may even push help away in their anger. Other families may come up with names of people who weren't previously thought of as supports. Some questions to ask:

- Do you have anyone to help you care for the children?
- Whom do you turn to when you have questions or problems?
- Whom do you trust?
- Who's your best friend?
- Are the people you live with helpful?
- Do you have relatives or neighbors who might help?
- Are any other health care professionals involved?

The more people you involve in supporting the family, the better. The family can rely on them for support after the crisis as well.

How have they coped in the past?

Determine how the family coped with stress before this. Ask: Have you ever had an experience like this before? What did you do? How do you usually relieve tension? Have you tried that method this time? If not, why? What do you think would reduce this stress?

Perhaps they used such common stress relievers as taking a walk, playing the piano, going away for the weekend, getting a babysitter more frequently, talking with a friend, painting, biking, or gardening. They may also remember methods of coping that they haven't used for years. Adaptive skills are very individual, so work with the family to determine what will best relieve stress for them.

A crucial part of your assessment is to discover any suicidal or homicidal tendencies. People in crisis do things they would never do normally. An abusing, alcoholic, addicted, or emotionally disturbed parent needs special attention.

Assess such a person carefully: Does he appear tearful, jolly, silly, indifferent? Can he express his mood openly, saying "I feel like..."? Does he appear not to care? Does he express aggression?

If you suspect a person is potentially suicidal or homicidal, ask directly: Are you planning to take your life? Have you ever thought of harming your children? Tell me your plans. How desperate do you feel?

Some people may express relief that you recognize their desperation. If appropriate, make a psychiatric referral immediately. If not, move on to intervention.

Intervention: Explore the options, then follow through

Your intervention will have two phases: a planning phase and an action phase. In the planning phase, determine how disrupted the family is and consider all the possible coping methods.

First, see if the family is continuing their

daily functioning of work, school, housework, and child care. How are other family members being affected? Are they also in crisis? Are the children receiving adequate emotional and physical care? Are they upset? You may find that a woman is so stressed by the care of her physically disabled child that she no longer cares for herself, the house, or the child. She'll require immediate intervention for child care and housework.

Consider the options

Next, investigate options open to the family to restore balance. These are usually methods they've used in the past. For example, the mother who feels like abusing her colicky baby might propose that she share the child's care with others until the colic passes. Or parents who feel their premature baby may die might choose to be told the exact status of their child and perhaps help in his care to alleviate some of their anxiety.

After you explore the possible options, put them to work. Your goals are:

- to help family members understand why they're in crisis
- to help them air feelings they've suppressed
- to explore new ways of coping
- to restore family functioning.

These goals are especially important if the family hasn't seen the relationship between the precipitating event and the crisis.

Of course, you can reduce tension by providing an opportunity to express feelings. Many people suppress their emotions of hate, grief, or guilt. This is especially true of parents who have a physically disabled child. They characteristically feel shock, denial, shame, envy, bitterness, and rejection. These feelings aren't readily admitted in our society, but they are real and must be aired to reduce anxiety. You might open a conversation such as this by saying: "People sometimes have difficulty accepting something like this. Many parents are angry (or bitter, shocked, envious, and so on). Do you feel that way?" Listen supportively and be prepared for the feelings that might be expressed.

Test the coping methods

Try to evaluate each different coping method after it's tried. If it wasn't successful, explore other options. For example, if a baby who fails to thrive makes his mother anxious because he doesn't respond to a specific formula, have her try another formula, nipple, or method of handling him during the feeding.

If a thorough assessment and adequate intervention are carried out, the coping methods tried during this phase may well be successful. And the family may then be more open to ideas about preventing future crises.

Resolve and reinforce

When the family in crisis realistically examines the problem, has adequate support, and is able to use old or new ways of coping, the crisis should be resolved within 6 weeks after the event. Evaluate at that time whether the family is beginning to function normally again. Look for a positive mood and a decrease in psychosocial symptoms such as depression, insomnia, crying, and headaches.

Finally, reinforce the family members' coping mechanisms by reviewing the experience and the action taken with them. Let them feel satisfaction with their progress in resolving the crisis.

And take personal satisfaction, too, for you've helped calm their storm and have made them better able to cope in the future.

UNIT SIX

Study questions

1. Using the approach described by Arnold and Boggs in "Self-Concepts in the Nurse-Client Relationship," how might a nurse adapt care for a toddler to maximize growth and development? For an adolescent?

2. According to "Human Interaction and Personal Boundaries" by Scott, how does the behavior of a client with opened boundaries differ from that of a client with closed boundaries? (Give five examples.)

3. In "Denial," Forchuk and Westwell suggest taking a "back door" approach when caring for a client in denial. What is this approach? Why is it more effective than direct confrontation?

4. Copel's article, "Loneliness: A Conceptual Model," describes stressors that can cause loneliness: feelings of lack of trust, shame, grief, alienation, social obstacles, cultural patterns, and pain. How do these stressors lead to loneliness? (Pick any three.)

5. "AIDS: Coping with the Fear" by Kennedy describes fear as the most "contagious" and debilitating effect of acquired immunodeficiency syndrome (AIDS). What steps can the nurse take to halt the spread of fear in the client with AIDS, the client's family and friends, other clients, and health care staff members?

6. In "Sorrow Has Many Faces: Helping Families Cope with Grief," Archer and Smith encourage the nurse to individualize care for a grieving client because no two people grieve in exactly the same way. Grief may prompt physical, emotional, mental, social, familial, or spiritual responses. How can the nurse recognize each of these responses?

7. According to Adams in "Drug Dependency in Hospital Patients," a drug-dependent client may buy drugs from a roommate, split the staff, and use other manipulative strategies to obtain drugs while hospitalized. How should a nurse deal with such a client?

8. Using the approach described by Runyon, Allen, and Ilnicki in "The Borderline Patient on the Med-Surg Unit," which nursing interventions might help a client who has a borderline personality disorder with a diagnosis of potential for violence?

9. In "At Risk for Suicide," Bydlon-Brown and Billman advise the nurse to watch a suicidal client for suicidal ideation; lack of rapport, compliance with the treatment plan, and socialization; hyperactivity or abrupt change in activity; and frequent changes in mood or constant feelings of anger or frustration. How does each behavior affect the nursing supervision of the suicidal client?

10. Hradek's "Crisis Intervention and Suicide" suggests a problem-solving method that the nurse can use in crisis intervention with a suicidal client. What are its six steps and how are they used?

11. According to "Helping the Family Through a Crisis" by Baird, which questions can a nurse ask to determine how the family perceives the problem?

UNIT SEVEN

Physiologic concepts in nursing

IN ITS DISCUSSION of psychosocial concepts, Unit Six investigated one aspect of holistic nursing care. Unit Seven explores another aspect: physiologic concepts. Significantly, a disruption in physiologic processes is the primary reason why people seek health care.

Unlike other health care professions, nursing is prinicipally concerned with the diagnosis and treatment of potential and actual human *responses* to illness — not illness itself. Therefore, the nurse does not act solely on physiologic problems, but rather on the health and lifestyle alterations caused by those problems. Thus, the nurse needs a thorough understanding of physiology and its disruptions to provide adequate care.

Physiologic concepts are more easily defined and measured than are psychosocial concepts. Knowledge about them, which comes from study of the body's normal functioning in health and its altered functioning in illness, is essential for the nurse. Yet these concepts are no more important than the more abstract ones in this book, such as psychosocial concepts. The nurse considers physiologic and psychosocial concepts, advocacy, therapeutic use of self, and various other concepts in planning and caring for a client.

Basic physiologic concepts

A client with a physiologic disruption may develop such problems as pain or alterations in nutrition, mobility, sleep, or sexuality. These problems can affect the client's psychosocial aspect (see Unit Six) and cause or exacerbate other physiologic problems. For example, pain can cause fear and anxiety, two common psychosocial concerns. It can also lead to alterations in mobility and sleep, which can be worsened further by fear and anxiety. Fortunately, the nurse understands basic physiologic concepts and can put them into practice to help the client overcome these problems. To prepare the student for this role, Section One investigates the physiologic concepts of pain, nutrition, mobility, sleep, and sexuality and describes how to relieve or prevent problems associated with them.

Physical protection

Infection control, a form of physical protection, is vital to the health of the client — and the nurse. The chain of infection consists of three basic links: a microorganism that causes the infection (an agent), a mode of transmission, and an organism (or host) susceptible to invasion by the agent. If any one of these links is missing, the chain remains incomplete and no infection can develop. The nurse can help prevent infection by using physical protection to eliminate the second link in the chain. By applying the physical protection concepts described in Section Two, the nurse can reduce the risk of infection to herself, the client, and other health care workers.

Application to practice

The articles chosen for this unit are not intended as a comprehensive review of all physiologic concepts. Rather, they are a selection of readings that illustrate the role of basic physiologic concepts in nursing practice. In fact, application to practice was a deciding factor in article selection for this unit because only through application can the nurse use physiologic concepts to improve client care. For more information about physiologic concepts, see the list of references at the end of the articles and section introductions.

SECTION ONE

Basic physiologic concepts

THIS SECTION HIGHLIGHTS several key physiologic concepts: pain, nutrition, mobility, sleep, and sexuality. It also investigates some nursing diagnoses commonly related to these concepts, including altered comfort, pain; altered nutrition, less than body requirements; impaired physical mobility; sleep pattern disturbance; and altered sexuality patterns.

Pain

Section One begins with a discussion of pain to emphasize the importance of this physiologic concept in nursing practice. To promote a therapeutic nurse-client relationship, as well as the client's health, the nurse must relieve pain. In fact, pain interventions are typically the nurse's first priority in dealing with various physiologic and psychosocial problems.

For the student, an understanding of pain holds special value for several reasons. First, it sheds light on the experience of pain, a complex physiologic process with many psychosocial implications. Second, it illustrates that pain can dramatically affect a client's interactions with the nurse, recovery from illness, and quality of life. Third, it helps the student realize the importance of an appropriate response to the client in pain to promote a therapeutic relationship and lay the groundwork for healing.

The first article, "Pain: Advances and Issues in Critical Care" by Harrison and Cotanch, provides a basic understanding of this physiologic concept. It explores the sources of pain in the critical care environment and explains several theories of pain. Then it investigates pharmacologic and other physical methods of pain relief as well as alternative therapies, such as hypnosis, relaxation techniques, and therapeutic touch. It concludes by describing how to combine these pain relief methods in a holistic (body, mind, and spirit) approach to pain management. Although this article focuses on nursing care for the critically ill client, its techniques can be applied to clients in various settings since pain is not limited to certain settings.

In any setting, however, the nurse faces two challenges related to pain: accurate pain assessment and appropriate use of analgesics (pain medications), especially narcotics.

To help the nurse assess pain effectively, Puntillo (1988) describes the following tools and their use in clinical practice:

> Pain rating instruments developed for clinical use include verbal descriptor scales and visual analogue scales to measure pain intensity. [Houde, 1982; Chapman, et al., 1985] Visual descriptor scales use words such as "no pain" and "agonizing pain" for quantification. Visual analogue scales ask patients to quantify their pain by placing a mark on a line drawn between word descriptors such as "no pain" and "worst pain." A magnitude estimation scale measures the intensity of pain exponentially by using the law of powers. [Melzack, 1975] Other scales, such as the McGill pain questionnaire, [Grinde, et al., 1984] measure additional components of the total pain experience: physiologic, emotional, and evaluative....

Appropriate analgesic administration also challenges the nurse because many health care professionals underestimate analgesia requirements, leading to inadequate pain control and prolonged client recovery. Watt-Watson (1987) explains this phenomenon:

> ...nurses and physicians fear that patients might become addicted to narcotics [Charap, 1978; Cohen, 1980]. Other clinicians feel that patients are given enough analgesia, despite those patients' reports of continued pain [Charap, 1978; Cohen, 1980; Rankin, 1982].

In effect, these health care professionals judge the client's pain by their own standards instead of the client's. To overcome this problem and relieve pain properly without overmedicating the client, the nurse should scrutinize personal views of analgesic administration, learn to assess pain accurately and objectively, and study the actions and effects of narcotics and other drugs.

Nutrition and mobility

Like pain, alterations in nutrition and mobility can affect multiple aspects of the client's recovery and can alter the nurse-client relationship. They also occur in a wide variety of settings. Unlike most instances of pain, however, they may be overlooked until they become severe.

Because most individuals easily meet their basic nutritional and mobility needs, they take those needs for granted. A client may not give nutrition or mobility a second thought until an illness or injury disrupts these normal processes. Then the nurse must be able to understand these concepts and intervene appropriately to build a therapeutic nurse-client relationship and move the client toward recovery.

In "Fulfilling Nutritional Requirements," Iverson-Carpenter et al. help the nurse do just that. They look at the assessment and etiologies of alterations in nutrition. They also explore factors that influence nutrition, signs and symptoms of undernutrition, and nursing interventions for undernutrition, including diet management, environmental structuring, client teaching, and monitoring and surveillance. The article includes a case study that shows how to apply concepts about nutrition and evaluate their effectiveness in nursing practice. Although the article focuses on alterations in nutrition in elderly clients, its principles transfer easily to clients of all ages.

The next article, "Impaired Physical Mobility" by Milde, points out that any illness or injury that restricts activity can impair the client's mobility. To help the nurse manage this potential problem, the article describes interventions designed to achieve three goals: maintenance of muscle strength, maintenance of joint flexibility, and development of an attitude that values preventive interventions. Using a case study of an elderly client with a nursing diagnosis of impaired physical mobility, the article shows how to plan, implement, and evaluate these interventions to correct the initial problem or prevent it from worsening.

Milde's article focuses on an elderly client, but any client whose movement is restricted by disease or trauma can suffer from impaired physical mobility and other problems. This article's importance is underscored by Rubin's (1988) discussion of the effects of forced bed rest:

> Skeletal muscles lose tone when the feet no longer bear weight. After just three days, a person on bed rest loses plasma and calcium, secretes less gastric juice, has less blood flowing through the calves, and shows some impairment of glucose tolerance [Greenleaf and Kozlowski, 1982].

Sleep

Although rest (a condition of altered activity) and sleep (a state of altered consciousness) are related, they are distinctly different. Their differences are readily apparent in their related nursing diagnoses: *Impaired physical mobility* deals with the physiology of rest; *sleep pattern disturbance* deals with the physiology of sleep.

Recent findings about circadian rhythms (patterns of bodily functions based on a 24-hour cycle) indicate that these rhythms keep bodily functions in balance and that disruption of these rhythms can directly affect the development, progression, and outcome of many disorders. Researchers have even demonstrated that chronic disruption of circadian rhythms can shorten the life of laboratory animals.

Unfortunately, the application of knowledge about circadian rhythms has been delayed because of the complexity of these rhythms and the difficulty in assessing them. However, many nurses are researching alterations in circadian rhythms and seeking ways to assess and treat them.

For example, circadian rhythm research at the National Institute of Mental Health prompted Ryan, Montgomery, and Meyers (1987) to describe this relationship between circadian rhythms and the client's affect:

> ...In the human body there seems to be a characteristic daily rhythm to virtually every function we can measure; e.g., the rate of absorption in the gut, intraocular pressure..., pupil size, secretion of various hormones, motility of the cilia in the respiratory tract, and the sleep/wake cycle. Although body rhythms are influenced by many factors, they are not just manifestations of external stimuli; when studied in constant environmental conditions, the rhythms persist, indicating that they are endogenous and self-sustained. These cyclic changes in the body's internal milieu...constitute a kind of temporal anatomy [that] little is known about....Biological rhythms [may] help us to adapt to our changing environment,... normal temporal anatomy may be essential to health, and...disturbances in biological rhythms [may] be consistent with illness (Wehr & Goodwin, 1981).
>
> While disturbances in biological rhythms have not been proven to *cause* affective disorders, there are substantial reasons to investigate the relationship of the circadian system to mood. Affective illness itself is inherently recurrent, with episodes often occurring and remitting spontaneously....Several classic symptoms of depression may indicate circadian rhythm disturbances, such as diurnal variation, early morning awakening, and other alterations in the sleep/wake cycle....

Normal sleep patterns contribute to the maintenance of circadian rhythms and other aspects of client health. The article, "Sleep Pattern Disturbance" by Barndt-Maglio, discusses these patterns, their causes, and nursing assessment of this condition. Then it describes how to formulate and evaluate a nursing care plan to minimize any sleep pattern disturbance and its consequences.

Although this article addresses the sleep needs of a pediatric client in a critical care unit, its principles apply to clients in other age groups and settings.

Sexuality

The last article in Section One explores human sexuality. Unlike pain, nutrition, mobility, and sleep, the concept of sexuality typically is subject to stereotyping, anxiety, and misunderstanding, especially when related to elderly clients.

In "Sexuality in Older Adults: A Continuing Education Concern," Glass and Dalton help the nurse overcome these hurdles by describing the physiology of sexuality and sexual behavior in elderly clients. They also discuss the nurse's role as sex educator, advising the nurse to examine personal views of sexuality closely before counseling others.

Sexuality can be difficult to discuss openly for the client — and for the nurse. This article's value lies in its presentation of information about sexuality that can help the nurse feel more comfortable in factual discussions, appreciate the client's concerns, and understand personal feelings that may affect the nurse-client relationship. It gives the nurse the necessary tools to assess the client accurately and intervene appropriately in this vital aspect of client health.

REFERENCES

Chapman, C., Casey, K., Dubner, R., Foley, K., Gracely, R., Reading, A. (1985). Pain measurement: An overview. *Pain, 22*, 1-31.

Charap, A. (1978). The knowledge, attitudes, and experience of medical personnel treating pain in the terminally ill. *Mt. Sinai J. Med.,45*(4), 561-580.

Cohen, F. (1980). Postsurgical pain relief: Patients' status and nurses' medication choices. *Pain, 9*(10), 265-274.

Greenleaf, J., & Kozlowski, S. (1982). Physiological consequences of reduced physical activity during bedrest. *Exerc. Sport. Sci. Rev.,10*, 84-119.

Grinde, J., Grina, R., Gallatly, T. (1984). Pain management by epidural analgesia: The challenge for nursing. *Heart & Lung, 13*, 105-110.

Houde, R. (1982). Methods for measuring clinical pain. *Acta Anaesthesio Scand, 26*, 25-29.

Melzack, R. (1975). The McGill Pain Questionnaire: Major properties and scoring methods. *Pain, 1*, 277-299.

Puntillo, K. (1988). The phenomenon of pain and critical care nursing. *Heart & Lung, 17*(3), 262-271.

Rankin, M. (1982). Use of drugs for pain with cancer patients. *Cancer Nurs, 5*(6), 181-190.

Rubin, M. (1988). The physiology of bed rest. *American Journal of Nursing, 88*(1), 50-55.

Ryan, L., Montgomery, A., and Meyers, S. (1987). Impact of circadian rhythm research on approaches to affective illness. *Archives of Psychiatric Nursing, 1*(4), 236-240.

Watt-Watson, J. (1987). What do we need to know about pain? *American Journal of Nursing, 87*(9), 1217-1218.

Wehr, R., and Goodwin, F. (1981). Biological rhythms and psychiatry. In S. Arieti and H.K.H. Brodie (Eds.), *American Handbook of Psychiatry* (2nd ed., Vol. 3). New York: Basic.

Pain: Advances and issues in critical care

MARGARET HARRISON, RN, MSN; PATRICIA H. COTANCH, RN, PhD

PHYSICAL PAIN AND ANTICIPATION of pain lead to increased discomfort for the already stressed, uncomfortable, critical care patient. Physical discomfort accompanies many treatment modalities and disease entities such as dressing changes for burned patients, deep breathing exercises for thoracotomy patients, and painful symptoms in ischemic cardiac disease patients. The critical care nurse must carefully assess the patient's pain and stress level as well as the causes of the pain and stress. The nurse must be knowledgeable about the pathophysiology of the patient's disease and potential treatment modalities. Interactions between the nurse, patient, environment, and any treatments must constantly be assessed and revisions made in the plan of care.

This article presents current knowledge in dealing with pain in the critical care patient. Current theories on pain are first presented followed by an overview of the critical care environment. Advances in pharmacologic and other physical methods of pain relief are reviewed. Alternative therapies such as hypnosis and therapeutic touch are briefly presented. Finally, these concepts are integrated into a holistic approach to pain management in critical care.

Critical care milieu

Perhaps one of most important challenges in dealing with pain in critical care areas is the fact that the patient is not always able to inform the nurse of pain. Thus assessment of indices such as facial expression, heart rate, and blood pressure are essential tools. The nurse also must be able to integrate these subtle observations with knowledge regarding possible causes of the patient's pain.

There are numerous causes of physical discomfort or pain in the critical care setting, either from iatrogenic means or because of the patient's disease process itself. The nurse must be aware of the causes in order to choose the best treatment. Surgical wounds are perhaps the most easily recognized as pain sources. Patients must not only deal with incisional pain postoperatively, but soreness from having been positioned in one place on the operating table for several hours. Invasive procedures such as central and peripheral intravenous line placement and Foley catheter insertion also can cause pain. In addition, positioning of the patient for these procedures can cause discomfort. Finally, patients, such as those suffering from a myocardial infarction or osteosarcoma, perceive pain as caused by their diseases.

There are additional factors consistent with the critical care environment that add to the patient's perception of pain. As will be discussed in the following section, emotions and state of mind affect pain perception.[10] Research indicates that the unfamiliar sights and sounds of critical care units create stress and increase discomfort in patients.[16] This psychologic stress adds to the physical factors creating a sensation of pain for the patient. Patients in critical care units lose the rapid-eye-movement sleep cycle, and thus become increasingly irritable, fatigued, and prone to pain.[13]

There are many unfamiliar stimuli in the critical care unit that may overwhelm the patient. Unpleasant tactile stimulation ranges from intravenous catheterizations to defibrillation. Unfamiliar noises and surroundings make it difficult to rest. Family and friends are able to spend only a small amount of time with the patient. Personal space is compressed, and privacy is minimal. These factors must all be considered in light of current theory on pain when planning appropriate interventions for the critical care patient.

Pain theory. Current theories on pain postulate that the peripheral sensations of pain are affected by the emotions and psychologic state of the person experiencing the pain. The most widely accepted of these theories are the gate control theory [14] and the influence of endogenous opiates or endorphins.

According to the gate control theory, the peripheral intensity of the pain can be modulated through cortical and spinal influence. Impulses from pain receptors travel via small (delta A) and large (C) diameter fibers to the substantia gelatinosa in the dorsal horn of the spinal cord. Here, the impulse is modulated by afferent stimuli from the brainstem, reticular formation, and cortex. Thus, information from the brain (memories, emotions, and situations) not only influences the perception and meaning attached to the afferent pain impulses but also affects the opening or closing of the "gate" in the spinal cord, thereby increasing or decreasing the actual transmission of the pain impulse.[14]

Recent research also indicates that substances produced in the gastrointestinal and central nervous system called endorphins play a part in changes in pain perception.[5] Enkephalin, part of the endorphin molecule, inhibits transmission of pain impulses in the spinal cord and intercepts afferent pain messages in the brainstem. Endorphin levels are increased with exercise, noxious states, labor, and delivery. Thus, altered physical and emotional states can affect the level of the pain threshold.[5]

Current theory suggests that there is an interaction of physical stimulus and psychologic or neurohormonal influences to produce the pain level as it is perceived by the patient. It must be emphasized that pain is a subjective sensation. Although there are several objective physiologic indicators often used to assess pain (such as heart rate, respiration, and blood pressure), they are not as reliable as the patient's subjective expression of pain.[10] Unfortunately, the critically ill patient is often unable to express pain or discomfort, and must rely on the nurse to anticipate pain, interpret pain signals, institute appropriate relief measures, and evaluate the degree of relief.

Advances in physical and pharmacologic pain relief

There have been several advances in pain therapy in the past decade, to block both the cause of the pain and the pain impulses before they reach the cortex. Cardiology has made several advances in relieving anginal pain at its source. Advances in modalities to block efferent pain impulses have led to the development and use of transcutaneous electrical nerve stimulation (TENS) and epidural and patient-controlled analgesia.

Advances in cardiology. Several new methods of treating blocked coronary arteries to relieve ischemic pain have been instituted in the past decade. Intravenous (IV) nitroglycerin (NIG) dilates coronary arteries in both healthy and ischemic cardiac tissue.[19] Intravenous streptokinase dissolves fibrin clots, thus opening the lumen of occluded coronary arteries.[15] Research in tissue-type plasminogen activator (t-PA) indicates that this substance is effective in dissolving coronary artery fibrin clots with less peripheral side effects than streptokinase.[4] The more invasive therapy of coronary artery angioplasty yields good results for a select group of patients without the hazards of surgery.[12]

TENS. Other recent advances in pain treatment seek to block the pain impulse before it reaches the brain. The TENS unit generates electrical pulses of adjustable frequency and amplitude, which interfere with the conduction of afferent pain stimuli to the spinal cord.

TENS has been used most widely with non-critically ill patients. However, this non-narcotic analgesia has the potential to alleviate incisional pain for postoperative patients in critical care units. Studies indicate that it may be used safely for patients with cardiac pacemakers.[18] The electrodes must be placed along the incision line so that efferent pain signals are blocked. This device is thus best used with patients who have pain of specific physical origin, so that the nerve tracts are more easily identified. The obvious advantage to this type of analgesia is pain relief without sedation.

Patient-controlled analgesia (PCA). Continuous intravenous infusions of small amounts of narcotics allow a more constant serum level of medication, and thus a more constant level of analgesia. PCA devices allow...patient[s] to administer small dosages of their prescribed medication when they feel the need.[2]....

Constant levels of the drug in the blood stream mean that lower levels may be used to obtain analgesia, thus decreasing the chances of sedation and other undesirable effects. Critical care patients eligible for this type of device are those who are alert, such as burn patients or trauma patients without head injury.

Spinal analgesia. Epidural anesthesia has been used for many years in surgery, as well as in labor and delivery. However, spinal analgesia has only recently been recognized as an option in pain relief. Several institutions have found this method of analgesia preferable for postoperative thoracotomy patients because it reduces the need for parenteral narcotics and improves the patient's ability to perform postoperative exercises.[7]

The level of analgesia allowed by epidural narcotics is greater than that of parenteral narcotics, without as severe a depression of the central nervous system.[11] Epidural analgesia does not block the sympathetic nervous system; therefore, problems with hypotension are rare. The major side effects are urine retention, nausea, vomiting, and pruritus. Respiratory depression is rare, but the patient must be monitored closely for any changes in respiratory pattern.[11]

Spinal/epidural analgesia is currently gaining popularity as a pain relief modality for critical care patients. Its advantages in patient care and pain relief are obvious....

Alternative therapies

Although some researchers have made advances treating the source of pain, or blocking efferent pain impulses before they reach the brain, other researchers have explored very different avenues for pain relief. Several of these techniques have been used effectively in other patient populations; however, very few critical care patients have had the opportunity to test them.

Hypnosis has been used successfully to treat chronic and acute pain states for many years.[1] Critical care patients are already in an altered state because of unfamiliar surroundings, pharmacologic therapy, and stress and would thus be susceptible to hypnotic suggestions for pain relief. Hypnotherapy for pain relief can be an effective, noninvasive method of analgesia for the critical care patient....

Muscle tension and anxiety have been implicated as causes of pain.[14] Research indicates that muscle relaxation and relief of anxiety can alleviate pain.[6] Postoperative cardiac surgery patients who were instructed in relaxation techniques demonstrated lower pain and distress levels on ambulation than those patients who received no relaxation instruction.[9] For critically ill patients who are able to understand instructions, this could be a valuable pain reduction tool, especially during unpleasant procedures such as cardiac catheterization and pacemaker insertion.

Finally, therapeutic touch has been used successfully to alleviate pain in critical care patients.[17] Therapeutic touch [is] a form of laying on of hands that redirects the energies of the client into a more heathful balance.... Studies indicate that this intervention is effective in reducing anxiety [8] and augmenting pain relief.[3] Although formal training in therapeutic touch requires workshop attendance and practice, nurses use some of the principles and techniques of therapeutic touch when administering back rubs, holding a patient's hand, or massaging a painful area. Whether guided by formal techniques or simply by a caring attitude, touch seems to assist the patient in coping with pain and anxiety.

Holism in pain care

As indicated previously, there are many methods of pain relief. The critical care nurse is in the unique position of coordinating the health care team's efforts to obtain pain relief for the patient. The nurse is at the bedside and is in the optimal position to assess the patient. This assessment should include physical, psychologic, and emotional causes of the pain, as well as the availability of support systems and significance of pain to the patient.

With these data, the nurse may then work with other members of the health care team to plan the most appropriate therapies for the patient. Pharmacists can assist in suggesting the most appropriate pharmacologic agents, as well as searching for any adverse drug interactions that may negate analgesic effects. Physical therapists can plan exercise programs and other therapies such as TENS or heat packs to alleviate pain. Whirlpool treatment will play a large role in the treatment of patients with burns. A clinical nurse specialist may be consulted for assistance with therapeutic touch or hypnotherapy if the bedside nurse is not skilled in these areas.

Although the critical care nurse may not provide all treatments for the patient, she or he retains the responsibility for monitoring the patient's overall response. Knowledge of each treatment modality is essential. The nurse must be familiar with methods of enhancing the particular methods used as well as monitoring any phenomena that would lessen their effect.

Pain relief involves not only administration of pharmacologic agents, but the creation of an atmosphere conducive to pain relief. This is difficult in a critical care unit, where stressors seem to surround the patient. However, the skillful critical care nurse can do much to overcome these obstacles with a careful mixture of technical as well as psychoemotional knowledge and skills.

Decreasing physical and emotional stressors through comfortable positioning of the patient, and visitation of family and friends can aid in pain relief. The latter can bring familiar objects such as a radio or tape-player, which should be checked for safety by hospital engineering before use by the patient. Music from a favorite radio station can be distracting and soothing, thus enhancing analgesia. In addition, planning care and altering the environment in order to allow for long sleep periods also can decrease perceived pain levels.

Finally, it is important to avoid any negative suggestions in conversation with the patient. Substitute "now this is going to hurt a little" with "this is going to help us care for you. You can feel more comfortable by taking slow deep breaths and concentrating on the music from the radio." The burn unit in one large teaching hospital has found that pictures of soothing scenes coupled with the patient's favorite music can assist in decreasing perceived discomfort during dressing changes.

Many of these interventions are very simple and do not require any extra training. However, positive suggestion, distraction, and relaxation can augment pharmacologic analgesia. These simple methods assist patients by closing the gate to pain impulses and increasing circulating endorphins.[1, 14] Providing measures for stress reduction through family input and familiar surroundings reduces anxiety, and thus pain.[5] The combination of stress reduction and pain relief through the methods discussed previously all contribute to decreased pain perception for the critical care patient whose environment is replete with stressors and painful stimuli....

REFERENCES

1. Barber J., Adrian C (eds): Psychological Approaches to Pain Relief. New York, Brunner Mazel, 1982

2. Bennett R, Griffen WO: Patient-controlled analgesia. Contemporary Surgery 23:83, 1983

3. Boguslawski M: Therapeutic touch: A facilitator of pain relief. Topics in Clinical Nursing 2:27, 1980

4. Brewer CC, Markis JE: Streptokinase and tissue plasminogen activator in acute myocardial infarction. Heart Lung 15:552, 1986

5. Dolphin NW: Neuroanatomy and neurophysiology of pain: Int J Nurs Stud 20:255-263, 1983

6. Flaherty GG, Fitzpatrick JJ: Relaxation techniques to increase comfort level of post-operative patients. Nurs Res 27:352-355, 1978

7. Grinde JW, Grina TA: Pain management by epidural anesthesia: The challenge for nursing. Heart Lung 13:105-110, 1984

8. Heidt P: Effect of therapeutic touch on anxiety level of hospitalized patients. Nurs Res 30:32-37, 1981

9. Horowitz BF, Fitzpatrick JJ, Flaherty GG: Relaxation techniques for pain relief after open heart surgery. Dimensions in Critical Care Nursing 3:364-371, 1984

10. Kim S: Pain: Theory, research and nursing practice. ANS 2:43-59, 1980

11. Lieb RA, Hurtig JB: Epidural and intrathecal narcotics for pain management. Heart Lung 14:164-174, 1985

12. Loan T: Nursing interaction with patients undergoing coronary angioplasty. Heart Lung 15:368-375, 1986

13. McCauley K, Polomako RC: Acute pain: A nursing perspective with cardiac surgery patients. Topics in Clinical Nursing 2:45-56, 1980

14. Melzack R, Wall PD: Psychophysiology of pain. Int Anesthesiol Clin 8:3-34, 1970

15. Nissen MB: Streptokinase therapy in acute MI. Heart Lung 13:223-230, 1984

16. Patacky MG, Gavin BJ, Schwirian PM: Intra-aortic balloon pumping and stress in the coronary care unit. Heart Lung 14:142-148, 1985

17. Quinn JF: Therapeutic touch as an energy exchange: Testing the theory. ANS 6:42-49, 1984

18. Shade SK: Use of transcutaneous electrical nerve stimulation for a patient with a cardiac pacemaker. Phys Ther 65:206-208, 1985

19. Vallardes BR, Lemberg L: Intravenous nitroglycerin in acute infarction: I. Heart Lung 11:383-385, 1982

Fulfilling nutritional requirements

MARTHA S. IVERSON-CARPENTER, RN, BSN, MA; DEBBIE HASKIN, RN, BSN; MERIDEAN MAAS, RN, PhD; MARY HARDY, RN, PhD; MARGARET BUTTON, RN, BSN

ALTERATION IN NUTRITION includes the concepts of malnutrition,[1-3] undernutrition,[4-6] overnutrition,[4-6] and starvation.[7, 8] Undernutrition, however, appears closely related to the nursing diagnosis of Alteration in Nutrition: Less than Body Requirements, which is defined by the North American Nursing Diagnosis Association (NANDA), as "The state in which an individual experiences an intake of nutrients insufficient to meet metabolic needs."[9]

Assessment and etiologies of alterations in nutrition

Nutritional assessment includes dietary history, physical examination, anthropometric (body) measurements, biochemical measurements, and socioenvironmental and functional abilities evaluation. From the assessment data, factors influencing the alteration in nutrition and diagnosis are determined. Good nutritional status improves other important patient outcomes. Quality patient care requires assessment of nutritional status, planning of intervention strategies, and monitoring of progress.

The assessment must be highly individualized, since elderly persons' abilities, capabilities, and levels of function vary widely. Intervening variables affecting alteration in nutrition include age, prior nutritional status of the client, food habits and beliefs, and the severity and duration of the antecedent conditions.

Factors influencing undernutrition

Any factor that interrupts or interferes with any stage of the nutritional process can result in Alteration in Nutrition. The Less than Body Requirements etiologies/related factors can be grouped into four categories: inadequate ingestion; increased need; inadequate digestion; and inadequate absorption. Each of these categories will be discussed as they relate specifically to the elderly [client]....

Inadequate ingestion. Both quantity and quality of food intake can be involved when the amount of nutrients ingested is a problem. Elderly persons with mechanical feeding problems such as difficulty chewing with dentures or poor condition of mouth or teeth may have difficulty maintaining an adequate food intake.[4] Dysphagia, difficulty swallowing, may result from a stroke[10] or other neurological disease.[11] Intake may be reduced because of a mechanical obstruction of the esophagus such as a tumor or a stricture[12] or the painful swallowing that accompanies esophagitis.[5]

Anorexia is another factor that often influences intake. Neural mechanisms located in the hypothalamus are responsible for hunger and satiety. Conditions related to anorexia may be disease related, drug related, or psychological.[13] Disease processes resulting in anorexia include cancer, fevers, and gastrointestinal disorders.[4] Liver dysfunction, a common secondary effect of alcoholism, also often results in anorexia.[14]

Drugs reported to alter taste include griseofulvin, Atromid-S, Lincocin, chloral hydrate, paraldehyde, vitamin B complex, and penicillin.[15] Psychological factors of emotions, stress, and alterations in body image can result in anorexia. Finally, confusion and social isolation that often accompany institutionalization of elderly persons increase distraction and lack of motivation for eating.

The quality of food intake can result in inadequate ingestion of nutrients. Factors involved include environmental constraints, food allergies, education, and sociocultural responses.[13] For the elderly who are more apt to be institutionalized and have higher instances of confusion and impaired mobility, these factors are especially likely to result in altered nutrition.

Hospital procedures that require fasting and prolonged use of glucose and saline intravenous feedings affect the quality and quantity [of] food intake.[8,16,17] Physical and social immobility in the elderly at home or in long-term care facilities can result in inadequate quality of food because of inaccessibility to food supply, difficulties of food preparation, and lack of interest in eating alone.[4]

Food allergies, commonly [to] wheat, milk, eggs, fish, shellfish, nuts, pork, strawberries, tomatoes, chocolate,[5,16] or artificial colors or additives,[5] can result in nutrient deficiencies if adequate substitution or supplements are not made. Knowledge the elderly client has about nutrition as well as religious, cultural, and economic factors[1] will affect the intake of food. Lack of education and poor nutritional status often co-exist.[1]

In addition, illiterate people or persons... who have not mastered English may not be able to read food product labels or directions found on food packages.[18] The amount of money available to purchase food and the facilities available for food preparation will influence nutritional intake.[1,5,18] Elderly on fixed public assistance, Social Security, and pension incomes are especially prone to economic factors that interfere with adequate nutrition.

Increased need. An increased need for nutrients can result from an increase in metabolism or from a loss of nutrients from the gastrointestinal tract. Because the elderly are more prone to chronic illnesses and effects of acute exacerbations, they are especially likely to experience undernutrition due to increased metabolism without a corresponding increase in nutrients. Fever, infections, surgery, stress, and burns all increase the need for nutrients.[19] Administration of sufficient intravenous solutions to meet daily caloric requirements may cause problems of fluid overload for many elderly [clients] who have compromised cardiovascular systems....

The body's store of glucose and glycogen [is] sufficient for only one day.[12] The body turns to protein catabolism to meet the requirements of glucose-dependent cells, such as brain and kidney cells.[6,17,21]
A well-nourished individual can endure semistarvation for three to four days, but after that period, muscle protein and subcutaneous fat are used for energy sources.[13] Patients with only saline and dextrose intravenous support for a period greater than five days are at risk for protein-calorie malnutrition.[22] A major surgery may result in six weeks of catabolism[17] and can result in muscle wasting, muscle weakness, weight loss, and increased excretion of urinary nitrogen.[12] These circumstances are often further compounded for chronically ill elderly [clients] who also require diuretic drug therapy.

An increased loss of nutrients results from vomiting, diarrhea, and increased food transit time through the intestinal tract. Diseases such as gastritis, irritable bowel, inflammatory bowel disease, and bacterial and viral infections can result in diarrhea.[5, 11] Intestinal obstruction,[12] prolonged pain,[23] and side effects of many drugs, especially chemotherapy,[5] are frequent causes of vomiting.

Vomiting and diarrhea also result from radiation therapy for cancer.[5] Overuse of cathartics, a common occurrence for many elderly persons, increases gastric motility and often results in diarrhea.[24] The dumping syndrome following gastrectomy increases food transit time and diarrhea results.[25]

Inadequate digestion. Inadequate digestion results in decreased utilization of food particles present in the stomach and the small intestine. Factors influencing digestion in elderly persons include drugs, diseases, and treatment regimens. Drugs that inhibit gastric acid in the stomach include diazepam, carbonic anhydrase inhibitors, cimetidine, vasopressin, and atropine.[11] Drugs interfering with bile and pancreatic enzymes include alcohol, neomycin, and cholestyramine.[5] Chronic pancreatitis and pancreatic cancer reduce the level of pancreative lipase and proteolytic enzymes, thus impairing fat and protein digestion respectively.[11]

Cirrhosis and/or obstructions in the hepatic-biliary systems reduce the amount of bile, thereby decreasing micelle formation[5] necessary for absorption of fatty acids, glycerol, and fat-soluble vitamins by the body. Liver dysfunction can result in faulty absorption, faulty metabolism, and faulty storage of nutrients.[14] Gastric resection and radiation of the stomach can reduce the formation of hydrochloric acid[11] necessary for protein breakdown.

Inadequate absorption. Inadequate absorption results in a decrease of amino acids, glucose, fat complexes, vitamins, and minerals available to body cells. Factors influencing absorption of nutrients for the elderly [client] are diseases, drugs, and surgical procedures. Diseases such as diverticulosis and chronic irritable bowel syndrome decrease absorption. Drugs known to interfere with nutrient absorption are colchicine, antacids, neomycin, pyrimethamine, and para-aminosalicyclic acid.[5] Intestinal procedures such as bowel resection and colectomy reduce the amount of available surface[25] for nutrient absorption. Decreased absorption of nutrients can result in weight loss, body atrophy, and vitamin deficiencies of A, B complex, and D.[12]

Signs and symptoms of undernutrition

Nutritional deficiencies are regarded as primary or secondary problems. Primary nutrient deficiency occurs from an inadequate ingestion of nutrients. Secondary nutrient deficiency results from inadequate digestion, absorption, or metabolism of nutrients.[2,5] The signs and symptoms of Alteration in Nutrition: Less Than Body Requirements fall into five categories: inadequate food intake, changes in serum and urine laboratory values, changes in body organs, changes in functioning of body systems, and disease states....

Inadequate ingestion. Inadequate ingestion of nutrients, [whether] quality or quantity, results in inadequate food intake for the body. Dietary standards such as the Recommended Dietary Allowances (RDA) provide a guideline and a measurement...for the people in the United States.[6] However,...these standards are developed for healthy individuals, [and]...the calorie requirements for [the] elderly (beyond 75 years) [are] reduced to 75-80% of that [for] young adults.[26] However, protein requirements increase slightly for the elderly [client]....

Laboratory values. Secondary deficiencies result in biochemical changes in urine and serum values.[5,6] A listing of some biochemical measurements for separate nutrients is found in Table 1. Serum albumin level and the total lymphocyte count are the most useful indices to assess nutritional status,[22] while creatinine height index may be the most sensitive measure.[27]

Body changes. Although a weight loss of greater than 10 lbs is a significant measure,[22] it is not an independent valid indicator of undernutrition. Elderly persons may experience muscle wasting and still be obese. The use of anthropometric measures can determine muscle wasting.[4,5,19] In general, women tend to be more prone to undernutrition with obesity than men. For both sexes, protein-calorie malnutrition can exist when weight status appears normal. It is important that the nurse, in consultation with the dietitian, carefully evaluate all the signs and symptoms of Alteration in Nutrition: Less than Body Requirements so that the diagnosis is not mistakenly assessed in the presence of no weight loss. A combination of weight history and measures of protein

TABLE 1. Biochemical measures of nutritional status

NUTRIENT	MORE SENSITIVE MEASUREMENTS	LESS SENSITIVE MEASUREMENTS
Protein	Plasma amino acids Hair root morphology Serum albumin Urinary creatinine height Urinary hydroxyproline	Total serum protein
Lipids	Serum cholesterol Serum triglycerides Lipoproteins	
Vitamin A	Serum vitamin A Serum carotene	
Vitamin D	Serum 25-OH-vitamin D_3 Serum alkaline phosphatase	Serum calcium Serum phosphorus
Vitamin E	Hydrogen peroxide erythrocyte hemolysis test Serum or plasma tocopherol	
Vitamin K		Prothrombin time
Thiamine	Urinary thiamine Erythrocyte transketolase activity	Blood pyruvate
Riboflavin	Urinary riboflavin Erythrocyte glutathione reductase	
Nicotinic Acid	N^1 methyl nicotinamide	Urinary pyridone
Vitamin B_6	Tryptophan load test (mg xanthurenic acid in urine)	Urinary pyridoxine (mcg gm creatine) Blood transaminase
Folic Acid	Red cell folate	Serum folate Bone marrow film Thin blood film Urinary FIGLU
Vitamin B_{12}	Serum B_{12} Serum thimidylate synthetase Urine methylmalonic acid	Bone marrow film Thin blood film Schilling test
Vitamin C	Serum ascorbic acid	Urinary ascorbic acid
Iron	Iron deposits in bone marrow Serum iron % saturation of transferrin	Hemoglobin Hematocrit Thin blood film
Iodine		Urinary iodine Tests for thyroid function
Zinc	Serum and plasma zinc	Hair
Magnesium	Serum magnesium	

status are the critical indicators for assessing nutritional status.

Functioning of body systems. Malnutrition can interfere with any body mechanism that acts to resist infectious agents.[28] Protein deficiency inhibits the immune response due to decreased production of lymphocytes and can result in susceptibility to infections[28,29] and delayed antibody response to antigens.[22,27,29] Wound healing is delayed in patients with nutrient alteration. Nutrients required for adequate wound repair include amino acids; glucose; vitamins C, D, E, K; zinc, copper, and iron; and essential fatty acids.[13,30-32]

Consolazio identified impaired work performance with a diet deficient in nutrients.[33] Physical immobility due to decreased energy, resulting from inadequate nutrition, was identified by Carnevali and Brueckner.[34] Kim and Moritz have identified alteration in nutrition as an antecedent in the following diagnostic categories: ineffective airway clearance, ineffective breathing patterns, and impairment of skin integrity.[35] Any physiological condition could be affected by nutrient deficiencies; thus additional categories could be included: decreased cardiac output; actual volume deficit; sleep pattern disturbance; alteration in tissue perfusion and alteration in bowel elimination; constipation; and diarrhea.

Disease states. Protein and caloric deficiencies are called marasmus and kwashiorkor in children but also occur in adults. Vitamin deficiencies result in diseases such as scurvy, lack of Vitamin C; rickets, lack of vitamin D; pellagra, decreased niacin; and pernicious anemia, lack of Vitamin B_{12}. Mineral deficiencies and associated disease states are calcium and tetany, iodine and goiter, calcium and phosphorus and osteoporosis, and iron deficiency anemia.[2]

Case study

Mrs. S, an 84-year-old widow[ed] for 15 years, was admitted to a long-term care (LTC) facility by her daughter. The daughter stated that the reason for Mrs. S's admission was that her mother was becoming more forgetful and had experienced a 25-lb weight loss during the past year. The daughter stated, "Mother just can't seem to sit still and seems to have lost interest in eating and life in general." The daughter also reported that she tried to provide three well-balanced meals each day, [but] her mother just couldn't sit still long enough to eat them. She also reported a deterioration in eating habits stating, "Mother often tries to eat food with her fingers, even food like mashed potatoes. She drinks well if I hand the glass to her frequently, but usually walks around when she eats."

Mrs. S especially likes fresh fruits and vegetables. The noon meal is her favorite, and she is used to light breakfast and supper. She has never been much of a meat eater, but likes fish and turkey. She is especially fond of coffee, tea, and fruit juice.

She drinks a glass of prune juice daily, which seems to keep her bowels regular. Her caloric intake has been about 1000 calories per day and her fluid intake has been 1000 cc. or less each day. Mrs. S's weight for most of her life was about 130 pounds and is now 95 pounds. She is 5'2" tall, indicating that she was somewhat overweight when younger, but is now below average for her age and build.

Mrs. S has always been healthy, according to her daughter, and currently takes no medication. Physical examination revealed no major medical problems other than unspecified dementia. She has had a recent vision exam and obtained a new pair of glasses which corrected her vision to 20/30 in both eyes. She appears to hear normal tones of voice, but has never had her hearing evaluated by an audiologist. She ambulates with no restriction of mobility and is very curious about her surroundings, exploring periodically during the interview and exam.

She is able to bathe, dress, and groom her-

> self if she is reminded. She toilets herself and has no incontinence. Mrs. S was unable to provide information herself, although she verbalizes and responds to questions. She is easily distracted by environmental stimuli. Her answers were often inappropriate and indicated disorientation to time, place, and person. She did, however, call her daughter by name.
>
> Mrs. S has her own teeth and none are chipped or cracked. She has had regular dental exams throughout her life. Oral mucosa is free of lesions, redness, or swelling. She is generally well groomed. Her skin is intact with dry, scaly skin noted on shins, forearms, and face. Her hair is gray with a straw-like texture. Recently, she had a cut on her leg that the daughter stated was very slow to heal. Laboratory results [showed] her hematocrit within normal limits, but her hemoglobin was 9 gm/100 ml. BUN was within normal limits. Skin fold measurements revealed less than 1/2 inch of body fat over the entire body. She is very frail looking and pale and appears to have generalized muscle wasting.

The nursing diagnosis inferred from the assessment data in the case study is "Alteration in Nutrition: Less than Body Requirements related to inadequate ingestion secondary to dementia, evidenced by 25-lb weight loss, inability to sit for eating meals, distractibility, low daily average caloric and fluid intake, and low hemoglobin level."

Interventions

Interventions are aimed at the factors judged to be related to or influencing the nutritional problem. Nursing interventions for the diagnosis of Alteration in Nutrition: Less than Body Requirements must focus on the individual signs and symptoms evidenced by the client. Two specific interventions, diet management and environmental structuring, are developed herein and applied to the preceding case study. Additional interventions that may be appropriate for undernutrition are summarized in Table 2.

Diet management. The nurse and the dietitian must collaborate to effectively manage the elderly person's diet. This begins with initiation of a food diary. The food diary not only tells the nurse and dietitian the amount of intake in 24 hours, but also will reveal what foods/fluids and patterns of intake are best received by the elderly client. This is epecially important for identifying the kinds of iron rich foods that are preferred, which are tolerated best, and what time of the day they are most often eaten. In collaboration with the dietitian, the nurse should capitalize on the food preferences that are identified and arrange for the provision of foods that are most apt to be eaten and that are [rich] in calories and iron....Once the beneficial foods and patterns of intake are selected, ongoing monitoring of intake, weight, and hemoglobin is necessary for evaluation of effectiveness.

Weight should be measured weekly at the same time and on the same scale. The food diary should be continued until the foods and times for ingestion are shown to be accepted by the client. Then the food diary should be kept at some appropriate interval for 24 hours to verify [that] foods and patterns of intake are still acceptable. Periodic follow-up with the food diary will minimize the burden of documentation for nursing staff and potentially increase accuracy of the measurement of intake, continuing to keep attention focused on the client's food and fluid intake.

Environmental structuring. Environmental structuring is prescribed to minimize the client's distractions from eating; increase the pleasure of eating; and capitalize on aspects of the setting, utensils, and assistance that will most likely result in increased eating time at the table for the client. Hall, Kirschling, and Todd found that neither the large group dining arrangement nor completely isolated dining were optimally effective for cognitively im-

TABLE 2. Interventions for alteration in nutrition: less than body requirements

Diet Management	Reduce or eliminate causative factors: -nausea or vomiting -swallowing difficulty -mechanical obstruction Vary liquids to allow for different textures and tastes Use commercially prepared or homemade high-protein calorie supplements Communicate likes to appropriate persons Provide one food item at a time Provide finger foods Serve small frequent meals Provide foods with a variety of textures Provide diet as tolerated with the exception of alcohol, coffee, meat extracts, cola drinks, black pepper No foods eaten 2 hours before bedtime Increase liquid intake with meals Wet foods to make up for lack of saliva or use artificial saliva Avoid eating only milk and milk products because they tend to cause tenacious mucous Provide food selection Grant special food requests Serve food for individual tastes
Environmental Structuring	Reduce or eliminate causative factors: -altered sense of taste or smell -social isolation -noxious stimuli Arrange pleasant surroundings while eating
Patient Teaching	Instruct or assist resident to keep a record of intake Teach techniques to maintain adequate nutritional intake and stimulate appetite Instruct to perform oral hygiene prior to eating Instruct to rinse mouth of debris, refresh, and lubricate mouth Teach side effects of drugs pertaining to dry mouth and decreased salivation Instruct to suck on lemon immediately prior to eating to increase salivation Promote independence in eating
Monitoring and Surveillance	Monthly weight, at least Regular monitoring of lab values Ongoing evaluation of tolerance to diet

paired elderly [clients].[36] Food items introduced one at a time, arrangement of medication administration, and other unit activities should be structured to not disrupt eating. For example, staff should not converse with one another, music if present should be soothing and subtle, and all staff should maintain an unhurried and supportive atmosphere. Food should also be delivered and served in the most attractive and respectful way possible.

If these prescriptions fail to increase the client's eating time and intake of essential foods, the nurse should arrange provision of supplemental foods and fluids so that it matches the nutritional needs and behavior of the client. Finger foods and fluids with high nutrient value can be prepared in advance to be given to the client to eat on the run.

Application to case study. Diet management and environmental structuring are interventions appropriate to Mrs. S's case because they focus on the inadequacy of her intake, inability to sit for eating meals, distractibility, low daily average caloric and fluid intake, and low hemoglobin. Specifically, the nurse should seat Mrs. S at a table with two to three other residents in a quiet, pleasant room. One food item at a time should be offered to Mrs. S to reduce distractibility. Also, when new items are offered, it helps focus the client's attention and extend interest in eating.

The nurse should also make arrangements so that medications are not passed when Mrs. S is trying to eat. Other unit activities should be structured to not disrupt eating. Mrs. S might further respond to the nurse sitting with her while she eats, prompting her to eat and drink, and providing other quiet conversation that refocuses Mrs. S's attention and interest on eating.

If Mrs. S gets up and walks around, the nurse should be prepared to accompany her in a nonthreatening way and redirect her to the table and her food. Food supplements appropriate for Mrs. S might be raisins, nuts, cheese, cookies made with grains, and juice in a non-spill cup that she could carry with her.

Evaluation

Evaluation is the process of measuring achievement of outcomes as a result of treatment. Expected outcomes from the nurse's intervention are the elimination or reversal of the signs and symptoms for the nursing diagnosis. Desired outcomes for the Mrs. S case study would include 1) weight gain of 3 to 5 lbs in three months; 12 to 15 lbs in one year; 2) increase hemoglobin to 10 gm/100 ml or above in six months; 3) increase in sitting time at meals to 15 minutes; and 4) increase [of] caloric intake to 1500 to 2000 calories and fluid intake to 2000 cc. (or whatever is appropriate). Ongoing and periodic measurement of achievement of these outcomes will determine the effectiveness of the above interventions and the changes necessary to meet the goals.

Summary

The critical role of nutrition for the well-being of older persons makes it imperative for the nurse to diagnose and intervene with nutritional problems. Alteration in Nutrition: Less than Body Requirements is one of the most prevalent nursing diagnoses among elderly persons in long-term and acute health care facilities[37] (Maas M, Hardy M, Akins J, unpublished data 1987), a diagnosis also prevalent among elderly persons who reside in their own homes.

REFERENCES

1. Loustau A: Nutritional Status, in Mitchell P, Loustau A (eds): *Concepts Basic to Nursing,* New York, McGraw-Hill, 1981.

2. Williams S: *Nutrition and Diet Therapy,* ed 4. St. Louis, CV Mosby Co, 1981.

3. Thiele V: *Clinical Nutrition,* ed 2. St. Louis, CV Mosby Co, 1980.

4. Caly J: Nutrition, in Burgess A (ed): *Nursing: Levels of Health Intervention.* Englewood Cliffs, NJ, Prentice-Hall, 1978.

5. Krause M, Mahan L: *Food, Nutrition, and Diet Therapy,* ed 6. Philadelphia, WB Saunders, 1977.

6. Green M., Harry J: *Nutrition in Contemporary Nursing Practice.* New York, John Wiley and Sons, 1981.

7. Moore F: *Metabolic Care of the Surgical Patient.* Philadelphia, WB Saunders, 1959.

8. Butterworth C: The Skeleton in the Hospital Closet. *Nutrition Today.* 1974; 9(2):4-8.

9. Kim M, McFarland G, McLane A: *Pocket Guide to Nursing Diagnosis.* St. Louis, CV Mosby, 1987.

10. Tilton C, Maloof M: Diagnosing the problem strokes. *Am J Nurs* 1982; 82:596-602.

11. Greenberger N: *Gastrointestinal Disorders,* ed 2. Chicago, Yearbook Medical Publishers, 1981.

12. Walter J: *An Introduction to the Principles of Disease.* Philadelphia, WB Saunders, 1977.

13. Howard R, Herbold N: *Nutrition in Clinical Care,* ed 2. New York, McGraw-Hill, 1982.

14. Fredette S: When the Liver Fails. *Am J Nurs* 1984; 84:64-67.

15. Lambert M: Drug and Diet Interactions. *Am J Nurs* 1975; 75:402-406.

16. Bodinski L: *The Nurse's Guide to Diet Therapy.* New York, John Wiley and Sons, 1982.

17. Steffee W: Malnutrition in Hospitalized Patients. *JAMA* 1980; 244:2630-2635.

18. Veninga K: Nutritional Assessment in Spradly B (ed): *Readings in Community Health Nursing,* ed 2. Boston, Little, Brown and Co, 1982.

19. Salmond S: How to Assess the Nutritional Status of Acutely Ill Patients, *Am J Nurs* 1980; 80:922-924.

20. Delaney R, Lapitan N, Askanazi J, et al: Nutritional Support of the Acutely Ill Patient. *Heart Lung* 1983; 12:477-480.

21. Forlaw L: The Critically Ill Patient: Nutritional Implications. *Nurs Clin North Am* 1983; 18:111-117.

22. Lang C, Cooning S, Newman S: Nutritional Support: A Foundation for Critical Care. *Critical Care Quarterly* 1982; 5(2):45-47.

23. Meinhart N, McCaffery M: *Pain: A Nursing Approach to Assessment and Analysis.* Norwalk, Connecticut, Appleton-Century-Crofts, 1983.

24. Black C, Popovich N, Black M: Drug Interactions in the GI Tract. *Am J Nurs* 1977; 77:1426-1429.

25. Hoppe M, Descalso J, Kapp S: Gastrointestinal Disease: Nutritional Implications. *Nurs Clin North Am* 1983; 18:47-55.

26. Worthington-Roberts B, Karkeck JM: Nutrition in Carnevali D, Patrick M (eds): *Nursing Management for the Elderly,* ed 2. St. Louis, JB Lippincott Co, 1986; 189-218.

27. Bistrian B, Blackburn G, Sherman M, et al: Therapeutic Index of Nutritional Depletion in Hospitalized Patients. *Surg Gynecol Obstet* 1975; 141:512-516.

28. Scrimshaw N: Nutrition and Infection. *Prog Food Nutr Sci* 1975; 1:393-340.

29. Keithley J: Infection and the Malnourished Patient. *Heart Lung* 1983; 12:23-27.

30. Keithley J: Wound Healing in Malnourished Patients. *ACRN J* 1982; 35:1094-1098.

31. Levenson S, Seifter E: Dysnutrition, Wound Healing, and Resistance to Infection. *Clin Plast Surg* 1977; 4(3):375-388.

32. Irwin T, Hunt T: Effect of Malnutrition on Colonic Healing. *Ann Surg* 1974; 180:765-772.

33. Consolazio C: Nutrition and Performance. *Prog Food Nutr Sci* 1983; 7:29-42.

34. Carnevali D, Brueckner S: Immobilization—Reassessment of a Concept. *Am J Nurs* 1970; 70:1502-1507.

35. Kim M, Moritz D: *Classification of Nursing Diagnosis.* New York, McGraw-Hill, 1982.

36. Hall G, Kirschling V, Todd S: Sheltered Freedom—An Alzheimer's Unit in an ICF. *Geriatr Nurs* 1986; 1986(3):132-137.

37. Hallal J: Nursing Diagnosis: An Essential Step in Quality Care. *J Gerontol Nurs* 1985; 11(19):35-38.

Impaired physical mobility

FRANCES KAY MILDE, RN, PhD

THE ABILITY TO MOVE freely and easily is a prized possession. The functioning of all body systems is directly or indirectly enhanced by periodic changes in body positions. Unfortunately, unrestricted mobility is not always possible. All disease and rehabilitative states involve some degree of immobility. With aging, potential for the occurrence of decreased mobility increases and the possibility of untoward outcomes also increases. Nursing management is central to maximize an individual's full mobility.

Impaired physical mobility may result quickly or insidiously. The duration may be time limited or chronic. One of the greatest tragedies occurs when an individual is impaired with an acute problem and later develops a chronic problem because of interactive effects and nursing management deficiencies. This article will address such a problem by presenting the onset and progression, through a case study, of an individual with a nursing diagnosis of impaired physical mobility. In addition, an explanation of the background of the problem and a prescription for interventions that effectively prevent or negate the pathological responses will be covered. The presentation will focus on the musculoskeletal system.

Onset: Case study

Alice P. is a 74-year-old female admitted to the hospital with acute abdominal pain. Prior to the onset of pain, she lived by herself and was very active ("I usually walk every day," "I do all my own house work"). Her younger sister, who lived two blocks from her, stated that "it's hard to keep up with her, she's always on the go." On admission, Mrs. P. had complete range of motion of all joints, except her right knee, which was limited from full motion from pain of arthritis. Her muscle tone and strength were good, but her movements were restricted because of pain.

Background

A nursing diagnosis of impaired physical mobility was made because of Mrs. P.'s reluctance to attempt movement (see Table). Voluntary curtailment of movement helps to control, relieve, or prevent pain; yet this curtailment of movement has serious implications for an older individual.

A period of decreased physical activity impacts on an already affected musculoskeletal system. Aging has been shown in both human and animal studies to directly or indirectly produce changes in muscles and joints. For example, peak muscle force and power are reached by early adulthood, after which there is a marked and steady decline in muscle strength.[1] Leg and back muscles have greater strength loss than arm muscles.[2,3] The decline is reflective of the changes that occur in both the fast twitch muscle fibers that produce power and strength and slow fibers that provide anaerobic endurance.[4] The greatest loss occurs in the fast twitch fibers; hence, strength is more affected than is endurance.[5-8]

Flexibility of joint movement is affected both by the length and composition of muscle fibers. With aging, the length of the fiber decreases[9] and collagen content of the connective tissue progressively increases.[10,11] The result is an increase in stiffness of tissue and a decrease in joint mobility.

TABLE. Mobility, impaired physical*

Definition
A state in which the individual experiences a limitation of ability for independent physical movement.

Defining characteristics
Inability to purposefully move
Reluctance to attempt movement
Limited range of motion
Decreased muscle strength, control, or mass
Imposed restrictions of movement
Impaired coordination

Functional level classification
1 = Requires use of equipment or devices
2 = Requires help from another person for assistance, supervision, or teaching
3 = Requires help from another person and equipment device
4 = Dependent, does not participate in activity

*Source: *Classification of Nursing Diagnosis: Proceedings of the Seventh Conference*, McLane, AM (ed). St. Louis: CV Mosby, 1987.

Interventions

Nursing care for the older adult with impaired physical mobility is directed towards neutralizing the deleterious effects by maximizing mobility within the limits of the individual's condition. The ultimate nursing goals are the maintenance of abilities and prevention of impairment.

Specific goals address three major areas. The first area is the maintenance of muscle strength and endurance, which involves: a) a daily conditioning exercise program [that] includes both isometric and isotonic muscle contractions and b) the promotion of protein anabolism. The second goal involves maintenance of joint flexibility. Interventions include range-of-motion exercises, proper positioning, and activities of daily living. The last goal relates to the attitudes or motivations of both the nurse and the patient. Attitudes of the nurse are important because unless the nurse values preventative interventions, none will be initiated. Unlike curative interventions, preventative interventions often do not have a high visibility factor.

Isometric muscle contractions. Isometric muscle contraction increases muscle tension without changing the length of the muscle or moving the joint. These tightening contractions help maintain the strength of muscle groups while not producing work or movement. Isometric exercises are particularly helpful in maintaining the strength of the quadriceps, abdominal, and gluteal muscles, which are needed for upright mobility.

Isometric muscle contractions are useful when it is essential to avoid increasing cardiovascular load. Isometric contractions produce elevation of both systolic and diastolic blood pressure; but this change persists only during the exercise period.[12] Additional stress to the cardiovascular system can result from the inadvertent use of the Valsalva maneuver, which increases the intrathoracic pressure by forcible exhalation against a closed glottis. The use of this maneuver can be prevented by having patients breathe through their mouth while exercising.

Isometric exercises involve alternately tightening [a] muscle as hard as possible and then relaxing the muscle. The stronger the contraction the greater the benefit. An exercise schedule of five maximal isometric contractions each held for six seconds with a two-minute relaxation period between contractions has been found to increase muscle strength in healthy young males.[13]

Isotonic muscle contractions. Isotonic muscle contractions change the length of a muscle without changing the tension. As muscles shorten and lengthen, work is accomplished.

Isotonic exercises can be accomplished by pushing or pulling against a stationary object. Examples for a bedfast individual include: pressing feet against footboard; lifting body off bed using a trapeze; pushing body to a sitting position; and lifting buttock off bed by pushing with the hands against the mattress.

Isotonic exercises produce cardiovascular changes. The systolic blood pressure becomes elevated during the exercise and the elevation persists after the contraction is completed. This exercise should be used with caution in patients with compromised cardiovascular status. Further stress may be produced by the inadvertent use of the Valsalva maneuver.

Promote protein anabolism. The promotion of protein anabolism involves conservation and replenishment of energy stores. Energy conservation results from a decrease in stressors, such as anxiety or elevated temperature. Replenishment of energy stores involves adequate intake of protein and calories. A primary indicator of an adequate intake is maintenance or increase in weight.

Positioning. Alignment of the body, regardless of the position, affects mobility. All positions should be evaluated with the normal upright standing position as the reference. The spine should be kept straight, the neck without lateral or anterior flexion, and the extremities in extension.

Range-of-motion exercise. Active and passive range-of-motion exercise provides different benefits for the immobilized individual. Active range-of-motion exercise provides joint movement and stress on the bones. Active motion is beneficial for the maintenance of joint flexibility, skeletal strength, and muscle strength. In contrast, passive range of motion, where the individual's joints are moved through their range of motion, provides only for the maintenance of joint flexibility.

Attitude. The patient's attitude regarding exercise is an important variable for the maintenance of an intact functional musculoskeletal system. Often an individual does not value the benefits of early and repeated exercise during a period of decreased activity. A general belief is that the need for exercise diminishes with age. A person is expected to "act his age," to "slow down a bit," or to "enjoy a well-earned rest." A second reason for devaluing behavior relates to the perception of the sick-role. That is, when individuals become ill they must rest to get well. Activity is viewed as detrimental to recovery.

To negate or overcome such attitudes, interventions may need a two-fold approach. The first relates to increasing the individual's cognitive base. Knowledge about the importance of exercise facilitates a more active, productive life as well as allows an individual to feel in control during the period of decreased activity. The second approach is the use of benchmarking, directing an individual's attention to specific abilities that have been retained or improved.

Progression: Case study

Two weeks after admission and after two surgeries, colon resection for ruptured diverticulitis and colostomy for bowel obstruction, Mrs. P. appears older than her stated age. Her muscular strength and endurance have decreased. She is not able to stand or ambulate without the assistance of two nurses. When she stands she cannot maintain a straight, upright posture, and her height appears to have decreased five inches. Her body is in a flexed position as she attempts to walk (shoulders hunched and rotated forward, upper body leaning forward, head lowered looking at floor, and hips and knees in flexed position).

Background

The nursing diagnosis of impaired physical mobility is still present. In fact, Mrs. P. now exhibits all the major defining characteristics (see Table). Her functional level classification has increased from one to three, requiring help from another person and equipment devices.

From the period of physical inactivity, Mrs. P. has incurred the two major complications associated with the musculoskeletal system: a loss of muscular strength and endurance, and a loss of joint mobility. Compounding the problem for Mrs. P. was an inadequate nutritional intake and an increase in energy requirements.

The decrease in caloric and protein intake resulted from the routine post-operative fluid maintenance while NPO. The increase in metabolic demand resulted from the stressors, such as surgery and an elevated temperature. The result was the endogenous catabolism of muscle protein to meet the body's needs.

Loss of muscular strength and endurance. Changes in muscular strength occur both in the aging adult and in the individual with impaired mobility. The common denominator for this ocurrence is a decrease or lack of physical activity. Muscular strength is dependent on the tension of frequent contractions of muscle fibers.[14] When tension produced within a muscle is decreased, a loss of muscle mass and a concomitant loss of muscle strength results.

Loss of strength was studied in a group of normal, healthy, young adult males who were maintained on bedrest for six weeks without an exercise program. The loss of muscle strength ranged from 0.04 to 5.5% per day. The greatest decrease in strength occurred during the initial period of bedrest. A plateau of muscle loss occurred as the period lengthened.[15]

No comparative study has been reported in older adults who already have decreased strength. It is theorized that the total loss of muscle strength will be less than a muscularly developed young adult. The impact of the loss, however, should be greater for the older adult both for the immediate effect on remobilization and for regaining strength to previous levels. Often compounding the problem for the older adult is a history of inadequate protein intake. This condition accelerates loss of muscle strength with inactivity and also hinders the body's ability to anabolize protein during the rehabilitative phase.

The rate of muscle strength loss is mainly dependent on the one factor of activity, muscle contraction with tension. The greater the amount of movement, the less the loss of muscle strength. Not all of the body's muscles are equally affected with impaired mobility.

Muscles most affected are [those that] facilitate locomotion and maintenance of an upright position.[16,17] These muscles include the gastrocnemius-soleus group, quadriceps, glutei, and erector spinae.

If muscle mass is lost, the return of muscle strength and mass is a slow process. When there is no planned exercise program, recovery of muscle strength will approximate the period of inactivity.[15,16,18] The slow twitch endurance muscle fibers recover faster than the fast twitch.[18]

As muscle strength and mass decrease, so does endurance. Muscles are less able to sustain activity without fatiguing. Muscular endurance is further reduced when the circulation is impeded. Nutrients cannot be supplied to the muscles, and waste products cannot be removed.

Loss of joint mobility. Motion in joints and soft tissue is maintained by normal movement of body parts, including joint capsules, muscles, tendons, and subcutaneous tissues through full range of motion. If, for any reason, range of motion is restricted, tightness develops, which restricts the arc of motion.

With reduced joint movement, ligaments and tendons shorten and composition of connective tissue changes. In animal studies, the connective tissue undergoes a marked increase in collagen; these changes occur very early.[19] Joint changes can be accelerated if pain, edema, inflammatory exudate, trauma, impaired circulation, spasticity, and degenerative joint changes are present.

Muscle weakness affects joint mobility. Both flexors and extensors have a reduction in muscular strength; the greatest loss occurs in the extensor muscles.[17,20] Flexion of the joint results as the extensor muscle becomes weak and fatigued.

Although all of the body's joints are susceptible to structural changes, the hip, knee, and ankle joints of upright mobility are most frequently affected. The hip joint becomes involved because full extension of the hip is difficult in all positions except during relaxed standing. In all other positions, partial flexion of the hip is always present. Even prone hip extension is still 10 to 20 degrees less than when upright.[21] Sitting, elevation of the headrest, use of pillows under the knee, or elevation of the legs all increase flexion of the hip.

Full extension of the knee while in bed seldom occurs without conscious effort. All positions, except prone, favor flexion. The dominant muscle of the lower leg, the hamstring muscle group, tends to draw the knee into flexion. Other factors contributing to flexion of the knee include use of pillows under the knee, painful disabilities, and stationary positions.

The ankle has a high risk for the development of flexion contractions (drop foot) because of the effects of gravity and the strength of the plantar flexor muscle group. In addition, the weight of the bed clothes contributes to fatigue of the dorsal flexor muscles. If flexion is maintained, reambulation is difficult if not impossible.

Interventions

Goals and interventions for an individual who has complications associated with the musculoskeletal system from decreased physical activity are the same as the interventions to prevent complications. Major differences are the need for greater commitment on the nurse's part to help the patient and for greater awareness by the nurse of the essential interactive factors.

Essentials to consider when selecting interventions for goal attainment are the pathological process precipitating the inactivity period, the concurrent limits imposed by medical therapy, and the individual's abilities and limitations. Likewise, the potential adverse effects of activity and exercise on all body systems must be assessed. Without this knowledge, inappropriate and potentially detrimental nursing care may be prescribed.

Evaluation criteria

The success of nursing interventions can be measured by evaluating the tone, strength, and size of muscles, endurance ability, and range of motion. To facilitate this evaluation, an initial collection of baseline information must occur as close to the onset of a period of decreased activity as possible. Maintenance or improvement of functioning is the measure of successful intervention.

To evaluate muscle tone, the indiviudal is observed in a relaxed, comfortable position. The tautness of relaxed muscle indicates tone. Greater reliability of such subjective measurement can be attained if the same person repeats the assessment. Strength can also be evaluated subjectively by the degree of resistance muscle groups afford or by strength of hand grip. A more objective measure of strength can be obtained by the use of an ergometer. Size can be evaluated via circumferential measurements of appendages. A prominent landmark affords a point of reference to ensure reliability of repeated measurements.

Levels of daily living activities can provide endurance indicators. Statements regarding weakness or tiredness reflect endurance patterns. In addition, the length of performance of a task can be used to measure endurance. When an activity is stopped earlier than previously due to fatigue, endurance may be decreasing. Objective evidence of decreased endurance is reflected by an increase in heart and respiratory rate during the activity.

Joint mobility can be evaluated subjectively by observation of activities of daily living. A more objective measurement of joint motion is obtained with the use of a goniometer.

Outcome

The nurse is the key to the planning, implementation, and evaluation of an intervention program for an individual with impaired mobility. Inherent in this program is the individual patient's motivation to gain daily adherence to an activity program. Without interventions, loss of muscular strength, endurance, and joint mobility will result. Early initiation and consistent application of an activity program has the power to negate or prevent the deleterious effects associated with decreased physical activity. In addition, such a program has the opportunity to help the older adult view exercise as an integral and essential component of an active life.

REFERENCES

1. Bosco C, Komi PV: Influence of aging on the mechanical behavior of leg extensor muscles. *Eur J Appl Physiol* 1980; 45(2):209-219.

2. Grimby G, Saltin B: The aging muscle. *Clin Physiol* 1983; 3:209-218.

3. McDonagh MJN, White MJ, Davies CTM: Different effects of aging on the mechanical properties of human arm and leg muscles. *Gerontology* 1984; 30:49-54.

4. McCarter RJM, Masoro EJ, Yu BP: Rat muscle structure and metabolism in relation to age and food intake. *Am J Physiol* 1982; 242(1):289-293.

5. Nelson RM, Soderberg GL, Urbscheit NL: Comparison of skeletal muscle motor unit discharge characteristics in young and aged humans. *Arch Gerontol Geriatr* 1983; 2:255-264.

6. Scelsi R, Marchetti C, Poggi P: Histochemical and ultrastructural aspects of M Vastus Lateralis in sedentary old people (age 65-89). *Acta Neuropathol* 1980; 51(2):99-105.

7. Sato T, Akatsuka H, Kito K, Tokoro Y: Age changes in size and number of muscle fibers in human minor pectoral muscle. *Mech Aging Dev* 1984; 28:99-109.

8. Sato T, Akatsuka H, Kito K, et al: Age changes of myofibrils of human pectoral muscle. *Mech Aging Dev* 1986; 34:297-304.

9. Hooper ACB: Length, diameter and number of aging skeletal muscle fibers. *Gerontology* 1981; 27(3):121-126.

10. Alnaqeeb MA, Al Zaid NS, Goldspink G: Connective tissue changes and physical properties of developing and aging skeletal muscle. *J Anat* 1984; 139(4):677-689.

11. Hamlin CR, Luschin JH, Kohn RR: Aging of collagen: Comparative rates in four mammalian species. *Exp Gerontol* 1980; 15(5):393-398.

12. Nutter DO, Schlant RC, Hurst JW: Isometric exercise and the cardiovascular system. *Modern Concepts of Cardiovascular Disease* 1972; 41:11-15.

13. Muller EA: Influence of training and of inactivity on muscle strength. *Arch Phys Med Rehabil* 1970; 51:449-462.

14. Kottke FJ: The effects of limitation of activity upon the human body. *JAMA* 1966; 196:825-830.

15. Dietrick JE, Whedon GD, Shorr E: Effects of immobilization upon various metabolic and physiologic functions of normal men. *Am J Med* 1948; 4:3-36.

16. Browse NC: *The Physiology and Pathology of Bed Rest.* Springfield, Illinois, Charles C Thomas, 1965.

17. Booth FW, Gollnick PD: Effects of disuse on the structure and function of skeletal muscle. *Med Sci Sports Exerc* 1983; 15(5):415-420.

18. Witzmann FA, Kim DH, Fitts RH: Recovery time course in contractile function of fast and slow skeletal muscle after hindlimb immobilization. *J Appl Physiol* 1982; 52(3):677-682.

19. Williams PE, Goldspink G: Connective tissue changes in immobilized muscle. *J Anat* 1984; 138(2):343-350.

20. Tomanek RJ, Lund DD: Degeneration of different types of skeletal muscle fibers: Immobilization. *J Anat* 1974; 118(3):531-541.

21. Kottke FJ: Therapeutic exercise, in Krusen FH, Kottke FJ, Ellwood PM (eds): *Handbook of Physical Medicine and Rehabilitation*, ed 2. Philadelphia, WB Saunders, 1971.

22 *Classification of Nursing Diagnosis: Proceedings of the Seventh Conference*, McLane AM (ed). St Louis, CV Mosby, 1987.

Sleep pattern disturbance

BONNIE BARNDT-MAGLIO, RN, MS

SLEEP IS A UNIVERSAL activity common to all living organisms. In humans, it is essential for physical, mental, and emotional well-being. It has long been believed that sleep is nature's mechanism for conserving and restoring energy for important survival activities. Persistent disturbance of a well-established sleep pattern often proves to be detrimental to the recovery of hospitalized patients. Lewandowski and Kositsky, reporting the results of a Delphi study, rank sleep pattern disturbance among critical care patients as the issue of greatest concern among critical care nurses.[1] This article will discuss the nursing diagnosis of sleep pattern disturbance, including the causative factors prevalent in the pediatric intensive care environment, and nursing interventions that prevent or treat this diagnosis.

In order to assess and diagnose sleep pattern disturbance accurately, it is important to define and understand sleep and the function it serves in the maintenance of health. Sleep may be defined as a natural, recurring state of altered consciousness that provides rest for the body, mind, and spirit, and is terminated by intrinsic or extrinsic stimuli. Implicit in this definition is the relationship between sleep and all components of human functioning.

The nursing diagnosis of sleep pattern disturbance includes a functional data base for assessment. Sleep pattern disturbance was defined by the Third and Fourth National Conference on Nursing Diagnosis as "a disruption of sleep time which causes patient discomfort or interferes with the patient's desired life-style."[2] This definition operationalizes sleep pattern disturbance by utilizing the criterion of the desired life-style as a standard of measurement. Defining characteristics (identified as cues) are used to objectively validate the diagnosis. Therefore, to diagnose the problem of sleep pattern disturbance accurately, the nurse needs to gather data regarding the patient's usual life-style, sleep pattern, and sleep rituals.

Assessing the child's sleep pattern disturbance

Admission is the ideal time to gather data about sleep pattern disturbance, but in the critical care unit this is often impractical. However, when the child and the situation stabilize, questions about the child's normal sleep pattern can easily be obtained with the usual admission questioning (Table 1). Too often, assessment data pertaining to sleep [are] limited to questions about what time the child goes to bed at night and awakens in the morning. Sleep assessment should include the developmental sleep needs of the child and the usual bedtime rituals that the child observes, predisposing him to sleep. Examples of rituals utilized by children include bedtime stories, a warm bath, prayers, lullabies or music, a security blanket nearby, or a beloved stuffed toy.

Daytime naps are a segment of a child's (or adult's) sleep pattern that is easily overlooked in the initial assessment. Naps provide invaluable restoration, both physically and emotionally, and should be encouraged by the nurse. Unfortunately, many school-aged children think of naps as an activity for babies only and are resistant to them. During the admission assessment, parents can provide successful strategies to overcome the child's reluctance.

TABLE 1. Sleep pattern assessment guide

1. What time does your child usually go to bed at night?
2. What time does your child usually arise in the morning?
3. What is your child's usual routine before retiring for the night?
4. Does your child have a special blanket or toy that he/she usually takes to bed with him/her?
5. How long does it usually take for your child to get to sleep?
6. In what position does your child usually sleep?
7. Does your child often wake up and have difficulty falling asleep? If so, how many times per night, per week?
8. What helps your child return to sleep once awake?
9. How well would you say your child sleeps at night?
10. Does your child take naps? If so, at what time of day does he/she nap?

Another area for assessment is habitual awakening during the night. Some children routinely awaken during the night at a special time and need a drink of water, a trip to the bathroom, or reassurance before returning to sleep. Other children sleep through the night and any awakening is an unwelcome intrusion into their sleep. For such a child, the awakening may be both a cause and a symptom of sleep pattern disturbance.

Simulating the child's home routine as closely as possible throughout the hospitalization provides comfort both for the child and his parents by creating an atmosphere of safety and stability. Restful sleep cannot be achieved until the need for security is met.

Causes of sleep pattern disturbance

Sleep pattern disturbance may be caused by a multitude of factors...as diverse and complex as the patients who are affected by them. Sleep, as discussed earlier, is interrupted by factors that are either external or internal in origin.

Internal factors. Internal factors that affect sleep patterns include the illness itself and psychological stress on the child. The child with asthma often has difficulty sleeping, yet requires the energy that stage 4 sleep provides.[3] Postoperative patients have difficulty falling asleep because of pain and stiffness from the surgery, and are frequently inhibited from assuming their normal sleep position. The painful joints of juvenile arthritis may awaken children frequently as they attempt to change their position during sleep.

Psychological stress nearly always accompanies illness and hospitalization. "First night syndrome" describes the phenomenon of disruptive sleep that occurs during the first night or two in an unfamiliar environment.[4] The characteristic sleep pattern is a longer sleep latency period (time it takes to get to sleep) and frequent awakenings throughout the night. Frequent awakenings cause a disproportionately large amount of sleep time to be spent in sleep stages 1 and 2, and a relatively small amount to be spent in the deep sleep of stage 4 and REM.[5] The child's normal pattern can be altered even when sleeping in a pleasant and desirable location, such as grandma's house, a friend's room, or on the family's vacation. The stress of being a patient in an ICU is likely to have an even greater effect on the child's sleep pattern.

External factors. Treatment protocols and environmental disturbances, such as routine care, medications, lights, and noise, are external factors contributing to sleep pattern disturbance. Research conducted in an intensive care unit with postoperative open heart cardiac adult patients documented the number of times sleep was disturbed by caregivers to be as many as 14 times per hour.[6] A similar study of infants in a neonatal intensive care unit concluded that the infants' sleep was by accident rather than plan.[7] The study recorded an average of 132 disturbances over a single 24-hour period, averaging 20 minutes per hour or 5.5 times per hour. Another significant statistic revealed in this study is that slightly over 79.2% of disturbances were by nurses. Clearly, while the restorative powers of sleep are particularly important during illness, sleep is often not part of the plan of care.

Sleep pattern disturbance is a frequent side effect of drugs prescribed for treatment or pain relief. A recently documented side effect of digoxin is violent nightmares.[8] In the pediatric population, nightmares may be intensified by separation from family and awakening in a foreign environment. Both meperidine (Demerol) and morphine decrease REM sleep.[9] Fortunately, meperidine's disruption is much less dramatic than that of morphine. Diazepam (Valium) decreases stages 3, 4, and REM sleep, an effect which is particularly devastating to the intensive care patient because stage 4 sleep restores the body and REM sleep allows the mind to put the day's events into perspective.[10] Chloral hydrate decreases REM sleep to a lesser degree than meperidine, facilitates relaxation, and eases the transition between waking, stage 1, and stage 2 sleep. Chloral hydrate is a particularly gentle and effective sedative for pediatric patients.

The light and noise that exist at all hours of the day and night in an ICU can cause children to become desynchronized. Although younger children cannot tell time, their days are synchronized by the activities and functions of those around them, especially their parents, as well as by the amount of light or darkness present. In the intensive care unit, the child's parents are not always with the child, and, when present, they are not performing their usual duties. Events that enable the child to gauge time are replaced by activities that are unfamiliar and meaningless to the child. For example, lab work or x-rays at six o'clock every morning mean nothing to the child except discomfort, even if his parents are with him. Activities of daily living are continued in the intensive care unit, but often at a time that is different from the routine for the child. At home he may have a warm bath every night before bed, while in the intensive care unit he is bathed at nine o'clock in the morning. Certain treatments that are carried out throughout the day and night, such as neuro checks and vital signs, are disruptive and confusing to the child as he attempts to differentiate day from night.

Another sleep distractor is the emotional effect of watching the treatment of other patients. The dramatic scenes played out in the care of other patients are difficult to understand, integrate, and accept, even for adult patients who have well-developed reasoning abilities. Children possess little knowledge or past experience that can facilitate their interpretation of scenes that may resemble nightmares.

In addition to psychological and environmental cues, there are also strong physiological determinents of sleep time.[11] Body temperature begins to rise around the usual time of awakening, peak in the late afternoon, and then slowly decrease as bedtime draws near. Cortisol secretion peaks during the time that early morning activities usually take place and dramatically decreases at bedtime. Desynchronization causes the mechanisms to adopt a different pattern, producing symptoms of fatigue, sleeping at inappropriate times, an inability to deal with stress, and a decrease in mental alertness.

Desynchronization is intensified dramatically in the critical care setting. Symptoms of desynchronization are accompanied by disorientation, combativeness, irritability, fear, and paranoia.[12] "ICU psychosis" is the term used by critical care health professionals to describe the desynchronization and behavior disturbances that result from frequent interruptions of the patient's sleep. When sleep is disturbed regularly, the amount of REM sleep is dramatically decreased, and stages 1 and 2 are increased. During REM sleep, the day's activities are reviewed and categorized for integration and storage. REM sleep is also important for psychosocial adaptation and learning.[13] REM debt is the loss of REM sleep over a period of consecutive days. Coincidentally, the symptoms of REM debt closely mimic those of ICU psychosis.

The severity of the child's illness may require frequent disruptions for monitoring and care while in the intensive care unit. Realistic goals in this instance may be to disturb the child only once an hour by grouping care tasks together or timing care around sedation.

The physical layout of the intensive care unit must be considered when formulating specific goals. If the unit is composed of one large room, the noise level will be extremely difficult to control without walls to buffer the sound. Other patients in the ICU need care that generates noise from personnel. The meaningless noise of monitors, ventilators, and other equipment is a constant backdrop in the ICU, making it difficult for patients to fall asleep. Loud conversation among the staff is another disruptive element inhibiting sleep. Bright lights both day and night not only discourage sleep, but confuse the child's day-night orientation.

Writing sleep goals for the PICU patient

Goals reflecting the need for adequate rest and sleep are an essential component of every nursing care plan. Generally, goals to insure adequate sleep and rest involve providing comfort, minimizing discomfort, and increasing the quality and quantity of sleep.[14] However, setting specific and realistic goals in the care plan for a child in intensive care requires expert problem-solving skills and creative strategies on the part of the nurse. Factors to be considered when formulating goals include the child's home sleep pattern, parental availability, necessary treatment regimen, environmental concerns, and age (Table 2).

Ideally, goals are set in collaboration with the parents or primary home caregiver. The assessment data enables the nurse to understand the child's normal daily routine. The willingness and availability of parents to be present at bedtime is a major factor to be considered. However, the needs of other children at home may not allow the parent to be with the sick child at bedtime.

The nurse is often restricted in the amount of control she has over her patient's situation when developing goals for preserving a patient's sleep pattern. For example, the design of the unit cannot be changed to meet the needs of every patient, silencing the alarms of all equipment is not appropriate or safe, and equipment can be restrictive, limiting the positions which a patient can assume....To identify realistic goals, the nurse must be able to distinguish between factors that can be controlled, minimized, or accepted. Some factors are fixed, and, therefore, cannot be controlled, while others fluctuate with the severity of the illness and/or the number of other patients in the unit. Appreciating the degree of possible impact of each factor can guide the nurse in the formulation of workable goals, and in the selection of nursing interventions.

Developing a plan of care

Interventions based on the assessment data and goals are individualized for the child and made workable for the nurse. Imitation of the child's usual wake-sleep routine is the basis of the plan. A schedule posted at the foot of the bed helps to alert other health caregivers to the child's routine and assists with the maintenance of uninterrupted rest periods....Adher-

TABLE 2. Sleep cycles of children

Full term infants
- Sleep time ranges between 10 and 23 hours per day, averaging 17 hours.
- Usually sleeps in periods of 3-4 hours.
- Night awakenings common through first year.
- NREM sleep is not differentiated into stages.
- May progress from wakefulness directly into REM sleep.
- 50-95% of total sleep time (TST) is spent in REM sleep.
- Usually begin to sleep through the night at 6-8 months.

1-year-olds
- Sleep about 12 hours per night with a morning and afternoon nap.
- NREM sleep begins to be differentiated into stages.
- Sleep cycles are 45-60 minutes in length.
- 30-40% of TST spent in REM sleep.

2- to 5-year-olds
- Sleep about 10-13 hours per night.
- Begin experiencing nightmares.
- Decrease in nap time to elimination after age 5.
- Sleep cycles are 45-60 minutes in length.
- Boys require more TST than girls.
- REM sleep time increases while time in stages three and four decreases.

8- to 12-year-olds
- Sleep between 8.5 and 10 hours per night.
- Generally play hard and sleep soundly.
- The 90-minute adult sleep cycle is firmly in place.

12- to 14-year-olds
- Sleep time is about 8.5-9 hours per night.
- Hormonal changes with growth spurts increase the need for sleep.
- REM sleep is 20% of TST.

15-year-olds to adults
- Sleep time is 7-8.5 hours per night.
- Adult sleep cycle fixated.
- Stage 1 is 5% of TST.
- Stage 2 is 50% of TST.
- Stage 3 is 10% of TST.
- Stage 4 is 10% of TST.
- REM sleep is 20-25% of TST.

Adapted with permission. From Bell LP. Sleep through the life cycle. Plastic Surgical Nursing 1983;3:11-12. Also from Kupfer DJ, Reynolds CF. Sleep disorders. Hospital Practice 1983;18(2):101-114.

ence to the schedule by the nursing staff encourages others to do the same. Planning activities of direct physical care for completion at a few central times and scheduling routine lab work and x-rays around sleep time are essential to promote uninterrupted sleep. If possible, allow 90-minute intervals to elapse between waking the child in order to allow at least one sleep cycle to be completed....Before awakening the child, observe the eyelids for movement that is indicative of REM sleep and, if possible, wait to wake the child until the movement stops in order to decrease REM debt.

Utilizing the assessment data of established bedtime rituals to plan care will allow the child to feel a sense of stability and security. A warm bath, prayers, and a story are activity cues for the child that it is "bedtime." Familiar objects, such as the blanket from his bed at home, pajamas, and a beloved stuffed toy, facilitate relaxation by making the environment more friendly and giving a sense of security.

Entertaining the child with play activities, stories, or television at least 2 hours before the scheduled sleep time facilitates relaxation.[15] This also provides an excellent opportunity for parents to actively participate in their child's care and reinforces the family bond....

The lighting in an intensive care unit is often very bright to enable accurate observations of subtle changes in the patient's color and condition. Unfortunately, bright lights disturb sleep by increasing sleep latency time, and can cause frequent awakenings once the patient is asleep. Dimming the lights around the patient enough to encourage sleep while providing enough light for accurate observation can be an effective compromise. A flashlight can be used for closer observation. Drawing the privacy curtain around all but one side of the child's bed decreases the amount of light and visual stimulation, while still allowing the nurse to observe the patient directly.

Controlling some noise in the unit, such as emergency admissions or resuscitation activities, is impossible. However, minimizing the noise caused by conversations and some activities of the staff is possible. Reinforcing the child's posted schedule with gentle reminders is all that is usually necessary. The multidisciplinary care conference is also an excellent forum to discuss the importance of sleep to the critically ill child, as well as strategies to decrease the staff-generated noise. The noise from monitors can be minimized by remaining in close proximity to the child and reducing the volume levels. When at the child's bedside, the nurse is also in a good position to reassure the child when he awakens and to intercept any intruders that would interrupt his sleep.

Some intensive care units are equipped with a limited number of private rooms for isolation purposes. It is important to consider the activity level of the ICU census before assigning the private rooms. For example, if the majority of the patients require continual care, the few whose conditions are less complex are good candidates for the private rooms.

Evaluating plan effectiveness

Evaluation criteria of the maintenance of an adequate sleep pattern are based on the measurable criteria stated in the goals, and should be documented every shift. Identifiable cues of sleep pattern disturbance include a sleep latency period of greater than 30 minutes, restlessness either while awake or asleep, inappropriate behavior while awake, less sleep than normally acquired at home, and dozing at unusual times, such as meals.[16] An older child's sleep pattern can be evaluated by discussing his subjective feelings of rest after sleep. A useful tool for daily evaluation of sleep pattern disturbance is the question: Does sleep pattern disturbance still exist, or does it potentially exist? A "yes" answer requires re-evaluation of the nursing care plan and its interventions. Often the measures to decrease discomfort must be enhanced. Parents, once again, are an excellent source of information regarding measures that will encourage sleep for their child.

Summary

Maintenance of a normal sleep pattern is an essential component of the restoration of health. A nursing care plan formulated from assessment data and based on realistic goals provides interventions that maximize sleep for children who need it critically. The primary nurse is the ideal communication link between the parents, child, and staff, to ensure that an adequate sleep pattern will be maintained throughout the child's hospitalization.

REFERENCES

1. Lewandowski L, Kositsky A. Research priorities for critical care nursing: A study by the American Association for Critical Care Nurses. Heart Lung 1983; 12:35-44.

2. Kim MJ, McFarland GK, McLane AM. Classification of Nursing Diagnosis: Proceedings of the Third and Fourth National Conference. New York: McGraw-Hill, 1982.

3. Kales A, Kales J. Evaluation, diagnosis, and treatment of clinical conditions related to sleep. JAMA 1970; 213:2229-2335.

4. Monroe LJ. Psychology of good and poor sleepers. J Abnorm Psychol 1967; 12:255-264.

5. Wotring KE. Using research in practice. Focus 1982;9:34-36.

6. Selulia AJ. Sleep deprivation and biological rhythms in the critical care unit. Critical Care Nurse 1981;1:19-23.

7. Korones SB. Disturbance and infant's rest: Iatrogenic problems

in neonatal intensive care. Report on the Sixty-Ninth Ross Conference on Pediatric Research. Columbus: Ross Laboratories, 1976.

8. Breziz M, Michaelis J, Hamburger R. Nightmares from digoxin. Ann Intern Med 1980;93:639-640.

9. Kales A, Kales J. Evaluation, diagnosis, and treatment of clinical conditions related to sleep. JAMA 1970;213:2229-2235.

10. Kleitman N. Sleep and wakefulness. Chicago: University of Chicago Press, 1972.

11. Lanuza DM. Circadian rhythm of mental efficiency and performance. Nurs Clin North Am 1976;11:583-594.

12. Helton MC, Gordon SH, Nunnery SC. The correlation between sleep deprivation and the intensive care unit syndrome. Heart Lung 1980;36:11-13.

13. Chuman MA. The neurological basis of sleep. Heart Lung 1983;12:177-183.

14. Carpenito LJ. Nursing Diagnosis: Application to Clinical Practice. Philadelphia: J.B. Lippincott Co., 1983.

15. Cluydts R, Visser P, Mood and sleep: Effects of aversive presleep stimulation. Waking and Sleeping 1980;4:199-203.

16. Kim MJ, McFarland GK, McLane AM. Classification of Nursing Diagnosis: Proceedings of the Third and Fourth National Conference. New York: McGraw Hill, 1982.

Sexuality in older adults: A continuing education concern

J. CONRAD GLASS, JR., EdD; JO ANN DALTON, RN, EdD

ALTHOUGH STUDIES OF SEXUALITY were revolutionized by the 1953 Kinsey report, there continues to be a dearth of information on the sexual attitudes, needs, and concerns of the older adult. Myths and stereotypes regarding sexuality in old age persist among older adults, their children, and, at times, among the health professionals who work with older adults. Nurses may assist older adults and their families to separate sexual fact from fiction. Such assistance may aid older adults in maintaining their sexuality.

However, many nurses are often uncomfortable discussing sexual issues with their patients, and particularly with older persons. Many nurses do not feel they possess the competence to discuss such issues....

Sexuality and aging

Prior to this century, individuals often did not live beyond the reproductive years; thus, sexuality of the older adult was not an issue. However, with the expansion of scientific knowledge and the advent of modern medicine, life expectancy has greatly increased. As the average life span has increased, so has the need for physiological and psychological adaptations, including adaptations in sexuality. Factors that affect aging and sexual behavior vary according to the physical condition of the individual, his/her personality and attitude, and the attitudes of others (Gadpaille, 1975, p. 10).

The physical condition of the older adult changes as a result of alterations in hormone levels. In the female, the cessation of menses, or menopause, is characterized by a decrease in estrogen production and atrophy of the reproductive organs. The vagina shrinks and loses some of its elasticity. There often is a decrease in vaginal secretions that may be accompanied by thinning of the tissues of the vulva and partial loss of the engorgement response. These physical changes may be associated with complaints of "hot flashes," occipital headaches, neck aches, chronic fatigue, irritability, and insomnia. The breasts undergo a loss of fatty tissue with the soft, glandular tissues being replaced by fibrous cords. These physical changes occur more rapidly between 40 and 60 years of age.

The older male does not experience a similar acute hormonal change, although he does undergo a decrease in testosterone throughout maturity (Delora & Warren, 1977, p. 229). He may experience some decrease in blood flow to the genitals and a disturbance of pelvic innervation. Changes in his sexual activity may be associated with the fatigue of chronic illness as well as with psychosocial factors.

In addition to these physiological changes, older females and males experience change in the sexual response cycle (SRC) which is slow and subtle, although males seem to experience more decline than females. During the excitation phase of SRC, the older male may require more time to achieve an erection, which may not be as full as those experienced by younger males. The female may not attain the same vaginal response of a younger woman due to the hormonally induced involution of the vaginal lining.

Older adults who abstain from sexual relations for an extended period of time may find that the male has increased difficulty achieving an erection, and the female experiences greater shrinkage in the size of the vagina, a problem sometimes labeled "disuse atrophy" (Kolodny, Masters, Johnson, & Biggs, 1979, p. 88). These problems are difficult to correct; therefore, it is easier to preserve sexual function than to restore it.

The plateau phase of the SRC may be lengthened in individuals. The older male may find that he does not experience the degree of intense urgency to reach orgasm that he once did, while a decrease in clitoris size and sensitivity can be responsible for change in the plateau phase of females. For the male, the orgasmic phase, which is dependent upon psychological readiness as well as recurring contractions of the prostate gland, is characterized by changes in rhythm and a decrease in the severity of the expulsive contractions which occur during ejaculation.

The older female may experience a shortened orgasmic phase. During the resolution phase, the older male experiences an increase in the refractory period, while the female may experience a decrease (Hendricks & Hendricks, 1979, p. 67).

Older adults may also experience some alteration in sexual response in association with various medical and surgical therapies. Many drugs taken by older adults, such as sedatives, narcotics, antianxiety agents, antidepressants, tranquilizers, antihypertensives, and antispasmodics, may cause a decrease in sexual response. Older males also may experience erectile dysfunction after a prostatectomy. Females may feel that a hysterectomy renders them sexually incompetent, although there is no physiological or anatomical reason for alteration in the female sexual response. After myocardial infarction, some older adults fear resumption of sexual activity, although resumption of this activity is part of the rehabilitation program.

As the older adult's body ages, pain and stiffness associated with musculoskeletal changes may affect intercourse. Such discomfort contributes to negative views regarding sexual performance (Calderone, 1968, p. 288). However, feelings that sexual intercourse should be discontinued should be explored so that aids to adaptation may be recommended. The use of positions other than the traditional "missionary position" for sexual intercourse should be encouraged. Side-lying or rear entry penetration can provide comfort and pleasure.

While the physical changes that occur with aging are real and may affect one's sexuality, social, psychological, and personal factors may be just as damaging to the individual's feelings regarding his/her sexuality, and, in the final analysis, may be more damaging. The mind of the older adult is an excellent medium for the development of personal feelings about sexual attractiveness or unattractiveness, sexual failure, and/or rejection. The physical changes that occur in the body can affect the older adult's sexual self-image. Sagging skin, skin discolorations, age spots, thinning of body and scalp hair, and new body odors may constitute serious impediments to a positive sexual self-image (Calderone, 1968, p. 288). The older adult may feel that his/her physical appearance is unattractive to persons of the opposite sex.

Sadly, many of the negative attitudes older adults have about their own sexuality are imposed by society. They are learned from what others say and how they act. Society sometimes reacts as if sex were a "fixed reserve" that can be used up, or that "age brings the older adult dignity which sexual activity would offend" (Diamond, 1980, p. 65). Friends and adult children perpetuate the concept of aging as a "sexless time" and in so doing impose feelings of guilt and moral decadence upon their peers, their parents, and other elders (Delora & Warren, 1977, p. 234). Society glamorizes vitality and idealizes the concepts of youth, health, and physical attractiveness; and, as a consequence, the older adult feels guilty or embarrassed about sexual excitation (Kolodny et al., 1979, p. 85). The sexually active older adult becomes a "dirty old man" or a "dirty old woman."

Society also has been responsible for the perpetuation of myths regarding the sexuality of the older adult, such as "too much, too early will leave the body depleted." However, studies have demonstrated that high sexual activity in early and middle life most often is followed by high sexual activity in later life (Delora & Warren, 1977, p. 234).

One author identified five myths and misconceptions that society has imposed on the older adult:

1. Sex isn't important and doesn't matter.
2. Interest in sex is abnormal for the elderly.
3. Remarriage should be discouraged.
4. Older women shouldn't become involved with younger men.
5. Institutionalized older adults should be segregated according to sex, and privacy should be prohibited (Hogan, 1980).

All of these myths seem to relate to the general misconception that for older adults "it's all over." Society obviously needs an education!

The age of 65 suggests retirement for many adults and, therefore, the withdrawal from many of life's activities — including sexual relationships. Studies have demonstrated, however, that while interest in sexual activities may exceed the incidence of sexual activities in older adults, the incidence is greater than the younger generation might presume. Although men report greater interest and activity, females tend to be more sexually durable. Older men and women agree that the decrease in frequency of intercourse is more often a reflection of male performance than female. It sometimes is associated with the "better to quit than to be fired" attitude!

For women, marital status appears to be a critical factor for continued sexual involvement because of the fewer number of sexual outlets for the single older female. There just aren't enough males to go around! The ratio of males to females aged 65 to 74 is 100:131; 100:180 for adults over 75; and 100:229 for the 85+ group. There are 5.3 times as many older widows as there are widowers. Data indicate that of older adults in the 65-to-74 age range, 8.5% of the males are widowers, while 40.3% of the women are widows. These figures change to 24.0% widowers and 67.4% widows for the over 75 group (Select Committee on Aging, 1982). One study reports that seven out of eight women age 50 engage in sexual activity, as do 70% of women age 60, and 50% of women age 65 (Hendricks & Hendricks, 1979, p. 66). However, other data indicate that only 48.1% of the females 65 to 74 live with husbands, and only 22.1% of the females 75 and over live with husbands, a fact that indicates a significant deficit in male sex partners (Select Committee on Aging, 1982, p. 27).

There is evidence that masturbation among older women in the 50-to-70 age range is increasing (Hendricks & Hendricks, 1981), a fact that suggests that masturbation is a significant part of sexuality and also may be a byproduct of the decrease in male partners. A healthy sexual relationship most often is associated with reasonably good health and an interesting, interested partner. The fact that older women outnumber older men is significant with regard to the expression of the sexuality of both men and women.

The sexual activities of the older adult male appear to decline less rapidly than the older female. Historically, this has been due primarily to the greater number of available partners for the male and also due to the socially accepted aggressiveness of the male and to the acceptance of his desire to seek younger women. The decline in male sexual activity may be associated with a variety of related factors such as excessive use of food or alcohol, monotony in the marital relationships, anger, and for those who may still be working, preoccupation with major work-related problems (Green, 1979)....

The nurse as sex educator

Nurses have an excellent opportunity to provide sexual education to older adults. However, before they can begin to provide education for others, it is imperative that they examine their own attitudes toward sexuality. If nurses have negative attitudes regarding their own sexuality, it may be very difficult for them to assist others to maintain a positive attitude toward sexuality. If nurses feel that expression of sexuality by older adults is wrong or unnecessary, if they feel that old age is a sexless time, they will be inefficient in helping older adults develop positive attitudes.

To serve as an effective educator, it is important for the nurse to establish a relationship in which the older adult feels comfortable talking about sexuality. As in any counseling situation, an atmosphere of trust and confidentiality must be developed.

The nurse should assess the older adult's current feelings and concerns regarding sex, and the degree of change that is desired. The nurse can assess and evaluate the dynamics of various types of relationships as well as the individual's level of self-esteem. The nurse can also determine the adult's level of knowledge of the normal physical changes occurring in his/her body and be prepared to offer suggestions as needed. Suggestions could include the use of hormonal replacement therapy or alternate styles and techniques of sexual behavior. The nurse can help the older adult prepare for bodily changes that result in decreased vaginal lubrication or lengthened phases of sexual response. The nurse can help the older male, and female, to anticipate and be comfortable with the fact that the older male may not ejaculate at each coital opportunity. Nurses can encourage older adults to engage in open communication with their partners regarding their feelings, needs, and likes and to enjoy rather than repress their own sexuality. The nurse must be careful not to impose practices that do not interest older individuals who are satisfied with their sexual life styles.

Society, also, must be educated to improve the quality of sexuality for the older adult. Nurses can contribute to the elimination of myths and stereotypes surrounding sexuality, including sexuality in old age. Negative attitudes can be corrected.

One place to start is with the families of older adult patients. Children of older individuals often have problems dealing with their parents' sexuality. Many children were uncomfortable with the idea that their parents were sexual beings when the parents were younger, but to accept such an idea now that the parents are older is even more difficult. The children may discourage a widowed or divorced parent from dating or meeting others. They may be reluctant to accept their parent considering remarriage and resuming sexual intercourse with a new partner (Walbroehl, 1984). Nurses can have the opportunity to educate adult children with accurate facts regarding the sexual needs and concerns of their aging parents.

Nurses often are invited to help other segments of society regarding sexual matters. Whether helping young children or youth to learn the correct labeling of organs and functions of the body, or helping middle and older adults to learn the kinds of bodily changes that occur in time, the nurse can help persons gain factual information, but also gain positive attitudes on how sexuality can enrich life throughout its entirety. Sexual behavior is learned, and must be perpetuated in its beauty throughout life.

Older adults must be given the kind of life style that allows them privacy as well as "social permission" to engage in sexual relationships. This atmosphere must exist in institutions housing older adults, as well as in community living. Sexuality, many times, is ignored in nursing homes and supervised retirement communities. The sexes are separated. Even married couples may be forced to separate. There is little opportunity for privacy. Closed doors are not respected by the staff, and no locks are available. This situation is receiving more attention lately, and some institutions are changing. The nurse can help change the practices of those institutions that do not recognize the existence of older adult sexuality or provide opportunities for expression of sexual needs. Healthy standards of living, including sexual standards, can contribute to good mental health, and good mental health can improve the older adults' feelings about themselves, and maybe even society's feelings about the older adult.

With the number of older persons increasing in this country every year, the nurse/older person contact will also increase. Nurses need to become more informed in all aspects of aging, including the sexual needs of older persons. Continuing education is needed to begin changing negative attitudes toward sexual desires and sexual expression, and to help nurses gain proper information about sexuality in older adults. Many practicing nurses were trained in an era in which human sexuality, and particularly sexuality in older adults, was not discussed to any great extent. Such nurses need to be educated if they are to feel comfortable in discussing sexual matters.

An individual's sex life need not end once he/she reaches a certain age. Individuals over 65 do not automatically become desexualized. There are innumerable false ideas surrounding sexuality in old age. Older adults need to be free of social and psychological pressures that can inhibit a fulfilling sex life. Nurses have a role to play in this fulfillment, and continuing education has a role to play in equipping the nurse for his/her task. Hopefully, both of these roles will be assumed!

REFERENCES

Calderone, M.S. (1968). *Release from sexual tension.* New York: Random House.

Delora, J.S. & Warren, C.A.B. (1977). *Understanding sexual interaction.* Boston: Houghton Mifflin.

Diamond, M. (1980). *Sexual decisions.* Boston: Little Brown & Co., p. 65.

Gadpaille, W.J. (1975). *The cycles of sex.* New York: Charles Scribner Sons.

Green, R. (1979). *Human sexuality.* Baltimore: Williams & Wilkins, p. 134.

Hendricks, J. & Hendricks, C.D. (1979). Sexuality in later life. In V. Carter & P. Liddiard (Eds.), *An aging population.* New York: Holmes & Meier.

Hendricks, J. & Hendricks, C.D. (1981). *Aging in mass society: Myths and realities* (2nd ed.). Cambridge; Winthrop, p. 357.

Hogan, R. (1980). *Human sexuality.* New York: Appleton-Century-Crofts, p. 396.

Kolodny R., Masters, W.H., Johnson, V.E., & Biggs, M.A. (1979). *Textbook of human sexuality for nurses.* Boston: Little Brown & Co.

Select Committee on Aging. (1982). *Every ninth American* (Comm Publication No 97-332). Washington, DC: U.S. Government Printing Office

Walbroehl, G.S. (1984). Sexual changes with aging. *Geriatric Medicine Today, 3*(9), 31.

SECTION TWO

Physical protection

THIS SECTION DEALS with an additional physiologic concept related to self-care — specifically, physical protection from infection. By following the principles discussed in this section, the nurse reduces risk of infection to herself, clients, and other health care workers.

Recently, the media have called national attention to infection control and physical protection because of acquired immunodeficiency syndrome (AIDS) and the fear it engenders. Yet physical protection always has been important to the nurse concerned with delivering the best possible care. For the nurse and other health care professionals, the current publicity does not reflect a new level of safety concern, but serves as a reminder to continue applying the basic principles that guide safe, effective care.

The first article, "Worker Exposure to AIDS and Hepatitis B: Facts for the Health Care Industry," describes these disorders, their means of transmission, symptoms, and methods of prevention. By emphasizing the seriousness of these infections and the urgent need for their control, this article helps the student understand why the Centers for Disease Control (CDC) revised its recommended practices for protection against occupational exposure to infections. It also sets the stage for the next article, which addresses these recommendations in detail.

Because most carriers of the human immunodeficiency virus or the hepatitis B virus do not know that they have it, the CDC now recommends that health care professionals take *universal* precautions when they are likely to come in contact with any human blood or body fluids or wastes. This means that the nurse must treat *all* blood and body fluids as infectious whether or not they come from a client with a diagnosis of an infectious disease.

The second article, "Why Not Treat All Body Substances as Infectious?" by Jackson et al., describes how to put universal blood and body-fluid precautions into action. Based on recommendations from the CDC, the American Hospital Association, and the Association for Practitioners of Infection Control, it provides practical guidelines that protect the nurse and the client from infectious diseases of any kind.

Worker exposure to AIDS and hepatitis B: Facts for the health care industry

The following article, presented by the editors of AAOHN, *was reprinted from the pamphlet* Worker Exposure to AIDS & Hepatitis B, *published by the U.S. Department of Labor, Occupational Safety and Health Administration, 1987. Excerpts (marked by ellipses) remove specific recommendations, which are covered in more detail in the next article.*

THE ACQUIRED IMMUNE DEFICIENCY SYNDROME (AIDS) and hepatitis B (HBV) viruses merit serious concern for workers, especially those in the health care industry.

Workers at risk of blood, body fluid, or needle stick exposures are at the highest risk of infection. They include, but are not limited to, nurses, physicians, dentists and other dental workers, podiatrists, laboratory and blood bank technologists and technicians, phlebotomists, dialysis personnel, medical technicians, medical examiners, morticians, housekeepers, laundry workers, and others whose work involves contact with blood or other body fluids, or with corpses. Other personnel, such as paramedics, emergency medical technicians, law enforcement personnel, firefighters, lifeguards, and others whose jobs might require first-response medical care and potential contact with blood or body fluids are also at risk.

AIDS was first recognized in the United States in 1981. As of August 1987, the Centers for Disease Control (CDC) have received reports of more than 40,000 cases of AIDS, including 23,000 deaths. An additional 1.5 million people are estimated to be carriers of the virus that causes AIDS, but have no symptoms of the illness. Experts predict that by the end of 1991, there will have been a cumulative total of 270,000 AIDS cases in the U.S., including 179,000 deaths. Infection with the AIDS virus in the workplace represents a small but real hazard to health care workers. Only a few such cases have been reported to date.

According to CDC surveys, an estimated 300,000 new HBV infections occur each year in the U.S., and nearly 10% of those infected (1 out of every 300 persons in the U.S.) become long-term carriers. Of the 300,000, almost one-fourth become acutely ill or jaundiced, about 15,000 are hospitalized, and several thousand die from acute and chronic disease. HBV infections occur in about 8,000 to 12,000 health care workers per year and result in over 200 deaths per year due to acute and chronic effects.

AIDS and HBV infections have been reported from every state. The seriousness and immediacy of the problem have prompted the Occupational Safety and Health Administration (OSHA), in cooperation with the U.S. Public Health Service, to provide workers with information on the CDC recommended practices to protect against occupational exposure to AIDS and HBV. The recommended practices include precautions for the appropriate handling of blood and other body fluids, as well as items soiled with blood and other body fluids. Following these precautions should help prevent the spread of these viruses in the workplace.

AIDS

What is AIDS/ARC? AIDS is a bloodborne and sexually transmitted disease in which a virus invades the body, damages the immune system, and allows other infectious agents to invade the body and cause disease. ARC (AIDS Related Complex) refers to a variety of conditions caused by infection with the AIDS virus. These conditions range from mild symptoms to life-threatening ones.

What causes AIDS/ARC? AIDS/ARC is caused by the Human Immunodeficiency Virus (HIV), formerly called Human T-lymphotropic virus type III/lymphadenopathy-associated virus (HTLV-III/LAV).

How is it transmitted? The AIDS virus is spread through body fluids, primarily blood and semen. Although other fluids have not been shown to transmit infection, all body fluids and tissues should be regarded as potentially infectious. AIDS is transmitted by sexual contact, by needle sharing, and through contaminated blood products. An infected woman can pass the virus to her fetus. The AIDS virus is not transmitted by casual contact, touching or shaking hands, eating food prepared by an infected person, or from drinking fountains, telephones, toilets, or other surfaces.

What are the symptoms? Persons who are infected with the AIDS virus may have no symptoms, may have ARC, or may have AIDS. Individuals with ARC may have enlarged lymph nodes and a fungal infection of the mouth (thrush), which may be accompanied by fatigue, weight loss, and some problems with the immune system. AIDS is frequently diagnosed when the patient develops an opportunistic infection (an infectious disease that is only likely to occur when the immune system is depressed), such as *Pneumocystis carinii* pneumonia, or malignancies such as Kaposi's sarcoma (a rare form of skin cancer).

Is there a vaccine for the prevention of AIDS? To date, no vaccine is available to prevent AIDS and no antiviral drugs are available to cure AIDS. Some drugs, however, have been found to inhibit the action of the virus and others are able to fight certain opportunistic infections. Research is currently underway to develop antiviral drugs and vaccines; however, prevention is currently the only approach to control the virus.

Hepatitis B

What is hepatitis? Hepatitis is an inflammation of the liver. It can be caused by infectious agents, medications, or toxins. There are several types of infectious hepatitis (A, B, non-A/non-B, and delta), but hepatitis B presents the greatest risk to workers in the health care industry.

How is HBV transmitted? Hepatitis B is transmitted by sexual contact, by needle sharing, and through contaminated blood or blood products. An infected mother can transmit the virus to her fetus.

HBV is not transmitted by casual contact, touching or shaking hands, eating food prepared by an infected person, or from drinking fountains, telephones, toilets, or other surfaces. Thus, the occupational risk of HBV infection directly relates to the extent of worker contact with infected blood or blood products. As with AIDS, all body fluids and tissues should be regarded as potentially infectious.

What are the symptoms? Many people who are infected with the hepatitis B virus never have symptoms. The usual symptoms of acute infections are flu-like and include fatigue, mild fever, muscle and joint aches, nausea, vomiting, abdominal pain, diarrhea, and jaundice. Severe HBV infections may be fatal. Chronic carriers of HBV may develop a chronic hepatitis that may progress to cirrhosis, liver cancer, or death.

Is there a vaccine for the prevention of HBV? A hepatitis B vaccine is available that is safe and effective in the prevention of HBV infection. This vaccine is recommended for persons at risk of HBV infection, including health care workers and emergency personnel....

Why not treat all body substances as infectious?

MARGEURITE M. JACKSON, RN, MS; PATRICIA LYNCH, RN, BSN; DIANA C. MCPHERSON, RN, BSN; M. JEANNE CUMMINGS, RN, BSN; NANCY C. GREENAWALT, EPIDEMIOLOGY TECHNICIAN

USING ISOLATION PRECAUTIONS only with patients diagnosed with infectious diseases misses the vast majority of people who may harbor infectious agents. It makes far more sense to treat *all* blood and body substances (feces, urine, wound drainage, oral secretions, sputum, emesis, and so on) as potentially infectious. So for some time we have used a body-substance isolation system with *all* patients at our hospitals, regardless of their diagnoses.

The CDC recommends that all blood and body fluids be treated as if they are potentially infectious. In June 1987, the American Hospital Association and the Association for Practitioners of Infection Control also recommended the practice of universal blood and body-fluid precautions.

Q. What about isolation precaution signs?
A. When blood, drainage, secretions, and excretions are always treated as potentially infectious, no additional precautions are needed when patients have blood-borne or enteric infections. So special signs are not needed.

A sign is placed on the door when a patient has an airborne infection, however. The sign tells people to see the nurse before entering the room. The nurse advises susceptible people not to enter the room. Or, when everyone is susceptible (for example, with meningococcal meningitis), the nurse instructs people to wear masks when they are in the room.

Q. What precautions do you use?
A. Wear gloves when it is likely that your hands will touch *any* moist body substance, mucous membranes, or nonintact skin. Always change gloves before caring for the next patient.

Also wear a disposable plastic apron or cover gown if it is likely that your clothing will be soiled with body substances. Protect your eyes and oral/nasal mucous membranes from splashed body substances by wearing masks, glasses, or goggles. Discard used needle-syringe units, uncapped, in puncture-resistant containers.

Wash hands between patients and wash hands immediately whenever you accidentally have contact with body substances.

Q. Do you wear gloves when bathing patients?
A. No. Gloves are not routinely needed for bathing patients who have intact skin. But when patients have open skin lesions or when you are cleaning rectal or genital areas, it is advisable to wear gloves.

Gloves reduce the risk of heavy soiling when bathing an incontinent patient and make later handwashing easier and more efficient. Sometimes you need to wear a plastic apron or cover gown when cleaning spills from incontinent patients or when changing their beds.

If you have cuts or dermatitis on your hands, wear gloves when bathing any patient.

Q. What do you do when suctioning?
A. Always wear gloves — on both hands — to suction. Most nurses who suction patients frequently have learned how to position themselves so that they are not splattered when patients cough. Use eye protection and mask only if spray to the face is likely.

Q. Do you wear gloves when starting an IV?
A. Not necessarily. Remember, the major risk in starting IVs and drawing blood is needlestick injury. So careful needle handling is the most important safety factor. You need gloves only if it is likely that blood will get on your

hands. Most people who are skilled at starting IVs or drawing blood do not need to wear gloves when working with cooperative patients. Until your skill is adequate to prevent blood spills, wear gloves. You may need to wear gloves when manipulating stopcocks or lines.

Q. What about urinary drainage bags?

A. Wear gloves when emptying the drainage from a urinary catheter. Do *not* empty several patients' urinary drainage bags wearing the same gloves because doing so could transmit organisms from one catheter drainage spout to the next. Discard the gloves and wash your hands before emptying a second patient's drainage bag.

Q. When are masks needed?

A. Wear a mask if it is likely that body fluids will splash into your mouth, such as when you are suctioning a patient with copious secretions. Many hospital personnel wear masks in the rooms of patients with airborne infections such as TB. But the ability of masks to filter inspired air is actually not known.

Q. Where are goggles available?

A. We keep disposable goggles in the utility room on each nursing unit. After use, the goggles may be washed and reused by the same caregiver. Remember, eyeglasses are usually an effective barrier.

Q. How do you label specimens?

A. Treat all blood and body substances as potentially infectious. Using a label such as "blood and body-fluid precautions" on some specimens conveys a false sense of security about unlabeled specimens. Therefore, many hospitals no longer put biohazard labels on any specimens, even specimens from patients with identified infections.

Q. What do you do with linen from patient rooms?

A. Handle all linen in the same way. Place linen in *single* leak-resistant bags (e.g., plastic or nylon-coated) and tie them securely. Do not overfill the bags.

Laundry workers must always wear gloves and cover gowns when handling soiled linen.

Q. How do you clean patient areas?

A. Daily and terminal cleaning is the same for *all* patient rooms. No extra cleaning is required for rooms of patients with diagnosed infections, even when they are discharged.

Cleanse articles soiled with moist body substances immediately. Wear gloves.

Q. Where do you dispose of used needles and sharps?

A. Discard needles and sharps immediately after use. We keep puncture-resistant containers in all patient rooms as well as in utility and medication rooms.

Do not recap needles after use. When recapping is necessary (for example, needles of vacuum blood-collection systems), use only one hand. (Place the cap on a surface and insert the needle into it. Do not hold the cap in your other hand.)

Q. How do you discard trash?

A. Each health care facility must work out details with the city, county, or state agency that has jurisdiction over trash disposal in its area because regulations vary. Infection control personnel usually work closely with their governmental services and housekeeping department to ensure that trash disposal and "infectious waste" procedures comply with the appropriate regulations.

We enclose small dressings inside the disposable glove used to remove the dressing. (Pull the glove off inside out, keeping the dressing inside the glove. Then discard the dressing and glove in the regular trash container in the patient's room.) We discard larger dressings and gloves in an impervious bag (for example, in a wax-coated brown paper bag) and then discard this bag in the regular trash container in the room.

Always wear gloves when emptying fluid-filled containers. If splashing is likely, wear an apron or cover gown and eye protection. In some hospitals, Pleur-Evacs, suction canisters, and Hemovacs are not emptied before being incinerated or discarded.

Q. When are private rooms necessary?

A. Use private rooms for patients who soil the environment with body substances and for patients who have airborne-transmitted infections.

Q. Do you use additional precautions when a person has AIDS?

A. No additional precautions are needed even if the person's blood is known to be infectious.

Q. Can you combine this system with a traditional isolation system?

A. In our experiences, it does *not* work well to have both types of system in place at the same time because it presents a mixed message to personnel. Since the body-substance isolation system is designed to reduce risk of crosstransmission of any infectious agent in any body substance, the diagnosis of the patient is irrelevant. In other words, if all patients are treated with the *same* standard of care, why would additions be needed for those *diagnosed* with infections transmitted by contact with body substances?

The only exception is for airborne diseases: the diagnosis initiates use of a private room, evaluation of caregivers' susceptibility, and, sometimes, use of masks.

Q. How different is this system from other precaution systems?

A. Both category-specific and disease-specific isolation precautions are systems that are diagnosis-driven. That is, the diagnosis of an infection prompts the implementation of efforts to interrupt nosocomial transmission.

The body-substance isolation system, however, does not place emphasis on people with diagnosed infectious diseases. It recognizes that feces, airway secretions, and wound drainage always contain large numbers of organisms and that blood and urine sometimes do. Thus, precautions are based on interaction with patients. And the strategies characteristic of each system of isolation precautions (gloves, gowns or aprons, and so on) are consistently applied in the same fashion for contact with body substances from all patients.

Q. What are the advantages of this system?

A. The system should more consistently interrupt both cross-transmission from patients who are colonized but not infected, and cross-transmission from infected patients. Thus, it provides broader protection for health care workers and patients. A secondary advantage is its conceptual simplicity.

Q. Does this system cost more than traditional isolation systems?

A. Costs will vary among hospitals. The use of gloves will rise and disposable plastic aprons may be purchased. Purchasing and laundering isolation gowns, however, can be reduced or eliminated. Isolation carts are not needed. Some costs for special handling of trash and linen may be reduced or eliminated.

UNIT SEVEN

Study questions

1. According to "Pain: Advances and Issues in Critical Care," the nurse should take a holistic approach and "coordinate the health care team's efforts" to relieve the client's pain. What specific actions can the nurse take to accomplish this?

2. The article, "Fulfilling Nutritional Requirements," states that the nurse can use assessment data to formulate a nursing diagnosis of alteration in nutrition: less than body requirements. Which assessment techniques supply the data that support this diagnosis? What nursing interventions may be used for a client with this diagnosis?

3. In "Impaired Physical Mobility," Milde suggests three major goals for an elderly client with impaired mobility: maintenance of muscle strength and endurance, maintenance of joint flexibility, and development of an attitude that values preventive interventions. To reach these goals, which nursing interventions are most useful?

4. Based on "Sleep Pattern Disturbance," which internal and external factors are likely to disturb a pediatric patient's sleep patterns in an intensive care unit? How can the nursing care plan help prevent or treat sleep pattern disturbances for such a patient?

5. The article, "Sexuality in Older Adults: A Continuing Education Concern," reports these common misconceptions about sexuality in older adults:

1. Sex isn't important and doesn't matter.
2. Interest in sex is abnormal for the elderly.
3. Remarriage should be discouraged.
4. Older women shouldn't become involved with younger men.
5. Institutionalized older adults should be segregated according to sex, and privacy should be prohibited.

What facts can the nurse use to help correct these misconceptions?

6. Based on "Worker Exposure to AIDS and Hepatitis B: Facts for the Health Care Industry," how would you compare the transmission, symptoms, and prevention of acquired immunodeficiency syndrome (AIDS) and hepatitis B?

7. According to the universal blood and body-fluid precautions described in "Why Not Treat All Body Substances as Infectious?" when should the nurse wear gloves? a mask? a cover gown or apron? Why?

UNIT EIGHT

Professional practice of nursing

THIS UNIT PRESENTS several topics of vital interest to the nurse: the nature of nursing practice, education for professional practice, and making the transition from theory to practice. Each of these interrelated topics has sparked controversy in the nursing community. To help the student understand these controversies and prepare her to assist in resolving them, Unit Eight takes an in-depth look at the issues surrounding them.

The nature of nursing practice

Perhaps the first controversy is the status of nursing as a profession. By classical definition (Greenwood, 1957), a profession is a group of individuals who come together to provide a service to the public. It usually has a unique body of specialized knowledge, community sanction, ethical codes, a specialized culture, and authority over practice decisions.

Although nursing possesses a unique body of knowledge, community sanction, ethical codes, and a specialized culture, it lacks complete self-regulation and authority in its primary practice setting, the hospital. Nearly two-thirds of all nurses practice in hospitals, and many of them express discontent that they have little autonomy over decisions that govern their practice.

This leads to another controversy: the conflict between the ideal practice of nursing as learned through formal education and the occupational practice of nursing as experienced in clinical settings.

The conflict is compounded further by the fact that three educational methods — baccalaureate degree, associate degree, and hospital-based diploma programs — currently are accepted as preparation for registered nurse licensure. These controversies explain why, in nursing literature, the phrases *professional nurse* and *nursing profession* may be used in two different ways — to refer to nurses and nursing in general *and* to nurses with baccalaureate or higher degrees and their practice.

Additionally, determining the nature of nursing practice affects other issues, such as career opportunities for nurses and the future of nursing education.

Education for nursing practice

Education for entry into practice is a hotly debated issue among nurses. The issue centers around the position of the American Nurses' Association (ANA), among other organizations, that a baccalaureate degree should be the minimum educational requirement for en-

Glossary

Bureaucratic model of practice: model based on the occupational practice of nursing learned through clinical experience.

Profession: group of individuals who come together to provide a service to the public. A profession usually has a unique body of specialized knowledge, community sanction, ethical codes, a specialized culture, and authority over practice decisions.

Professional model of practice: model based on the ideal practice of nursing learned through formal nursing education.

Professional nurse: one who engages in nursing practice which, according to ANA recommendations, would require a baccalaureate degree. Also called registered nurse.

Socialization: process of learning and internalizing the expectations and demands of the professional or occupational role.

Technical nurse: one who engages in nursing practice which, according to the ANA recommendations, would require an associate degree.

try into professional nursing practice.

In a related decision, the ANA also recommended two levels of nursing practice and titles, requiring two levels of educational preparation: professional nursing practice would require baccalaureate degree preparation and carry the title of registered nurse; technical nursing practice would require associate degree preparation and carry the title of associate nurse.

These recommendations, too, have created controversy. At times, the debates over entry into practice and two-level titling have been public and heated. Some nurses view such debate as a sign of weakness in the profession. Others see it as an indication of the profession's health and the strength of its conceptual bases.

In fact, thoughtful discussions about educational preparation do not diminish the intelligent and caring practice of nursing. Rather, they indicate the robust health of a profession that struggles not for its existence, but for clarity of focus and unity.

Other educational issues that concern nurses include mandatory continuing education, effective use of staff development (or in-service) programs, and appropriate use of computer-assisted instruction.

Socialization: Making the transition from theory to practice

Issues related to preparing nursing students for the expectations and demands of their occupational roles are based in educational controversies. How are schools to prepare their students for the transition from classroom to the hospital or other occupational setting? Without successful preparation, the student will experience *reality shock* — the disparity between what the nurse *learns* in school and what she or he is expected to *do* at work.

Here are some of the debated questions: What are the best methods to prepare students for nursing realities *before* they graduate? How can the nursing student learn a specialty needed on the job when educational programs are geared to provide general knowledge and skills? What does a student need to learn about nursing management? What effect would the recruitment of male nurses have on the profession?

Debate and opinion

The articles in this unit build a foundation for understanding some of the difficult professional issues that confront contemporary nurses. Because these issues are complex, the articles cannot provide simple answers. Instead, they define the issues clearly and review the history of the debates.

When reading and discussing these articles,

the student should remember that thoughtful debate can promote intelligent and reasoned responses to the problems that nursing faces. Such debate will help prepare the student to fill the role of the reflective, caring nurse by providing an understanding of the impact of such issues on nursing practice and nursing care.

REFERENCES

Greenwood, E. (1957). Attributes of a profession. *Social Work* 2(3), 45-55.

SECTION ONE

Nursing practice

FOCUSING ON ISSUES of nursing practice, Section One begins by examining the relationship between nurses in academic and practice settings. Just because all registered nurses receive the same license, they do not necessarily share the same goals for their clients and their profession.

Nurse educators typically believe in a professional (ideal) model of nursing practice. They may differ on several issues with those nurses in clinical practice who follow a bureaucratic (occupational) model. This difference in approach has caused conflict between nurses with divergent aspirations for themselves and the profession. The conflict is fueled further by the diversity of nursing education programs, which typically espouse different goals for nursing education and practice.

The first article, "Nursing Education and Nursing Practice: The Need for Consensus" by Elliott, takes a close look at this conflict. Written by a former director of the U.S. Public Health Service Division of Nursing, it takes a positive, holistic approach to the debate between nurse educators and nurse clinicians by highlighting their areas of agreement, their successes, and the unresolved areas that require further dialogue. The author offers suggestions for resolving disagreements so that nursing can continue to grow. Throughout, Elliott lays the foundation for understanding many of the practice issues in this unit.

Just as Elliott's article describes the diversity of opinions in nursing education and nursing practice, the next article demonstrates the diversity in nursing practice itself. In "Other Options: Great Opportunities Outside the Hospital," Sandrick illustrates a wide range of nursing careers in various settings. (For more information on practice settings, see Unit Five.)

Although hospital nursing remains the profession's mainstream, Sandrick reports that many nurses are moving beyond the role of the hospital-based, bedside nurse, expanding the range of client services and the traditional limits of nursing practice. She examines the careers of ten nurses who work as independent practitioners, entrepeneurs, genetics consultants, business managers, and in other nontraditional roles. Although their careers are diverse, these nurses all have one thing in common: They use their nursing knowledge and skills to improve their clients' health and welfare. For the nursing student, their stories are particularly relevant because they offer new role models and show how to provide valuable nursing services while meeting personal goals.

However, some authors feel that one who does not care for clients directly is no longer a nurse. Wintz (1987) disagrees, arguing for a broader definition of nursing that includes nurses in various nontraditional careers, such as software designers for nursing care plan programs or health care policy analysts. Wintz writes:

> When is a nurse no longer a nurse? Lillian Wald established the first settlement house. Elizabeth Kinney founded the discipline of physical medicine. These nurses saw a need and used their nursing knowledge and experience to fill that need. Did these innovations make them ex-nurses? Florence Nightingale did not stop considering herself a nurse when she began the discipline of biostatistics. Mod-

> ern nurse pioneers will not only define but expand the boundaries of nursing. You can take the nurse out of the profession, but it seems unlikely that you can take the profession out of the nurse.

Even though new career paths are opening up for nurses, many still prefer to give direct client care in a hospital-based career, which has traditionally offered limited career advancement. Yet these nurses have the same need for reward, recognition, and career advancement as other individuals. Roberts and Fisher (1988) summarize this dilemma:

> In the past, staff nursing has been regarded as a dead-end job [that] frustrated the nurse who faced the dilemma of wanting to remain at the bedside while still desiring career advancement. All too often, this image and this dilemma hinders recruiting talented practitioners and drains away staff nurses' desires to take on greater responsibility in practice and to excel in nursing. Ultimately, this also partly explains turnover as nurses "float" from one position to another in search of more "interesting" work or a more satisfying environment.

Roberts' and Fisher's institution overcame this problem by developing a clinical ladder (a system for recognizing and promoting nurses who demonstrate advanced clinical knowledge and skills). But other solutions also can be effective.

"An Expanding Universe: Professional Career Opportunities," by Sossong and others, looks at another hospital's method of creating opportunities for advancement while allowing the nurse to engage in traditional client care. It describes previous career paths, cooperation between the institution and the nurses in developing the new program, and the program's positive effects.

Models of practice like this one suggest ways to enrich the daily practice of client care, expand nursing practice to meet the increasing demand for nursing services in hospitals, and minimize conflicts between the ideals of nursing education and the realities of nursing practice.

REFERENCES

Roberts, M., & Fisher, M. (1988). Establishing a clinical ladder: The process. *Nursing Management 19*(5), 86.

Wintz, L. (1987). Career paths of nurses: When is a nurse no longer a nurse? *Journal of Nursing Administration 17*(4), 33-37.

Nursing education and nursing practice: The need for consensus

Jo Eleanor Elliott, RN, AM, FAAN

The nursing profession is extraordinarily diverse: educationally, politically, economically, and experientially. Such diversity provides excitement and challenge; however, it can also stimulate conflict and dissension. This article will take a holistic approach to the profession by looking at its areas of consensus and its areas or issues in flux. Nursing's successes will also be explored to provide the balance and optimism so necessary to continued growth.

Agreements

One area of agreement is that the patient or client, whether that client be defined as an individual, family, or community, is the focus of the discipline of nursing. A patient needing care is the reason for our existence as a profession. Everyone who needs health and illness care should have access to that care; such access increasingly can be supplied by nurses. For example, nurse-run clinics are increasing in this country, as is nurse-managed geriatric care in nursing homes. The nurse practitioner and nurse midwife are also providing primary care and health maintenance.

The quality of nursing care, regardless of how it is measured or observed, is paramount. Care provided must be both cost-effective and efficient. A corollary is that nursing education must be cost-effective and efficient. Nurses have talked less about what will be done to make nursing education more cost-effective than about making nursing practice more cost-effective. With the reduction of resources at local, state, private, and federal levels, it is incumbent upon nursing educators to address themselves to cost-effectiveness and efficiency. Simply saving money is not enough; the educational process must also be efficient.

Another area of agreement is that nursing education exists to prepare students for nursing practice. New nurses must have preparation to undertake staff level positions. Staff nurses — direct care nurses — are the backbone of nursing care delivery and must be a constant focus for controlling our future and gaining consensus. Nurses warrant or merit salaries commensurate with academic preparation and responsibility. An additional benefit of matching salary levels with academic preparation and responsibility is the sense of self-worth and competence that comes from being recognized and rewarded. Matching salaries with preparation therefore must be addressed.

In the practice arena, we can agree that a variety of patient care sites and settings requires a broad array of nursing competencies and considerable depth of knowledge. The increasing acuity of illness of hospitalized patients and the increasing complexity of nursing in home care and long-term care facilities present much more complicated problems than existed five to seven years ago.

Successes

Nursing, like all professions, needs to regularly reflect upon and build on its successes to shape a preferred future. It is a success of nursing's educational programs and practice arenas that more nurses are licensed to practice today than ever before. There are 1.5 million nurses working, and 1.9 million nurses licensed to practice. The 1984-1985 nationwide graduating class of 82,000 students was the largest in nursing's history. The participation rate, or the number of nurses working, is 78 per cent.[1] For a predominantly female field, this is an excellent participation rate.

Unfortunately, many people, including some of our legislators, still believe that there are vast numbers of nurses out there who are not currently practicing nursing, and that if they could be encouraged to return to nursing, one of the current problems — the nursing shortage — would be solved.

One group of nonpracticing nurses is mothers with children. They comprise 22 per cent of the nonpracticing nurse population; they might be considered the revolving door group. They are going to come back to nursing when their children go to school. There are also nurses who are over 50, retired, but who maintain their licenses. These nurses are *not* potential returnees to the high-energy, high-stress areas of ICU and CCU. So, one must remind oneself: vast numbers of nonpracticing nurses simply do not exist "out there." This myth must be put to rest.

Not only are there more nurses, but more nurses are working in hospitals than ever before. There are *not* fewer nurses working in hospitals; over two-thirds (68 per cent) of nurses working are in hospitals.[1] However, the need for nurses has expanded beyond our apparent capacity to meet those needs. Nearly one-third of nurses work part-time. In the early 1980s, when the nation was experiencing a nursing shortage, some part-time nurses converted to full-time, and nonpracticing nurses came back to work. The profession may want to consider the potential in such a strategy. The supply of nurses could increase considerably if a certain number switched from part-time to full-time status.

Another success story is that the academic preparation of nurse leaders, both in education and service, has risen steadily over the past 20-30 years. It is reassuring to see the rapidly growing strength in nursing service leadership, which is now on a par with nursing education. In fact, the nurse educator may have to run like the dickens to keep up with the nurse administrator.

Another related success is the excellent example of collaboration between service and education provided by the joint statement from the American Organization of Nurse Executives (AONE) and the American Association of Colleges of Nursing (AACN) on graduate education in nursing administration.[2] The statement says, "Educational preparation for nurse administrators should take place within collegiate schools of nursing offering specialized graduate programs in nursing administration." This statement should now become the criterion measure for organized and new nursing administration programs.

The number of nurse researchers and the quality and quantity of nursing research has been increasing, a fine success. The potential exists for practice or curricula to be changed only as a direct result of research. A research project done at George Washington University with a nurse as co-investigator demonstrated that the quality of nursing care is the most important factor affecting the survival rate of patients admitted to intensive care units. Many more projects like this are needed to demonstrate to funders the need for increased nursing research support.

Another success story is the report from AACN on the "Essentials of College and University Education for Nursing."[3] This report should become a hallmark for existing and future programs because of its potential to influence the quality of nursing education and eventually effect changes in the first professional degree in nursing.

Nurse-midwifery practice has greatly increased, partly because different sections of the population are seeking this specialty care. For most of their existence, nurse midwives did their work in low income areas such as the ghettos, the hills of Kentucky, and the barrio. Now, because of their increasing popularity, nurse midwives are competing with physicians for health care dollars. Middle- and upper-middle-class women are beginning to recognize the benefits of using nurse midwives. This growing interest in nurse-midwifery is healthy and should be supported. Nurse midwives also need collegial recognition and support.

It is a success story that nurses are quickly learning to become entrepreneurs as a way of making sure services are available to those needing them. At least three local visiting nurse services have taken a page from hospitals' books. They have begun their own practices, they provide care, and they get reimbursed by Medicare and Medicaid. Nurses will need to learn competitiveness, particularly if Visiting Nurse Services (VNAs) are to survive. Keeping the VNAs alive is very important, because once the reimbursement runs out patients will be sent to whoever is there to take care of them, i.e., the VNAs.

Nursing has learned to mobilize clout and exercise influence at the federal level; that is a real success story. The Nurse Training Act of 1964 and its subsequent renewals have resulted in an enormous contribution to nursing. Most of the nursing school buildings built in the late 1960s and 1970s were built with federal participation....

The Nurse Training Act and its current Nurse Education Amendments also [have] been tremendously influential in providing support for graduate students as well as establishing new graduate and doctoral programs. Nursing should take great credit for these accomplishments. The continuing need for such legislation was especially noted in the Institute of Medicine study on nursing.[4]

The National Center for Nursing Research is clearly a creation of the nursing profession. Rarely has nursing been so united as during the struggle to establish the Center. President Reagan vetoed the bill; Congress overrode the veto — one of the few vetos that has been overridden in the President's terms.

Increasing numbers of nurses are in policy-making or policy-influencing positions. The number of nurses on senate and house staff rosters is increasing. Deborah Turner was a staffer on the Senate Labor and Human Resources Committee chaired by Senator Hatch (R-UT). She nurtured the present Nurse Education Act through Congress....

Carolyne Davis was Director of the Health Care Financing Administration for several years....

Other notable nurses in influential positions include Gloria Smith, nurse and director of the Michigan State Health Department, and Marilyn Goldwater of Maryland, who has been appointed liaison to the federal government for the Maryland State Health Department. Goldwater was an advocate of health issues and a strong friend of nursing when she served in the Maryland legislature.

The military has nurses in key policy positions who have had an impact on nursing's role in the Armed Forces. Leadership and policy-making positions are logical and important for nurses to assume. Nurses in these positions provide visibility and credibility for the profession.

The Robert Wood Johnson Fellows program provides marvelous opportunities to excite nurses with the possibilities of making and influencing policy. Nurses have also been White House Fellows. Charlene Connolly Quinn started as a White House Fellow and is currently working with Dr. Bowen (DHHS) on such issues as catastrophic insurance....

One success that hasn't been given much play recently is the Commission on Graduates of Foreign Nursing Schools. The Commission was created about 10 years ago to provide English and nursing knowledge and skills tests to nurses from around the world who wanted to come to the United States to work. The data show that, before the Commission was established, only about 15 per cent of the nurses emigrating to this country passed state boards.

The percentage has risen to about 85 per cent. Foreign graduates should be welcome in the United States, but they should be expected [to] meet the same standard as American graduates.

Areas in flux

The final section of this article addresses "areas in flux." That term has been chosen because it suggests unresolved issues or issues whose pros and cons are almost equally strong rather than issues that are potentially divisive.

The first area in flux is the *nursing shortage,* or at least, the discussion about a nursing shortage. A shortage of nurses does exist *in some settings....*The last data collected by the Division of Nursing were in 1984. The pattern of how events have influenced the nursing supply hasn't been tracked and analyzed, although the Division is working on it. Materials are being prepared for a report to Congress to address the issue of nursing shortage.

The following are what people have specifically identified as areas of need: experienced nurses seem to be in short supply, intensive care units are short-staffed, as are acute care units and rural hospitals; certain geographic sites have been short-staffed for some time. Whether or not a national shortage exists is difficult to ascertain because requirements for nursing personnel have increased so much.

A final visit to the shortage of the early 1980s will serve as a reminder that, in response to the shortage, the American Hospital Association (AHA) launched the National Commission on Nursing, the Division of Nursing funded a study to look at supplementary nursing services, and suddenly there were all these new nursing services. Then, within two years, the shortage was over. Thus, when addressing the shortage issue, all the variables must be examined.

Enrollments are decreasing, numbers of college-bound students are decreasing, and it is likely that this trend will continue until about 1994 at which time higher education will experience a turn-around. Nursing education has not recruited students nationally and systematically for at least 10 years. The profession is going to have to learn a great deal about recruiting, and whom to target for recruiting efforts. Nursing will have to attract nontraditional populations such as ethnic minorities. The two fastest growing segments of the population in this country today are Hispanics and Blacks. Young people from these populations are a valuable resource for nursing.

As a field that has traditionally been female, nursing must work harder at recruiting men. The profession must look at graduates of other disciplines, and at the educationally or economically disadvantaged as potential nursing students.

Certainly exit standards should not be lowered, but admission standards should be re-examined. The availability of federal money in the 1970s was a highly successful source of funding for special programs that permitted broader access into nursing and that supported students in many ways. However, that changed the minute lots of potential nursing students started knocking at the door; requirements went up and special programs closed down. Creative ways must be found to bring students in and keep them moving through the programs, not only up to graduation, but through taking and passing NCLEX-RN.

Salaries are another area in flux. The profession needs to address what might be done if salaries were increased substantially, and how to bring this about. Also, the profession has not really given broad consideration to the general perception that salaries are just that, and not wages. Nurses generally are not now seen as earning a salary; nurses earn an hourly wage. To what extent should we consider the relationship between being seen as professionals and the ways we are paid?

A further area in flux is *image*. Some of us

think large well-planned media campaigns will change the public's perception of the profession. However, it is equally true that what nurses do every day on the job conveys the image of nursing. Perhaps what is needed is to exhibit nursing as a field that deserves the best and brightest. Such an approach could not only improve nursing's image but also attract the kind of students the profession needs to maintain and expand quality standards of care.

Mentoring has been a well-discussed issue. The best case to be made for mentoring uses the following definition: giving support and help through a personal relationship. The definition implies a supportive socializing process that is crucial in such a diverse profession. Discussion with a staff nurse a generation or so ago often went like this: Upon being asked if she would be willing to have a student work with her, she responded, "If I had wanted to be a teacher, I would have gone into teaching." Nursing cannot afford that kind of attitude. Nurses, particularly in service settings, must develop the notion that each nurse should be a mentor and provide welcoming support. Mentoring can really transform the culture of nursing.

A Passion for Excellence, by Tom Peters and Nancy Austin, has a section that describes what the authors call "skunk works": little pockets of highly innovative people who are involved in slightly eccentric activity, and who operate at the edges of the corporate world.[5] If innovative solutions are needed, then nursing may wish to facilitate its own skunk works. Clusters of creative staff or head nurses or faculty could generate marvelous new ways of being cost-effective and efficient.

Peters and Austin also described the people in skunk works as having fun, and experiencing zest and enthusiasm.[5] Nursing needs to generate, cultivate, and encourage these qualities. The profession takes itself too seriously.

It is not the purpose of this article to judge whether nurses tilt toward agreement and consensus or toward diversion. Clearly agreement exists on some issues and disagreement on others. As nurses must develop perspective, creativity, humor, and enthusiasm, so must we maintain an open mind....

REFERENCES

1. Moses EB: 1984 Registered Nurse Population. USBHHS PHSHRSA BMP Division of Nursing June 1986, p3, 9

2. American Association of Colleges of Nursing: Indicators of quality in doctoral programs in nursing. J Prof Nurs 3:72-74, 1987

3. American Association of Colleges of Nursing: Essentials of College and University Education for Nursing. Washington, D.C., AACN, 1987

4. Institute of Medicine, Nursing and Nursing Education: Public Policies and Private Actions. Washington, D.C., Committee on Nursing and Nursing Education, 1983

5. Peters T, Austin N: A Passion for Excellence. New York, Random House, 1985, p xiii, 116-160

Other options: Great opportunities outside the hospital

KAREN M. SANDRICK

MORE NURSES ARE WORKING in the United States than ever before, but they aren't working exclusively in hospitals. Of the nearly 1.9 million RNs in the country, about 78 percent are currently employed; about 68 percent are practicing in hospitals. The remaining 10 percent are working outside hospitals.

The noticeable movement of nurses from hospital settings into nonhospital ones is a relatively recent phenomenon. It probably has more to do with the increasing opportunities for nurses in other health care or business fields than with any problems in hospitals. "Hospital nursing has always been pressure filled and stressful," explains Connie R. Curran, vice-president for nursing, American Hospital Association in Chicago. "And although hospitalized patients' acuity levels have risen, I still don't think pressure on nurses is causing them to leave hospital nursing. I think most nurses who leave are doing so because they can see the rewards of taking another career direction."

Nurses have never had more directions to choose from. As the nursing profession has broadened its horizons in recent years, so have many nurses. Nurses can help develop or sell the latest medical equipment. They can advise insurance companies to better meet patients' needs. They can work in hospices or home care agencies or open up whole new specialty areas — in genetics or organ transplantation. They can even put out their own shingle or start up a brand-new business.

Sounds exciting, doesn't it? But what's behind all the excitement? What's it really like to be a corporate manager? Or a flight nurse? How does a hospital product manager spend a typical day? How does a nurse practitioner juggle patient care and her personal finances? What are the challenges? And yes — what are the advantages over hospital nursing?

Recently, we asked 10 nurses in new and challenging nursing careers to talk about their work. Here's what they told us.

Independent nurse practitioner

Eileen Zitzer, RN, MSN, Philadelphia, Pennsylvania. The number of nurse practitioners in the United States grew from 9,000 in 1977 to nearly 25,000 in 1986. And although most nurse practitioners work in hospitals, preferred provider or health maintenance organizations (HMOs), home care agencies, or industrial settings, some have their own offices. Eileen Zitzer is one of them.

Zitzer opened her nurse practitioner office in 1984 to provide primary care and traditional nursing services, such as teaching, counseling, and medical screening. She says she wanted to "take nursing to patients on my own terms."

Zitzer, an adult nurse practitioner, and her associates — a pediatric nurse practitioner and a nurse therapist — offer a full range of primary care services, including preventive care, counseling in weight loss and smoking cessation, and continuing care. They currently see 150 patients a month and have referral arrangements with doctors who'll admit their patients if necessary.

Although Zitzer and her associates don't provide home care, they do make house calls. "We'll go out and do blood testing, blood pressure monitoring, or other testing if someone can't come to us," she says.

By leaving the hospital and setting up her

own nurse practitioner office, Zitzer gained autonomy but temporarily lost her financial footing. The office is financially secure now, but the nurse practitioners still can't rely on patients' standard insurance coverage to meet costs. "Smaller carriers have reimbursed us. But the large insurance companies and HMOs don't," she says. Most patients pay out of their own pockets or else barter their services.

Some health care experts believe the growing doctor surplus may put the squeeze on nurse practitioners. But Zitzer thinks doctors will drift away from primary care toward subspecialty care — opening this arena to nurses.

"Eighty percent of what people need is primary care," she says. "When you match that statistic with the consumer outcry for informed decision making and for medical personnel who give personal attention, there will always be a place for nurse practitioners."

Organ transplant coordinator

Mary Hoffman, RN, BSN, Musculoskeletal Transplant Foundation, Chicago, Illinois. Until recently, Mary Hoffman was organ transplant coordinator for Rush-Presbyterian-St. Luke's Medical Center in Chicago.

Paradoxically, an organ transplant coordinator's job swings from *death* to *life*. "On one side of the transplantation cycle, we see a dying or dead patient," explains Mary Hoffman. "But on the other side, we see a patient who owes his life to that first patient."

"Most transplant coordinators are called in when someone has been declared brain-dead or has had a neurologic injury and may donate visceral organs, or when someone has died of a myocardial infarction or respiratory arrest and may donate tissues, such as skin or corneas," she says.

After the death, information on a potential donor organ is forwarded to a computerized organ-transplantation information system in Virginia. Then, to make sure the organ is well perfused and oxygenated, the coordinator maintains the donor's blood pressure, input and output levels, and so on. Finally, she arranges for the surgical team to retrieve the organ and may assist in the operating room.

"Being an organ transplant coordinator is hectic and demanding work," Hoffman comments. "At any time, I may have to drop everything and go to a hospital to talk to a family."

There are about 160 transplant centers in the country, each with from one to five coordinators. "So, transplant coordination isn't a huge field," she admits. But it's growing by leaps and bounds. Rush-Presbyterian-St. Luke's Medical Center alone added two coordinators to its staff only last year.

In her present position as director of the Musculoskeletal Transplant Foundation, Hoffman teaches health care professionals about tissue and organ donation. "Most seminar participants are nurses," she says, "because they're most involved in obtaining donations.

"Many nurses still find it difficult to approach families of potential organ donors because they feel they're imposing on the relatives at a time of grief. But in many cases, organ donation is a consolation. Our responsibility is to be family advocates in this situation, to give the relatives the option and let them make the decision."

Hospital product manager

Kris Barlow, RN, Methodist Hospital's Women's Health Connection, Omaha, Nebraska. Five years ago, if someone had told Kris Barlow she'd be doing hospital marketing, she'd have said, "No way. I'm a nurse." But now, as product manager for the Women's Health Connection at Methodist Hospital, Omaha, she conducts marketing of women's medical services, including direct sales and advertising.

Although her work seems far afield from nursing, Barlow says she uses her tried-and-true nursing skills every day. "Whether assessments are being done from a nursing or a marketing viewpoint, the process is the same," she says.

Boiled down, product management is "keeping in touch with what consumers need and determining how the hospital can meet that need," she says.

One way Barlow and her team of nurse-marketers keep in touch with women consumers is through a toll-free telephone service. The telephone service allows local women to air complaints, ask questions, and request follow-up or referrals, and it helps Barlow plan educational events and special support programs.

"After learning that the needs of postmastectomy patients weren't being met, we developed a program with the American Cancer Society that gives volunteers 16 hours of training to create an ongoing support group for those patients," she explains.

In the current competitive health care environment, marketing hospital services to attract patients is vital, and more hospitals are asking nurses to be their marketers.

That makes sense to Barlow. "Nurses know what patients like and dislike, and they have the maturity and ability to deal with many types of people. Plus, nurses know about communicating with patients, about doctors' relationships with each other, and about issues of confidentiality and ethics. These are the basics of nursing, but they're also the basics of marketing and consumer relations."

Nurse-entrepreneur

Elizabeth Dayani, RN, MSN, Founder, American Nursing Resources, Kansas City, Missouri. Although nearly 19,000 people start new businesses each year, only half last 5 years, and only one out of five lasts 10.

So what makes Elizabeth Dayani, founder of a multimillion-dollar, nationwide chain of nursing placement agencies, successful? Her use of business as "a vehicle to give nurses more autonomy," she says.

With an initial investment of $1,500,000, Dayani, her husband, and three other nurses built American Nursing Resources into a $30-million operation by "finding the right nurse" for the local branches of the chain. The right nurse executive is one "who is committed to quality, is willing to bend over backward to serve clients, and is committed to working hard," she says.

For many years, Dayani felt that nurses could own and operate their own businesses and provide better-quality services. "In our company, we say, 'Okay, nurse, go for it. Treat it as your own business. We'll mentor you and give you the financial support you need to be successful, but you can develop your agency around your own areas of expertise.'"

Dayani's commitment to nurse ownership and management has led to a string of 24 placement offices from Hartford, Conn., to Los Angeles.

The American Nursing Resources' corporate offices in Kansas City, Mo., provide centralized payroll, billing, and accounting, plus fiscal training and guidance programs for the nursing directors of the placement offices. But in keeping with the company's philosophy of nurse autonomy, the business office is more of a support and educational center than a corporate headquarters.

Dayani stresses one major principle: "Health care is a business, and its survival depends on our understanding the proper management of resources. We have to take the best part of business — efficiency, marketing, and responsible service — and marry that to health care's commitment to quality."

Genetics counselor

Julia Mahon, RN, MSN, Memorial Hospital of South Bend's Regional Genetics Center, South Bend, Indiana. As a genetics counselor,

Julia Mahon does much more than explain the risks of genetic diseases to pregnant women and their husbands. She sees many other types of patients, too. "We also counsel patients who are finding out for the first time that they have a genetic disorder, such as Marfan's syndrome," she says.

In the center, which is affiliated with the Indiana University School of Medicine, Indianapolis, Mahon is called in by doctors to suggest proper diagnostic studies and to offer opinions on the possible causes of genetic disorders in newborns. She also coordinates genetics clinics, scheduling and interviewing families with hereditary diseases who've been referred there, and she participates in community education.

But she spends most of her day counseling families. "I meet with pregnant women who are age 35 or older and who are concerned about various genetic defects, particularly Down's syndrome. I see families with hereditary problems and talk with them about the kinds of prenatal testing available and whether they should pursue further testing. And I explain things in an understandable way to patients who have genetic problems and who often are afraid to ask questions," she explains.

Besides Indiana University's genetics program, there are three other regional genetics centers in Indiana (most states have at least one center). Mahon thinks that those are only a beginning. Clinical genetics centers are going to multiply as the demand for genetics counseling increases. "And the demand for services is going to expand because of dramatically new technology," says Mahon.

"We're increasingly able to locate the genes that cause disease. So, before a couple even considers pregnancy, we can pinpoint if they're carriers of a certain disease. The field of genetics counseling is just getting started."

Critical care consultant

Linda Buschiazzo, RN, CEN, CNA, BSN, Emercon Associates, Cheltenham, Pennsylvania. In 1984, after working as a manager in emergency nursing for many years, Linda Buschiazzo went into business for herself because she was "already doing a lot of consulting on a piecemeal basis," she says.

Her reputation grew by word of mouth, and today Buschiazzo's business, Emercon Associates in Cheltenham, Pa., employs two full-time and several part-time emergency and critical care consultants.

Buschiazzo conducts management consultations for hospital administrators and emergency department staffs on topics such as organizational operation, staffing and scheduling, computerized information systems, and program development. She and her associates also teach seminars and write articles on emergency nursing, critical care, trauma, and management.

Being a management consultant in critical and emergency services keeps Buschiazzo one step ahead of the field. For example, when she saw that there was nothing published on patient classification systems for emergency departments, she developed her own system, which is now being used in more than 150 hospitals in the United States and Canada.

And she needs to create educational and management programs that are right on the cutting edge. "Guest relations and marketing programs seem to be very high in importance right now as emergency departments try to increase the in-hospital census by building up the emergency department census and by increasing emergency admissions to the hospital," she says.

Finally, Buschiazzo helps emergency departments integrate good business practices into basic health care. "Many hospitals still don't have triage programs; in the 1980s, that doesn't make sense. I get the hospitals started, help them get their triage programs going, then let them take it from there."

Buschiazzo sees a bright future for nurse

consultants in many areas of health care management. "We find that many hospitals are looking to the outside for educators, consultants, and new programs."

Insurance company nurse consultant

Ruth Wintle, RN, BS, Aetna Insurance Company, San Diego, California. In the past year, Ruth Wintle has saved the company where she works over $12 million. How? By finding the best treatment options and the lowest-cost care for patients.

Wintle coordinates the Individual Case Management Program, established by Aetna Insurance Company in 1984 to smooth the transition of patients from hospitals to alternative care arrangements. "This program reduces hospital days, decreases overall health care costs, and helps patients recuperate faster," she explains.

Wintle has found major cost savings without sacrificing patient care by coming up with creative solutions to problems. For example, she arranged for Aetna to pay an LPN to care for her own husband at home following a stroke. Although the insurance company ended up paying the woman for working at home, it saved money in two ways — by getting the patient out of the hospital and by avoiding nurse placement agency charges. Results for the patient and his family: The woman could continue to support her family, the patient got individual attention in his own home so he could have more control over his care, and the family could maintain a stable home life.

Working closely with hospital administrators, Wintle tries to alter insurance policy provisions to reduce costs and gives advice on keeping costs down. With patients, she explains technicalities of insurance coverage and various treatment options. With both, she tries to prevent unnecessary admissions and reduce unnecessary hospital days while at the same time helping people get necessary health care. Being a nurse helps her balance these priorities.

She admits: "Sometimes I'm accused of trying to give away the store. But I want to give everyone a fair shake — to be cost-effective and to provide needed care. And to do it all from the heart."

Home hospice nurse

Dana Clark, RN, Hospice of Santa Barbara, Santa Barbara, California. Dana Clark came to Hospice of Santa Barbara 2 $^{1}/_{2}$ years ago to get away from high-tech care. A nurse for 15 years, 8 in critical care, she decided she needed a change because she was "too focused on computers and machines and tubes."

Although Clark still performs technical nursing, her goal now is to make the dying patient's life easier by accommodating medical treatment into his life-style. "I go in with the attitude of serving him the best I can, according to his environment," she explains. That means keeping intrusive medical equipment to a minimum, reinforcing the patient's own habits and customs — and sometimes even incorporating folk medicine into the hospice care regimen.

Many of Clark's patients come from the area's Hispanic population and have relatives from Central or South America who prepare poultices or herbal teas for dying patients. "We're dealing with deep-rooted customs and beliefs," she says. "So unless we feel a home remedy is actually going to harm a patient, we don't discourage the patient from trying it."

Clark normally has a caseload of 7 to 12 patients who have a wide variety of problems: cancer, acquired immune deficiency syndrome, stroke, heart disease, or end-stage renal failure. During her visits, she arranges for "whatever treatment the patient needs for comfort." Most often, however, she simply tries to do the "small things that make a difference," such as making a personalized medication list so a patient can remember when to take his pills, or sitting down and eating some pudding with him.

For Clark, hospice care is uplifting. But it's also highly stressful. With an average career span of only 3 years, the specialty has a higher burnout rate than many others.

The nurses who stay in hospice care longer, says Clark, have "found the key to taking care of themselves. They have an awareness of how important it is to nurture themselves so they'll be able to nurture others."

Corporate manager

Susan Smith, LPN, Cooper Lasersonics, Santa Clara, California. "Giving my current job description would be almost impossible because every day I get involved in something new," says Susan Smith, a corporate manager for the largest laser manufacturer in the country.

Indeed, as director of education and marketing services, Smith performs a wide variety of duties. Primarily, she directs a group of field nurses who train doctors and hospital technicians in laser technology. "When we sell a laser, one of our nurses spends a few days teaching staff members how to operate the equipment and helping them write appropriate policies and procedures."

With a budget of more than $1 million, she also coordinates workshops to introduce doctors and nurses to the new equipment and handles presentations at professional conventions. She helps develop corporate educational materials, too.

An LPN, Smith provides input on marketing Cooper's product lines and on the design of experimental laser models. "For a long time, medical equipment was designed by engineers who had no idea how the equipment would be used," Smith says. "Many simple design flaws caused problems. For example, a piece of equipment might not have handles to push it around with. So now I get involved in customer-oriented design elements — even in determining how big the wheels are for better maneuverability."

The customer-oriented aspect of her work is most satisfying to Smith. "Our industry must realize that it can't be successful unless it's attuned to the customer — who he is and what his needs are."

So, Smith sees great opportunities for nurses in medical manufacturing. More than anyone else, nurses know the equipment's users — doctors and other nurses. "Hiring a nurse who knows the jargon and what the customer needs is a real advantage to any medical manufacturing company," she asserts.

Flight nurse

Amy Tomecko, RN, CCRN, BS, Samaritan Air Evac, Phoenix, Arizona. When Amy Tomecko gets a "scramble call," she has only 3 minutes to respond to one of many critical care situations. She may be flying to the site of a multivehicle accident...or moving a transplant donor or recipient across the state...or transporting a critically ill cardiac patient from a general community hospital to a heart center.

For the past 6 years, Tomecko has been a flight nurse for the nation's first and busiest hospital-based emergency air transportation program. "We're called in to provide rapid transport of patients from the outskirts of Phoenix to Level I trauma centers in the middle of the valley. We're also called in to provide quick advanced life support to patients in rural communities," she says.

Tomecko is one of a growing number of flight-trained nurse specialists in the rapidly expanding field of medical air-rescue services. In 1978, there were only about 12 air-rescue operations in the country; now there are 136 hospital-based services and another 30 or more police and rescue squad programs.

Owned and operated by Samaritan Health Service, a multihospital system in Phoenix, Samaritan Air Evac has been offering 24-hour medical emergency air service since 1969. It currently employs nearly 1,500 flight nurses who each year direct the air transport of over 4,000 medical and trauma patients in and around Arizona and other parts of the continental United States, Canada, and Mexico.

Tomecko manages 31 full-time and 5 part-time flight nurses, but her primary duty is to act as chief medical officer during air transports. "Every flight is different," she observes. "We have to be skilled not only in performing life-support procedures but also in managing different types of patients — medical, trauma, and pediatric patients."

Although flights can be traumatic and tense, they're rewarding, too. "You get a sense of satisfaction when everything goes properly and you know you've made a real difference in a patient's life."

An expanding universe: Professional career opportunities

Ann Sossong, RN, MEd, CNA; Marteile Benson, RN, CNA; Paula Ballesteros, RN, CNA; Sharon Dauphinee, RN; Penelope Dolley, RN, CNA; Evelyn Garrick, RN, CNA; Patricia Gray, RN, CNA; Dawn P. Couch, RN, MN; Patricia Miller, RN, MA; Amy Pollard, RN, CNA, BSN; Catherine Smith, BA, MLS

This article shows how creative managers in one institution developed a stimulating environment for pursuing a nursing career. The key to their program's success was recognizing the staff nurse as the center of nursing services. Note: Summaries (shown in bracketed italics) condense extensive background material.

Eastern Maine Medical Center (EMMC), a 431-bed regional medical center, cares for the rural population of northern Maine far from the great metropolitan centers of educational and career opportunities. Still, the corporation [that] manages EMMC strongly supported enriching nursing careers to keep a more stable, more satisfied work force.

Time for change

EMMC had been operating under the traditional nursing services hierarchy [that] locked staff nurses in a system of tasks and routines. Specialization and automation were reducing the meaningfulness of staff nursing. There were only two ways for a nurse to be promoted. She could either become an instructor in the School of Nursing or climb the ladder of nursing supervision. Unfortunately, these conventional alternatives could lead very effective clinicians to become less effective managers or educators in the name of advancement. These prospects and arrangements certainly did not encourage trying the new concepts of nursing practice and different approaches to delivering health care [that] a burgeoning nursing literature was advertising. Beyond this, social changes in the 70s and 80s were reshaping nurses' career desires.

To recruit competent nurses and to retain them, we would have to change our perceptions of the potentials in staff nursing. We aimed at total development [that] would integrate efforts of nursing management, education, practice and research to enrich careers in the Center itself as much as possible. To do this, the Center would have to make further education more accessible, to open more assignment and career options within its organization, and to develop progressive salary scales for increasing competence in those options.

[Program development and implementation

To plan the program, the Center formed a Career Opportunities Task Force that included all head nurses and several key EMMC administrators. The task force met weekly to develop plans that would uphold this nursing philosophy: "Nurses must be provided with opportunities to advance professionally and financially and to participate in decisions affecting nursing practice and standards."

To accomplish this, the task force had to shift its perspective. At first, it viewed the nurse at the bottom *of a hierarchy with four distinct paths that led up to top clinical, educational, nursing practice, or administrative positions. This view, however, segmented nurses' career development and could foster individual competition. So the task force developed a model that placed the nurse in the*

Exhibit 1

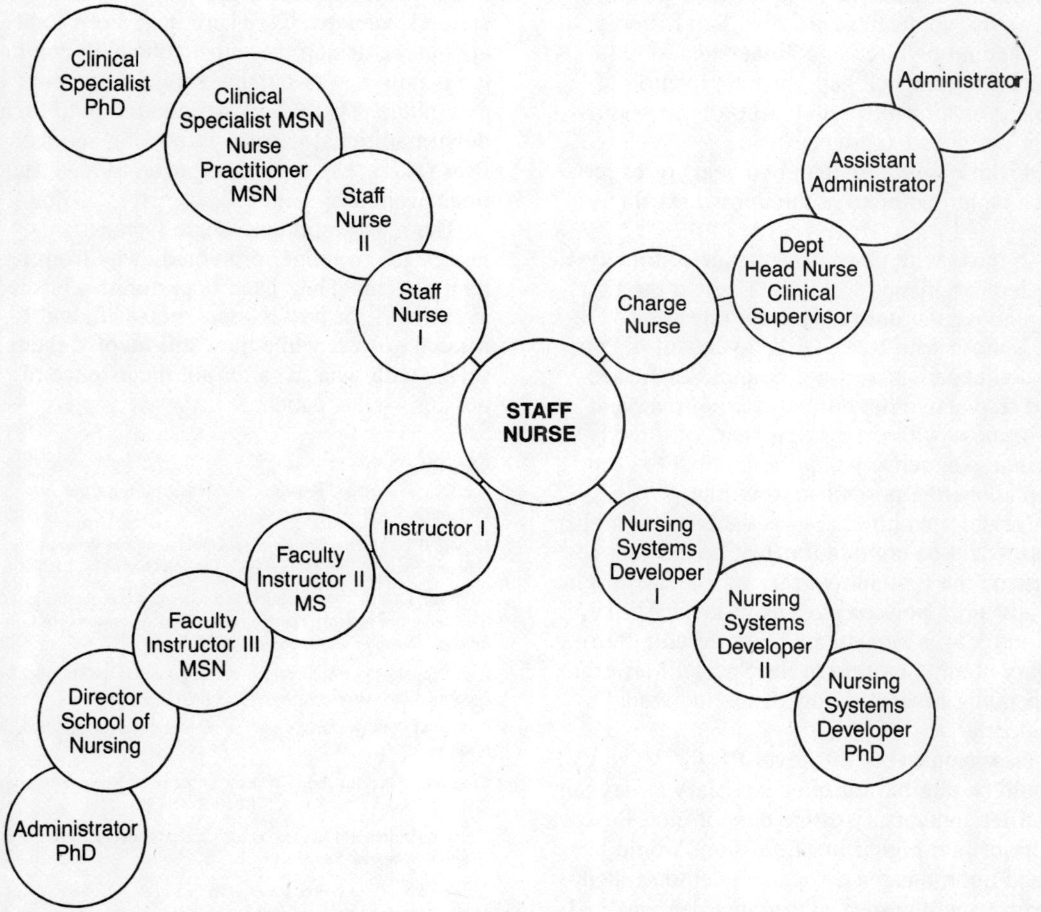

center *of a universe of relationships and functions to which she or he could aspire. (See Exhibit I.) This view would bind the nurses together in service and could foster mutual respect.*

After agreeing on this model, the task force defined each position, determined education and experience requirements, and wrote performance standards. It also made opportunities available for qualified staff to obtain the certification or advanced degrees required for the advanced positions.

When managers first introduced the program, they met some resistance in nurses who believed that experience should count more than education or certification. The benefits of the program to consumers and the nurses soon overcame this resistance. Many nurses sought certification or advanced degrees, and the institution gave them financial support.]

Rewarding competence in salary

Applicants for Level I and II positions could be hired at the starting rate for their position. However, applicants for Level I and II positions could be hired at a higher step, or advanced to a higher step upon completion of their probationary period, according to pertinent previous experiences:

1. those with less than two years of experience would be hired at the normal starting rate;
2. those with two to five years of directly related experience would be hired at the first step above the normal starting rate;
3. those with five to seven years of directly related experience would be hired at the second step above the normal starting rate; and
4. those with over seven years of directly related experience would be hired at the third step above the normal starting rate.

New nurses hired at or advanced to a higher step would be eligible for their next salary review on the first anniversary of the date of hire or advance. New employees in Level III, IV, V, and VI positions would be offered a starting salary at any point up to the Special Merit rate, depending upon a review of the individual's credentials.

New employees for Level III, IV, V, and VI would be eligible for the next salary review on the first anniversary of the date of hire. Promotions into higher level positions would be based upon budgeted vacancy, demonstrated performance, proper educational degrees, and the recommendations of current department head and nursing administrators. For a promotion of one level, the employee's salary would normally be increased by a percentage of applicable rate.

Since our program has been instituted, turnover has dropped and interest in educational programs and opportunities has increased dramatically. There have been joint appointments and the nurse education committee is now a joint nursing service-education committee. These work as integrators to break down traditional barriers in nursing service. Peer review has been recognized to have functional validity.

The most important single factor is that nurses are no longer promoted away from patient contact. They have opportunities onsite, at EMMC, for professional, personal, and financial growth while they still involve themselves with what is, after all, the essence of nursing — the patient.

REFERENCES

Alt, J.M., *et al.* "New Hope for 'Hands-on' Nurses: Clinical Promotions." *RN.* 43:6:49-53.

Brown, B.J. "The Role of Nursing Administrator in Patient Care Delivery Systems." *Nursing Administration Quarterly.* 1:Fall:1-6.

Callahan, J., *et al.* "Processing a Task Group: A Continuing Educaton Committee at Work Planning a Conference." *Journal of Continuing Education in Nursing.* 2:5:8-15.

Christman, L. "The Autonomous Nursing Staff in the Hospital." *Nursing Administration Quarterly.* 1:Fall:37-44.

Colton, M.R. "Cost Analysis of Career Mobility Programs." *Supervisor Nurse.* 10:7:20-28.

Courtade, Sister Simone. "The Role of the Head Nurse: Power and Practice." *Supervisor Nurse.* 9:12:16-23.

Meintel, Patricia and Rhodes, D.E. "Clinical Career Ladder RNs." *Hospital Progress.* 58:8:36-41.

Nursing Service Division. *Philosophy of Nursing.* Eastern Maine Medical Center. October, 1979.

Olson, E.M. "Strategies and Techniques of the Nurse Change Agent." *Nursing Clinics of North America.* 14:323-336.

Styles, M.M. and Wilson, H.S. "The Third Resolution." Nursing *Outlook.* 27:1:44-47.

Welch, L.B. "Planned Change in Nursing: The Theory." *Nursing Clinics of North America.* 14:307-321.

SECTION TWO

Education for professional practice

LIKE NURSING PRACTICE CONCERNS, nursing education issues have witnessed lively debate recently. Also, nurse educators and nurse clinicians have shown the same healthy signs of intelligently considering the issues. To help the student understand the debate, Section Two addresses two of the most controversial issues: education for entry into practice and continuing education for nurses.

The first article in this section, "Entry into Practice: The Continuing Saga" by Dunbar, looks at an issue that nurses have debated for decades — that of the appropriate educational preparation for the beginning nurse. It reviews this complex issue thoroughly, identifying several key questions and discussing the impact of two levels of titling (professional nurse and associate nurse) on critical care nursing practice, education, and certification. Written by the former president of the American Association of Critical-Care Nurses (AACN), this article emphasizes the importance of defining the scope of practice and competency for two levels of nursing before developing curricula. For only when nurses are clear about the expected competencies of the entry-level nurse will they be able to define the appropriate educational preparation for practice at any level.

No matter what level of practice a student wishes to pursue, this article is useful because it illustrates the complexities for practitioners, lawmakers, and the public in trying to redefine requirements in a profession.

But education does not end when the student becomes a nurse. To be effective, the nurse must keep abreast of practice issues and new technologies. One way to do this is to take part in continuing education programs. These formal, organized programs promote the knowledge, skills, and professional attitudes of nurses. They are usually short-term and specific and may offer a certificate or confer continuing education units (CEUs) for program completion.

In some states, continuing education is so important that nurses must participate in it for relicensure. In "Continuing Education Requirements by State," Foss examines the issue and summarizes requirements for relicensure by state.

Although almost all nurses agree that continuing education is important, some, such as Cooper (1973), argue against mandatory continuing education for nursing relicensure. Cooper gives these reasons:

1. Educational resources are inadequate.

2. Problems of accrediting or approving suitable offerings have not been solved.

3. Measuring the effectiveness of continuing education is inadequate.

4. Legal requirements tend to be inflexible and rigid and do not allow for differences in learning.

5. Legal requirements always are minimal requirements.

6. You cannot force people to learn.

On the other hand, many nurses affirm mandatory continuing education. Allison (1973) believes that, by making educational activities mandatory, the profession can ensure their use. Ayers (1973) suggests that mandatory continuing education could help forestall nursing malpractice. McGriff (1973) believes that the issue of professional competence is too important to be left to the individual nurse.

Although a literature review by Weiss-Farnan and Willie (1988) found widespread acceptance of mandatory continuing education in 1983, they predict that the debate will be rekindled. They report that:

> ...the benefits of mandatory education are still unknown...the debate [probably] will continue until evidence rather than belief is presented that mandatory continuing education not only insures practitioner competence and performance, but also improves patient health.

One form of continuing education is the staff development (or inservice) programs provided by a hospital for its staff. Foglesong, Lambert, and Emerick (1987) have investigated if such programs improve client care. Surprisingly, they found that the effect of staff development programs on nursing practice depended primarily on the degree of nursing autonomy: Greater autonomy was associated with greater change in practice and improved client care.

In baccalaureate or continuing education for nurses, the computer is a valuable tool. In a summary of 11 independent studies of computer-assisted instruction, Belfry and Winne (1988) report:

> ...computer-assisted instruction is an effective method for teaching nursing students. [It] is most effective for student[s] when it...supplement[s] other forms of instruction. In addition, students may learn...in less time. The technology can adapt instruction to individual learning needs and allows students to learn at their own pace and at a convenient time. The positive attitudes that nursing students develop toward this form of instruction...may increase motivation to learn and, as a result, the amount of learning that actually takes place.

However, Belfry and Winne believe that further research is needed into how to use computers even more effectively for instruction. They suggest investigating the most appropriate types of computer-assisted instruction for meeting different learning objectives and student needs, the degree of retention of knowledge and its application in practice, and variables such as learning styles and attitudes that influence the effectiveness of computer-assisted instruction.

REFERENCES

Allison, E. (1973). Should continuing education be mandatory? Yes. *American Journal of Nursing, 73*(3), 443.

Ayers, R. (1973). In California continuing education will be mandatory. *AORN Journal, 18*(3), 487-493.

Belfry, M., & Winne, P. (1988). A review of the effectiveness of computer assisted instruction in nursing education. *Computers in Nursing, 6*(2), 77-85.

Cooper, S. (1973). Continuing education should be voluntary. *AORN Journal, 18*(3), 471-478.

Foglesong, D., Lambert, J., & Emerick, J. Variables which influence the effect of staff development on nursing practice. *The Journal of Continuing Education in Nursing, 18*(5), 168-171.

McGriff, E. (1973). Mandatory continuing education for nurses. *AORN Journal, 18*(3), 480-484.

Weiss-Farnan, P., & Willie, R. (1988). Mandatory continuing education: The discussions a decade apart. *The Journal of Continuing Education in Nursing, 19*(2), 73-75.

Entry into practice: The continuing saga

SANDI DUNBAR, RN, DSN

Background

RECENT TITLING RECOMMENDATIONS by the American Nurses' Association (ANA) for two levels of nursing practice have created much fervor, controversy, and debate both within and outside the nursing profession. The ANA position recommends that the title "registered nurse" be retained and used exclusively for nurses with educational preparation at the baccalaureate level. Thus "registered nurse" and "professional nurse" would be synonymous. The title "associate nurse" would be used to describe nurses prepared at the associate-degree level thereby making "associate nurse" and "technical nurse" synonymous. The ANA position further recommends congruence between the scope of practice and the educational preparation for the two proposed licenses for nursing practice.

As states move to implement this position, legislative action, changes in rules and regulations, or both are required, since the title "registered nurse" is currently encompassed in law. Ideally the nursing profession would, from a united position, accomplish these changes expediently and appropriately. However, there continues to be much dissension within nursing as the 120-year-old debate on entry into practice continues.

As critical care nurses address the issue of titling for licensure, many questions have been, and will continue to be, raised and discussed. In this message, I will identify several key questions and provide an overview of the impact of two-level titling for licensure of critical care nursing practice, education, and certification.

Titling for licensure issues

Scope of practice. At the heart of the controversy is the implicit need to define the scope of practice and competency statements for two levels of nursing. This complex and emotionally charged issue is central in analyzing the titling for licensure position. Several projects are under way to develop and research distinct competency statements for the two levels.

Two schools of thought appear to be emerging. One position holds that the associate nurse would function in staff positions defined as we currently practice nursing, and the registered nurse would fulfill job competencies that have a broader scope than we currently expect. The other school of thought distinguishes the two levels of nursing according to practice settings, roles, types of patients, and knowledge base. This perspective recommends that the professional nurse function as the coordinator of care for patients who need complex care in both structured and unstructured settings. The associate nurse, on the other hand, would focus on clients with predictable or stable conditions, implement protocols developed by the professional nurse, and assist in collection of assessment data.

Currently, several projects are under way to refine these scope-of-practice recommendations and to test their implementation. One such project has been undertaken by an ANA task force that is defining the scope of practice by building on the Social Policy Statement and previous documents that detail the role of the nursing profession. This group has just completed the first draft of its proposal and has circulated it to other nursing groups for feedback and suggestions.

Another important project is the National Commission of the Nursing Implementation Project (NCNIP), funded by the Kellogg Foundation. The purpose of the NCNIP is to coordinate the implementation of key recommendations outlined in 1983 by the National Commission on Nursing by identifying areas of consensus and developing strategies for change. One work group is focusing on education and titling for entry into practice and has proposed moving from four to two levels of entry by 1995. This group has identified several competencies on which there is consensus regarding the different roles filled by nurses with an associate degree in nursing (ADN) and by those with the degree of bachelor of science in nursing (BSN).

Another project, entitled "Defining and Differentiating ADN and BSN Competencies," is sponsored by the Midwest Alliance in Nursing and is also funded by the Kellogg Foundation. In this project, job descriptions that represent different competencies for the two proposed levels of nursing are being pilot-tested. To date, the results of the test indicate that the job descriptions "work" in the practice arena.

The Integrated Competencies of Nursing Project is in process on several nursing units at Yale-New Haven Hospital. Teams consisting of two associate nurses and one professional nurse work together. Some similar interventions, such as direct patient care and communication, are performed by all team members. However, the professional nurse admits patients, performs the initial nursing assessment, and formulates a nursing plan of care. Professional nurses are salaried and receive no overtime pay.

These projects are exciting and each demonstrates momentum in answering vital questions about two levels of practice. Each will also provide results that will be invaluable in achieving consensus on the scope of practice and competencies for two levels of nursing practice. Such consensus is, and will continue to be, essential for educators to prepare nurses for successful implementation of two levels of practice in the service setting across the nation. Additional and immeasurable benefits will be obtained if such consensus leads to greater unity between nursing service and education. The claim that "nursing education does not prepare nurses for the real world" and the response that "graduates are prepared adequately but are not used appropriately in entry-level positions" are tiresome, derisive, and damaging. In addition, success in approaching legislative bodies *depends* on consensus regarding the scope of practice.

Variability in implementation of titling for licensure. Changing regulations governing nursing will require state-level legislation or rulemaking. It is anticipated that such activity and change may take 10 years or longer to accomplish. Compounding the situation are the high variability in the time when the changes become effective and the variation by state in the selection of titles for the technical nurse. Although ANA went on record in favor of "associate nurse" as the preferred title for the technical nurse, states have needed to implement a title that best suits their individual situation.

To date, two states have either legislated change or adopted rules to implement the titling for licensure position creating two levels of nursing. The North Dakota Board of Nursing adopted revised rules requiring nursing education programs, beginning in 1987, to offer a curriculum leading to an associate degree for licensed practical nurses (LPNs) and a baccalaureate degree for registered professional nurses. Several diploma schools of nursing had, however, obtained a temporary injunction that halted implementation efforts pending resolution of legal action against the North Dakota Board of Nursing. The North Dakota Supreme Court recently upheld the revised rules and affirmed the legal authority of the state board to set nursing education standards.

The state of Maine adopted legislation revising its nurse practice act. The revisions stipulated that by 1995, there will be two levels of nursing: one requiring an associate degree and the other requiring a baccalaureate degree. Other states are currently examining strategies for implementing two levels of nursing practice.

Grandfather clause. Misconceptions abound regarding the issue of the grandfather clause in proposed legislation. Many nurses oppose the titling for licensure recommendations on the false premise that their current nursing status would change. Ironically, the use of a grandfather clause seems to be the one area of general consensus in the titling recommendations. That is, most support grandfathering current registered nurses to the professional level, with the attendant scope of practice, *regardless of educational preparation.*

The same right is not as clear for the LPN. Although the 1986 ANA House of Delegates adopted a resolution supporting grandfather rights of LPNs to placement at the associate level, state approaches to this issue differ. Some states favor a grandfather clause for LPNs, whereas others suggest competency examinations. It has also been suggested that nurses currently licensed as LPNs be retained at the present title and scope of practice but that there be no additional LPN graduates.

As changes are implemented at varying times in the various states, nurses will be confronted with the simultaneous existence of both new and old titles. Nurses with the same educational preparation may be eligible to be registered nurses in one state and associate nurses in another. Hospital recruitment may take different approaches on the basis of which nursing level is involved. Confusion on the part of consumers of nursing services, including both the employers and patients, will definitely be a visible issue during this time of transition.

Implications for critical care nursing practice

The predominant question to be answered regarding the implementation of two levels of nursing practice centers on how nurses placed at these levels will function in critical care settings. As is true throughout all of nursing, the dimensions of practice and the competency statements regarding the two levels of nursing will need to be studied, analyzed, and tested in critical care settings.

Currently, critical care nurses who are registered nurses are responsible for the same level of practice regardless of educational preparation. What would be the impact of having two levels of nursing practice in critical care? How would one level versus two levels of nursing affect costs, patient outcomes, patient and family satisfaction, and quality of care? Should there be only one level of nursing in critical care? Should only the professional registered nurse provide care for critically ill patients? What will be the impact of our current critical care nurses' shortage on implementing one or two levels in critical care?

At present, we are facing a shortage of qualified critical care nurses, and it is increasingly clear that this is not a short-term phenomenon. I have recently heard of institutions that rely on LPNs to provide the majority of care for critically ill patients. Until adequate numbers of qualified registered professional nurses are available, we will continue to be confronted with supply-and-demand dilemmas and nurses with varying levels of educational preparation in critical care.

Implications for critical care nursing education

To develop nursing curricula that are consistent with the scope of practice for each of the two recommended levels of nursing practice, educators will need to achieve a considerable amount of reorganization. Many will actually welcome this opportunity to refine nursing education and develop strategies for reality-based education. If the professional registered nurse is to be designated to care for critically ill patients, then the inclusion of critical care content at the undergraduate level will be essential.

In addition to a redefinition of nursing curricula, greater career mobility must be developed to provide access to educational opportunities for nurses. Even though registered nurses will benefit from the grandfather clause, there will continue to be a great need for nurses prepared at the baccalaureate level to meet the needs of an increasingly complex patient population and health care system. Barriers to baccalaureate education (such as scheduling, expenses, and academic credit for experience) must continue to be identified, reassessed, and overcome.

Implications for specialty nursing certification

Certification for specialty practice adds another dimension of complexity to the titling issue. The role of a professional association is to set standards and advance the *profession*. The role of certification, on the other hand, is to test competence according to current practice expectations for the protection of the *consumer*. This inherent difference in focus may at times create conflicting positions.

AACN has a position statement in support of the BSN degree as the requirement for entry into professional practice; however, a BSN degree is *not* required by the AACN Certification Corporation to be eligible for CCRN certification. Explanation of the rationale for this apparent discrepancy is frequently sought by both AACN members and nurses who have obtained the CCRN. Until different job descriptions, different licensing examinations, and different scopes of practice are developed and implemented for different educational and practice levels of nursing, *or* until the majority of the nurses in critical care have BSN preparation, it would not be reasonable to require a BSN degree for CCRN certification.

Variability of timing in implementation of the titling for licensure recommendations may complicate the issue further. If a registered nurse license remains part of the certification eligibility requirements, then eventually only those nurses who have been grandfathered into the professional level or those with a baccalaureate degree will be eligible. Depending on the scope of practice for the associate nurse, would a second-level certification examination be needed? There is, once again, the potential for inconsistency in terms of who would be eligible because of the variability among the states. The key to coping with this dilemma is to remember that CCRN certification is for the protection of the consumer.

There is also the potential for the CCRN credential to have even greater meaning and value to consumers — both patients and administrators. During this period of transition, the CCRN may be the credential of competence that remains stable while educational requirements and titles are in a state of flux.

Summary

In this message, I have tried to outline the critical care issues involved in implementing the titling for licensure position. Now, more than ever, a unified nursing profession is needed to address these issues. Misconceptions about disenfranchising some nurses must be laid to rest. We must continue to ask what is best for our patients, society, and the nursing profession.

As I have met critical care nurses throughout the nation during this year, I have found very few who do not believe that someday we will all need to be better educated. Critical care nurses have also indicated to me their perceptions and beliefs about the increasing complexity of nursing and the fact that entry levels of today may not be appropriate for the twenty-first century. In the practice arena, critical care nurses apply special practice skills to anticipate and respond to rapidly changing patient needs. These same attributes and skills make critical care nurses especially equipped to cope with the ambiguity of the upcoming years of transition.

In 1979, AACN adopted a position statement that supported the baccalaureate degree in nursing as the minimal preparation for entry into professional nursing practice. The position is not inconsistent with the titling recommendations. However, the titling issue and the questions addressed in this message are currently being, and will continue to be, addressed by AACN because it is the role of our professional association to set standards for critical care and to respond to society's needs. As Merton has so clearly stated: "Professions do not stand still. The issue...is whether a profession, or an occupation moving toward professional status, will wait until changes in the society of which it is a part compel it to reluctant change or whether it will try to anticipate the changes now in the making and be prepared to meet them. The issue is of a choice between passive accommodation and active anticipation."[1] Which will we choose for critical care nursing?

REFERENCES

1. Merton R. Issues in the growth of a profession. In: Proceedings of the forty-first convention of the ANA. New York 1958:296.

Continuing education requirements by state

JODY FOSS, RN, MS

ENSURING THE CONTINUED COMPETENCE of the registered nurse is a difficult and sometimes complicated process. Even though state boards of nursing interpret and use measures of competence in nursing practice differently, they share a common goal — making sure that licensed registered nurses are competent to practice nursing.

Professional nurse competency is monitored through peer review, client review, periodic refresher courses, competency examinations, minimal practice requirements, and continuing education (CE). AORN [Association of Operating Room Nurses] provides CE through its accreditation by the American Nurses' Association (ANA) as a provider/approver of continuing nursing education offerings. This accreditation is accepted in most states that require CE for relicensure. Four states (Florida, Iowa, California, and Kansas) require AORN be accredited at the state level to offer programs in that state as a provider/approver. AORN is accredited as a provider in Florida, Iowa, and California.

Relicensure requirements

The AORN credentialing division surveyed state registered nurse licensing agencies in November 1987, to update the state licensing rules. Twelve states reported that they require continuing education for relicensure. States that require CE as a demonstration of competency reported that a nurse must complete course hours ranging from 15 hours in a two-year renewal cycle to 45 hours in a three-year renewal cycle. States requiring continuing education are listed in Table 1. Mandatory CE has been dropped as a licensing requirement in Washington state.

Of the 39 states that do not require CE for relicensure, three require employment practice hours for relicensure. Mississippi requires 1,440 employment practice hours every five years; North Dakota requires 500 employment practice hours every five years; and Vermont requires 120 employment practice days every five years.

Alaska enacted legislation in 1988 that requires a nurse to complete two of the three following conditions for license renewal: (1) 15 hours of continuing education every two years, (2) 15 hours of professional activity every two years, or (3) 320 employment hours as a registered nurse every two years. Alaska defines professional activity as volunteer activities that affect the health of individuals or the community.

Five boards of nursing reported that legislation on mandatory CE for relicensure was being reviewed, proposed, or in process in 1988. Delaware is proposing that continuing education for relicensure begin in 1991. New Hampshire's proposed nurse practice act includes a continuing education requirement that would take effect in 1988. In Michigan, members of the Board of Nursing are currently writing rules that would require 18 hours of CE every two years. The Boards of Nursing in Mississippi and in the District of Columbia are reviewing rules on mandatory continuing education.

Most states using refresher courses as criteria for relicensure require a nurse to complete a refresher course if the nurse has not practiced nursing during the previous five years.

TABLE 1. **Requirements for relicensure**

STATE	CE HOURS	EMPLOYMENT PRACTICE	OTHER
Alaska	15 hr every 2 yr	320 hr every 2 yr	15 hr professional activity
California	30 hr every 2 yr	—	—
Colorado	20 hr every 2 yr	—	—
Florida	24 hr every 2 yr	—	—
Iowa	15 hr every year	—	—
Kentucky	30 hr every 2 yr	—	—
Massachusetts	15 hr every 2 yr	—	—
Minnesota	30 hr every 2 yr	—	skill demonstration
Nebraska	20 hr within preceding 5 yr	200 hr practice every 5 yr	—
Nevada	30 hr every 2 yr	—	—
New Mexico	30 hr every 2 yr	1,000 hr every 5 yr	—
Wyoming	20 hr every 2yr (or)	500 hr every 2 yr, (or) 1,600 hr in 5 yr	—

States that use minimum employment practice criteria require a nurse to work from 320 hours in a two-year period to 1,600 hours in a five-year period to maintain licensure.

Instructor requirements

Even though most states follow the criteria for CE activities established by ANA, two states have proposed language that further defines instructor qualifications. California is proposing that nurse instructors have a baccalaureate or higher degree *in nursing*. [A] nonregistered nurse instructor must be licensed or certified in his or her area of expertise, hold at least a baccalaureate degree in [the] area of content he or she is teaching, and show evidence that he or she collaborated with a registered nurse who has expertise in the subject. Kansas has recommended that 50% of the course content be taught by an RN qualified in the subject.

SECTION THREE

Entry into nursing practice

SECTION THREE ADDRESSES the seemingly diverse topics of preceptorships — direct supervision by an experienced nurse — for student nurses, generalist and specialist preparation for nursing practice, methods of learning about nursing management, and the recruitment of men in nursing. Yet these topics reflect a common theme: how nursing education and nursing practice work together to influence the culture of nursing.

As described in the unit introduction, a specialized culture is one of the defining characteristics of a profession. Nursing's culture includes the ethics and mores of organized nursing, the commitment to professionalism in practice, and nurses' expectations of their own and their peers' image and practice style. Upon entry into nursing's culture, the new nurse learns and internalizes the expectations and demands of the professional role.

This transition is not always as easy as it sounds. Typically, the demands of the nurse's occupational role conflict with the ideals learned as a student. To complete the transition into nursing practice, the new nurse not only must learn the expectations of the occupational role, but also resolve any conflict between the professional (ideal) and bureaucratic (occupational) models of nursing.

The first article, "The Senior Preceptorship as a Method for Anticipatory Socialization of Baccalaureate Nursing Students" by Dobbs, describes one way to ease the transition from nursing student to working nurse. It researches the effectiveness of a pregraduation preceptorship in promoting preservice indoctrination in the demands, expectations, and values of the working role. It also underscores the importance of close cooperation between nurse educators and nurse clinicians to smooth the transition. This article will help the student understand one proven way to bridge the gap from student to practitioner.

In "Specialization Meets Entry into Practice," Bajnok considers another way to bridge the gap. For years, baccalaureate nursing education has provided a broad overview of nursing, giving the student a core of *general* knowledge, skills, and attitudes that can be used in diverse practice settings. Over those years, however, nursing practice has come to rely increasingly on *specialized* clinical knowledge and skills. This recent divergence between the generalist approach in education and the specialization in practice has compounded the new nurse's problems. To help the student — and the profession — narrow the gap between education and practice, Bajnok explores the issues and suggests innovative ways to resolve them.

Not only may Bajnok's recommendations help the student make the transition from education to practice, but they also may make the new nurse more valuable to employers and help resolve the entry-into-practice debate. (See Section Two).

As part of the transition to practice, the student typically is allowed to practice direct patient care in a supervised clinical setting. Another approach is to expose the student to the nurse manager's role. This exposure helps the student appreciate the challenges facing the nurse manager and the forces that can affect client care.

The article "Learning About Nursing Management" by Davis describes one university's approach to understanding nursing management. It explains how one class planned their ideal hospital and used it to discuss seminar topics in nursing management. The fantasy-realism approach gave the class opportunities to apply theories and ideas to practice and helped them develop a realistic view of nursing management. The article underscores the dual aspects of the nurse manager's role: advocate for the professional caring practice of nursing and advocate for cost-efficient, time-saving practice in the employing institution.

The last article, "Should Men Be Actively Recruited into Nursing?" by London, takes a different view of the culture of nursing. After characterizing nursing as having a female nature, the author tries to predict the effects of male nurses on the profession by investigating the results of increased male recruitment in teaching (another predominantly female occupation) and of the large percentage of male nurses in Great Britain. The author presents some of the pros and cons of actively recruiting men into nursing, but this complex and emotionally charged issue remains open for debate.

The senior preceptorship as a method for anticipatory socialization of baccalaureate nursing students

KATHLEEN K. DOBBS, RNC, PhD

This article reflects nursing research into the effectiveness of pregraduation preceptorships — coaching by nurse practitioners — in anticipating the professional nurse's working role. It describes a study that was conducted before and after the students' final clinical course. Note: Summaries (shown in bracketed italics) condense extensive methodological descriptions.

FOR MANY NURSES, the most stressful time of their career was the period immediately after graduation. A difficult period of transition from student to practitioner is not unique to nursing. But it seems to be more of a problem for baccalaureate nurse graduates than for other nurse graduates (Schmalenberg & Kramer, 1979).

Pregraduation preceptorship is an increasingly popular approach for dealing with this problem. While nursing education, service, and students applaud the preceptorship experience as easing role transition, there is little research data to document this belief.

Literature review

The new graduate's inability to function immediately as a competent professional nurse seems to be the result of inadequate socialization to the professional role, rather than inadequate theoretical knowledge (Benner & Benner, 1979; Blanchard, 1983). Inadequate socialization refers to the limited understanding of the total demands and expectations of the working role. The graduate lacks experience in dealing with a) bureaucratic needs of the organization; b) the unwritten rules of the work group; and c) various professional and organization personnel (Schmalenberg & Kramer, 1979). As a result, the new nurse is unable to make satisfactory compromises between what is perceived to be conflicting role demands in the work environment, those of accomplishing bureaucratic goals and maintaining practice standards.

The graduate experiences frustration when unable to fulfill both personal and organizational practice expectations. The internal response felt by the nurse when there are situational limitations to role enactment is called role deprivation (Kramer, 1966). If the resulting stress remains elevated, the individual eventually experiences "reality shock" (Kramer, 1974).

When new graduates are not assisted with socialization to the working role, they frequently resolve the perceived role deprivation in a negative rather than a positive manner. This outcome usually results in one of two adaptive modes: a) values prizing patient care and high professional standards are diminished or discarded; or b) values prizing accomplishment of bureaucratic goals are discarded and active practice is abandoned (Kramer, 1974).

Resolution of perceived role deprivation in a positive or productive manner stems from the deliberative intermeshing of the three role values: a) *service* — the degree of commitment to the patient, humanity, and altruism; b) *bureaucratic* — the degree of loyalty to the hospital administration and nursing care delivery within the organization; and c) *professional* — the degree of dedication to knowledge, continued learning, and the nursing profession (Kramer, 1974). Studies have shown that the most productive nurses for both the health-care organizations and the nursing profession are those nurses who prize all three types of role values (Hollefreund, Mooney, Moore, & Jersan, 1981; Holloran, Mishkin, & Hanson, 1980; Schmalenberg & Kramer, 1979). By deliberately intermeshing the values, these nurses can accomplish bureaucratic goals while maintaining professional standards and quality patient care.

Several practice disciplines, namely medicine, pharmacy, and the ministry, have used a period of guided-practice to help ease the new practitioner into an active professional role (Backenstose, 1983). The goal of this strategy is anticipatory socialization.

Anticipatory socialization has been defined as the preservice role-learning involving the process of being indoctrinated in what is important to the job (Simpson, Back, Ingles, Kerckhoff, & McKinney, 1979). The individual is aided in achieving membership in the work group by understanding and being able to function with the beliefs and values held by that group (Bond & Bond, 1980).

Anticipatory socialization to the professional nurse role is the goal of a senior preceptorship experience. This experience allows the student to practice in the role of a graduate nurse under the direct supervision of an experienced professional nurse and the "mentor" type guidance of a faculty advisor. As the student becomes competent in the work culture, values learned during school are reinforced (Chickerella & Lutz, 1981).

Experiential learning such as the preceptorship experience involves the whole person of the learner. The role of faculty is to assist the learner with the reorganization and transferral of what has been learned to new and changing circumstances (Warner, 1976). As knowledge is integrated with personal experience, the student reinterprets existing facts and beliefs to create a more useful and applicable framework from which to act.

The student develops values by actively formulating beliefs through interaction with the environment (Czmowski, 1974). The faculty advisor maintains the value-development process and acts as a "sounding board" for the student. This added dimension makes experience-based learning a significant learning process beyond the experience of work (Warner, 1976), and different from nursing's apprenticeship approach to education.

During the preceptorship, a student is assigned to a specific role within an organization. Dewey stressed that the role an individual is assigned in an environment [and that] what one is permitted to do is what one learns (Warner, 1976). The student's role is guided by the preceptor, who is a member of that organization. The preceptor serves as a role model, resource person, consultant, and supervisor for the student (Suess, Schweitzer, & Williams, 1982).

The student indirectly experiences the preceptor's role through observations and constant verbal and nonverbal clues (Douville, 1983). Role functions specific to the skills being learned are incorporated into the learner's self-image. As the student practices the professional nursing role and demonstrates desired role values, the student is rewarded for this behavior.

As a result, the student internalizes role values compatible with the role of a practicing professional nurse. Specifically, the student learns to adapt conflicting role values to maintain quality care and professional standards while meeting the bureaucratic needs of the workplace.

Role expectations alter as role values change. As the student adapts his or her role expectations, the change in self-image from that of a student to that of a practicing professional occurs. According to Douville (1983), integrating one's self-image and one's role expectations is essential in initiating goal-directed professional development.

Internalization of values also occurs through identification with a role model. The modification of role expectations and self-image is reflected by a concurrent change in the type of role model esteemed by the student (Olsen & Whitaker, 1968). The new role model exhibits behavior and attitudes closely resembling those now valued by the student.

In summary, a student who graduates having learned to cope with differing role values should experience less role deprivation during the first job. Attitudes [that] prize the ability to accept and adapt conflicting role values within the same environment can be learned through anticipatory socialization in a form of experience-based learning.

Preceptorship experiences provide the opportunity to practice in the work role of a professional nurse, but do the experiences actually promote anticipatory socialization to the role? For this study, the occurrence of anticipatory socialization was evidenced by changes in self-image and in role expectations. These changes were indicated by a decrease in perceived role deprivation and a change to a work-centered role model.

[The study

Before their preceptorships began, 103 baccalaureate nursing students took a test (Corwin's Nursing Role Conception Scale, 1961) that measured three components of their role values: service, bureaucratic, and professional. In the test, the students were asked to rank hypothetical situations by how close each is to the ideal and by the extent to which each exists in nursing practice. Differences between the "ideal" and "actual" ratings provided role deprivation scores.

Then each student began a preceptorship, working in a clinical area for eight weeks for at least 28 hours per week. Each selected the clinical area from various types of health care facilities and developed behavioral objectives with the assigned preceptor and faculty advisor. The preceptor was a registered nurse with a baccalaureate degree in nursing, appropriate skills and attitudes, and at least one year of work experience.

After the preceptorship, the students were retested and their pre-test and post-test scores were compared. Test results revealed a decrease in perceived role deprivation, indicating that the students had learned to cope with different role values in the work setting. The results also identified an increase in a work-centered role model, suggesting changes in the students' self-image and role expectations.]

Discussion

The senior preceptorship experience is effective in promoting anticipatory socialization as evidenced by changes in role expectations and in self-image. Students experienced a significant decrease in perceived role deprivation and a significant increase in the number of work-centered role models.

The preceptorship experience exposed students to positive conflict resolution behavior. The majority of students incorporated this perspective into their role expectations, as reflected by the decrease in perceived role deprivation. As these students became more competent in the work subculture, they retained their values from the school subculture, as evidenced by the relative stability of role conception scores.

When student role deprivation scores were compared by role model changes, the impact of anticipatory socialization became apparent. Students who experienced the greatest decrease in perceived role deprivation were those who changed their role models to work-centered nurses.

It can be reasonably expected that these graduates, who have learned to make satisfactory compromises between differing role values, should experience less role deprivation during their first job. It cannot be concluded that these students will not experience reality shock, for they have only partially experienced their role models' jobs. All of the ramifications of the working role will not be felt until these new graduates have become full-time employees.

Summary

This study supported the effectiveness of the preceptorship as a method for promoting anticipatory socialization to the working role of a professional nurse. It is a strategy to increase the beginning competency of baccalaureate graduates functioning in health-care organizations. By facilitating adjustments prior to graduation, education and service's joint efforts increase the likelihood of graduates finding their new jobs rewarding and vehicles that can be used for continual learning (Douville, 1983).

REFERENCES

Backenstose, A.G. (1983). The use of clinical preceptors. In S. Stuart-Siddall & J. Haberline (Eds.), *Preceptorships in nursing education* (pp. 9-27). Rockville, MD: Aspen Systems.

Benner, P., & Benner, R.V. (1979). *The new nurse's work entry: A troubled sponsorship.* New York: Tiresias Press.

Blanchard, S.L. (1983). The discontinuity between school and practice. *Nursing Management, 14*(4), 41-43.

Bond, J., & Bond, S. (1980). In touch with reality. *Nursing Mirror, 150*(9), 27-30.

Chickerella, B.G., & Lutz, W.J. (1981). Professional nurturance: Preceptorships for undergraduate nursing students. *American Journal of Nursing, 81*, 107-109.

Corwin, R.G. (1961). The professional employee: A study in conflict in nursing roles. *American Journal of Sociology, 64*, 606-608.

Czmowski, M. (1974). Value teaching in nursing education. *Nursing Forum, 13*(2), 192-206.

Douville, L.D. (1983). Positive aspects of working with a preceptor. In S. Stuart-Siddall & J. Haberline (Eds.), *Preceptorships in nursing education* (pp. 121-126). Rockville, MD: Aspen Systems.

Hollefreund, B., Mooney, V.M., Moore, S., & Jersan, J. (1981). Implementing a reality shock program. *Journal of Nursing Administration, 11*(1), 16-20.

Holloran, S.D., Mashkin, B.H., & Hanson, B.L. (1980). Bicultural training for new graduates. *Nurse Educator, 5*, 17-24.

Kramer, M. (1966). Some effects of exposure to employing bureaucracies on the role conceptions and role deprivation of neophyte collegiate nurses. *Dissertation Abstracts, 27*, 2425B-2426B, (University Microfilms No. 66-14, 683).

Kramer, M. (1974). *Reality shock: Why nurses leave nursing.* St. Louis: C.V. Mosby.

Olsen, V., & Whitaker, E. (1968). *The silent dialogue: A study in the social psychology of professional socialization.* San Francisco: Jossey-Bass.

Schmalenberg, C., & Kramer, M. (1979). *Coping with reality shock: The voices of experience.* Wakefield, MA: Nursing Resources.

Simpson, I.H., Back, K.W., Ingles, T., Kerckhoff, J., & McKinney, J.C. (1979). *From student to nurse: A longitudinal study of socialization.* New York: Cambridge University Press.

Suess, L.R., Schweitzer, B.J., & Williams, C.A. (1982). Nursing students experiment with reality. *Nurse Educator, 7*, 28-33.

Warner, A.R. (1976). *Clinical experiences and clinical practice in professional education.* Houston, TX: University of Houston, Teacher Center.

Specialization meets entry to practice

IRMAJEAN BAJNOK, RN, BScN, MScN

THE CHOICE OF a baccalaureate in nursing or a specialty certificate presents a challenge to nurse educators in undergraduate programs and to diploma-prepared nurses seeking further education. Yet, the question should not be "baccalaureate or specialty?" Why not baccalaureate *and* specialty?

By simply replacing that "or" with "and," we discovered the true challenges. How can an experienced, diploma-prepared nurse obtain a degree and feel ready to practice in a specialty area? How can undergraduate degree programs incorporate situation-specific content and practice? How can specialty certificate programs be related to baccalaureate education? How can we facilitate the achievement of two goals: baccalaureate as entry to practice, and graduates prepared to work in settings where unique knowledge and skills are needed? Employers, educators, and nurses see the specialty issue as one of the most critical in nursing today.

Traditionally, nursing practice and education have been at opposite poles in relation to the generalist-specialist issue. Employers hire nurses to work in particular settings; job descriptions rarely say "generalist practitioners needed."[1] Employers want some evidence of the graduate's commitment to and confidence in one area of practice.[2]

Nurse educators, on the other hand, want the graduate to have a broad education, including elements of liberal studies as well as core nursing knowledge. They want to provide the graduate with the flexibility to work in a variety of settings.

Because educators' aims differ so much from employers' goals, the generalist-specialist dichotomy was born. Employers are not alone in thinking the educational programs do not prepare practitioners for the specific practice setting. Many nursing graduates feel the same way. Hence, many nurses, whether educated at the degree or diploma level, study specialty courses.

With the move toward the baccalaureate as the minimum level for entry to the practice of nursing, many initially thought the problem of specialization was being solved. But current programs contain no link between a baccalaureate and specialization. As employers and nurses recognize this lack, support wanes for the entry to practice position and nurse educators are charged with ignoring the problems of the work setting. There is much that can be done to relieve problems of the work setting and advance the realization of a baccalaureate for all, if we recognize that baccalaureate education and specialization are not mutually exclusive. They can be linked, and it is time nurse educators began forging that link.

Generalists and specialists

Generalists are nurses with a common core of knowledge, skills, and attitudes relevant to working with clients in any setting.[3] Specialists have narrowed their focus to a particular area of practice; a broad range of theories are applied to selected phenomena within nursing practice. A nursing specialty is a defined area of clinical and functional nursing with a narrowed, in-depth focus, ensuring the safe delivery of the full range of services within that area of nursing.[4]

Specialization can take place at different levels and in different degrees.[5] At least one author believes that as more and more nurses specialize, the generalist — with an overall comprehension of nursing practice — will surpass the specialist, whose focus is narrow.[6] But just how broad and thorough is the generalist's knowledge? Another author defines specialization as the opportunity to acquire beginning skill in a unique setting.[7] Obviously, "generalist" and "specialist" are not simple concepts, easily defined.

Generalist and specialist knowledge is needed at all levels of nursing education — baccalaureate, post-baccalaureate, and graduate. Only the proportion of general to special education should vary with each level.

Baccalaureate education should consist of core knowledge basic to the understanding and practice of nursing. It should also provide the opportunity to increase skills and expertise in a specialty area.

Post-baccalaureate specialty education should include in-depth knowledge in one area plus general core knowledge. The general education should focus on contextual variables related to how and when to use the advanced knowledge.

Graduate education should provide both specialty and generalist knowledge. The specialty area should be the focus, with such generalist skills as consultation, research, leadership, and negotiation included to assist the graduate in the role of specialist consultant. Some graduate programs could even focus on generalist practice as the specialty area.

The ideal near future of nursing contains four elements:

- All baccalaureate programs offer students the opportunity to focus on one clinical major, allowing additional theory and practice.
- All specialty certificate courses are offered at the post-degree level. In other words, baccalaureate would be the minimum requirement for specialty practice in nursing. (The American Nurses' Association Certification Registrar now requires a baccalaureate in nursing for a number of specialty certificates.)
- A closer link exists among baccalaureate, post-baccalaureate, and master's programs in relation to specialty content. There is progression and credit from one level to the next.
- The baccalaureate nurse, that is, one in first level practice, is a generalist in a specialty area. The post-baccalaureate-educated nurse, in specialty practice, is a specialist in a specialty area. Nurses with graduate degrees, in advanced specialty practice, are generalists and specialists in specialty and general areas.

Baccalaureate programs that provide opportunities for in-depth focus in a specialty area will better prepare nurses to be generalists. These nurses will feel comfortable and confident carrying out their generalist skills in specialty areas.

Post-baccalaureate specialty certificates would allow educators to meet the immediate need for specialized practitioners. These certificates would enable nurses to practice as specialists in specialty areas.

Graduate education could prepare nurses with both specialist and generalist knowledge. Depending on the focus of their programs, graduates would be prepared to work as advanced specialists in specialty or generalist areas, or to work as generalists in both specialty and generalist areas.

Responding to the challenge

Nurses currently seeking to upgrade their education must consider not only the choice between different types of education, but also the previous time spent studying, finances, values, and family and work constraints. Educators seeking changes to deal with the issue of specialization in nursing must therefore consider six criteria.

First, educators must be able to help nurses with career choices in realistic ways, ways that acknowledge their lifestyles and aspirations. Second, repetition and duplication in nursing education must be avoided. It costs the student time, money, and energy; it costs the system money; it costs the profession time lost when practitioners could be contributing to the field and developing new skills instead of repeating old lessons. Third, baccalaureate education and specialization must not be considered mutually exclusive. Fourth, educators must promote...the baccalaureate level entry to practice goal. Fifth, practice needs of specialty nurses must be met. Finally, short-term actions must not jeopardize long-term goals.

The preferred course of action also includes six points. Educators and counselors must be aware of the long-term effects of career counseling. Registered and aspiring nurses need to know the implications of their decisions on career planning and nursing education.

Post-baccalaureate specialty education must be achieved. In the short term, specialty certificate programs should include degree credit courses. Similarly, degree programs must contain some courses that can be credited toward a specialty certificate. Nurse educators from colleges and universities need to begin work in this area immediately....

University education must acknowledge the need for specialty education, incorporating such courses and programs into the credit stream. Ideally, baccalaureate courses would link to post-baccalaureate certificates, which, in turn, would provide some credit toward master's studies.

Universities and health care agencies must work together to link the needs of particular settings with course offerings that have credit toward degree education. Examples of this collaboration already exist in the critical care field: the University of Alberta works with Misericordia Hospital, and Ryerson works with Toronto General Hospital.

Specialty practice must move away from medical model designations to a classification system that accurately describes the fields of nursing. Educators must exercise caution: when this reclassification was attempted in baccalaureate programs, medical model terminology was often replaced with meaningless titles.

Because separate post-RN degree programs still exist, university educators must consider how these programs can help nurses to gain specialty nursing education. A number of options could be explored: freedom in choice and focus of clinical practice, so [that] a student can operate as a generalist in a specialty area; courses in the program's final year that could lead on to another year of study giving the student a post-baccalaureate certificate; or specific clinical electives including both theory and practice, enabling the student to focus on a particular area. Though the baccalaureate practitioner should be prepared at the generalist level [and be] able to function in beginning practice positions, a number of post-RN students already have many years of practice. They have often advanced to different levels and areas of focus in nursing. A baccalaureate for such nurses must help them build on their practice and facilitate their career development.

The generalist-specialist dichotomy is false. The baccalaureate level entry to practice can be achieved with careful decisions today. The time is ripe for educators to seek creative approaches to the long overdue changes in nursing education and practice.

REFERENCES

1. Mantle, J. Generalist-specialist: A false dichotomy. In *Baccalaureate nursing education for the 80s*. Proceedings of the 1983 Western Region, CAUSN, 1983, University of Alberta, Edmonton, Alberta.

2. Pick, J. Specialization in nursing: Will we find a way to meet the need? *The Canadian Nurse,* 80 (5), 1984, 22-23.

3. Mantle, *Op. cit.*

4. Canadian Nurses' Association. *Credentialing in nursing,* 1982, Ottawa.

5. Gray, A. Specialization at the baccalaureate level: Occupational health nursing. In *Patterns of specialization: Challenge to the curriculum,* National League for Nursing, 1985, New York.

6. Pick, *Op. cit.*

7. Gray, *Op. cit.*

Learning about nursing management

GAIL C. DAVIS, RN, EdD

NURSING MANAGEMENT PROVIDES myriad challenges to those involved in it, for guidelines affecting the nurse manager's decisions are changing almost daily. The realities of the present day include such factors as increasing supply costs, tightening budgets, staffing for a fluctuating patient census, and the morale of nursing staff. Given their lack of experience, how can senior baccalaureate nursing students be expected to grasp these realities? Although students are exposed to current issues and trends affecting nursing practice and health care throughout their baccalaureate education, their focus is primarily on the actual nursing care of a small number of patients. As new graduates, however, they need to be able to shift their focus to management practices that encourage the best possible care of a group of patients and, at the same time, to derive satisfaction from providing that care. An understanding of the pressures and challenges faced by nurse managers is also important to the process of adapting to the work setting. Such understanding can only lead to better appreciation of the forces that affect practice.

A group of 12 senior students at Texas Christian University found an innovative approach for their own learning. These students were concurrently registered in a 3-semester-hour class and a 5-semester-hour practicum in nursing management. The 6-week practicum included a seminar that met 4 hours a week to help them integrate theory and practice. The specific seminar topics were to be selected by the students. In the process of selection, one student suggested that the students plan an ideal hospital as they discussed their topics, and the others supported the idea. As topic selection continued, it was influenced by the suggested approach. For example, the students decided that the first two sessions would be devoted to community assessment and planning the physical facility, topics that would have received hardly any attention otherwise. The approach of mixing fantasy and realism was evolving.

The students selected a county about 75 miles from a major metropolitan area for their hospital. They looked at such population statistics as urban versus rural, median age, number of residents under 17 years of age, number of births per year, percentage of residents with health insurance, and income levels. In addition, they researched the number of licensed physicians and registered nurses currently residing in the area. Based on these data, they decided to continue planning. The hospital would be divided into specific numbers of medical-surgical, pediatric, intensive care, obstetric (labor, delivery, and recovery), and surgical recovery beds. In addition, there would be an emergency room (with four treatment rooms), a home health service (with office space in the hospital), a holding area for day-surgery patients, and a fitness center for use by patients, staff, and community.

The stage, then, was set and actually became the basis for the continuing seminar discussions. How exciting could it be to discuss the planning of a physical facility? The group's animation in planning the physical layout of the building answered that question. Discussion revolved around some of the following concerns: What services should be in close proximity? What should be the ratio of semiprivate to private rooms? Where should visitors' areas be put? What types of storage would be needed? There was not enough time to achieve a final scale drawing of the facility, but the "rough picture" in everyone's mind did assist in later discussions.

Subsequent discussions covered the topics of nurse recruitment, staff development, career ladders, budget, staffing, home health services, committees, care planning and documentation, and characteristics of a professional environment. One advantage of the "fantasy-realism" approach that immediately became evident was that the students were considering facets of each topic that most likely would not have surfaced had we not been attempting to make an actual application. In addition, none of the topics could be discussed in isolation from the others. The focus on application aided in the realization that each of these areas affected all others. Each seminar involved some reference to a prior discussion; previous decisions were sometimes altered or changed.

The two dominant goals that emerged from the discussions were: management that supports good patient care, and management that provides a professional and satisfying work environment for nurses. These themes provided an informal framework for content, integrating a professional work environment with quality nursing care.

Support of good nursing care

The students made a number of management decisions that supported good nursing care. These began with the mutual acceptance of a philosophy of nursing based on several available models, as well as on ANA's *Nursing: A Social Policy Statement*.[1] Much of the discussion revolved around the definition of nursing taken from the ANA document. The group agreed that nursing is the diagnosis and treatment of human responses to health problems (actual and potential). In accepting this definition, the students also made a commitment to use the list of accepted nursing diagnoses compiled by the North American Nursing Diagnosis Association (NANDA).[2]

The group was well aware that budget and staffing decisions affected the quality of nursing care. They adopted a decentralized nursing service organization in which there was an assistant hospital administrator for nursing, two directors of nursing (inpatient services and home health services), and four head nurses who were responsible for hiring, staff evaluation, budget, staffing, etc., in their respective areas. They chose an organizational approach that blended primary nursing and total patient care for the ideal hospital, with a desired nurse-patient ratio of 1:6 on the medical-surgical and pediatric units. However, the group did not view some aspects of primary nursing, such as 24-hour accountability, as attractive. Only RNs would be used in special care areas; initially, at least 80 percent of the staff in all other areas would be RNs, with an eventual goal of 100 percent. Although an 8-hour work day (40-hour work week) would be used primarily, some flexibility would be offered to those who preferred working 10-hour overlapping shifts — e.g., 7-5, 1-11, 9-7.

A discussion of the budget was actually based on figures provided to the students by a local hospital that was planning to build a 100-bed facility. This helped students to consider the expense of such items as employee salaries and benefits, equipment, supplies, staff education, and public relations. These considerations were real eye openers. Some of the decisions based on this discussion were to: contract for child-care services with an established agency; contract with a larger hospital 35 miles away for use of the CAT scan; and sell bonds as the major method of funding, to be subsidized by other sources. Although such budget decisions do not belong entirely to

Desirable characteristics of the ideal hospital

1. Benefits: insurance, paid vacation, anniversary raise (starts at 6 months), paid moving expenses
2. Availability of a child care center
3. Salary differential: educational preparation, shift
4. Clinical ladder
5. Decentralized organization with staff active in decision making
6. Supportive administration
7. Professional accountability and autonomy
8. Good communication:
   a. Expectations communicated
   b. Staff meetings for information sharing with director attending frequently
   c. Directors [who] work on clinical unit at least once per month
   d. Directors [who] hold meetings with *all three* shifts
9. Rewards and recognition offered in variety of ways
10. Orientation: comprehensive initial orientation with shorter annual update
11. Continuing education: four required in-service education programs to be offered by the hospital annually with additional paid educational days for study in particular area of interest
12. Good supplies and equipment, along with good maintenance services
13. Committees, with nurse participation
14. Good quality assurance program
15. Nursing philosophy based on caring
16. Low nurse-patient ratio
17. Nursing image that reflects respect and caring attitude
18. Flexible staffing and scheduling
19. Organization of care: total patient care (incorporating some aspects of primary nursing)
20. Predominantly RN staff

nursing, discussing such factors brought out essential aspects of the total management process in which nursing should be involved.

The group discussed both nursing and hospitalwide committees in relation to their effects on the quality of patient care. Of the 12 committees to be established, all except one (physician credentialing) included nurses. The students decided that there would be one hospitalwide quality assurance committee encompassing consideration of all services to patients. Task forces could be appointed from this group as needed. They paid much attention to establishment of nurse-physician committees for each major area of the hospital. Each of these informal committees would include several nurses and physicians selected to serve for a given period of time. Meetings would be structured in a somewhat informal environment with group leadership rotating between a nurse and a physician member. The major purpose would be to maintain open, honest communication.

The group decided to discuss the home health service to be provided by the hospital because the students had had little previous exposure to that concept. Because there are no other home health services easily accessible to persons in the same county as the ideal hospital, those services would probably expand quickly. The hospital would attempt to locate some nurses who would be willing to work part-time and/or might consider rotating between inpatient services and home health. The scope of services to be offered throughout the county included patient and family teaching; home health aides to assist with daily care; RNs to plan and evaluate care and give care as appropriate to patient needs; and coordination of patient care with other community agencies.

The group agreed to discuss documentation and care planning after some gentle prodding. Their reluctance perhaps reflected the care plan burn-out syndrome that can result from using the written care plan as a teaching methodology. Given the opportunity of planning the ideal procedure, they were at least willing to discuss it. The group confirmed its commitment to using NANDA's accepted list of nursing diagnoses and decided that the use of nursing diagnoses would be a part of the orientation program for all new nurses, and that all RN job descriptions would include the function of care planning using nursing diagnoses.

The actual patient care plan would be partially standardized, allowing for individualization. This semistandardized care plan would be stored on computer files for easy access. The care plan would become part of the patient's permanent record. While discharge planning should be reflected in the long-range goals on the care plan, there would be a separate discharge plan form, which would be completed just before the patient's dismissal from the hospital, outlining all instructions. Copies would go to the patient, the hospital (patient's chart), and the home health service, if appropriate. The group agreed that good communication between the physician and the nurse regarding the patient's post-hospital care was essential.

Documentation would combine the use of narrative notes with flow charting. The information on the flow chart would be limited to that identified as routine for patients in that particular area; thus it would vary between the medical-surgical units and the intensive care unit. Computerizing the documentation and care planning in a combined form as soon as possible would be a high priority. This would be done immediately if acceptable software could be identified.

Support of a professional work environment

The topics of staff development, recruitment, and characteristics of a professional environment all helped the students articulate some of their own expectations as professionals. Early in their discussions, they identified the following factors as important to recruiting nurses: inservice education; part-time and flexible scheduling; good benefits (health and life insurance, retirement plan); other fringe benefits (gym or fitness center, an arrangement with a licensed child-care facility at reduced prices); and organization of patient care, using a modified primary-total patient care approach.

Some of the same factors were discussed at a later meeting on characteristics of a professional environment. The 20 characteristics that the students identified as making the ideal hospital a good place to work are very similar to those identified by nurses in the *Magnet Hospitals* study.[3]

The group was concerned that the ideal hospital have a positive image in the community from the outset, so they developed some public relations approaches to create and foster the desired image. They felt that it was important that any activity involving nurses should demonstrate a professional nursing image. Their ideas included screening programs provided as a community service by nursing staff members, a county health fair planned and coordinated by nurses, and health teaching programs prepared for local cable television and for inhouse use by patients.

Summary

Summaries of the discussions were compiled in a booklet. The group then expressed an interest in getting some feedback on their decisions from nurse managers, so a meeting was arranged in the hospital where they were completing their nursing management practicum. The prepared booklet was distributed to each nurse manager attending the meeting: several head nurses, the director of medical-surgical nursing, and the assistant vice president for nursing. The resulting discussion provided a good summary and an opportunity for testing ideas. The interest and feedback of these nurses were very encouraging to the students.

Overall, the mix of fantasy and realism provided a successful way of helping students gain a realistic view of nursing management. An understanding of and identification with the issues faced by today's nurse manager should help new graduates to appreciate and adapt to the realities of the clinical setting, regardless of their position.

REFERENCES

1. American Nurses' Association. *Nursing: A Social Policy Statement.* (Publ. No. NP-63) Kansas City, MO, The Association, 1980.

2. North American Nursing Diagnosis Association. *Classification of Nursing Diagnosis: Proceedings of the Seventh Conference*, ed. by A.M. McLane St. Louis, C.V. Mosby Co., 1987.

3. American Academy of Nursing, Task Force on Nursing Practice in Hospitals. *Magnet Hospitals: Attraction and Retention of Professional Nurses.* (Publ. No. G-160) Kansas City, MO, The Association, 1983.

Should men be actively recruited into nursing?

FRAN LONDON, BA, BSN

MANY OF NURSING'S PROBLEMS have been attributed to the predominantly female composition of the profession. Sexism and oppressed group behavior have been blamed for nursing's low pay, low status, lack of leadership, and lack of unity. It has been suggested that these problems could be eliminated by actively recruiting men into nursing, thereby removing the causative factor.

This article explores the assumption that more males in nursing would solve the profession's problems. Two related situations are examined: the impact of an increase in males in another traditionally female occupation, teaching, and the status of nursing in Great Britain, where there is a larger percentage of men. Data from these situations indicate that the active recruitment of males into nursing at this time is not as advantageous for the profession as is generally thought.

Female character of nursing

In the United States today, 97 percent of all registered nurses are female.[1] Roberts argues that nursing's style of leadership has evolved because nurses are primarily female and they are an oppressed group, controlled by societal forces.[2] She cites many parallels between the behavior of nurses and oppressed groups. Nurses tend to exhibit self-hatred, lack self-esteem, and internalize the values of dominant groups such as physicians. Their lack of participation in professional organizations can be viewed as evidence of a lack of pride in nursing and a desire not to be associated with it. Nurses have difficulty unifying because their aggression toward their oppressors is channeled into a safer release of tension, infighting. Roberts also states that fear of success prevents positive change, and nurses consider positive change to be impossible. Nursing leaders are generally ineffective because they have often been promoted for their allegiance to maintenance of the status quo.

Roberts believes most of nursing's problems are related to its dominant female character, and she is not alone. Many authors carry this a step further and promote the advantages of encouraging males to enter nursing. All but two of the articles reviewed on this subject support the recruitment of men.

Men are more willing to work longer hours than women, and are more career oriented.[3] They would offer greater stability to nursing because they are more apt to make an active lifetime professional commitment.[4] Women, on the other hand, tend to place their concerns for their families ahead of their jobs. They leave work to have children, and if they return, they return with decreased flexibility in scheduling. While female nurses are often tied geographically to their husbands' careers, male nurses have the same career mobility as men in general.[5]

Effect of male nurses on the profession

The mere presence of men in nursing is said to increase its recognition as a profession. Male nurses could positively affect physicians' attitudes toward nurses, because they would not be intimidated by physicians as easily as females might be.[6] Men would bring increased status, pay, and benefits to the profession, because they are better able to bargain competitively and appear more power oriented in their coalition strategies than women.[7] In addition, men in nursing are less likely to accept poor salaries and working conditions.[8] Consequently, male nurses can be used as measuring sticks by which equal pay for equal work claims can be made.[9] Men would also bring to the profession administrative abilities, supervisory skills, leadership qualities, drive, initiative, ambition, and independence of thought.

A 1968 editorial in *Hospitals,* the official journal of the American Hospital Association, stated that men are generally preferred, even by women, for supervisory and administrative positions.[10] Hardy stated that it is a commonly held belief that even capable women do not make good supervisors because workers would be uncomfortable with a female boss.[11]

Image of nursing

Minnigerode, Kayer-Jones, and Garcia reported that an expressed interest in nursing is a feminine indicator on the Masculinity-Femininity scale of the Minnesota Multiphasic Personality Inventory (MMPI), one of the most frequently used psychological tests. Their empirical research has shown that, despite this image, the skills actually needed in nursing require both masculine and feminine characteristics. Depending on the situation, nurses may need to be assertive or yielding, instrumental or expressive. Therefore, nursing should satisfy this need for balance by finding ways to attract more men to the profession.[12]

Fottler believes that the overwhelmingly feminine image of nursing is the only factor that discourages sexual integration.[13] Silver and McAtee suggested that nursing change its name to "health care practice."[14] This would eliminate the female identification of the profession and remove the major barrier that keeps men out.

Treatment of male nurses

Although male nurses are in a definite minority, they are not treated with the social isolation, performance pressure, and role entrapment typically associated with powerless tokens. A study by Snavely and Fairhurst found that in nursing, token dynamics do not apply when the tokens are members of the socially dominant white male group. They determined that male nursing students have high status and operate from a power base that resists majority group assertions of control.[15]

Actually, sexism within nursing tends to favor the male nurse. A survey of male nursing students has shown that they perceive that they get more respect from instructors and are treated better than women students.[16] Only 27 percent of male nurses feel they have ever experienced discrimination by female nurses.[17] Etzkowitz stated that even if male nurses are discriminated against in isolated instances by individual female nurses, they tend to get preferential treatment from hospital administrators.[18]

The American Nurses' Association (ANA) and the National League for Nursing (NLN) have both spoken in support of male nurses. In 1966 the ANA pressured the military to award their mandatory commissions to male nurses in the service.[19] In 1967, an editorial in *Nursing Outlook,* the official journal of the NLN, praised the stability and reliability of males in nursing. The piece urged that any residual discrimination against men be eradicated, for the good of the profession.[20] Clearly, there is overwhelming support for an increase in the percentage of men in nursing. But what would such a change actually accomplish?

Effect of male teachers on teaching

It is possible to predict what might be expected in nursing by looking at teaching, an occupation that has evolved from an all-female profession to a sexually integrated one. Less than two centuries ago, teaching was male dominated, because females were thought to be noneducable and all teachers and students were male. As females infiltrated the student ranks, the status of teaching declined and males left the profession.[21] Since the Civil War, women have predominated as school teachers.[22]

At the end of World War II, the Government Issue (GI) Bill made it possible for more young men to attend college. Many majored in education, taught in public schools, and were quickly promoted into administrative positions where salaries were higher.[23] In the mid-1970s teaching had another influx of males who wanted to avoid the draft and the Vietnamese struggle.[24] As the percentage of men in education increased, the percentage of women in administration decreased.

Administration. In the 1955-56 school year, more than 88 percent of elementary school teachers were female. Yet females held only 38 percent to 62 percent of the principalships, depending on the size of the district. In that same period, 50 percent of the secondary school teachers were female, yet only 9 percent of the junior high school principals and 5 percent of the high school principals were women.[25] Seventeen years later, in 1973, elementary school principals were only 23 percent female, and secondary school principals only 3 percent. Less than 1 percent of all school supervisors were female.[26] Eight years after that, in 1981, although 80 percent of all elementary school teachers were female, women held less than 20 percent of the principalships.[27]

Salaries. In the 1970-71 school year, the average salary of male teachers was $2,000 higher than female teachers. In addition, males advanced faster and further.[28] By the 1979-80 school year, salary discrepancies between men and women in the same roles in education were negligible. However, females in administration disproportionately occupied the lower-paying administrative positions and consequently made an average of $5,000 less annually than male administrators.[29]

Recognition and control. The disadvantage of being a woman in education was expressed in other ways, too. As late as 1973, no females were admitted into Phi Delta Kappa, the professional honor society for education.[30] As of 1976, no woman had served on the Executive Committee of the American Association of School Administration in 25 years.[31]

It appears that, although females remain the major constituency within elementary and secondary education, males dominate the administration and control of the profession. Despite the rise of the women's liberation movement, the proportions continue to become more and more skewed in favor of males.

The education literature includes a great many articles that attempt to trace the source of this situation to determine ways to change it. They almost always come to the same conclusion: Research shows no valid reason for the decrease in the number of women in administrative and supervisory positions other than the sexist attitudes of hiring committees.[32] Men are simply preferred for leadership positions in this society.

This is particularly significant in light of evidence from Taylor,[33] who cites a number of studies that indicate that women make good educational administrators and in many cases are better than men. Women outscore men on ability to work with objectives, and they possess a greater knowledge of teaching methods and techniques. In addition, women tend to use a democratic style of leadership while men prefer an autocratic style. Douglass states that a democratic leadership style yields high productivity and is the most desirable form of management in a wide variety of work situations.[34]

Implications for nursing. Did the increase of men in teaching improve the lot of all teachers, or did it only succeed in limiting potential professional growth for the female majority? The answer to this question has important implications for nursing.

One argument for actively recruiting men into nursing is that their ability to organize and bargain collectively would improve the lot of all nurses. The correlation between the presence of men in education and the rise of teachers' labor unions is viewed as proof of this assertion. However, a study of the differences in attitudinal militancy between teachers and nurses has disputed this assumption. Attitudinal militancy was operationally defined as being approving of unions, collective bargaining, and strikes by professionals. The researchers found that sex was not a significant attitudinal correlate. Male teachers were no more likely to be militant than female teachers, but both were significantly more militant than nurses of either sex. The study concluded that teachers are more likely to join forces than nurses due to self-selected personality factors, characteristics of the work, or characteristics of the occupational group.[35]

Sexual integration of nursing: Implications for the profession

Perhaps teaching and nursing cannot be compared fairly. The condition of nursing in Great Britain, where sexual integration is a step ahead of the United States, may be a more appropriate comparison. In the early 1970s, 17 percent of the nurses in Great Britain were male. At that time, men held one-third of all the top nursing posts in British hospitals. By 1984, men held one-half of all top hospital posts.[36]

British nursing literature shows much the same response to this skew as the education literature expressed. How did this happen? What are the implications? How can nurses get more women into management?

One extreme series of articles went so far as to blame the situation on the increased scientific foundation of nursing. Austin argued that men were presumed better at scientific thought than women, and consequently men were more likely to move ahead in modern nursing. She then proposed that, to discourage men from taking over, nursing should return to its prescientific, task-oriented base.[37, 38]

In the United States today, male nurses are moving toward greater representation in the better-paying and policy-making positions. In 1980, males comprised 3 percent of the registered nurse population, but held 4 percent of the administrative and supervisory positions. More impressive is the fact that 25 percent of all nurse anesthetists that year were male. In 1984 the average yearly salary of a nurse anesthetist was $12,000 more than that of a staff nurse.[39]

Men may gravitate toward these better paying jobs not only for the obvious economic benefits, but also to reduce uncomfortable sex-role strain. Men in nursing tend to specialize in anesthesiology, psychiatric nursing, or administration. Each of these specialties requires a minimum of physical intimacy and escapes explicit identification as a nurse by avoiding the nurse's traditional uniform.[40]

Why should the domination of nursing by men be an issue of concern, especially when men could balance the profession and contribute unique qualities that would grant nursing the influence it deserves? This question can be answered by looking at the arguments that support the active recruitment of men into nursing. They are based on circumstantial evidence. They assume that if male-dominated professions are more powerful than female-dominated professions, more males in nursing would make nurses more powerful. But the evidence from teaching in the United States and nursing in Great Britain suggests that the male power base is so strong that when males are introduced into a predominantly female profession, they tend to rise to the executive positions. The disadvantages of a male-dominated nursing profession have not yet been addressed by nursing literature in the United States.

A large proportion of men at the top would tend to be self-perpetuating. Once this domination was established, it would be very difficult for women to regain leadership roles. A number of factors would contribute to this problem: (1) the sexist hiring criteria that pervades society dictates that the more demanding the job, the more males are preferred over females for the position [41]; (2) men refer other male associates to jobs [42]; (3) fewer women may become interested in leadership positions because of a loss of female role models; and (4) men at the top may not choose to be mentors to women, consequently limiting female nurses' opportunity to have this crucial developmental relationship. [43]

If men dominated the leadership, the oppressed group behavior currently keeping nursing in its submissive place would be internally reinforced. This would serve not only to minimize the political effectiveness of female nurses, but also to stymie the development of the whole profession. At a time when nursing would seriously need quality leadership, the pool for leadership development would be reduced to the male nurse minority, and women's potential for growth would be severely limited.

Future of nursing

Nursing is an intrinsically female profession, based on female values and morals and a holistic world view. [44] What impact would imposing a male-dominated leadership have on the nature and direction of the profession? Although Austin urged a return to unsophisticated nursing, the real concern is not that women will lose this last bastion of territory. Rather, it is for the future of nursing itself, in its role as a unique contributor to health care.

Because the skills needed in nursing require both masculine and feminine characteristics, nursing has a choice. Responsibilities could be delegated by sex, or the best qualities of both...could be developed in nurses of both sexes to maximize the resource pool. Nursing could greatly benefit from full sexual integration on all levels, and this is an admirable goal for the profession. Although the active recruitment of men into nursing superficially appears to be the simplest method to achieve this goal, the experiences of teaching in the United States and nursing in Great Britain should be heeded in the transition.

The male power base in society is incredibly strong. Male nurses are not treated as powerless tokens, but are looked to as saviors of the profession. Yet evidence indicates that when the male minority in a female profession approaches 20 percent, administrative control of the profession shifts to that male minority. Research has also shown that male nurses are no more likely to bring a unifying attitude to the field than female nurses do. Attitudinal militancy with regard to collective bargaining, which is generally attributed to men, may not be significantly present in male nurses.

It appears that actively recruiting men at this time may not provide what nursing is looking for. However, this does not relegate nursing to a future of sexually segregated, semiprofessional limbo. Nursing can become sexually integrated, if it is patient and remains on its current course.

Sex roles in society are slowly changing. Women and men are in the process of learning how to deal with one another as equals. Nursing is in a position to take full advantage of this evolution. It is moving away from its traditional image, even though it is still 97 percent female. It is well on its way to establishing a unique scientific base and full professional status. Nursing is becoming a progressive, profitable contributor in a redefined health care system. As this change develops, men will naturally gravitate toward the field, because the only factor keeping them away is nursing's traditional image.

As nursing evolves, so will female nurses. The women in nursing will have developed enough confidence in their own expertise that they will be able to accept entering men as equals and not as superiors.

By starting from a strongly female base at this stage of social history, nursing can accomplish what no other profession has. It can effectively demonstrate that men and women can work together as true equals in a scientific business. Nursing has the potential to become a discipline that all of society can emulate.

REFERENCES

1. American Nurses' Association. *Facts about Nursing: 84-85*. New York: American Nurses' Association, 1985.

2. Roberts, S. "Oppressed Group Behavior: Implications for Nursing." *Advances in Nursing Science* 5, no. 4 (1983): 21-30.

3. Fottler, M.D. "Attitudes of Female Nurses toward the Male Nurse: Study of Occupational Segregation." *Journal of Health and Social Behavior* 17 (1976): 98-110.

4. Silver, H.K., and McAtee, P. "Health Care Practice: An Expanded Profession of Nursing for Men and Women." *American Journal of Nursing* 72, no. 1 (1972): 78-80.

5. Christman, L. "Let's Have More Men in Nursing (Or, At Least, More Career-Oriented Women)." *Nursing '74* 4, no. 5 (1974): 16-17.

6. Vestal, C. "Men Nurses: Who Needs Them?" *Vermont Registered Nurse* (July 1983): 9-11.

7. Williams, A. "Characteristics of Male Baccalaureate Students Who Selected Nursing as a Career." *Nursing Research* 22 (1973): 520-25.

8. Fottler, "Attitudes of Female Nurses."

9. Bush, P.J. "The Male Nurse: A Challenge to Traditional Role Identities." *Nursing Forum* 15 (1976): 390-405.

10. "Men in nursing." *Hospitals* 42, no. 9 (1968): 41.

11. Hardy, L.K. "The Emergence of Nursing Leaders —A Case of In-spite of, Not Because-of." *International Nursing Review* 31, no. 1 (1984): 11-15.

12. Minnigerode, F.A., Kayer-Jones, J.S., and Garcia, G. "Masculinity and Femininity in Nursing." *Nursing Research* 27 (1978): 299-302.

13. Fottler, "Attitudes of Female Nurses."

14. Silver and McAtee, "Health Care Practice."

15. Snavely, B.K., and Fairhurst, G.T. "The Male Nursing Student as a Token." *Research in Nursing and Health* 7 (1984): 287-94.

16. Vestal, "Men Nurses: Who Needs Them?"

17. Greenberg, E., and Levine, B. "Role Strain in Men Nurses." *Nursing Forum* 10 (1971): 417-30.

18. Etzkowitz, H. "The Male Sister: Sexual Separation of Labor in Society." *Journal of Marriage and the Family* 33 (1971): 431-34.

19. Vestal, "Men Nurses: Who Needs Them?"

20. "Are Men Nurses Really Accepted?" *Nursing Outlook* 15, no. 5 (1967): 27.

21. Whittemore, M.L. "Males: The Second Sex in Elementary Education." *The Journal of Teacher Education* 24 (1973): 317-18.

22. Neidig, M. "Rise and Decline of Women Administrators." *National Elementary Principal* 56 (1976): 53-54.

23. Dale, C.T. "Women Are Still Missing Persons in Administrative and Supervisory Jobs." *Educational Leadership* 31 (1973): 123-27.

24. Palmieri, P., and Shakeshaft, C.S. "Up the Front Staircase: A Proposal for Women to Achieve Parity with Men in the Field of Educational Administration." *The Journal of the Association of Women Deans, Administrators and Counselors* 39 (1976): 58-65.

25. Simpson, R.L., and Simpson, I.H. "Women and Bureaucracy in the Semi-professions." *The Semi-professions and Their Organization,* edited by A. Etzioni. New York: Free Press, 1969, pp. 196-265.

26. Taylor, S.S. "Educational Leadership: A Male Domain?" *Phi Delta Kappan* 55 (1973): 124-28.

27. Futrell, M.H. "Female Leadership and the Future of Education." *Educational Horizons* 63 (1985): 20-21.

28. Taylor, "Educational Leadership."

29. McCarthy, M., and Zent, A. "School Administrators: A Profile." *The Education Digest* 47 (1982): 28-31.

30. Taylor, "Educational Leadership."

31. Collins, L. "About Those Few Females Who Scale the Heights of School Management," *American School Board Journal* 163 (1976): 24-27.

32. Dale, "Women Are Still Missing Persons in Administrative and Supervisory Jobs."

33. Taylor, "Educational Leadership."

34. Douglass, L.M. *The Effective Nurse: Leader and Manager*. St. Louis: Mosby, 1984.

35. Aluto, J., and Belasco, J. "Determinants of Attitudinal Militancy among Nurses and Teachers." *Industrial and Labor Relations Review* 27 (1974): 216-27.

36. Hardy, "The Emergence of Nursing Leaders."

37. Austin, R. "Sex and Gender in the Future of Nursing, Part 1." *Nursing Times* 73, no. 34 (1977): 113-16.

38. Austin, R. "Sex and Gender in the Future of Nursing, Part 2." *Nursing Times* 73, no. 35 (1977): 117-19.

39. American Nurses' Association, *Facts about Nursing*.

40. Greenberg and Levine, "Role Strain in Men Nurses."

41. Clement, J.P. et al. "No Room at the Top?" *American Education* 13 (1977): 20-23.

42. Taylor, "Educational Leadership."

43. Hardy, "The Emergence of Nursing Leaders."

44. London, F. "Why Choose Nursing?" *American Journal of Nursing* 85 (1985): 114.

UNIT EIGHT

Study questions

1. In "Nursing Education and Practice: The Need for Consensus," Elliott identifies three major unresolved issues: the nursing shortage, salaries, and the image of nursing. What are Elliott's recommendations for resolving these issues? Do you believe they will be effective? Why?

2. Sandrick discusses the nontraditional careers of 10 different nurses in "Other Options: Great Opportunities Outside of the Hospital." Pick one career and compare it to a career in hospital nursing, noting their similarities and differences. Which of these careers is more appealing to you? Why?

3. According to "An Expanding Universe: Professional Career Opportunities," managers should recognize the hospital staff nurse as the center of nursing services. Why? What career paths can the staff nurse take?

4. Based on "Entry into Practice: The Continuing Saga," nursing must define the scope of practice for the professional nurse and associate nurse. How would you define their scopes of practice? Do you think a particular type of education is best for contemporary nursing? What arguments would you use to support your position? How will the entry-into-practice debate help shape nursing's role in the health care delivery system?

5. Foss summarizes the legal requirements for relicensure in "Continuing Education Requirements by State." In some states, continuing education is mandatory; in others, it is not. Which arguments support mandatory continuing education? Which arguments oppose it? What do you believe is the role of continuing education in nursing?

6. According to "The Senior Preceptorship as a Method for Anticipatory Socialization of Baccalaureate Nursing Students," what are the benefits of a successful transition into nursing practice? How can a preceptorship help?

7. In "Specialization Meets Entry into Practice," Bajnok calls for a stronger link between general nursing education and specialization in nursing practice. How would a combination of generalist and specialist education benefit the nurse? How can it be achieved?

8. Davis's "Learning About Nursing Management" describes how a student can be oriented to the nurse manager's role and the work setting. In the project it describes, how did the students combine fantasy and realism to learn about nursing management in a hospital? What did they select as representative desirable characteristics of the ideal hospital? (Name five.) Do you agree or disagree with their selections? Why?

9. In "Should Men Be Actively Recruited into Nursing," London cites the pros and cons of this issue. Based on these data, would you support active recruitment of men into nursing? Why?

UNIT NINE

Current patterns of nursing and health care

PREVIOUS UNITS FOCUSED either on the nature and definition of nursing or on issues of direct patient care. Unit Nine explores the relationship of nursing to the broad societal forces confronting all health care professions and health care providers, regardless of educational preparation, type of specialty practice, or client setting. This unit presents a brief overview of nursing theory development and nursing research efforts, looks at the economic forces that are dramatically altering contemporary health care (and thus nursing), and addresses the additional challenges to nursing that technological advancement and increasing competition among health care providers may bring. The unit identifies, therefore, many of the issues and trends that offer nursing in the 1990s its greatest risks and greatest opportunities. The status of nursing in the twenty-first century may well depend on nurses' knowledge of and ability to respond to these issues and trends.

Nursing theory

Debate continues over the role that nursing theory should play in the classroom and in clinical practice. Some argue that the work of nurse theorists is not based on the same realities as those encountered by practicing nurses and that the theories do not provide the practicing nurse with sufficiently concrete information to manage problematic conditions. And if these theories hold little relevance to the experienced nurse, of what value are they to the student nurse who will soon be required to face the same problematic conditions?

Proponents insist, however, that the nursing theories of Orem, Neuman, and Roy, among others, not only advance the scientific basis of nursing practice but also help the nursing student and novice nurse to develop sound judgment skills as they progress from competence to proficiency to expertise. Furthermore, these theories can enhance clinical practice by providing the veteran nurse with advanced scientific bases for nursing actions. The clarity, applicability, and use of nursing theories in clinical practice will be benchmarks by which nursing will be judged in the future.

Nursing research

Nursing research, meanwhile, has played an increasing role not only in validating nursing actions but in testing nursing theory in the practice setting. Such research requires collaboration between nurses in service and academic settings who are educated and trained in the conduct, dissemination, and evaluation of

Glossary

Diagnostic Related Groups (DRGs): classification system that organizes clients into groups based on homogeneity of resource consumption. The system has 23 major diagnostic categories and 467 subdiagnoses.

Nursing diagnoses: theoretical formulations that link the nurse's knowledge with the client's health state and needs.

Nursing process: systematic method of collecting and analyzing client data to arrive at one or more nursing diagnoses, a plan of care, implementation of the plan, and evaluation of its effectiveness.

Nursing theory: statement of the definitions and interrelationships between concepts of an abstract nature and their more concrete meanings in an effort to describe the nature of nursing practice.

Prospective payment system: method of payment for hospitalization (or other health care costs) based on predetermined payment-rate guidelines tied to the client's disease or disorder, age, and subsequent complications (if any)

clinical research. Identifying research priorities, testing nursing theory in the practice setting, refining the delivery of expert, scientifically based nursing care, and documenting the economic and social value of nursing services constitute the principal objectives of all nurse researchers in the United States today.

Contemporary nursing

Perhaps the most profound effect on contemporary nursing has been the recent implementation of Diagnostic Related Groups (DRGs) and a prospective payment system to finance health care. Drastic reductions in federal payments, based largely on normal lengths of hospital stay for a patient condition rather than on the care the patient receives during hospitalization, have increased the frequency of early discharges and outpatient treatments and lowered hospital occupancy rates.

Although recent evidence suggests that most clients are no less happy with the quality of care they now receive, nurses have typically given the new payment system mixed reviews. Cost-effective decentralization of departments has led to increased specialization of skills, which has improved nurses' knowledge, autonomy, and self-esteem. However, increasing paperwork, staff reductions, and fluctuations in the client census have combined to disrupt nurse-client continuity. Most nurses are no longer able to spend as much time working directly with their clients as they believe is necessary. As a result, at a time when their knowledge is increasing and their profession is gaining greater prominence in the scientific community, hospital nurses' job satisfaction remains low.

The future of nursing

Traditionally, the nursing profession has moved in directions that ultimately benefit the client. With foresight and dedication, the profession can continue this pattern. Increased efforts in nursing theory and research will be needed to help nurses control costs while providing their clients with the highest quality of care. Movements to standardize nursing education, increase specialized clinical knowledge among nurses, and improve computer applications to record, monitor, and analyze patient data will further these causes.

The topics addressed in this unit help form links between nursing and the scientific community, nursing and the health care delivery system, and nursing and the consumers and regulators of nursing practice and education. The ability of nursing to shape its own future depends on how well nurses understand the role these forces play in nursing and in the larger social, political, and economic arenas.

SECTION ONE

Theory and research in nursing

THIS SECTION EXPLORES the ways in which the work of nursing theorists and researchers affects the student nurse and the practicing nurse.

"Bridging the Gap: Theory to Practice — Part I, Clinical Applications" examines the use of nursing theory in the clinical setting. Christmyer et al. describe how nursing theories have been used at the Francis Scott Key Medical Center to develop a conceptual framework for providing and evaluating nursing care and for staff education and research.

In "The Impact of Nursing Theory on the Clinical Decision Making Process," Field also explores how theory influences the delivery of client care. She demonstrates how selected nursing theories apply to the nursing process and to nursing diagnoses. Field believes that current nursing theories improve nursing practice, but she argues that nurses must receive appropriate training — and be willing to gain the experience that comes only with time — before they can become competent, proficient, and, ultimately, expert in applying theory to practice.

Theory development, with its concurrent evolution of metaparadigms and taxonomies, has been difficult for many practicing nurses to accept and incorporate into patient care. The uneasiness with which they view nursing theory, however, seems to result not only from its specialized language or complexity but also from the uncertainty inherent in creation and change. What they may not realize is that application of unique and specialized theories to nursing is a sign of a healthy and vibrant profession willing to mature. These theories were essential to the professionalization of nursing and will continue to influence nursing education, research, and practice. Nursing's evolution — its willingness to mature — has enabled those now entering the profession to be regarded as an essential part of the health team and a distinguished member of the scientific community.

The evolution of nursing research, like theory development, has had a rapid and significant effect on the nursing profession. Over the past 30 to 40 years, nursing research has played an increasing role in testing nursing theory in the practice setting; refining the delivery of expert, scientifically based nursing care; and documenting the economic and social value of nursing services. By testing nursing theory and validating caring aspects of nursing practice, research has helped establish nursing as a unique and essential scientific discipline.

"The National Center for Nursing Research [NCNR]: Challenges and Initiatives" outlines the national program initiatives for nursing research. Hinshaw, the NCNR's director, discusses such topics as continued development of the depth of nursing science, development of a larger pool of nurse scientists, and improvements in the ways nurses disseminate and use research results in clinical practice. The author focuses on the role of the NCNR in developing a national nursing research agenda that will meet the health care concerns of society while providing for the continued scientific development of the profession. The NCNR, product of an intense political struggle in the mid-1980s, provides an avenue for federal funding of nursing research and a forum within the scientific community for conducting basic and applied nursing research.

"Use of Research-Based Knowledge in Clinical Practice" offers practical solutions to the problems of implementing research findings within the practice setting. Goode et al. illustrate how the staff at a rural acute care hospital in Iowa applied research findings to improve and refine their delivery of patient care. The authors cite many of the obstacles they had to overcome, chief among them a staff with little experience in reading, critiquing, and using research. Further, they describe two research projects conducted at the hospital, the systems theory they used, and the policy changes that resulted from the studies.

Bridging the gap: Theory to practice—part I, clinical applications

CAROL S. CHRISTMYER, RN, MS; PENNY M. CATANZARITI, RN, MS, CCRN; ANITA M. LANGFORD, RN, MS; JUDY A. REITZ, RN, MSN, SCD

Although schools of nursing use conceptual frameworks to develop curricula, until recently, hospitals and other health care institutions rarely used such frameworks to guide program development. In the following article, the authors describe their experience at the Francis Scott Key Medical Center in Baltimore. They contend that using a conceptual framework to guide clinical practice, staff development, quality assurance programs, and nursing research can help bridge the gap between — and thus strengthen — nursing theory and nursing practice. Note: In this article, summaries (shown in bracketed italics) and excerpts (indicated by ellipses) condense extensive background information.

[The Framework for Nursing Practice, formulated by Reitz in 1982, incorporates the concepts of health and nursing and acknowledges the relationship between the two: health requires continuous adaptation to stressors, and nursing supports the patient's adaptive processes, helping him maximize changing states of wellness to achieve equilibrium. According to the framework, health has two primary dimensions — consisting of 7 biophysical and 4 behavioral health parameters — as detailed in Figure I. This structure allows the nurse to analyze and categorize patient needs and the nursing interventions that can address those needs. The following sections discuss how the framework is applied to four major components of nursing service: quality assurance, clinical practice, staff education, and research.

Quality assurance

The first step in developing a quality assurance program was to identify nursing practice standards. From the definitions of the 11 functional health parameters, specific standards for each parameter were developed, and each standard was structured according to the nursing process. Thus, assessment standards delineated the data to be collected on admission and during hospitalization. Planning standards reflected critical elements in patient care. Intervention standards were related to the identified assessment criteria. Evaluation standards included process and outcome criteria. Next, a quality assurance measurement tool was designed to ensure that the nursing practice standards and quality assurance criteria were compatible with the conceptual framework. The next step was to develop documentation tools for our clinical information system.]

Clinical information system

The conceptual framework provides a comprehensive, systematic and logical approach to developing nursing documentation tools. The core of our clinical information system includes an admission data base, care plan, progress notes, and discharge summary.

The first documentation tool developed, the admission data base, organizes assessment information according to the 11 functional health parameters. The data base provides a baseline description of the patient on admis-

FIGURE I. **Dimensions of health: Conceptual framework**

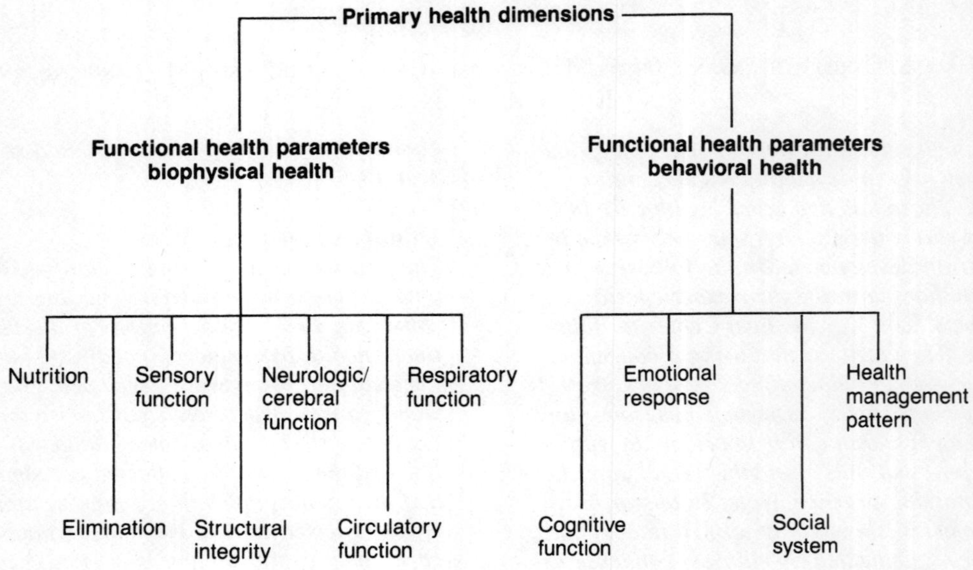

sion and is the initial phase of the nursing process. The admission data base includes the patient's 1) initial admission demographic data and 2) biophysical and behavioral health status. Within each health parameter, assessment information important to each is identified. An example of the cognitive parameter assessment information is shown in Figure II.

The next forms developed were the nursing discharge summary and the nursing transfer summary. The discharge summary is a tool which documents the patient's health status related to the major health problems identified during hospitalization. This form is less structured than the data base; each functional health parameter is followed by cues which identify important aspects of that paramenter (Figure III). In completing the form, the nurse addresses the nature, magnitude, and complexity of nursing actions. The tool is used to communicate important information to health care agencies involved in the care of the patient following discharge. The transfer summary is similar; it is used when the patient is moved to another unit within the medical center. A comparison of the discharge or transfer summary with the admission data base clearly demonstrates changes in the patient's health status documented according to health parameter as a result of nursing intervention.

The final major piece of the clinical information system, the nursing care plan, also incorporates the framework for nursing practice. The care plan illustrated in Figure IV identifies parameters relative to the given patient problem.

Implementation. The process of implementing

FIGURE II. Cognitive response

Language: Speak ________ Read ________ Write ________________________________

Education: ____

Ability to understand plan of care: ________________________________

Problem-solving ability: ____

Ability to understand routine teaching: ____________________________

Other conditions pertinent to this parameter: ________________________

a comprehensive clinical information system included three phases utilizing three inpatient nursing units: 1) a general surgical nursing unit with a high percentage of orthopedic patients; 2) a general medical unit with a large number of elderly patients and 3) a newly opened Center for Chemical Dependency (CCD). The medical and surgical units were selected because their patient populations were diverse. The CCD waus selected both because it was a specialty discipline and because it was a new unit where nurses had no prior experience with the previous documentation system.

The first phase of implementation consisted of educational programs to introduce the framework and documentation system. Education included both formal classes and informal consultation by nurse clinicians. After a pilot period of two months, revisions were made based on feedback of staff nurses on pilot units. The second phase of implementation was the adaptation of the data base to specialty areas. Our neonatal intensive care unit, psychiatric unit, and pediatrics unit have developed data bases suited to their patients' unique needs.

The final phase, still incomplete, consists of revising the nursing progress notes to reflect parameter-specific information. Both the Subjective-Objective-Assessment-Plan (SOAP) format and parameter assessment format are being piloted. Development of a clinical information system based on the framework for nursing practice is an ongoing process. The goal of this process is to achieve a relevant, practical, and conceptually sound system of documenting patient care.

Clinical practice — triage

The Emergency Department at this medical center serves a very large inner-city community. Large numbers of patients are seen daily and the Emergency Department staff determined that an effective method of triage, or prioritization of treatment urgency, would improve patient flow. A task force was formed to develop a triage system that would meet patient needs.

The task force visited several area hospitals to evaluate existing triage programs and reviewed the literature to identify new trends in nursing triage. Two similarities were seen: 1) all triage systems were based on medical models, although consistently performed by registered nurses and 2) triage decisions were based solely on chief complaint, often with little or no written criteria describing the degree of severity of the chief complaint.

Task force members agreed that written protocols were needed to ensure consistency, and that a nursing model would be most useful. Because patients express physical or emotional complaints when presenting in the ER in

FIGURE III. **Nursing discharge summary**

Address nature, magnitude, complexity of nursing actions in all areas:

BIOPHYSICAL HEALTH

Nutrition (Diet, fluids, weight, nausea, vomiting, appetite, assistance needed, etc.)

Elimination (Bowel & bladder habits, abdomen, independence in elimination)

Sensory function (Gait and balance, deficits, pain)

Structural integrity (Mobility, exercise, infection, muscle strength, skin)

Neurologic/cerebral function (Sleep patterns, behavioral, thought content, memory, speech)

Circulatory function (Pulse, rate and quality, edema)

Respiratory function (Breath sounds, cough, oxygen support)

FIGURE IV. **Nursing care plan**

	Primary nurse												
Review of care plan Date & initial													

Date	No.	Functional health parameter	Nursing diagnosis/ patient problem	Goal	Nursing intervention	Date goal achieved	Initial

Nurse's signature				Nurse's signature			
Init.		Title		Init.		Title	

a way unique to the individual, it was difficult for the task force to assign triage decisions based on the severity of the disease process. Some persons may come to the Emergency Department with minor lacerations, but so emotionally upset that they are unable to follow treatment instructions while waiting to be seen by a physician. Others may come with complaints of mild epigastric discomfort. Although all physical indicators may be stable, the nurse may believe that serious cardiac alterations are present. Both of these patients should be treated more rapidly than physical signs would indicate, yet traditional triage programs lack the documentation system necessary to validate this type of triage decision.

The task force decided that nursing assessment, based on the Framework for Nursing Practice, would allow for a holistic approach to triage decision making. The 11 functional health parameters were used to categorize a number of patient complaints and symptoms. Each parameter was divided into four categories of treatment, each color-coded, as shown in Figure V. The triage nurse classifies the chief presenting complaint and assesses the patient using the nursing triage indicators relative to each of the health parameters. High scores in more than one area may make it necessary to expedite patient treatment.

The use of a framework for triage assessment was new to the Emergency Department. Therefore, several steps had to be taken before the triage system could be implemented: 1) an eight-hour educational program was developed to introduce the use of the framework in triage; emphasis was placed on the use of the framework and nursing triage protocols; 2) the tool was piloted by RNs for six months and 3) all completed triage documentation was reviewed by the task force; the triage tool was then modified, based on input from staff nurses who had participated in the project. The pilot supported the viability of the triage tool as a useful prospective aid for triage decision-making. Since the tool provided assessment parameters in subjective as well as objective physical findings, documentation was enhanced as well.

[Staff education and nursing research

We used the Framework for Nursing Practice in the staff education program for the first time to complete an annual needs assessment survey, categorizing items according to the 11 functional health parameters rather than to the predetermined prioritization scheme used in earlier surveys. The nutrition parameter, for instance, incorporated such topics as hyperal-

FIGURE V. **Emergency department nutrition sheet**

CATEGORY I: GREEN	CATEGORY II: YELLOW	CATEGORY III: RED	CATEGORY IV: (No color) ESCOR
Known diabetic: Requests serum glucose check Requests insulin prescription	Known diabetic: Gradual loss of appetite; fatigue; complains of weakness; hx of vomiting and/or diarrhea for several days	Known diabetic: Insulin dependent; feels "shaky"; vs stable, hx of skipped meals or increased exercise	Known diabetic: Insulin dependent, with sudden change in mental status; respiratory rate decreased; Kussmul respirations
Vomiting/Diarrhea VS wnl—adequate fluid balance	Abdominal pain with vomiting and/or diarrhea—VSS—no orthostasis	Abdominal pain/vomiting/ diarrhea; VS wnl but orthostasis changes or other clinical signs of dehydration, e.g., poor skin turgor	Hematemesis with/ without abdominal pain
		Vomiting with or without diarrhea with or without abdominal pain—insulin dependent diabetic took insulin and unable to tolerate food—not symptomatic	
Dysphagia—no acute onset—no drooling nor sore throat nor enlarged lymph nodes; loss of appetite (adult)		Dysphagia (index of suspicion-foreign body) no respiratory distress—NAD—within 24 hrs.	Dysphagia with respiratory distress (also respiratory)
		Vomiting, febrile, dysuria, and/or urgency, with or without abdominal pain (also GU)	
Abdomen distended (chronic)	Abdomen distended, poss. cirrhosis	Abdomen distended, peripheral edema, fine rales (bases only) no respiratory distress (see also cardiac)	Abdomen distended, respiratory distress, CHF-pulmonary edema (aiso cardiac) Abdomen distended—unable to void (also GU)

imentation and special diets; the cognitive parameter included topics on patient teaching and adult learning principles. Survey results were analyzed within major clinical practice settings and aggregated across all nursing divisions. The results allowed nurse educators to determine the parameters most frequently identified. Thus, educators could now design specific programs to address specific practice settings (such as pain relief methods used during labor and delivery).

The staff education department then adopted the framework for curriculum development, restructuring workshops according to the functional health parameters rather than to the customary disease-process model. For example, the physical assessment course now has classes on nutrition and elimination rather than on the GI and GU systems.

The Nursing Research Committee at the Francis Scott Key Medical Center subsequently used the framework to help determine research priorities, underscoring the clinical practice model's relevance to nursing research.]

The impact of nursing theory on the clinical decision making process

PEGGY ANNE FIELD, RN, PhD

In the following article, Field explores the concepts of the nursing process and nursing diagnosis and examines the relationship of nursing models to the nursing process. The author concludes with a presentation of Benner's work (1984), offering suggestions on how nursing students and novice nurses can learn to make decisions based on theory and to translate that theory to the practice setting.

Nursing process

TO BE SUCCESSFUL, nurses need knowledge of and skills in the cognitive process of problem solving, commonly referred to as the nursing process, an understanding of the parameters of the care situation (that is the nurse, the client, and the setting), and the theoretical knowledge base needed in order to solve the problem.

The nursing process is a special case of problem solving using the logical-deductive mode. The steps of the process are no different from those used by the scientist embarking on a research project or a physician making a medical diagnosis. It is a systematic way of collecting information, which is then analyzed in order to arrive at some tentative hypotheses about what the client/patient needs, so that a plan of nursing care may be drawn up and implemented and an evaluation of the effectiveness of the intervention carried out. Virginia Henderson (1982) has asked the question, "Is the title right?" She argues that there is a danger that the nursing process is becoming seen as the only approach to problem solving in nursing and, secondly, that it is being used as a definition of nursing, negating the need for the theory base which must underlie any problem solving process.

Henderson points out that Nursing Practice Acts in the United States required a definition of nursing and that in some cases the nursing process was used to supply this definition. As the role of the nurse as a primary contact in the health care system developed, a second movement also evolved that had as its aim the establishment of nursing as independent from medicine. The nursing process and...nursing diagnosis were seen as ways of describing an independent role for nursing *vis à vis* medicine. Henderson argues that the nursing process is only one way of problem solving, the deductive mode. Ignored, in Henderson's view, is intuitive judgment, which is derived from clinical knowledge, not process, a point supported by Benner (1984) in her careful description of the evolution of the nurse from novice to expert.

The influence of the nurse's own emotional or subjective response to a situation also needs to be considered in relation to decision making. Nurses are not value free; they have biases, development from experience, that must be explored and examined. Unexplored prejudice in relation to age, sex, race, religion, alcoholism, [and] senility...may cloud or influence a nurse's judgment in unsuspected ways, no matter what techniques, such as the nursing process and/or nursing diagnoses, are employed.

Problem solving is an attempt to focus on nursing as a science, but nursing as an art is of equal importance. The sort of person that we are may substantially influence our relationships, our communication skills, [and] the way in which we care for another, and these in turn may influence our ability to nurse, but they are not part of the cognitive process of problem solving *per se*.

All health care workers, including nurses, operate within some sort of establishment that puts limits or boundaries on their practice. For example, the primary nurse practitioners are governed by societal laws that put limitations on their area of practice. These dimensions go beyond the conventional considerations inherent in the usual description of the nursing process, yet are a critical factor that must be considered by nurses as they make decisions about care. Knowledge of nursing and of such contextual factors as ethics and law [is] critical to nursing decision making.

Nursing diagnosis

Nursing diagnosis was first written about as early as 1953 (Fry 1953). However, it was not until the 1970s, in a further effort to differentiate the practice of nursing from the practice of medicine, that nursing diagnoses evolved as the end result of data gathering and analysis within the nursing process. To arrive at a nursing diagnosis, the nurse must make judgments about relationships within the data and arrive at conclusions. The purpose of a nursing diagnosis is to allow groups of signs and symptoms of interest to nurses to be classified or named (Ziegler *et al.* 1986). This can be construed as first level theory development. The diagnostic process described by Ziegler *et al.* (1986) includes determining cues by comparing the data to norms and standards suggested by theory and research findings; clustering of related cues into patterns using nursing knowledge, labelling the patterns; drawing conclusions about unhealthful patterns; relating cause to unhealthy responses; and combining responses and etiology into a nursing diagnosis. One difficulty with the current taxonomy, and this may be vested in the nomenclature of "diagnosis," is that it directs no focus towards the individual's *strengths* or the factors that might mitigate the severity of the diagnosis. This is particularly a problem when considering nursing practice in the community setting.

In one study (Field 1983) it was found that nurses...frequently collected data but failed to examine the relationships so that often they made poor judgments or did not arrive at appropriate conclusions. Tracing the roots of this situation, it seemed that either nursing educators were not moving students from the assessent to the analysis and hypotheses phases of problem solving or that nurses were unwilling to make judgments based on the data they had collected. While the current system of nursing diagnoses still has areas that need testing and may need expansion, its use can force neophyte nurses to consider patterns of behavior and force them to make conclusions based on the assessment they have made.

Nursing and medical diagnoses. Although nursing diagnoses and medical diagnoses are "independent" of one another, they are interrelated and should not be considered in isolation from one another. If the physician considers the patient to be dying, a diagnosis not included within the nursing framework, nursing diagnoses should reflect the patient's status, interpreted through the nurse's knowledge of the psychological needs of those who are dying. Interfacing of nursing knowledge, the nursing process, and nursing diagnosis will result in a defined body of knowledge, accountability on the part of caregivers, and...the provision of individualized care (Ziegler *et al.* 1986). Textbooks aimed at this type of synthesis are [beginning to] identify nursing interventions based on nursing diagnosis (Bulechak & McCloskey 1986). Thus, one sees an orderly progression toward a framework of diagnosis and intervention that can be evaluated for effectiveness. However, nursing diagnosis and intervention have been developed without due consideration of the need for a macro-theory of nursing. It is necessary to consider how proposed macro-theories interface with the nursing process and how they structure "nursing knowledge."

The relationship of the nursing process to nursing models

Theory is a powerful tool for explaining and predicting which allows a systematic examination of events. If one establishes casual relationships between events one comes "to know that" one event is related to another (Kuhn 1970, Polyani 1962). "Knowing that" and "knowing how" are two different types of knowledge. We have many skills in the "know how" category that are acquired without "knowing that" *x* or *y* is the reason we do the skill in a particular way. Such common activities as putting food into our mouth, walking, or riding a bicycle are examples of this fact.

Nursing theorists, in developing models of nursing, are attempting to provide nurses with tools which can be used to allow a systematic examination of events. Fawcett (1984) outlines four concepts common to all models: the person receiving nursing; the environment within which the person exists; the health-illness state of the person; and nursing actions. She argues that these are the elements of a metaparadigm of nursing, that is, they are the concepts central to the discipline of nursing. From this one metaparadigm several models of nursing have evolved. Kuhn (1970) describes multiple models as being typical of a preparadigm state within a discipline, and it has been argued that this is the current state of theory development in nursing (Conant 1986). The metaparadigm is emerging but is not yet sufficiently tested to be a stable theory.

To examine the four concepts described by Fawcett (1984), a nursing assessment would have to include the person, the environment, and the health status of the client; nursing actions would include the assessment, diagnosis, plan of care, intervention and evaluation of that care. The process of arriving at a nursing diagnosis can be applied to the metaparadigm, and as long as the theories of nursing include the four elements plus a mode for systematic problem solving then the classifications of the nursing diagnosis taxonomy should be applicable regardless of the particular model involved.

Data base. What will change from model to model is the way in which the data base is organized. For example, the focus of Orem's (1980) Health Care Systems Model is stressors that cause instability in the physiologic, psychologic, sociocultural and developmental subsystems of the client, while the focus of Roy's (1976) model is adaptation.

If one [were] collecting information on a presenting health problem using Orem's model, the nurse would collect information about the universal, developmental, health deviation self-care requisites and self-care deficits. For Neuman's model, the nurse would collect information or data as they relate to the physiologic, psychologic, sociocultural and developmental subsystem responses to stressors. If the model used was Roy's, the nurse would collect information about physiologic needs, self-concepts, role mastery and interdependence adaptive modes, as well as related stimuli.

If the client [were] a postpartum mother, the nursing diagnosis based on the North American Nursing Diagnosis Association taxonomy (Hurley 1986) might be: "Knowledge deficit in relation to breast feeding." In Orem's model the deficit would be noted in relation to the self-care agents knowledge base; in Neuman's model lack of knowledge would be a stressor in the physiological subsystem; in Roy's model the problem might occur in role mastery or in relation to the physiological system. Using the three models, one should arrive at a similar nursing diagnosis, although the way in which it is stated will differ.

With Orem's model the nursing diagnosis

statement would be couched so as to reflect an inability on the part of the client to meet a self-care demand, which would be related to self-care deficit. For example, "an inability of the self-care agent (client) to breastfeed due to a lack of knowledge related to breast feeding."

Neuman's diagnosis would reflect the client's actual or potential subsystem response to a related stressor. It would reflect both the potentially unhealthy response and the etiology. For example, "Potential failure of breast feeding due to the mother's lack of knowledge about the breastfeeding process."

Roy's statement would reflect the ineffective adaptive behavior in one adaptive mode. "Decreased ability to breast feed related to lack of awareness of the physiological adaptations related to breast feeding." This diagnosis is somewhat more specific than the others. Using Roy's model the statement of the diagnosis could equally reflect a way of developing one or more "means to an end," that is "lack of awareness of the techniques of breast feeding," the *techniques* being the means by which breast feeding is achieved. It appears that Roy's model may force the nurse to identify priorities in her diagnosis to a greater extent than Neuman or Orem, where a more general diagnosis is more likely to be attained

Criticisms of nursing models. In a recent article, Hoon (1986) criticizes the use of nursing models on the grounds that they are incomplete. This indeed presents difficulties when one or more models are used as the basis for curriculum development. No one will deny that models are currently incomplete and that they lack adequate testing and refining but to negate the role they can play in providing a useful framework for assessment and nursing intervention is an unfortunate — if not uninformed — attitude. One major criticism of nursing models is that they all have a major focus on a goal of "health" and that they tend to ignore the inevitability of "death." This is indeed an area of weakness that should be remedied. Testing of models, or parts of models, through research, will help to verify or negate their usefulness, but it is consistent testing in practice that is specially critical for future development. Both Orem and Roy have modified and extended their initial models based on feedback from practice settings.

The nursing theorists are...thinkers who, based on years of practical experience, have tried to identify the components necessary for a nursing interaction....Nurses...must translate the "know that" of the model into the "know how" of practice. Clark (1982) shows how models can be used by nurses as a practical tool to analyze their own practice, in particular to assess needs, and to plan, implement, and evaluate care. She states:

> ...it is important to recognize that any attempt to construct a model of nursing, however poor and inadequate the model may turn out to be, makes explicit the notion that there is something called nursing which has an identity of its own, distinct from other similar activities (Clark 1982).

She notes that the idea of a separate identity is not acceptable to those who still see nursing as a collection of tasks, initiated and directed by doctors for the sole purpose of assisting the medical function. Clark believes that models and theories...will make a significant contribution to professional nursing and are essential for the identification of both the independent and collaborative aspects of the nurse's role.

Nursing knowledge and skills

Models and theories, by themselves, do not provide a sufficient base of knowledge for nurses to make judgments. They only indicate the area of practice which is nursing as distinct from that of the other health related professions such as medicine, social work, or physiotherapy. Knowledge from other disciplines such as the sciences or behavioral sciences is also needed, but will need interpretation by the nurse if the knowledge is to be useful for nursing. If the parameters of nursing are clear, the selection and application of models from other disciplines becomes easier.

It is obvious that within the health discipline there is a need for practitioners to have knowledge in common and many shared skills if each profession is to collaborate in the provision of health care. A sound base in anatomy and physiology is required by nurse, physician, and physiotherapist. A nurse and a physician both need to understand and carry out aseptic techniques. A nurse and a physiotherapist both need to be able to do postural drainage. A social worker and a nurse both need to be able to assess the family support available to the client. However, the purpose for which the knowledge and skill is used may differ for each group.

The goal of the physician is generally curative, the goal of the physiotherapist is generally restorative. The physician will order the client physiotherapy. The physiotherapist prescribes the amount and duration of postural drainage, and evaluates the long-term effectiveness of that intervention. The nurse undertakes postural drainage as part of the client's treatment and evaluates the immediate effectiveness of the intervention, information needed by the physician and physiotherapist for evaluating the effectiveness of that type of treatment. The nurse will evaluate the treatment in terms of the client's well-being. Is the process excessively tiring? Does the postural drainage have a negative or positive effect on the patient's respiration? Does the patient expectorate? Nursing diagnoses following intervention might include the following: "decrease in rhonchi in left upper lobe following percussion" or "lethargic and listless following treatment, appears fatigued."

The nursing decision must balance the effectiveness of the treatment in clearing the lungs with the degree of fatigue observed. Decisions may need to be made on ways in which fatigue can be reduced. The nurse's goal is to carry out the required treatment while obviating or reducing factors which decrease the well-being of the client. These types of decisions require practice and experience — how can they be taught?

Benner (1984), in her description of the development of the nurse from novice to expert, provides insight into the ways in which decision making skills develop. She describes how nurses move from their initial theory base to become experts in practice.

Learning to use theory

Benner (1984) argues that "perceptual awareness" is crucial to good judgments and that judgment for experienced nurses begins with vague hunches and global assessments that initially bypass critical analysis. With experienced nurses, conceptual clarity follows rather than precedes the diagnosis. This appears to be the same process that Henderson (1982) referred to when she spoke of the use of intuition. The experienced nurses in Benner's study referred to this as a "gut feeling" or a "feeling of uneasiness." It appears to be a process of "gestalt" where the individual sees the situation as a whole, and only later do the parts become evident.

In translating theoretical knowledge to practical knowledge, students must learn to distinguish [among] subtle forms of the same event. For example, theoretical knowledge can teach us that the uterus following delivery will be hard but that a bleeding uterus will be "boggy." In practice there is a qualitative distinction between "hard" and "boggy" that must be learned. How do we encourage students to develop perceptual awareness — the ability to become aware of subtle differences and to relate these differences to one another? Such learning is acquired through experience, but are there ways that experience can be helped?

In relation to perceptual skills we know that

simulations can shorten learning time. Audiovisual aids can be used to present some contrasts, for example visual images of wounds and wound healing. In one school of nursing, I observed some excellent simulated case studies, using the model, Mrs. Chase, complete with wound, drainage tubes, and intravenous infusion. The focus of one simulated case study was the relationship [between] fluid intake and output. Intravenous input, respiratory rate, wound drainage, and urine output were all included in the case study along with relevant laboratory reports. This allowed students to pattern data and make judgments in a low-anxiety situation. However, by itself the simulated experience is insufficient. For example, in this situation other central aspects of dehydration (the furred tongue, sunken eyeballs, and lack of tissue turgor) were absent.

When I was a student nurse we had to take the ward sister (head nurse) on patient rounds and describe each patient's condition, complete with current signs and symptoms. Can we extend the knowledge of the nursing student and novice nurse through the use of rounds, the focus of which is to compare and contrast symptoms? Such comparisons are indeed frequently made in conferences following clinical experience, but students only *hear* the description of differences, they do not observe those differences for themselves nor do they necessarily articulate or explicate those differences.

The development of judgment. Using interview and observation, Benner (1984) studied practicing nurses to determine how they developed from novices into experts. She defined the novice as a nurse who had no experience with the situations in which she was expected to perform. Benner concludes that novices operate from a set of rules which are taught in a context-free situation. The nursing process can be considered as one such set of rules. A model of nursing also provides rules about the participants involved, the context and the data to be gathered. When the novice enters a new situation, she exhibits rule-governed behavior and is extremely limited and inflexible because her only experience is the information she has read or been told about in a context-free situation.

We have all seen nursing students follow a skill procedure step-by-step and have recognized the difficulty they had in adapting skills from [the] hospital to the home setting. In the same way, students tend to use the phases of the nursing processes as steps which must be rigidly followed in order to access, plan, and implement care. It is my experience that many graduate students revert to the novice mode of action when they are initially required to use a nursing model in their practice. However, they soon operate in a different way, tending to switch over to the competent or expert clinician mode in which they intuitively assess the immediate situation and only later analyze the patient encounter in terms of the model. What the use of the nursing model achieves is to make explicit the basis for their judgments, knowledge which previously had been intrinsic and hard to explain to others.

It is evident that clinically experienced masters' students can go beyond diploma or baccalaureate students in the use of a nursing model. At the novice level, most senior undergraduate nursing students can...apply theory to practice [only] in a rule-operating fashion. In graduate programs requiring previous professional experience, the master's level student already has context-dependent skills learned in "real" situations, and therefore has less need for rules. Thus, the graduate students can use models to start to discover the theory (the "knowing that") underlying their practice (the "knowing how").

Advanced beginners

Advanced beginners have coped with enough real situations to note the recurring components of clinical situations. In the maternity department, for example, they will begin to recognize that a mother's withdrawal into herself, shaking of the extremities, and an increase in blood-stained show all herald the transitional phase of labor. No longer are these separate attributes, but factors which begin to form a meaningful pattern for the nurse.

In my observation of community health nurses at work (Field 1983), a lack of ability to pattern data on the part of the relatively inexperienced nurse frequently led to erroneous or missed diagnoses. One classic example is related to a nurse who could be classified as an advanced beginner. The situation was one in which a 21-month-old girl was brought in for immunization by her obviously pregnant mother. The child, a redhead, was pale with dark circles under her eyes. The nurse remarked how active she was; the mother responded that she tired easily. The interview progressed with the nurse asking about the child's development and the mother's pregnancy. The mother commented that she had trouble making ends meet and that frequently by the end of the week they only had cereal and bread and jam to eat. When the nurse came to give the immunization, the mother remarked that her daughter hated needles since the doctor had taken blood. The nurse kept directing the conversation to the mother's pregnancy and made several attempts to get the mother to come to prenatal classes, despite the fact it was her third pregnancy. When the interview was over the researcher confirmed that the child had blood taken because she was anemic. The nurse was relatively inexperienced, she used her perception of the rules and regulations of the agency for guidance, focusing on the mother's pregnancy, the child's development and the immunization, ignoring information which she regarded as being extraneous to her perception of the agency's goals.

An instructor can help the advanced novice identify patterns by saying, "Did you notice how pale the child was and how the mother remarked on her loss of energy — what might this mean? What other information which was given in the interview might make you want to confirm your suspicions?" Students need this kind of help in [recognizing] relationships [among] different aspects of a situation. At this level the nurse generally does not have the experience to enable her to choose appropriately among priorities. If the nurse, at the level of an advanced beginner, believes the agency expects that the nurse will encourage all pregnant mothers to attend prenatal classes she will attempt to achieve this and may ignore more serious concerns that surface within the situation.

In [the] hospital, if the advanced novice nurse is told to get a laboring mother up to walk she will likely do so, ignoring the fact that the mother has told her she has not slept all night. She will likely give medications to relieve pain because the cervix is only 4 cm dilated, not realizing that the previous history of a rapid labor should be considered. The advanced beginner must still concentrate on rules; the teacher's role is to help the beginner weigh the different aspects inherent in the situation. "Generally it is acceptable to give pain medication when labor is this far advanced but what about the previous history and what has happened to her contractions in the last 15 minutes that may make you reconsider medication for pain relief?" The teacher moves the student within problem solving from data gathering to patterned analysis. The advanced beginner needs help in moving from linear thinking toward the first stages of perceptual gestalt.

It is at this stage that comparison between signs and symptoms exhibited by different clients can be of value in enhancing the nurse's ability to discriminate between degrees of severity of a symptom or to assess improvement in the client's condition or situation.

Here, wound healing could serve as an example.

Competence. Competence is typified, according to Benner, by the nurse who has been on the job in the same or similar situations for 2-3 years. It develops when the nurse begins to see his or her actions in terms of long-range plans or goals of which he or she is consciously aware (Benner 1984). Benner argues that such a plan is based on considerable conscious, abstract, analytic contemplation of the problem. Because the planning is still conscious and deliberate at this stage, the competent nurse lacks the speed and flexibility of the proficient nurse but is better able to identify priorities and is more flexible and less reliant on rules than the advanced nurse.

The process of becoming competent can be enhanced if students and beginning practitioners are given the opportunity to participate in decision making games and simulations that give them opportunity to practice planning and coordinating multiple, complex patient care demands. Board games, with cards for patient characteristics and situational (or context) characteristics, is one approach that can be used. However, if we are to reinforce the model in use and the appropriate nursing diagnoses, these too should be incorporated into the game. Another potential learning tool that can be used to enhance decision making is computer simulation. While simulation cannot substitute for experience it has been shown that pilot training and driver training can both be shortened considerably if simulated experience precedes reality. This mode of acquiring abstract knowledge through active practice with the decision making process can help to build a solid bridge into the domain of practical knowledge.

Proficiency. The proficient nurse perceives situations as wholes rather than in terms of separate selected aspects. Decisions are based on the nurse's perceptions of the situation which are developed through experience and recent events (Benner 1984).

Inservice educators could play a useful role in helping nurses reach the stage of proficiency. If inservice teaching was taken out of the classroom and put back into the clinical setting, nurses could have the opportunity to develop cross-patient comparisons under guidance.

For example, a teacher or a clinical mentor could select three patients with differing degrees of bronchiectasis and their symptoms. She could then encourage those patients to describe the limits of their activities and their concerns about their illness. If this type of approach was utilized, nurses could more rapidly develop the ability to discriminate among degrees of respiratory discomfort, to identify differences among clients, and to recognize relationships [among] symptoms. It is probable they would thus be able to more readily move to the stage where they could make patterns out of data. This level of clinical functioning differs from the nurse's earlier efforts to develop abilities to discriminate in that many factors rather than a single factor are considered. The proficient nurse develops a set of expectations as to what will happen to patient X given treatment Y, but she also recognizes that plans may have to be modified in response to specific events. Using clinical specialists to work with other staff members in the role of clinical mentors can be of particular help to nurses in this phase of development.

A nurse who is used to employing a nursing model, and who is encouraged to continue using it in the practice situation, is more likely to consider the interrelationships of data. If she systematically considers the patient (as man), the context (as environment), the steps needed to promote health, and the role of the nurse in achieving that goal, she will have a logical base from which she can operate in her passage from novice to expert.

Expertise. The expert no longer relies on an

analytic principle (the nursing process, guidelines, maxims, models of nursing) to connect her understanding to an appropriate action. The process has become internalized and her actions appear to the observer to be intuitive. The expert nurse can identify the problem without consideration of unfruitful diagnoses (Benner 1984).

However, currently, many "expert practitioners" cannot explain the basis for their actions. One nurse who was extremely successful in getting the baby to the breast when the mother was having difficulty could not explain what it was that she did that accounted for her success. A series of videotapes showed that she encouraged the mother to play with the baby until relaxation and nipple erection occurred. Although the nurse was unaware of the fact, she observed for this nipple erection as the sign that the mother was ready to nurse. She "knew how" but lacked the theoretical "know that," therefore she could not explain her success to other nurses and was not able to expand the understood practice base of nursing.

The nursing process, nursing diagnosis, and models can be considered the "training wheels" of the nursing profession. They give the guidance and direction needed by the novice who is dependent on rules for her practice, but [they] are not the needed everyday tools of the expert. However, the nurse who has used such training wheels and who has developed her expertise through consciously melding her theoretical base with her practical base should be able, as an expert, to stand back and analyze the reasons underlying her apparently intuitive decisions and subsequent actions. Such explanations from expert nurses can strengthen the desirable practice base of the discipline.

Conclusion

Decision making in nursing is a complex process. The nursing process, as a problem solving process, helps the novice develop a style of thinking that leads to judgments, in the form of nursing diagnoses. Nursing models give shape to the components, begin to define nursing, and direct the goals of nursing care. The educator has a role in moving the student from the stage of the novice towards becoming a competent nurse, remembering that in a strange context the nurse will most likely revert to being a novice, relying on rules until the requirements of the situation become clear. Clinical mentors and inservice educators have a role to play in helping novice nurses become proficient in making judgments.

Strategies that educators can use to move nurses along the path to becoming expert decision makers include techniques for enhancing discrimination across observations and events, judicious questioning which helps the learner establish relationships between events, simulations, ward rounds, and buddying with a clinical mentor. These have all been suggested as ways in which the acquisition of decision making skills can be enhanced so that nursing theory can be translated into practice theory in the clinical situation. It must be recognized that an expert cannot be produced in the classroom, for it is the melding of theory with experience that produces the expert. Conversely, a nurse who does not have a sound knowledge base, and who continues to rely on rules and regulations in the work setting, may become highly skilled in the technological sense but will never become a truly "expert nurse."

REFERENCES

Benner P. (1984) *From Novice to Expert.* Addison-Wesley, Menlo Park.

Bulechak G.M. & McCloskey J.C. (1986) *Nursing Interventions: Tratment for Nursing Diagnoses.* Saunders, Philadelphia.

Clark J. (1982) Development of models and theories on the concept of nursing. *Journal of Advanced Nursing* **7**, 129-134.

Conant L.M. (1986) Closing the practice theory gap. In *Perspectives on Theory Development* (Nicoll L.H. ed.), Little, Brown & Co., Toronto, pp. 419-423.

Fawcett J. (1984) *Analysis and Evaluation of Conceptual Models of Nursing*. F.A. Davis, Philadelphia.

Field P.A. (1983) An ethnography: four public health nurses' perspectives of nursing. *Journal of Advanced Nursing* **8**, 3-12.

Fry V.S. (1953) The creative approach to nursing. *American Journal of Nursing* **53**, 301-302.

Henderson V. (1982) The nursing process—is the title right? *Journal of Advanced Nursing* **7**, 103-116.

Hoon E. (1986) Game playing: a way to look at nursing models. *Journal of Advanced Nursing* **11**, 421-428.

Hurley M. (1986) *Classification of Nursing Diagnoses*. C.V. Mosby, St. Louis.

Kuhn T.S. (1970) *The Structure of Scientific Revolution*. University of Chiciago Press, Chicago.

Neuman B. (1980) The Betty Neuman health care systems model: a total person approach to patient problems. In *Conceptual Models for Nursing Practice*, 2nd edn (Riehl J.P. & Roy C. eds), Appleton-Century-Crofts, New York.

Orem D.E. (1980) *Nursing: Concepts of Practice*, 2nd edn. McGraw-Hill, New York.

Polyani M. (1962) *Personal Knowledge*. Routledge and Keegan Paul, London.

Roy C. (1976) *Introduction to Nursing: An Adaptation Model*. Prentice-Hall, Englewood Cliffs.

Ziegler S.M., Vaughn-Wroble B.C. & Eielen J.A. (1986) *Nursing Process, Nursing Diagnosis, Nursing Knowledge: Avenues to Autonomy*. Appleton-Century-Crofts, New York.

The National Center for Nursing Research: Challenges and initiatives

ADA SUE HINSHAW, RN, PhD, FAAN

THE NATIONAL CENTER FOR Nursing Research (NCNR), through its extramural programs, focuses on the promotion of excellence in science for the discipline and facilitation of a national research environment. Excellence in science has been a hallmark of nursing's research programs, with an emphasis on scientific rigor merged with societal relevance. The NCNR is committed to continuing and strengthening this tradition. Nurturing the development of a strong national environment for the support of nursing research and the profession's scientists is critical to the generation and testing of accurate, rich, and relevant information from which to guide nursing practice.

A series of program initiatives have been formulated for NCNR. These include the development of a National Nursing Research Agenda (NNRA), a career trajectory program in research training and career development, a models for collaboration program for research support and research training, an international program and an intramural program. The program initiatives for NCNR reflect the focus on scientific excellence and several identified challenges confronting the discipline's research endeavors.

The challenges ahead

Several challenges must be confronted if the nursing discipline is to actualize the potential of the current research programs and fulfill the promise of its evolving nursing science base. These major challenges include the delineation of priorities for nursing research, the pursuit of strategies that will allow for the development of depth in our science, and the dissemination and use of the evolving body of research findings.

Nursing research priorities. The need to target certain high-priority health care concerns of society for the discipline's scientific endeavors would allow focusing a portion of nursing resources on relevant areas in which the profession is judged to have the strongest influence. Over time, the targeting of specific research priority areas will also deepen the nursing science base in the targeted substantive fields. Given the breadth of nursing research, if the profession wishes to be societally relevant as well as build excellence in science, both the scientific endeavors and resources need to be partially focused on major areas of research priorities determined by the nursing scientific community.

Depth in nursing science. A number of strategies can be used to systematically develop depth in nursing science. These strategies include the development of individual investigator programs, promotion of critical masses of scientists working in the same or similar substantive areas of study, and the concept of research training as a career trajectory.

Individual investigator programs. Research should be thought of as a program of study by nurse scientists. Nursing history indicates that a shotgun approach was used early in the science. A research program is a continuing line of study consisting of multiple interlocking investigations that build on each other. The issue being raised is that nurse investigators must look at research programs in phases or stages, and at each research program as a number of research investigations. As one phase of an investigation is finished, it is wise to be ready to plan and implement the next stage. The strength of this particular mode of thinking for the development of nursing science is in the ability of individuals to build on their prior work, to substantiate and replicate that work, and to add other aspects that are congruent with the central phenomenon and the evolving base of findings. In such a way, depth of knowledge is developed in a substantive area of study.

Critical masses of scientists. Another strategy for developing depth in nursing science is to begin to build a critical mass of investigators functioning in the same common area of research and pursuing a line of research in tandem, either within one site or across several sites. In this way, scientists are able to build on each other's work and to understand multiple findings from various perspectives in a substantive field of study. Many of the universities have built solid research scientific communities. It is now being recommended that one further step be taken and that subgroups be formed within in these communities in common areas of research. This would have implications for both the resources and strategies needed for funding as well as for the way in which faculty and predoctoral and postdoctoral students would be recruited into positions and programs (e.g., recruited partially on the basis of their research and identified areas of scientific expertise or interest).

Career trajectory for research training. Research training for the scientific role is a career commitment. It is important that nurse researchers commit themselves to a life-style of periodic retraining or education. No one understands better than finishing doctoral students that the earned doctorate is only the beginning of a research career, in terms of both the conduct of research and the continual fine tuning needed for research. Thus nurse scientists must give considerable thought to points in individual careers when additional research training is required, based on the current line of study or the proliferation of information in a field of investigation. To ease periodic reentry into the training mode, programs and awards must be developed, not only for postdoctoral study but also for career development study for midcareer and senior level scientists.

Dissemination and use. The process of disseminating and using information that has been generated and tested by nurse researchers is extremely important in the nursing profession. Both basic and clinical research programs are pursued because they can ultimately be used to improve patient care and guide practice.

This problem is complex because of the breadth of the research field and the diverse nature of the information. For example, dentistry has done an outstanding job of generating research on oral hygiene and disseminating that information to decrease dental caries and the incidence of actual oral disease. Dentistry has developed a number of strategies for marketing its information on health care of the mouth to both dentists and hygienic practitioners, as well as to consumers. However, nursing has an additional problem because of the breadth of the discipline's research and the diversity of the information that must be disseminated. Different diffusion and utilization strategies may be needed for different types of practitioners in various settings to whom the information must be targeted.

Further initiatives of the NCNR

The NCNR staff has advanced several initiatives to promote the growth and excellence of nursing science. These initiatives are intended to provide leadership in terms of research priorities and guide the allocation of federal resources for the profession's developing science.

National nursing research agenda. The objectives of the National Nursing Research Agenda include providing structure for selecting scientific opportunities and initiatives, promoting depth in developing a knowledge base for nursing practice, and providing direction for nursing research within the discipline. The research agenda encompasses several components: identification of major program areas of study for nursing research, development of program priorities, projection of resources needed to put the program priorities into practice, and specification of an evaluation and update plan for the growth and scientific advances of the program areas. NIH bureaus, institutes, and divisions (BIDS) are required to submit a five-year plan and annual review of program priorities to guide funding decisions for their programs. The national nursing research agenda will provide the guidance needed for the creation and implementation of such a five-year plan for the NCNR.

The national nursing research agenda, particularly the identification of research priorities, will be established in collaboration with the nursing scientific community. The process will be guided by a steering committee that will include representatives of the NCNR staff and NCNR advisory council members. A number of seasoned investigators in the discipline will be involved in the identification and consideration of priorities to guide the targeting of part of the federal resources used for research support and research training.

Research training trajectory programs. In response to the challenge of considering research training as a career commitment for nurse scientists, the National Center for Nursing Research will promote the ability of individual investigators to obtain initial and periodic research training and career development support. A number of National Research Service Award mechanisms and career development opportunities. These will include both individual and institutional predoctoral and postdoctoral opportunities as well as mid-career and senior scientist alternatives.

Increased collaboration with other disciplines. A number of strategies for promoting collaboration with other disciplines are being explored for both research support and research training. Several strategies, such as cooperative agreements co-funded with other institutes, have been used to encourage the co-funding of research projects with institutes such as the National Institute on Aging and the National Institute of Child Health and Development. An announcement has called for applications for postdoctoral research training with intramural programs in NIH. In addition, a career development award (i.e., clinical investigator award) has been suggested as a strategy for individual nurse scientists interested in working in the NIH General Clinical Research Centers with other disciplinary investigators. These are examples of strategies that can be made available to the nursing scientific community for collaborative research support or research training.

Intramural research program. An intramural research program will be a major initiative for the National Center for Nursing Research in the next several years. This intramural program will include both basic and clinical research, which could be actively conducted both at the Clinical Center and with other health care agencies. Generally the intramural research programs at NIH are either based in the intramural laboratories of the individual institutes or are part of the intramural clinical research primarily conducted at the Clinical Center. However, the National Center may also wish to conduct its intramural program in diverse health care settings such as the home health care environment, skilled nursing homes, community hospitals and public health care agencies. Thus, the intramural program may actually reflect a "without walls" organizational concept that would encourage investigations that could be conducted in different types of agencies and promote research on movement and outcomes for clients as they are discharged from one kind of care and admitted to another.

International programs. With the discipline's emphasis on the cultural aspects of nursing care and the influence of such factors on practice, an international program seems natural for the National Center for Nursing Research. Access to multiple populations from diverse cultures would allow for the generation and testing of nursing science from various perspectives. Interaction with colleagues from other countries would provide a rich context for the generation and dissemiantion of research issues....

Use of research based knowledge in clinical practice

Colleen J. Goode, RN, MS, CNAA; Marilyn K. Lovett, RN, BSN; Jo E. Hayes, RN, BSN; Lori A. Butcher, RN, BSN

In the following article, the authors describe two research utilization projects that used a knowledge-driven approach to nursing practice. The projects required nurses to identify and critique clinical research, to develop protocols for use in guiding clinical practice, and to evaluate the implementation of and patient outcomes associated with the protocols. The authors describe the institutional and individual commitments necessary to such projects. Although the article focuses on a small community hospital, the elements of the process of research utilization are universal in their application. Note: In this article, summaries (shown in bracketed italics) and excerpts (indicated by ellipses) condense extensive background information.

[At a time when most nurses working directly with patients do not use research findings in their work,[1-6] demands are increasing within and outside of nursing for the profession to demonstrate the scientific basis for its practice. The staff of our 42-bed acute care hospital in rural Iowa attempted to address this issue by initiating two projects. Our first obstacle was lack of research experience: no nurse researcher was on staff to serve as a resource person, and no staff nurse had any experience in reading, using, or critiquing research. We did have a nursing administrator with basic research knowledge and a keen interest in using research at the facility and a group of professional nurses willing to undertake the challenge of developing the projects.

First, we organized a research committee, whose main goal was to encourage the use of research-based knowledge in clinical practice. This committee reviewed previous work on the utilization of nuring research and relied on the work of the Conduct and Utilization of Research in Nursing (Curn) project, carried out in the mid-1970s under the auspices of the Michigan Nurses' Association.[7] Secondary goals included learning to read research reports, reviewing and evaluating their findings, and recommending ways to use the research at the hospital.

Next, we adopted Haller, Reynolds, and Horsley's [8]criteria for determining whether research can be used in practice:

- *need for replication to provide greater confidence in reliability and validity of findings*
- *examination of each study's scientific merit in terms of reliability, generality, and statistical significance*
- *determination of potential risk to patients.*

Finally, the committee established the main activities involved in using research in practice:

- *dentifying problems that occur in the clinical area*
- *providing the nurses with adequate knowledge to read research studies critically and understand their implications*
- *gathering useful and relevant information from the studies to solve the problems*
- *devising ways to transform the knowledge so that it can be used in the clinical setting*
- *defining the expected patient outcomes*

• providing the education and training needed to implement the practice change into the system

• evaluating and possibly modifying the new practice protocol.

Staff nurses selected clinical practice problems for study. Two examples of completed research utilization projects follow.]

Temperature study. We wanted our first research utilization project to be an aspect of patient care to which all of our nurses could relate. Directed by hospital policy, temperature measurements were taken twice daily and were yielding many low readings. Electronic thermometers had just been purchased. There was some concern about the basis of the low readings and this encouraged us to study our technique for temperature taking as the first project. As a result of review and evaluation of the research literature, we found substantial support for making the following changes in both policy and procedures.

1. Oral temperatures may be taken on all patients receiving oxygen by prongs.[9-11]

2. Rectal temperatures may be taken on the acute myocardial infarction (MI) patient if an oral temperature cannot be taken accurately. We learned that the repositioning technique is more critical in cardiac rate change than the stimulation of a rectal temperature probe.[12-15]

3. We now wait 15 minutes to take an oral temperature if the patient has just smoked or had a hot or cold drink. If the patient has been chewing gum we wait 3 minutes.[12] The time that our routine temperatures were taken was changed so that temperatures were not taken before oral care or food intake.

The committee learned from this project that just because "that is the way we've always done it" is not reason enough to explain our practice. Previous to this, we did not take oral temperatures on patients receiving oxygen and we had a policy forbidding taking rectal temperatures on coronary care unit patients. Several weeks after implementation of the research finding for temperature taking, an audit of 25 charts revealed that we were indeed observing higher morning temperatures and probably more accurate readings. We continue to monitor both temperature taking techniques and temperature reading by time of day.

Breastfeeding study. The need for a standardized teaching program on breastfeeding was perceived when, on follow-up visits, mothers expressed exasperation because "one nurse told me one thing, another nurse told me something else, and the doctor told me the exact opposite."

We had nurses who had breastfed their own babies and who had helpful ideas and good intentions; and we had physicians who tried their best to be of assistance but who were not always knowledgeable about current literature on breastfeeding. All staff needed assistance with a step-by-step program based on current research on breastfeeding.

To develop the teaching program (Figure 1), we used three textbooks, *The Womanly Art of Breastfeeding,*[16] *Nursing Your Baby,*[17] and *A Practical Guide to Breastfeeding,*[18] to bring committee members up to date on current ideas regarding breastfeeding. A review of current research on breastfeeding was the next step. A bibliographic computer search was completed and articles were selected and reviewed by the nursing administrator and one of the committee members who worked in the obstetric unit and had knowledge about breastfeeding. Appropriate research articles were then distributed to committee members to read and critique. Through group discussion, information concerning breastfeeding was compiled and used to develop a standardized teaching program on breastfeeding.

Among the reports of research, Cohen[19] demonstrated the positive effect that a postpartum teaching session about breastfeeding can have on the subsequent use of milk supplements and duration of breastfeeding. In 1976, Johnson...[identified] that successful

FIGURE 1. **Excerpt from teaching protocol**

TEACHING CRITERIA	DATE & INITIAL	PATIENT UNDER-STANDING	EXPLANATION GIVEN TO PATIENT
Physiology of lactation			Milk is produced in response to baby's sucking, the more he suckles, the more milk you produce.
Let down reflex			Stimulated by sucking, felt as a light or strong tingling in breasts about a minute after baby starts sucking. It's caused by oxytocin hormone, causing milk ducts to contract and eject milk so it's available to baby. Milk may run from opposite breast. Initially it may happen even between feedings or if you just think of your baby or hear him or another cry. It may take until you get home to become established. Occasionally mother never feels this let down but still can nurse successfully.
Colostrum			Present in last weeks of pregnancy. Very important for immunologic properties. 7% glucose solution—acts as a laxative to rid baby of initial meconium and bilirubin—lowering jaundice. Small quantity—great quality. Baby is born with water surplus and colostrum is sufficient until milk comes in.

breastfeeding at 1 hour of age was an important factor in overall success...[and] demonstrated the importance of the nurse's role in the breastfeeding experience.[20]

A frequent point of conflict has always been "how long should a breastfeed last?" A 1980 study by that title and six other studies on the subject led to the recommendation for unlimited suckling and illustrated the positive role frequent suckling plays in diminishing nipple soreness, diminishing incidence of engorgement, and decreased milk supply — all factors that contribute to unsuccessful breastfeeding experiences.[21-27]

Other problems frequently discussed by nursing and medical staff included those experienced by the working breastfeeding mother and management of jaundice occurring in the breastfed infant. Recent studies in both areas, as well as studies on biologic benefits of human milk, suggested new approaches to management.[21, 28-31]

By following the teaching program, all breastfeeding mothers were given the same information by all obstetric nurses. Follow-up telephone interviews with patients have indicated that mothers who participated in the teaching program were knowledgeable about breastfeeding and that they perceived the teaching they received to be helpful....

A systems theory model for research utilization

Based on our experience, systems theory assisted us in depicting the process we used in the knowledge-driven approach to nursing practice. Theorizing that all systems interact with their environment in the form of input, transformation, and feedback,[32] the model depicts an open system with interaction between

FIGURE 2. A system theory model for using new research-based knowledge

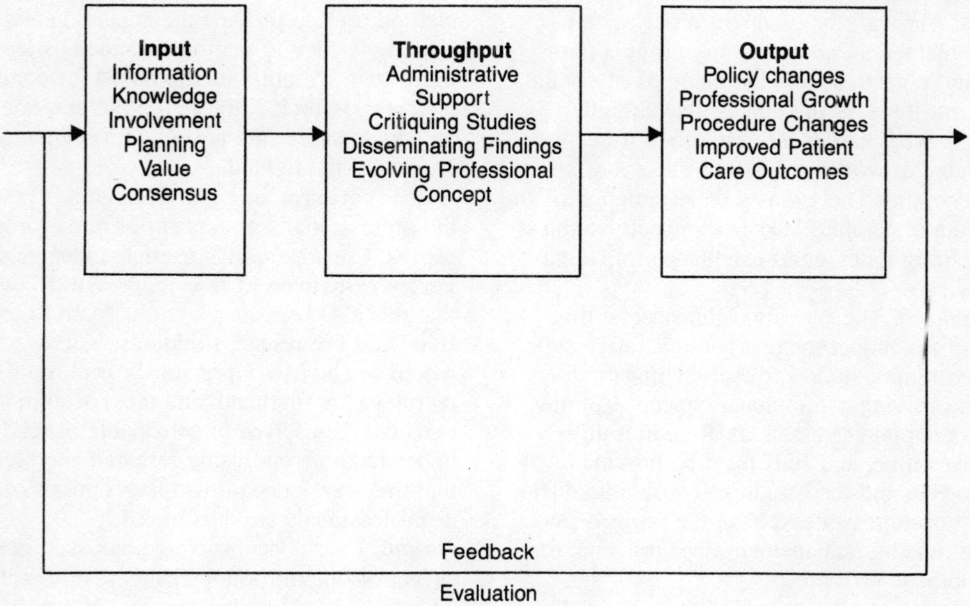

the system and the environment. Parts of the system are always in the process of adjusting to the changes taking place as the system receives energy from the environment, transforms the energy into usable form, and discharges transformed energy back into the environment (Figure 2).

The model contains a number of concepts that need to be considered and clarified if an organization is planning to use research based knowledge in clinical practice.

Input. Six concepts were considered to be part of input: information, knowledge, involvement, planning, value, and consensus. Input information was supplied to the staff through a literature search that identified pertinent reports of research. Three new journals were added to the hospital periodical subscription file: *Nursing Research, Research In Nursing and Health,* and *Advances in Nursing Science*. The staff already had...*The Journal of Nursing Administration, Nursing Management, Nursing Outlook, The American Journal of Nursing, Nursing, Nursing Administration Quarterly, The American Journal of Maternal Child Nursing, Birth,* and *Critical Care Nurse*. Because there is no University Library available in our rural setting, by using the State Library of Iowa and interlibrary loan services, we were able to obtain most of the research reports we needed. Knowledge was gained through reading and discussion, a practice that produced more and more involvement from committee members. Mutual sentiments and beliefs about the need for a research utilization project began to emerge. Nurses often discussed the need to deliver "quality" care. Research utilization was seen as a key to quality in the practice of nursing. A consensus evolved that we were engaged in important worthwhile work. Planning was essential to ensure success of the project. Through the planning process, committee members understood the group's purpose and objectives and the methods of obtaining them. Because the nurses placed high value on what they were doing they were stimulated to work hard and to make the project successful. There was a belief among Committee members that research utilization would bring a degree of excellence to patient care....

Throughput. The concepts addressed at this stage of the model include administrative support, critiquing studies, disseminating findings, and an evolving professional concept. Administrative support is essential. Research utilization takes time, and staff must be provided time to find and read studies. It would be difficult if not impossible to have the project succeed if nursing management does not support development activities.

Because not *all* nursing research is good research and not all research findings are applicable to the small rural acute care hospital, critiquing reports of research is a major function of the research utilization committee. The committee is attuned to the fact that changes cannot be based on the results of one study, with one small sample. The committee reviews and discusses findings from current research and makes recommendations regarding the quality of the research and its use of the findings. The committee also encourages other staff members to bring research studies to the committee's attention. In our experience new BSN graduates who have some research knowledge are the first to do just that.

A monthly staff inservice meeting is the channel through which research findings are disseminated and changes are planned and communicated. One committee member takes the responsibility for presenting each research utilization project at an inservice meeting. The committee member gives a summary and critique of each study used to support the utilization project. The inservice meeting is the method used to provide the education and training needed to get the practice change into the system. Another method used for communicating research is through a bulletin board on which studies are posted with segments of the study highlighted.

It is not surprising that through this process the professional self-concept of nurses improves. Conway speaks to such a change when nurses participate in research.[33] We believe that this also happens as nurses learn to understand and use research findings. Nurses for whom research was previously irrelevant see its relevancy firsthand, and those who did not perceive themselves to be capable of reading, understanding, and using research soon learn that they can indeed do so. Perceptions of self as professionals are thus raised.

Output. Four concepts were addressed as an aspect of output: policy changes, professional growth, procedure changes, and improved patient outcomes. As research is replicated and findings validated the scientific basis of practice emerges, obviating policies and procedures governing patients and delivery of nursing care based on tradition rather than on empirical evidence. As we learn more from research and use of research findings, we discover that tradition alone is not adequate to explain our practice. In some cases our range of interventions [is] increased or more finely defined. The research process thus becomes a method to obtain new knowledge or validate old knowledge. Evaluation to determine if patient care outcomes have improved involves both the process and outcome components. In terms of process, the committee evaluates to ensure that the innovation has been implemented accurately. The outcome component involves collecting and analyzing data to determine if the predicted outcomes did in fact occur. In any event the quality of nursing care is improved. Nurses involved in research utilization grow professionally. The research skills of registered nurses are enhanced as they work on these projects. Staff nurses develop and maintain a seriousness about research and lose many of their fears. As critical reading and thinking skills develop, nurses are motivated to higher levels of thinking. Finally, involvement in research is considered an expectation of the practicing professional nurse.

Feedback. An ongoing process of evaluation is necessary to determine whether the policies and procedural changes improved patient care outcomes. Feedback from peers and colleagues is essential. Moreover, to ensure that the change or transformation has not extended beyond the limits of the research base, we evaluate the effects of the innovation once a clinical protocol has been implemented [4] through audit studies and patient interviews.

Conclusion

The success of research utilization depends on organizational cooperation as well as the skills and motivation of nursing staff members. [34] Nursing in clinical settings needs a practical, systematic approach to the process of research utilization. Only then can we hope to effect research-driven change to our practice.

In today's technological world we talk about computers and programs that are "user friendly," meaning easy to use. We would like to see research that is "user ready," meaning already critiqued by experts and found to be "good" research and ready for use. As a committee, it would then be our responsibility to study the research to understand its implications and to determine if it fits our clinical setting. Perhaps more nurses would become involved in research utilization if this were accomplished.

As we carry out more research utilization projects, we acknowledge that we continue to increase our depth of knowledge. We are in our fifth year of work and the number of utilization projects [is] increasing. The audit/research committee has become a prestigious committee within our organization because of the important work of its members. Staff nurses volunteer to serve on this committee; however, we are reluctant to change the membership because of the amount of knowledge required of committee members and the amount of time it takes to acquire this knowledge.

We hope this article encourages nurses to begin research utilization projects. There is nothing more rewarding than instituting a protocol based upon research that improves patient outcomes....

REFERENCES

1. Crane J. Using research in practice-research utilization: theoretical perspectives. West J Nurs Res 1985;7(2):261-267.

2. Kirchoff KT. Using research in practice: teaching research utilization. West J Nurs Res 1984;6(2):265-267.

3. Horsely J. Using research in practice: the current context. West J Nurs Res 1985;7(1):135-139.

4. Stetler CB. Research utilization: defining the concept. Image 1985;17(2):40-44.

5. Duffy ME. Research in practice: the time has come. Nursing and Health Care 1985;6(3):127.

6. Duffy ME. Research utilization: what's it all about. Nursing and Health Care 1985;6(9):474-475.

7. Horsely J, Crane J. Using research to improve nursing practice: a guide. New York: Grune & Stratton, 1983.

8. Haller KB, Reynolds MA, Horsley J. Developing research based innovation protocols: process, criteria, and issues. Res Nurs Health 1979;2:45-51.

9. Grass S. Thermometer sites and oxygen. Am J Nurs 1974;74(10):1862-1864.

10. Levy F. The effect of oxygen inhalation on oral temperatures. Nurs Res 1982;31(3):150-152. 10. Nichols GA, Kucha DH. Oral measurements. Am J Nurs 1972;72(6):1091-1094.

11. Nichols GA, Kucha DH. Oral measurements. Am J Nurs 1972; 72(6):1091-1094.

12. Blainey CG. Site selection in taking body temperature. Am J Nurs 1984;74(10):1859-1861.

13. Gruber PA. Changes in cardiac rate associated with the use of the rectal thermometer in the patient with acute myocardial infarction. Heart and Lung 1974;3(2):288-292.

14. Mathewson M. Nursing rule: rectal temperatures should not be taken on a patient with coronary disease. Crit Care Nurse 1983;3(1):49.

15. McNeal GJ: Rectal temperatures in the patient with an acute myocardial infaction. Image 1978;10(1):18-23.

16. The womanly art of breastfeeding. Franklin Park, Illinois: LeLeche League International, 1981.

17. Pryor K. Nursing your baby. New York: Harper & Row, 1973.

18. Riordon, J. A practical guide to breastfeeding. St. Louis: CV Mosby, 1983.

19. Cohen SA. Postpartum teaching and subsequent use of milk supplements. Birth and the Family Journal 1980;7(3):163-167.

20. Johnson NW. Breastfeeding at one hour of age. Am J Maternal Child Nurs 1976;1:12-16.

21. Carvalho M, Klaus MH, Merkatz RB. Frequency of breastfeeding and serum bilirubin concentration, Am J Dis Child 1982;136: 737-738.

22. Carvalho M, Robertson S, Friedman A, Klaus M. Effect of frequent breastfeeding on early milk production and infant weight gain. Pediatrics 1983;72(3):307-311.

23. Cerutti ER. The management of breastfeeding. Birth and the Family Jounral 1981;8(4):251-256.

24. Egli GE, Egli NS, Newton M. The influence of the number of breastfeedings on milk production. Pediatrics 1961;27:315-317.

25. Howie PW, Houston MS, Cook A, Smart L, McArdle T, McNeilly AS. How long should a breastfeed last. Early Human Development 1981;5:71-77.

26. L'Esperance CM. Pain or pleasure: the dilemma of early breastfeeding. Birth and the Family Journal 1980;7(1):21-26.

27. Slaven S, Harvey D. Unlimited suckling time improves breastfeeding. Lancet 1981;1:392-393.

28. Carvalho M, Hall M, Harvey D. Effects of water supplementation on physiological jaundice in breastfed babies. Arch Dis Child 1981;56:568-569.

29. Maisels MJ. Breastfeeding and jaundice. Birth and the Family Journal 1981;8(4):245-249.

30. Auerbach, KG. Employed breastfeeding mothers: problems they encounter. Birth 1984;11(1):17-20.

31. Mata, L. Breastfeeding: main promoter of infant health.Am J Clin Nutr 31:2058-2065.

32. Richl JP, Roy C. Conceptual models for nursing practice. New York: Appleton-Century-Crofts, 1980.

33. Conway ME. Clinical research; instrument for change. J Nurse Adm 1978;8(12):27-32.

34. Krone KP, Loomis ME. Developing practice relevant research: a model that worked. J Nurs Adm 1982;12(4):38-41.

SECTION TWO

Contemporary nursing and health care

Section two examines ways in which economic forces have dramatically altered contemporary nursing and health care and addresses the challenges to nursing that technological advancement and increasing competition among health care providers may bring.

Under the Prospective Payment System (PPS) instituted in 1983, hospitals are reimbursed for services based on the client's diagnosis, age, and disease complications (a prospective approach). Before 1983, fees were not tied so closely to a specific diagnosis but to all aspects of care (a retrospective approach). Using reimbursement schedules based on categories of illness (known as Diagnostic Related Groups, or DRGs) and average costs per category, the PPS has significantly influenced client care and the way nurses view themselves within the health care system.

In their two-part article, "Magnet Hospitals Talk About the Impact of DRGs on Nursing Care," Kramer and Schmalenberg reveal how DRGs have affected clients, nurses, and the nursing profession. The authors analyze the advantages and disadvantages that have resulted from the PPS, including early client discharge, increased cost consciousness by hospital personnel, improved self-esteem among nurses that contrasts with growing job dissatisfaction, and staff reductions — issues of vital concern to all nurses. Clearly, nursing students and practicing nurses should become familiar with major aspects of health care financing if they want to understand and influence a significant aspect of their careers.

"A Challenge for the Future" discusses the impact of the use of nursing diagnoses on nursing decisions and client care. This system of classifying the assessments that guide and direct nursing actions has become an integral part of nursing practice in the past two decades. In their article, Maas and Hardy note the importance of nurses' involvement in validating and refining diagnostic categories to identify appropriate client outcomes and to assess the quality of care that nurses provide.

In "Computer-Assisted Care in Nursing: Computers at the Bedside," van Bemmel reveals how computers are increasingly used for diagnosing clients' conditions and monitoring their progress. The author suggests that nurses do not need to fear using computers; on the contrary, nurses are successfully using much of today's computer technology in day-to-day nursing activities. The article explores not only the technology but also the implications of computer use for the caring profession.

Magnet hospitals talk about the impact of DRGs on nursing care — part I

MARLENE KRAMER, RN, PhD; CLAUDIA SCHMALENBERG, RN, MSN

In 1982, the American Academy of Nursing conducted a nationwide survey to locate hospitals that had been particularly successful in attracting and retaining qualified nurses.[1] The survey identified 41 "Magnet Hospitals" with predominantly professional nursing staffs (with at least 85% of all budgeted RN positions filled), high patient occupancy rates, and well-educated nursing leadership. To determine the impact of Diagnostic Related Groups (DRGs) on nursing care, an in-depth study of 16 of these hospitals was begun in the fall of 1985. More than 1,600 nurses at all levels within the nursing departments were interviewed.

In the following article, the authors review prospective payment legislation that led to the creation of DRGs in 1983, outline the potential effects of DRGs as predicted at that time, and reveal the initial results of the 1985-1986 study, including the actual effects of DRGs on patient outcomes. The impact of DRGs on nurses and nursing departments is covered in Part II. Note: In this article, summaries (shown in bracketed italics) and excerpts (indicated by ellipses) condense extensive background information.

"DRGs CREATED AND SANCTIONED a business mind about health care." This major effect, noted by one of the Associate Directors of Nursing interviewed in this study, was echoed by hospital nursing staff at all levels. It is this "business mind" which has led to a shift in emphasis for many nursing departments — a shift from a goal-driven concept of nursing services to a resource-driven model; a shift from "quality at all costs" to "How much quality can be given with the resources available?" Whether the prospective payment system of the future will be a continuation of DRGs or a shift to a total capitation system, the revolutionary changes brought about by prospective cost payment demand that we assess the effects of Prospective Payment Systems (PPS) on nursing care and nursing delivery systems *now*. To what extent are nurses at all levels feeling the impact of Prospective Payment Systems? To what extent are they making the shift to a "business mind"?...

Prospective payment legislation

The Tax Equity and Fiscal Responsibility Act and the Omnibus Reconciliation Act of 1982 were the beginnings of sweeping changes in the health care field. While TEFRA provided for specific cost-cutting measures in Medicare and Medicaid, perhaps the single most significant change was the mandate for the development of a prospective payment proposal. By 1983, the mandate was realized, with the selection of DRGs as the prospective payment methodology, and the amending of the Social Security Act to provide for prospective payment for Medicare inpatient services.

PPS went into effect as of October 1, 1983. The system provided for:

1. Transition to prospective payment with "blended" rates for the first three years, with the fourth year being 100 percent, based on a national DRG rate. Regional wage adjustments, urban-rural designation, and teaching versus non-teaching institutions would account for variation in the national rate.

2. DRG rates [to be] applied to Medicare patients only, with no co-payment or deductibles charged beyond what was permitted by law. Cost and length of stay outliers would be reviewed for reimbursement.

3. Capital costs to be reimbursed on a reasonable cost basis for the first three years, with prospective payment beginning October 1, 1986.

4. Direct and indirect teaching costs [to be] excluded from prospective payments related to DRGs and separate arrangements provided for handling these costs.

5. Hospitals...to contract with a Professional Review Organization (PRO) for the review of quality of care, appropriateness of admissions, and appropriateness of care to designated outliers.

6. Psychiatric, long-term care, children's and rehabilitation hospitals (and distinct units) [to be] excluded from DRG payment and [to] continue on a cost system.

7. [Limitations to] the reimbursement of hospital-based physicians...[3-5.]

It was predicted that these 1982-83 legislated changes would have profound effects on hospitals, nursing, and health care within a very short period of time. The effects were expected to alter both financial and practice aspects of care. For many hospitals, the PPS changes and corresponding effects would occur before hospitals had recovered from the economic conditions of 1981, during which occupancy rates had plummeted. For other hospitals, notably those in the "oil company" states, the compounding effects of PPS and economic recession would be delayed until 1984-86. To understand better the impact of PPS on nursing and health care, it is wise to examine the DRG system for classification of patients, which is the basis for PPS.

Diagnostic Related Groups (DRGs) is a classification system with 23 major diagnostic categories and 467 subdiagnoses. The system organizes patients into groups based on homogeneity of resource consumption. The major factor underlying the use of resources in this system is length of stay of the patient. Each patient is assigned a DRG upon discharge from the hospital. The discharge summary serves as the basis forclassifying patients according to the following major variables: use of the operating room; discharge diagnosis; age; existence of complications or significant comorbidities; and length of stay. Once the DRG is assigned, the hospital receives the reimbursement set for that DRG. If a patient exceeds the expected length of stay or is within the length of stay but exceeds cost, he becomes defined as an outlier and is reviewed by the PRO for reimbursement.

PPS is expected to provide positive incentive to hospitals to cut costs. With this system, if patients are discharged with a decreased length of stay (when compared to means established through DRG data), the hospital profits. However, if patients have long stays and overutilize services and resources, the hospital is expected to absorb the losses. With most services included under DRG payment, the system is expected to decrease the use of unnecessary tests and services to patients, thus decreasing overall costs.

While DRGs initially applied only to Medicare, it has been stated that "We want to prospectively price out only Medicare services but eventually Medicaid and all personal health care services regardless of provider or setting."[2] It is expected that eventually the DRG system of PPS will directly or indirectly affect all medical and health care practices.

Various studies have been done to ascertain whether DRG reimbursement rates reflect nursing costs.[6-11] Findings indicate that for some DRGs, the patient's DRG classification is *not* an adequate measure for determining, assigning, or allocating nursing costs within the institution. The literature warns that hospitals that do not track actual nursing costs risk unanticipated cost overruns. New Jersey led the way in the development and testing of Relative Intensity Measure (RIMs), a method designed to incorporate a sensitivity to nursing resource use in the DRG payment mechanism. RIMs, however, have been roundly criticized for methodological failures and for the assumption that care delivered equals care required.[12-13] While the jury is still out on these two major approaches, virtually all hospital nursing departments have or are instituting some method of classification or acuity system to determine nursing costs and to describe and/or predict utilization of nursing resources.

Predicted effects of DRGs and PPS

[The] effects...anticipated as a result of the movement to prospective payment...included the following:

1. There was immediate concern about the financial viability of hospitals which cared for large percentages of the Medicare and Medicaid populations.

2. Hospitals were expected to examine their programs and admission policies and to shift to those patients and programs which spelled greater profitability.

3. Since length of stay would be the major consideration in profit and loss, there was concern about patients being discharged before they were ready.

4. Since hospitals would attempt to shorten length of patient stay, the volume and complexity of case-mix would increase, not only in hospitals but in home health agencies and extended care facilities as well.

5. The necessity of decreasing operating costs would force examination of supply and manpower expenditures. Quality of care was viewed with anxiety! As hospitals cut costs, labor-intensive departments such as nursing would suffer massive reductions in staff.

6. There would be increased emphasis on outpatient treatment and teaching programs.

7. Increase in competition between hospitals for the "profitable" patient would occur.

8. While DRGs were questioned as the appropriate method for the PPS by many, nursing administrators doubted the ability of DRGs to predict the intensity of nursing care.

9. Everyone, especially third party payors, expressed concern about massive cost shifting. As a result of cost shifting, the end result of DRGs would be to increase health care costs for everyone else. Ultimately this would result in having more individuals who could not afford or could not gain access care.

10. Changes in the character of the nursing work force were predicted, with two quite different pictures emerging. One scenario called for the demise of primary nursing because of the high cost of a complete or high-ratio RN staff. There would be an increased use of ancillary workers, thus further eroding quality care. Retention and recruitment of professional nurse staff would become difficult, due to decreased satisfaction in the work place. The other scenario called for marked shifts to an all-RN staff, thus augmenting the practice of primary nursing. There would be a corresponding decreased utilization of non-professional staff (LVN and nurse aide), because of increasing "down" time with more acutely ill patients. Registered nurse job satisfaction would increase because of more direct nurse involvement in patient care and less time spent supervising non-professional workers.

11. There was much concern as to the adequacy of the recording and coding systems, since accurate documentation and accurate assigning of DRGs to cases would be absolutely essential. Overall, the atmosphere of the health care world became charged with insecurity and anxiety.

Have the predicted effects of the new health care legislation come true? Which of these concerns materialized? And to what extent have practicing hospital nurses adopted a "business mind" or resource-driven models to accommodate these revolutionary changes in health care economics?...

[Results

The hospitals reported a reduction in the number of operating beds, from 6,454 in 1982 to 5,542 in 1985. The reduction was attributed largely to the closing of patient care units because of decreased occupancies in 15 of the 16 hospitals. Occupancy rates in 1982 ranged from 72% to 98%, with a median of 84%. By 1986, the range had dropped to 40% to 92%, with a median of 78%. Despite this decrease, the number of patients treated increased during the same period, with some nurses reporting that as many as three patients occupied the same bed in a 24-hour span. Thus, the decrease in occupancy rate resulted directly from a decrease in length of patient stay.

Although the nurses did not report any significant shift in the kinds of medical conditions for which patients were being hospitalized, they consistently validated the prediction of increased outpatient care and treatment. Patients who previously would have been admitted to the hospital for a procedure or surgery were instead being treated as outpatients. While favoring outpatient treatment when appropriate, the nurses usually expressed reservations about patients for whom outpatient care was perhaps unsafe and about hospitalized patients who were discharged early. Interestingly, although most nurses reported increased dissatisfaction with the quality of care they were providing, the patients at all 16 hospitals consistently indicated they were highly satisfied with the care they received.]

REFERENCES

1. McClure, Margaret *et al.*, *Magnet Hospitals*, (Kansas City, Missouri: American Nurses' Association, 1983).

2. Newman, Margaret and Sharon Autio, *Nursing in a Prospective Payment System Health Care Environment*, (University of Minnesota: School of Nursing, 1986).

3. Grimaldi, Paul L., "Regulations Proposed for Second PPS Year," *Nursing Management*, 15(9):60-62, 1984.

4. Maraldo, Pamela J., "The Challenge: Health Care in Crisis," in Shaffer, Franklin A. (Ed.), *DRGs: Changes and Challenges*, (New York: National League for Nursing, 1984), pp 9-14.

5. Shaffer, Franklin A., "DRGs: History and Overview," in Shaffer, Franklin A. (Ed.), *DRGs: Changes and Challenges*, (New York: National League for Nursing, 1984), pp 15-34.

6. Franz, Julie, "Challenge for Nursing: Hiking Productivity without Lowering Quality of Care," *Modern Health Care*, September 1984, pp. 60-64.

7. Mowry, Mychelle and Ralph Korpmann, "Do DRG Reimbursement Rates Reflect Nursing Costs?," *JONA*, 15(7,8): 29-35, 1985.

8. Piper, L.R., "Accounting for Nursing Functions in DRGs," *Nursing Management*, 14:46-48, 1983.

9. Reschak, Gary *et al.*, "Accounting for Nursing Costs by DRG," *JONA*, 15(9): 15-20, 1985.

10. Schaefers, Vicki, "A Cost Allocation Method for Nursing," in Shaffer, Franklin A. (Ed.), *Costing Out Nursing: Pricing Our Product*, (New York: National League for Nursing, 1985), pp. 69-84.

11. Urosevich, Patti, "How Nurses are Learning to Live with DRGs," *Nursing Life*, 4(2):64-66, 1984.

12. Grimaldi, Paul L. and Julie A. Micheletti, "A Defense of the RIMs Critique—RIMs Reliability and Value," *Nursing Management*, (14):40-41, 1982.

13. Grimaldi, Paul L. and Julie A. Micheletti, "RIMs and the Cost of Nursing Care," *Nursing Management*, 13:12-22, 1982.

Magnet hospitals talk about the impact of DRGs on nursing care — part II

MARLENE KRAMER, RN, PhD; CLAUDIA SCHMALENBERG, RN, MSN

The following article continues the discussion of the 1985-1986 Magnet Hospitals study described in Part I. In Part II, the authors reveal how nurses and nursing departments have been affected by DRGs. Summaries (shown in bracketed italics) and excerpts (indicated by ellipses) condense extensive background information.

[NURSES AT ALL LEVELS within the profession reported seven primary effects of DRGs:

Increased cost consciousness. *Nurses became involved in explaining costs to patients, a role that had been assumed entirely by the business office. Some hospitals even provided nurses with specific classes on how to do this. Most nurses indicated they were still somewhat uncomfortable with this new role, primarily because of their inexperience.*

Increased emphasis on documentation. *Clear, concise, and complete documentation of the patient's condition, treatments used, and the patient's response to those treatments became more critical. Although nurses understood the value of such documentation, many expressed frustration at being "tied up with paperwork" and having less time to spend directly on caring for their patients. The most common complaint — and the most vehement — involved written nursing care plans. The nurses did not object to planning patient care or communicating the plan orally to other nurses, but they strongly objected to the "drudgery, repetition, and time-consuming writing out of a plan of care."*

Decreased quality, quantity, and availability of supplies. *Lower inventories on the units caused delays in getting needed supplies for patient care.*

Increased specialization. *As hospitals reorganized units around specific patient problems to become more cost-effective, nurses became more specialized in their knowledge. Many hospitals provided programs for certification of nurses in their new specialty. With the increased knowledge came increased autonomy for decision making and new confidence in and respect for one another.*

Increased job dissatisfaction. *Ironically, at a time when their knowledge and confidence were growing and their role was clearly becoming more important, most nurses perceived a decrease in the quality of care they were providing; this perception tended to lessen the satisfaction they took from their work. With a greater emphasis on outpatient treatments and early discharge, the nurses usually saw the patient only at his worst; they seldom saw the fruits of their labor — the patient getting well.*

Increased value of teaching and discharge planning. *With briefer hospital stays, patient and family teaching became more critical to the patient and more difficult for the nurse. Nearly 50% of all preoperative patients were being admitted the morning of surgery, making it difficult to prepare them properly. As one nurse said, "Oftentimes we are teaching the patient and his family as the patient goes out the door." Another stated, "I've given up teaching the patient; you have to concentrate on the family. The patient simply isn't conscious long enough or ready to learn while he is here."*

Staff reductions. *The decreased occupancy*

rates (discussed in Part I of this article) led to staff reductions, accomplished primarily by terminating or reassigning nursing assistants and LPNs and by reducing or eliminating evening and night supervisors and assistant or clinical directors. Additionally, many staff members who resigned or retired were not replaced. Layoffs of RNs occurred at only 2 of the 16 hospitals. Staff reductions and reassignments led to the breakup of well-established working teams and caused a severe or moderate degree of job insecurity among nurses at 6 of the 16 hospitals.

Effects on nursing departments

Most of the nursing departments at the Magnet Hospitals reported significant changes in the following areas:

Decentralization. *In 10 of the 16 hospitals, the supervisory or assistant director level was eliminated, with the head nurse being elevated either officially or by default. Eliminating one or more levels in the organization increased decentralization of responsibility and decision making.*

Staffing patterns. *Because of decreased occupancy rates and wider fluctuations in the patient census, most hospitals increased the number of part-time staff, the number of in-house float nurses, or both; these measures usually resulted in a loss of work group cohesiveness. All hospitals also noted a movement toward all-RN staffing despite — or perhaps because of — the need to cut costs.*

Nursing care delivery systems. *At the time of the 1982 Magnet Hospital study, the predominant delivery system was Primary Nursing (characterized by case method of assignment, caregiver to caregiver reports, decentralized decision making, 24-hour accountability, and nurse-patient continuity). By 1986, the dominant system was either 8-hour Total Patient Care or a variation of the "modified team" approach. The new systems, for the most part, still incorporated the first three characteristics, but 24-hour accountability was no longer a factor in 14 of the 16 hospitals and nurse-patient continuity was virtually nonexistent. Shortened length of stays, increased use of part-time staff, and voluntary or mandatory furloughs on low-census days disrupted continuity of care. "How can we practice Primary Nursing," the nurses asked, "when neither the patient nor the nurse is present for several continuous days?"]*

Conclusions and discussion

This follow-up of the 1982 Magnet Hospital study was designed to get an answer to the question, "What impacts have PPS and DRGs had on hospital nurses and nursing care?" Magnet Hospitals were chosen to obtain the answer because they are perceived generally as being among the leading hospital nursing departments in the country, and because some comparative data prior to PPS were available. With or without the coexisting economic conditions, PPS seems to have had it greatest impact in the following areas:

1. While nursing and patient care may still be of the very highest quality (and Patient Satisfaction questionnaires would seem to validate that this is so), nurses don't *feel* as good about the quality of care that they are giving now because they don't *see* patients getting well.

Undoubtedly, this is a problem that is not going to go away and must be dealt with. Many nurses expressed the concern that it was all right if *they* did not actually nurse the patient back to a higher level of wellness, but they wanted to be assured that someone who was competent did so. Three of the Magnet Hospitals studied had in operation programs specifically aimed at dealing with this problem. One had instituted a decentralized home care program in which the staff nurse, in the role of Case Manager, worked directly with the hospital-employed home care nurses in seeing to it that the patient continued with the home care needed. Another hospital had a separate department of Continuity of Care whose Clinical Nurse Specialists worked with the primary nurses on the unit in planning and delivering care to patients in their homes. The third hospital had a highly effective and operative primary nursing system wherein the primary nurses directly planned and made arrangements for the continued post-discharge care of their patients. Alleviating the anxiety of nurses for their patients after discharge is something that would do a great deal to reestablish for a nurse the job satisfaction that comes from seeing and knowing that her patient is doing well....

2. Nurses at all levels in the organization are becoming more cost conscious. They definitely have begun to develop a "business mind."

While nurses generally saw the necessity of developing a business mind, they were quite resentful of physicians (and to a lesser degree, other department personnel) who were not made to play by the same rules. In a few instances where nursing and hospital administration insisted that the medical staff work with nurses in cost containment, a much more collaborative relationship between nurse and physician was established. For the most part, nurses are looking forward anxiously to the day when medical price tags will be regulated; they believe that this will encourage physicians to cooperate more with cost containment measures.

3. ...More and more acute care hospitals are moving toward all-RN staffing. Whether this is possible or desirable is beyond the scope of this article. But...staff nurses, head nurses, and nurse administrators are [convinced] that...the most educated nurse is the one best able to provide the needed care and...the most cost effective. The use of nursing assistants, who assist the nurses rather than giving direct care to patients, seems to be an established practice that is continuing.

4. With the "sicker, quicker, and early discharge" phenomenon, some established nursing care practices, such as primary nursing and written, detailed nursing care plans, may need to be altered somewhat, without losing sight of the desired goal.

In all likelihood, staff nurses themselves will work out the delivery system that works best for them. Many are very clear about principles and about the type of care they wish to achieve — continuous, planned, comprehensive, and non-fragmented. Also, they are very flexible adapting daily to the system of care that best fits the resources available for that day. The kind of help needed will be assistance in holding on to the principles, while working within a resource-driven model, to effect the best delivery system possible.

Written, individualized nursing care plans were developed by nurse educators for the education of the student. For this purpose, they work quite well. They have never been embraced enthusiastically by the majority of nurses at the bedside. Part of this is because many nurses do not see the NEED for them; part is because they are not USED by other nurses; part is because in many instances they are not part of the permanent record; part may be because some nurses are not comfortable in doing them. But perhaps the biggest impediment to the written, detailed nursing care plan is a negative cost-benefit analysis. In a resource-driven market, the nurse practitioner has to decide: "Given the limited amount of time and the many patient care needs, what are the most important things for me to do with the time available?" The documentation aspect of nursing care planning is understood clearly and strongly ascribed to: it is the advanced writing out of the plan that brings resistance. It was quite evident in the present study that computerization of nursing care plans greatly overcomes resistance; in fully activated systems, care planning and documentation can be done simultaneously.

5. The PPS may change over time, but clearly the dollars for inpatient health care will continue to be restricted. Clinical research is needed to determine which treatment modalities are most beneficial, from a cost-benefit perspective.

Through the years, nurses have developed a variety of different treatment modalities for nursing problems such as decubiti or incontinence. As yet, there has been minimal research done to determine which methods produce the best results — let alone which methods produce the best results at the lowest cost. Scientific studies to look at nursing treatments does not necessarily mean that just because a treatment is costly, it will be abandoned. However, where possible, the most effective treatment for the least cost should be our aim.

6. Some positive features emanating from PPS are recognized: increased specialization has led to increased taking of responsibility for health care by the patient and his family. More and more families are learning to provide health and illness care in the home. What is learned in one illness episode can be utilized by the family in caring for family members in subsequent episodes.

Because of the crucial role the nurse plays in getting the patient ready for discharge, the nurse role has become more powerful in the inpatient setting. The opportunities and necessities for collaboration with medicine and other members of the health care team have increased. There can be no summary better than that expressd by one of the staff nurses interviewed. "Sure, since DRGs, the nursing role has changed somewhat. I've certainly become more conscious of cost and length of stay, and outliers. But the nurse role has become more powerful and more important also. The most important thing for me to do now is to develop the confidence to respond with independent thought to the interdependent relationships in which I find myself."

REFERENCES

McClure, Margaret, *et al.*, Magnet Hospitals, (Kansas City, MO: American Nurses' Association), 1983.

A challenge for the future

MERIDEAN MAAS, RN, PhD; MARY HARDY RN, PhD

THE USE OF NURSING DIAGNOSES to describe the health problems that nurses treat has increased substantially since the early 1970's, largely due to the work of the North American Nursing Diagnosis Association (NANDA). Nursing diagnoses provide a standardized terminology of names for clusters of signs and symptoms of specific conditions and their etiologies and thus focus the treatment that nurses can use to reverse the etiologies and achieve desired outcomes.

Maas described a number of advantages: [1]

> Nursing diagnoses...promote autonomy, accountability, and participation of nurses in the achievement of clinical and organizational program objectives. Nursing diagnoses aid the delivery of quality nursing care and the building of meaningful research, quality assurance, and staff development programs. Nursing diagnoses provide a mechanism for costing out nursing services, implementing computerized information systems, and promoting collaboration. Nursing diagnoses are a vehicle to enhance the power, influence, and marketability of nursing service (p 39).

Thus, it is important that nurses...expand their knowledge about nursing diagnosis and use nursing diagnoses in their practice. Expanding knowledge and use of nursing diagnoses should include increased understanding of diagnostic concepts, interventions, and outcomes; data about the incidence and accuracy of diagnoses of clients in their settings as well as others; and an awareness of developments in the profession toward building an intellectual basis for nursing practice.

The purpose of this article is to promote sharing of clinical use and research of nursing diagnoses among nurses who work with elderly and long-term care clients. This article briefly reviews the results of five studies of the prevalence of nursing diagnoses among elderly and long-term care populations. Diagnoses presented in this article were selected from those that were prevalent in the five epidemiological studies. [2-6] Studies that assess the reliability and validity of these nursing diagnoses in elderly and long-term care populations are also reviewed. Future directions for research to test nursing interventions for these diagnoses are outlined. The remainder of this issue is devoted to sharing knowledge about selected nursing diagnoses which are prevalent among elderly and long-term clients.

Epidemiological studies

Gordon and Sweeney note the need for epidemiological studies of nursing diagnoses in a variety of settings and populations. [7] These studies are needed for early detection of problems that nurses can treat or prevent. Gordon notes that these studies increase nurses' awareness of signs and symptoms in certain populations that may indicate a high probability that certain diagnoses exist. Further, studies are needed to determine specific diagnoses that are more apt to be prevalent in groups of persons because of their age, length of stay, medical diagnosis, and other factors.

Five epidemiological studies of nursing diagnoses among elderly and long-term care populations were found in the literature....

Nursing diagnoses which were prevalent (occurred in at least 10% of the subjects) in all of the five epidemiological studies of elderly and long-term care populations/samples were: Self-care deficit: Total; Impaired physical mobility; Alteration in thought processes; Impaired skin integrity; Alteration in comfort: Pain; Alteration in nutrition: less than body requirements; and Alteration in bowel elimination: Constipation.[2-6] Alteration in urinary elimination: Incontinence; Sensory perceptual alteration; and Potential for injury were prevalent in four of the five studies....

Diagnoses that were prevalent in all five studies were also prevalent for both males and females....

Overall, the prevalence of diagnoses was also consistent among age groups: young (less than 65), young-old (65-79), and old-old (80 and older). The prevalence of Sensory perceptual alteration and Alteration in fluid volume: excess among the old-old; Disturbance in self-concept in the young group; and Alteration in nutrition; less than body requirements in the young-old were exceptions.

Self-care deficit, Impaired physical mobility, and Alteration in thought processes were prevalent in each of the five length of stay groups: less than 1 year; 1 year to less than 3 years; 3 years to less than 10 years; 10 years to less than 20 years; and more than 20 years. For residents grouped by the intensity of nursing care that they required (Category I = most intense, Category IV = least intense), Alteration in thought processes and Alteration in health maintenance were prevalent in all four groups.

The prevalence of diagnoses was most consistent among the three groups requiring the most nursing care. Ineffective coping: potential and Disturbance in self-concept were prevalent only in the group that required the lowest intensity of care, who were mostly residents living in the residential care area. These results illustrate the importance of epidemiological studies that report the incidence of diagnoses by age, gender, and other characteristics. Results of studies in a variety of settings can then be compared and generalizations regarding diverse elderly and long-term clients can be prevented. Considerable replication of findings between the studies also provides evidence that the NANDA taxonomy has validity for describing the responses to acutal and potential illness that nurses treat among elderly and long-term care clients, and provides a framework for further research.

Validation studies

Validation research sets out to determine the extent [to which] defining characteristics of selected nursing diagnoses are nearly always or frequently present when clinicians make the diagnoses in a practice setting.[8] ...Creason, Pogue, Nelson, and Hoyt conducted a study to validate the etiologies and signs and symptoms of Impaired physical mobility in a sample of rehabilitation patients using a retrospective audit of nursing process papers, of students in an RN baccalaureate degree completion program.[9] Seventy-five percent of the defining characteristics were included in four broad categories: inability to perform self-care; decreased muscle strength, control, mass; limited range of motion; and other functional alterations. The most frequent etiologies identified were neuromuscular impairment, musculoskeletal impairment, and medical diagnoses. Investigators questioned whether Self-care deficit was often a more appropriate diagnosis with an etiology of Impaired physical mobility in order to focus interventions on compensation of mobility limitations to promote maximum functional abilities.

McShane and McLane reported the results of a validation study of Altered bowel elimination: constipation.[10] Results of this study are discussed by the investigators in their article on constipation, along with additional work which has been done to validate the diagnosis. Coffman studied Altered bowel elimination in a sample of 33 children with meningomyelocele in an outpatient clinic.[11] While the subjects for this study were children, etiologies found for these long-term care clients (decreased activity, not enough roughage, inadequate fruits and vegetables in diet) may also be relevant for the elderly.

In her article, *Alteration in Urinary Elimination: Incontinence,* Tunink reviews studies by Voith, Madson, and Smith and Youngbauer[12] to validate six specific incontinence diagnoses. Tunink also discusses additional work by Specht, Tunink, Maas, and Bulechek[13] to specify and validate types of incontinence in the elderly.

Proceedings of the Seventh National Conference of NANDA contains several studies reporting validation of nursing diagnoses discussed in this volume, including Impaired skin integrity; Self-care deficit; Impaired physical mobility; Alteration in comfort: pain; Alteration in urinary elimination; and Alteration in nutrition; less than body requirements.[14] A variety of methods were used for validating these diagnoses, their etiologies, and defining characteristics.

There are also a number of validation studies in the literature of diagnoses that occur among the elderly, other than those discussed in this issue....Clearly, there is need for many more studies to validate diagnoses among the elderly. These efforts should be focused on the nursing diagnoses reported as most prevalent in epidemiologial studies of elderly and long-term care clients.

Future directions

Too few epidemiological studies in elderly and long-term care populations have been reported for conclusions to be drawn about the incidence of nursing diagnoses. Therefore, many more studies of the prevalence of nursing diagnoses in this population should be completed and reported. Examination of the methods used in the five epidemiological studies reported here, as well as others, will assist clinicians in doing and reporting prevalence studies. Nurses can use these findings to arrange further research, education, and practice priorities.

Validation of diagnoses, etiologies, and signs and symptoms in elderly and long-term care populations is another priority need. The prevalence of nursing diagnoses in specific populations and settings is a rational basis for arranging priorities to study their validity. Methods of validation have been described by Gordon and Sweeney[7] and Fehring.[15] One volume of *Nursing Clinics of North America* has been devoted to reports of research to validate specific diagnoses.[16] Thus, a variety of methodologies are available for nurses to use to validate diagnoses in diverse clinical settings. The NANDA Board of Directors is currently discussing the need for a conference on the subject of validation of nursing diagnoses. The involvement of nurses in clinical settings is critical for the effort to validate and refine diagnostic categories and their critical indicators. This is especially required for the identification of appropriate outcomes and for the assessment of the quality of nursing care.

Evidence of the validity of diagnoses is essential for further research efforts. Assessment tools can then be tested for reliability and validity. Outcome standards can be systematically defined, and the effects of interventions to achieve the outcomes can be analyzed. Identification of interventions to treat specific diagnoses is a critical need[17] and will be enhanced.

Historically, nursing has been task-oriented and has lagged in the development of treatment concepts. The result is that few interventions, explicitly defined and linked to diagnoses, have been developed and clinically tested. Accountability to clients demands that nurses correct this deficit.

Refinement and validation of diagnostic skills are other research priorities that will be facilitated by epidemiological and validation studies of diagnoses. If nursing diagnoses are to guide practice, and serve as the definition of nursing, diagnoses and diagnostic reasoning must be reliable and valid. Ethical issues associated with nursing diagnosis and treatment of specific problems must also be assessed.[18] In an environment of cost effectiveness and containment, nurses cannot ignore accountability for accurate judgments and ethical actions.

Further, costs of treatment compared to effectiveness can be examined. The work can be communicated to the nursing public through the nursing literature and at local, regional, and national nursing diagnoses meetings. These activities should encourage funding of research and support the communication of findings by NANDA and other nursing and health-related organizations.

Finally, nursing must continue to develop and validate a standard nomenclature for diagnoses and interventions so that information can be documented and processed efficiently. Computer technology has revolutionized the storage, analysis, and retrieval of information to the advantage of those who are prepared to use it. However, nursing information has not been in a form easily adapted for computer processing.

To a great extent, nurses remain disadvantaged by manual documentation, analysis, and retrieval of clinical data. Furthermore, nursing care problems and treatments have not been included in institutional or national minimum health data sets. The result is that nursing information has typically been underrepresented in the review of health needs and trends for policy decisions and resource allocation at institutional, state, and federal levels.

Diagnoses presented in this special issue are brief accounts of the diagnostic concepts and interventions that nurses use to treat the diagnoses. The authors have attempted to provide research based content wherever possible. Much of this knowledge is derived from theory or based on the experiences of clinical nurses. The content is intended to assist nurses to care for their clients.

The focus on nursing diagnoses...prevalent among elderly and long-term care clients will hopefully promote their use and testing in clinical settings, [foster the conducting] of research to describe their incidence in a variety of elderly and long-term care client groups, and encourage sharing of these results. The issue is a challenge to nurses in gerontological and long-term care settings to use nursing diagnoses in their practice, conduct research on nursing diagnoses, and report their clinical research experiences.

REFERENCES

1. Maas M: Nursing diagnoses in a professional model of nursing: Keystone for effective nursing administration. *J Nurs Adm* 1986; 16(12):39-42.

2. Hallal J: Nursing diagnosis: An essential step to quality care. *J. Gerontol Nurs* 1985; 11(19)35-38.

3. Leslie, FM: Nursing diagnosis in long term care. *Am J Nurs* 1981;81(5):1012-1014.

4. Rantz, M, Miller T, Jacobs, C: Nursing diagnosis in long term care. *Am J Nurs* 1985; 85(5):916-926.

5. Rantz M, Miller T: How diagnoses are changing in long term care. *Am J Nurs* 1987; 87(3):360-361.

6. Hardy M, Maas M, Akin J: The prevalence of nursing diagnoses among elderly and long term care residents: A descriptive comparison. *Recent Advances in Nursing* 1988; (in press).

7. Gordon M, Sweeney M: Methodological problems and issues in identifying and standardizing nursing diagnoses. *Advanced Nursing Science* 1987; 1(2):1-15.

8. Vincent K: The validation of a nursing diagnosis: A nurses consensus survey. *Nurs Clin North Am* 1985; 20(4):631-640.

9. Creason N, Pogue N, Nelson A, Hoyt C: Validating the nursing diagnosis of impaired physical mobility. *Nurs Clin North Am* 1985; 20(4):669-684.

10. McShane R, McLane A: Constipation: Consensual and empirical validation. *Nurs Clin North Am* 1985; 20(4):801-808.

11. Coffman S: Description of a nursing diagnosis: Alteration in bowel elimination related to neurogenic bowel with myelomeningocele. *Issues Comp Pediatr Nurs* **1986; 8:179-191.**

12. Voith A, Smith D, Madson, L. Youngbauer, P: Validation of nursing diagnoses regarding alterations in urinary elimination in McLane AM (ed): *Classification of Nursing Diagnoses: Proceedings of the Seventh National Conference.* St. Louis, CV Mosby, 1986, p 281.

13. Specht J, Tunink P, Maas M, Bulechek G: Alteration in urinary

elimination: Incontinence, in Maas M, Buckwalter K (eds): *Nursing Diagnoses and Interventions for the Elderly*. Menlo Park, Califonia, Addison-Wesley, in press.

14. McClane AM (ed): *Classification of Nursing Diagnoses: Proceedings of the Seventh National Conference*. St. Louis, CV Mosby, 1987.

15. Fehring R: Validation, in Hurley M (ed): *Classification of Nursing Diagnoses: Proceedings of the Sixth Conference*. St Louis, CV Mosby, 1986, pp 183-190.

16. Symposium on nursing diagnosis, Dougherty C (ed). *Nurs Clin North Am* 1985; 20(4).

17. Bulechek GM, McCloskey JC: Nursing diagnoses and intervention, in Bulechek G, McCloskey J (eds): *Nursing Interventions: Treatments for Nursing Diagnoses*. Philadelphia, WB Saunders, 1985.

18. Gordon M: Issues in nursing diagnosis, in McLane AM (ed): *Classification of Nursing Diagnoses: Proceedings of the Seventh National Conference*. St. Louis, CV Mosby, 1987, pp 17-20.

Computer assisted care in nursing: Computers at the bedside

JAN H. VAN BEMMEL, MSc, PhD

In the following article, van Bemmel discusses two applications of computers in direct patient care: diagnosis and monitoring. The author explores the advantages of computer-assisted electrocardiogram interpretation and examines some of the ways in which nurses are using computers to enhance patient health in intensive care units. Note: In this article, excerpts (indicated by ellipses) condense extensive background information.

AFTER THE LEGENDARY "Lady with the Lamp," nursing has gradually become more and more professional and specialized. Like physicians, nurses have also provided themselves with methods and techniques to operate efficiently and adequately. "The lamp" was extended with a thermometer and blood pressure gauge. Nurses now play a key role in the administration of drugs. Some nurses specialize in areas that require advanced education and experience with complicated equipment. In many countries inservice training is no longer considered sufficient for modern nursing education. The profile of the profession is changing.

During the last few years the computer has been added to the already existing methods and techniques, giving extra possibilities and offering new challenges (Ball & Hannah, 1984). The "Lady with the Lamp" with her comforting hand, could, as some may think, become the "Professional with the Terminal," with a hand operating a keyboard. The issue if whether the nurse will become one of the many specialists around the patient's bed, or whether nurses will be able to devote more time, assisted by today's new systems, to what is the core of the profession: caring for patients. New possibilities are on the horizon; it is important to be engaged in the changes, rather than being surprised by them. The lamp, thermometer, and syringe are being extended with terminals, display units, and printers. They should be used properly....

Computers in nursing practice

More and more, nurses are confronted with computerized processing and interpretation of information that (directly or online) originates from the patient.

Diagnostic applications. The use of computers for diagnostic support (the first stages of the cycle of information processing) concerns the stages of information processing and data analysis. Few computer applications offer a complete diagnosis. Moreover, the final diagnosis can only be reached if the entire patient history and the results of medical examinations and laboratory analysis are available.

Gradually, more instruments are using microcomputers for the processing, analysis, and classification of the acquired data. Examples are electrocardiographs, spirographs, and audiologic or ophthalmologic equipment. Computer support of the diagnosis can also be seen in areas of image acquisition and processing systems such as in scintigraphy, radiology, ultrasound, and the catheterization laboratory.

The following discussion will be restricted to the processing of signals: data as a function of time. Electrocardiogram interpretation was chosen as an example because it represents signal processing and is oriented toward diagnosis (Kors, Talmon, & Van Bemmel, 1986).

Computer assisted electrocardiogram interpretation. The electrocardiogram is one of the most frequent diagnostic examinations. It is used in outpatient clinics, in departments of cardiology, during preparations for major surgery, to exclude certain cardiac diseases, and in all areas of medicine from general practice to occupational medicine. Electrocardiogram interpretation requires thorough training; however, some computerized electrocardiographs offer a complete interpretation to the user. In such systems an electrocardiogram interpretation program has been implemented that contains the expert knowledge of a cardiologist and that can make diagnostic statements about the type of infarction, hypertrophy, conduction disturbances, ischemia, arrhythmias, or other disorders.

Computerized analysis is not only performed for the interpretation of resting electrocardiograms but also during physical exercise and for ambulatory patients (Holter electrocardiograms). Electrocardiogram analysis is also used in coronary care.

Like many other signals used in medicine, present-day computer-assisted analysis of the resting electrocardiogram involves a number of stages.

Electrocardiogram acquisition. In electrocardiogram systems, 10 electrodes are applied to the extremities and chest to derive the Einthoven (I, II, III), the augmented (aVR, aVL, aVF), and chest leads (V1...V6). In some systems other electrodes are used to derive the vectorcardiogram (X, Y, and Z). Such systems record all electrocardiograms (12 or 15 simultaneously during about 10 sec).

The most important tasks of the computer during data acquisition include checking the electrode applications (impedances), possible leads interchange, and checking disturbances). If an error is detected during acquisition, it is signaled directly to the technician who makes the recording. If everything is done correctly, the entire electrocardiogram is stored in the computer that samples the signal at 500/sec with an accuracy of about 12 bits. This offers maximally for 10 sec signal and 12 leads the storage of 10 x 12 x 500 = 60,000 12-bit samples. The person who makes the recording must check the quality of the signal because even computers can derive no reliable diagnostic information from signals that are incorrect or distorted. If the reading is done correctly (the procedure is explained to the patient and the patient is reassured) the rest of the analysis is done automatically.

Electrocardiogram analysis. After the data are acquired, complex operations are performed on the signals by programs that may contain more than 100,000 statements.

After the disturbances are checked, the signals may be corrected. Any different wave shapes in the 12 or multiple electrocardiogram leads are detected, such as the QRS complex, the P-wave, and the T-wave. Disturbances are also detected. All wave shapes are labeled by a number according to wave form type, such as dominant QRS complexes and premature ventricular beats. The same labelling is done for the ST-T complex. This stage of the processing is also call typification.

On the basis of the results of the preceding stages the dominant electrocardiogram complex (PQRST) is determined and it is assumed to represent the normal cardiac cycle. In this dominant complex pattern recognition methods are used to determine the onsets and endpoints of the P-wave, QRS complex, and T-wave to permit measurement in the electrocardiogram complex. This estimation of onsets and endpoints is done for all leads separately.

In the next stage it is necessary to acquire measurements or parameters by which the final electrocardiogram diagnosis can be made, such as the duration of waves, amplitudes, and relations between measurements from different electrocardiogram leads. This provides approximately 12 x 50 = 600 measurements.

However, such measurements have only limited accuracy, determined by the character of the signal, the disturbance that is always present, and the accuracy of the ADC.

The next stage of the interpretation program deals with the classification of the electrocardiogram in different types of arrhythmias and types of electrocardiogram complexes. Many diagnostic statements and combinations are possible, as well as grades in the different categories. At the same time a probability index is added to each statement such as certain, probable, or possible. Some electrocardiogram systems also make a serial comparison with an earlier recorded electrocardiogram.

The last stage of the processing is documentation, which is usually done both graphically and alphanumerically. Modern electrocardiogram interpretation systems print the report directly after the recording on a direct writer built into the recording equipment. This shows the electrocardiogram results, the selected complexes with indications of onsets and endpoints of the wave shapes, the significant measurements (wave durations, amplitudes), and the classification and should become part of the patient's medical record. Some systems allow the electrocardiogram data to be stored digitally on disk for comparison with later data.

Such systems offer reliability, speed, uniform interpretation, documentation, and evaluation of medical care. As the cost of such systems decreases, they will be used in more outpatient clinics and departments of cardiology, internal medicine, and pediatrics.

Medical and nursing records will contain more and more computer-processed documents such as the electrocardiogram as well as laboratory results. Eventually, all medical and nursing records may be stored on computers. However, before this is possible many decisions must be made about the types of systems that are required, nomenclature and coding, and accessibility.

Despite technological advances, nursing must not become merely digital patient care; the "Lady with the Lamp" must remain visible.

Another area in which computers are used at the patient's bedside is intensive care.

Intensive care. Intensive care may include critical care, coronary care, and patient monitoring. In this area, nurses are commonly confronted both with a patient in critical condition and with very advanced equipment. Typically, the patient in intensive care is connected to instruments by means of tubes and wires. Fluids are automatically withdrawn or administered.

Computers perform many functions in intensive care. They organize the data and observations that are generated. Most monitoring equipment now contains built in microprocessors.

Medical decisions are increasingly based on objective and numerical information rather than purely subjective impressions. Computerizing part of the decision-making process leads to the creation of protocols that clearly delineate the appropriate care and interventions and reduce the risk of human error.

There is a growing need for documentation, reports, planning, and evaluation of activities in intensive care. Such documents and reports can be generated alphanumerically and can be useful for medical audits or peer reviews.

Finally, computers can be used cost-effectively to keep records, freeing nursing time available for the human aspects of intensive patient care.

Computer-assisted intensive care concerns a wide area of functions, data, and purposes. Many body functions can be monitored by computers, in particular: cardiovascular, respiratory, and renal function, renal secretion, central nervous system function, body fluid levels, electrolytic balance, and blood gas values. Table 1 summarizes these functions.

TABLE 1. Types of data and domains that one could encounter during intensive patient care*

DOMAIN	CONTINUOUS DATA (SIGNALS)	SAMPLED DATA (e.g., MANUAL)	CODED DATA (MANUAL)
Circulatory	ECG, blood pressure, heart rate, VES	Blood pressure (cuff)	Color defibrillation
Respiratory	Respiratory rate, volume, flow, respiratory gases		Artificial respiration
Neurologic	EEG, EOG		Reflexes
Secretion	Urine infusions	Urine infusions	
Biochemical	pO_2, pH	Urine, blood, feces	Pain, anesthesia
Various	Temperature	Temperature	Drugs, treatment, pain
Computer input	Mostly via A-D conversion	Often via keyboard	After observation, via coding and keyboard

*Continuous data (signals) are usually automatically entered in a computer (via an ADC); the other data are, for example, manually sampled and/or coded and entered via keyboard.

Following is a discussion of some systems currently in use. Several systems are available commercially.

Postoperative care. One of the earliest systems for intensive care was developed in Alabama (Sheppard, 1979). It offers closed-loop control of the fluid balance. Infusions, drains, and urine secretion are automatically determined and weighed. Based on the results, the computer determines the amount of infusion that is necessary and alerts the nurse if this balance is disturbed, for instance, by internal bleeding. It is important for such systems to generate accurate patient reports so that nurses can use them to determine at a glance how a patient's condition has changed over time.

Coronary care. For patients who enter the hospital with an impending infarction it is important to react immediately to situations that may be life-threatening, such as ventricular fibrillation or cardiac arrest. Early detection of the symptoms that may lead to such situations is essential. Computers can effectively detect the signs that characterize such conditions as shortening RR intervals and runs of extrasystoles. Computers may also be used to evaluate the effects of drug therapy in an objective and quantitative manner.

The nurse in a coronary care unit may be assisted by systems that offer such parameters as a function of time computed from the electrocardiogram. The necessary information may be displayed on a video terminal, which reduces the data to trends and reports. Such systems can be installed for each bed. The computer-generated alarms are reliable.

It is important to remember that computer systems are not infallible. Certain events may be missed (false negative, FN) or may be seen incorrectly (false positive, FP). One can only be reduced, at the cost of the other because the relation between FP and FN is fixed for a certain processing system. Formally, this can be expressed as a receiver operating characteristic that shows that if the FP decreases, the FN increases....In an intensive care unit the receiver operating characteristic should be constructed in such a way that the ideal setpoint, FP=FN=0, is approximated as closely as possible. In a coronary care unit the FP will probably be somewhat higher than the FN.

Systems for the analysis of ambulatory or Holter electrocardiograms follow the same processing principles as for coronary care. Such systems usually process two electrocardiograms simultaneously. For Holter electrocardiograms, portable systems are available, including a microprocessor that performs the data processing online.

Perioperative care. The care of patients during major surgery differs slightly from that in other areas of intensive care mentioned above because the patient is unconscious. This type of intensive care is similar to process control as it is performed outside medicine as well. The anesthetist plays the key role in making decisions, such as the administration of drugs on the basis of measurements that were taken online.

Intensive perioperative care is needed during heart surgery (Pronk & Simons, 1983). The heart and lungs can no longer function naturally because of perfusion and artificial respiration, and the patient's temperature is also artificially controlled. One of the few vital functions that is still naturally regulated is the brain function, which is why it is monitored continuously by electrocardiogram.

The systems described in this article are among the most advanced. They are also commonly encountered by nurses, and illustrate the complexity of the medical/nursing activities that will increasingly be seen in many areas of patient care.

System requirements and advantages

Systems used for patient monitoring must be able to collect all necessary information at the patient's bedside; must have, in addition to bedside, decentralized systems, a central system for easy communication with users; must provide documentation and trend analysis; must be able to communicate with other systems in the hospital, such as the laboratory; and must be suited for the evaluation of patient care and research.

Patient monitoring systems provide nurses with more time for direct patient care; allow decisions to be made that are less intuitive and more objective; permit closed-loop therapy; allow faster stabilization of the patient's condition; allow earlier transfer of patients to areas of less intensive care; and provide better quality care through greater organization and definition of responsibilities....

Conclusions

This article gave an overview of some of the clinical uses of computers in hospitals. Computers are valuable tools and their use among nurses is expected to continue to increase. However, it is important for nurses to use this new technology to enhance, not replace, personalized patient care.

REFERENCES

Ball, M.J. & Hannah, K.J. (1984). *Using computers in nursing*. Reston, Virginia: Reston Publishing.

Kors, J.A., Talmon, J.L. & van Bemmel, J.H. (1986). Multilead ECG analysis. *Computers and Biomedical Research, 19*, 28-46.

Pronk, R.A.F., & Simons, A.J.R. (1983). Processing of the electroencephalogram in cardiac surgery. In Van Bemmel, J.H., Ball, M.J. & Wigertz, O. (Eds.), *MEDINFO 83* (pp. 764-767). Amsterdam: North-Holland.

Sheppard, L.C. (1979). The computer in the care of the critically ill. *Proceedings IEEE, 67*, 1300-1306.

UNIT NINE

Study questions

1. In "Bridging the Gap: Theory to Practice — Part I, Clinical Applications," the authors discuss two primary dimensions of health. What are they? What is the significance of each?

2. Describe the relationship of the nursing process to Neuman's Health Care Systems Model as detailed by Field in "The Impact of Nursing Theory on the Clinical Decision Making Process."

3. Enumerate and explain the major objectives of the National Center for Nursing Research as outlined by Hinshaw in "The National Center for Nursing Research: Challenges and Initiatives."

4. Describe the systems theory model used by the authors of "Use of Research Based Knowledge in Clinical Practice."

5. In "Magnet Hospitals Talk About the Impact of DRGs on Nursing Care — Part I," Kramer and Schmalenberg list 11 predicted results of DRGs and prospective payment systems. According to the authors, how have DRGs affected patient outcomes?

6. The authors outline some positive results of DRGs in Part II of their "Magnet Hospitals" article. In which ways have nurses benefited?

7. Maas and Hardy, in "A Challenge for the Future," outline both epidemiological and validation studies of nursing diagnoses. In conducting validation research of nursing diagnoses, what does the nurse set out to do?

8. In "Computer Assisted Care in Nursing: Computers at the Bedside," van Bemmel shows how nurses can use computers to enhance personalized patient care. Discuss five ways in which nurses now use computers in intensive care settings.

UNIT TEN

Leadership for change

UNIT NINE EXPLORED ways in which nursing theories and research efforts are influencing contemporary nursing and health care and how they might also help shape the future of nursing. In focusing on key aspects of leadership, Unit Ten demonstrates that nursing's future also depends on the emergence of leaders who can devise and implement effective solutions to today's serious problems. Many of these problems, as detailed in Unit Nine, have no easy answers.

Profession in transition

In response to escalating hospital costs, federal regulation of health care services has often resulted in dire consequences for the patient and the nurse. Most patients are hospitalized for a shorter time than they would have been before the federal regulations took effect; thus, today's nurses are caring for greater numbers of patients who are more acutely ill while hospitalized and who are sometimes ill-prepared for discharge.

The current nursing shortage underscores the difficulties nursing leaders face in recruiting and retaining qualified nurses. Nursing school enrollments have declined, and job switching is common among novice nurses, many of whom may be reacting to work loads that exceed their expertise or ability to function safely. While taking on duties previously assigned to nonnursing personnel and with limited support from the administration, many nurses spend less time working directly with their clients. Nursing care under such conditions becomes task-oriented rather than client-oriented — a troublesome and frustrating irony for most nurses, who typically list "caring for clients" and "making life better for others" as reasons for making a professional commitment to nursing.

If nursing is to survive and flourish as a profession, nurses at every level must be willing to accept the responsibility of improving their working conditions while ensuring the highest standards of care for their clients. Knowledge of traditional and emerging leadership concepts can help prepare the nursing student for such responsibility.

New leadership in nursing

A central theme of Unit Ten is the need for new leadership in nursing to address the problems mentioned above. Leadership traditionally has been regarded as the capacity of one individual to influence others — through example, intimidation, persuasion, or charisma — to achieve a specific goal. However, effective leadership is more than a composite of personality traits. Ideally, leadership causes interaction among people that increases knowledge and effects desired change. Leadership can empower others to reach their highest potential. Enlightened leaders not only articulate the needs of the group, take risks to achieve desired results, and develop innovative solutions; they also inspire creativity, motivation, and collaboration among the group's members.

Fortunately, as the articles in Unit Ten suggest, such leadership appears to be developing within the nursing profession. Nurses at all levels are being encouraged to play more significant roles in decision making, to further patients' rights, to collaborate rather than compete, to persuade rather than intimidate. Because health care management and the quality of patient care are integrally related to legislative action, more nurses are active in federal, state, and local politics.

Nursing leaders must have a keen understanding of their profession and a clear vision of the direction it should take. They also must be willing to acknowledge this irrefutable truth: creating a more effective working environment for nurses ultimately benefits the patient — the person for whom the science of caring exists.

SECTION ONE

The leadership role

SECTION ONE EXAMINES qualities and values needed to be an effective leader, addresses the question of who should assume such leadership, and provides constructive suggestions for all nurses who want to assume leadership responsibilities in their practice.

Effective nursing leadership comes from those with a strong sense of purpose and a commitment to fundamental values of the profession. Without such values, nursing is fragmented and meaningless. What are some of these values? In the first article, "Values and Professional Behaviors," the American Association of Colleges of Nursing (AACN) outlines seven essential values of the professional nurse: altruism, equality, aesthetics, freedom, human dignity, justice, and truth. The article also provides examples of attitudes, personal qualities, and professional behaviors that reflect a commitment to these values. For instance, the nurse who values justice would report unethical practices objectively and factually; the nurse who values truth would obtain sufficient data before reporting infractions of organizational policies. The AACN does not assign a ranking to these values; the nurse should prioritize them within specific contexts.

Diers and Evans begin the second article, "Excellence in Nursing," by examining stereotypical — and sometimes contradictory — views of excellence and nursing. The authors then explore seven facets of nursing practice on which excellence might be determined. Not surprisingly, the authors include discipline, responsibility, caring, and perseverance, all of which traditionally have been regarded as hallmarks of the nursing leader. But equally important, according to the authors, are three facets of nursing practice that most people — and perhaps many nurses — do not associate with the profession: choreography, skepticism, and passion. Nurse as choreographer? Skepticism as a valued trait? Passion as an integral component within the objective, clinical setting? Yes, claim the authors, and their article can provide the nursing student with valuable insights into nursing excellence.

The third article focuses on who should assume nursing leadership positions. In "Leadership and the Caring Role," Poulin proposes that to be a leader is not merely to seek higher positions within an organization. Rather, leadership is a requisite to the caring role. At the heart of such leadership is accountability to the patient, the profession, and the employer. In this context, leadership is not for the chosen few but for all nurses. And if nurses are accountable first and foremost to the patient, then they can best demonstrate leadership by functioning as patient advocates — willing to face controversy, exercise autonomy, and deal with adversity, if necessary, to enhance clients' rights.

The section concludes with two readings — one addressed to the novice and the other to the nurse executive — that focus on constructive applications of leadership in nursing practice. Lee distinguishes between old and new styles of leadership in the section's fourth article, "Leadership in Practice." The author first refutes several traditionally held notions of what constitutes effective leadership and then offers concrete suggestions for the novice nurse who wants to develop potential and skills as a leader.

The concept of "new leadership" is also the

central theme of the section's final article, "The Challenge for Innovation: A New Leadership." Because of changing social values, technological advancements, and a cost-containment environment that has made the health care system increasingly competitive, nursing leaders face the challenge of maintaining stability within their organizations while promoting changes to keep pace with society's changing health needs. Ryan and Walker propose that the new leader must foster a climate of innovation, restructure the organization to shift more authority and decision making to lower levels, and serve as an effective facilitator and communicator rather than an autocratic problem solver. The leader must articulate the goals and direction of the organization and then encourage its members to help define and shape its future.

Values and professional behaviors

AMERICAN ASSOCIATION OF COLLEGES OF NURSING

COLLEGE AND UNIVERSITY education for professional nursing includes processes that foster the development of values, attitudes, personal qualities, and professional behaviors. Values are defined as beliefs or ideals to which an individual is committed and which guide behavior. Values are reflected in attitudes, personal qualities, and consistent patterns of behavior. Attitudes are inclinations or dispositions to respond positively or negatively to a person, object, or situation, while personal qualities are innate or learned attributes of an individual. Professional behaviors reflect...commitment to specific values.

Nursing has been described as a cultural paradox. The professional nurse must adopt contemporary characteristics, such as independence, assertiveness, self-esteem, and confidence, as well as those of a more traditional nature, such as compassion, acceptance,...and

Values and professional behaviors

ESSENTIAL VALUES*	EXAMPLES OF ATTITUDES AND PERSONAL QUALITIES	EXAMPLES OF PROFESSIONAL BEHAVIORS
1. Altruism Concern for the welfare of others.	Caring Commitment Compassion Generosity Perseverance	• Gives full attention to the patient/client when giving care. • Assists other personnel in providing care when they are unable to do so. • Expresses concern about social trends and issues that have implications for health care.
2. Equality Having the same rights, privileges, or status.	Acceptance Assertiveness Fairness Self-esteem Tolerance	• Provides nursing care based on the individual's needs irrespective of personal characteristics.** • Interacts with other providers in a non-discriminatory manner. • Expresses ideas about the improvement of access to nursing and health care.
3. Esthetics Qualities of objects, events, and persons that provide satisfaction.	Appreciation Creativity Imagination Sensitivity	• Adapts the environment so it is pleasing to the patient/client. • Creates a pleasant work environment for self and others. • Presents self in a manner that promotes a positive image of nursing.

continued

*The values are listed in alphabetic rather than priority order.
**From CODE FOR NURSES, American Nurses' Association, 1976.

Values and professional behaviors *continued*

ESSENTIAL VALUES*	EXAMPLES OF ATTITUDES AND PERSONAL QUALITIES	EXAMPLES OF PROFESSIONAL BEHAVIORS
4. Freedom Capacity to exercise choice.	Confidence Hope Independence Openness Self-direction Self-discipline	• Honors individual's right to refuse treatment. • Supports the rights of other providers to suggest alternatives to the plan of care. • Encourages open discussion of controversial issues in the profession.
5. Human dignity Inherent worth and uniqueness of an individual.	Consideration Empathy Humaneness Kindness Respectfulness Trust	• Safeguards the individual's right to privacy. • Addresses individuals as they prefer to be addressed. • Maintains confidentiality of patients/clients and staff. • Treats others with respect regardless of background.
6. Justice Upholding moral and legal principles.	Courage Integrity Morality Objectivity	• Acts as a health care advocate. • Allocates resources fairly. • Reports incompetent, unethical, and illegal practice objectively and factually.**
7. Truth Faithfulness to fact or reality.	Accountability Authenticity Honesty Inquisitiveness Rationality Reflectiveness	• Documents nursing care accurately and honestly. • Obtains sufficient data to make sound judgments before reporting infractions of organizational policies. • Participates in professional efforts to protect the public from misinformation about nursing.

*The values are listed in alphabetic rather than priority order.
**From CODE FOR NURSES, American Nurses' Association, 1976.

kindness. Adoption of the essential values leads the nurse to a sense of commitment and social responsibility, a sensitivity and responsiveness to the needs of others, and a responsibility for oneself and one's actions.

We recommend that the following seven values are essential for the professional nurse. Examples of attitudes, personal qualities, and professional behaviors are included that reflect a commitment to one or more of these values.

The professional nurse assigns priorities to these values within specific decision-making contexts in the application of essential knowledge and practice. The nurse, guided by these values, attitudes, and personal qualities, demonstrates ethical professional behavior with patients/clients, colleagues, and others in providing safe, humanistic care focused on health and quality of life. Values, attitudes, personal qualities, and consistent patterns of behavior begin to develop early in life, but also are fostered and facilitated by selected educational strategies and the process of socialization to the profession.

Excellence in nursing

DONNA DIERS, BSN, MSN; DAVID LINN EVANS, BA, MA

"EXCELLENCE IN NURSING" is almost a contradiction in terms.

Nursing, it is said, is a set of simple routine activities for which a minimum of training is required if the nurse is just a good person — nice, kind, motherly person with a big heart and warm hands. To produce nurses, the legend goes, just take nice people and turn them loose. In this context, to be excellent would mean to be a better human being than anybody else, surely an assignment to break the morale of the best nurse.

Nurses deal with the most basic of human needs: feeding, heartbreak, warmth, elimination, suffering, loneliness, birth, and death. Our hands get dirty, our uniforms stained, and our psyches eroded by daily contact with human beings in need — people crying, immobilized, angry, frightened, depressed, and only occasionally joyful. We live with the outrage of the diagnosis made or missed; the crisis of faith in a higher being or a physician; the knowledge of decline, disability, permanent change, death, and the consciousness of our own mortality. We must be graceful over vomitus and effluvia, and dignified as we change the dressing, pack the wound, debride the decubitus, and give out the bad news. With our hands and eyes we touch the lives of others and are admitted to the privacy of their inner space without even asking.

For people who do such things, there can be no thing like excellence, so the story goes, because excellence only applies to matters of a higher order, not to the basic realities of life, living and dying.

There is another way in which the concept of excellence is foreign to nursing. Excellence means to excel, to surpass, to be the best, and there is in nursing the tradition of women's subservience that rarely allows us to grant differences in quality to one another. Besides, what would it be to excel in nursing? To do one's work faster, or more accurately? Never to make a mistake in assessment or treatment? To listen more deeply and carefully, to pick the right words to comfort or cleanse? To successfully manipulate the physician or the administrative hierarchy to bring one's services to the patient when and where he needs them? To involve the patient fully in his care and treatment and not steal his personhood or power?

And even if it were possible to excel in all these ways, and even if such surpassing quality were called excellence, who would know? For nursing is so personal a service, so private an experience, so invisible alone in a room with a patient that no one will ever know it fully except the individual nurse.

Perhaps it is only reasonable right now that the nursing activities that become public and applauded are the political and educational ones for there are still serious political and educational wars to be fought. But to restrict one's notion of excellence in nursing to activities outside the practice field is to draw attention away from our central values and reason for being.

John Gardner says it this way:

> We must learn to honor excellence (indeed to demand it) in every socially accepted human activity, however humble the activity, and to scorn shoddiness, however exalted the activity....An excellent plumber is infinitely

> more admirable than an incompetent philosopher. The society which scorns excellence in plumbing because plumbing is a humble activity and tolerates shoddiness in philosophy because it is an exalted activity will have neither good plumbing nor good philosophy. Neither its pipes nor its theories will hold water (Gardner, 1961, p. 102).

The stereotypes of nursing we began with are, of course, wrong. Here are some other facets of nursing practice upon which definitions of excellence might depend. which definitions of excellence might depend.

Discipline

There is, first, the notion of **discipline**. In nursing, discipline is what gets us up at strange hours of the morning or night, makes us put on even stranger attire and come eagerly to a place of work filled with demand and decision. Discipline is what makes a nurse check a medication three times even when it's the three-thousandth medication she's given. Discipline is what makes a nurse practitioner repeat laboratory tests because she knows the lab makes mistakes and the patient cannot suffer because an important bit of information is inaccurate. Discipline is what makes a psychiatric nurse watchful and alert as a patient stares fixedly into the middle distance, predicting an epileptiform seizure. Discipline is remembering that an I.V. down the hall is getting low and discipline is what makes one return to a patient to try one more time to offer succor when one's own strength is lagging, and when the patient is shy or hostile or simply scared.

Discipline makes one practice, as dancers or opera singers or actors do, to achieve a perfection of thinking and of activity, for the tools of the nurse are not the voice or the movement of the body, but the exercise of intellect and wisdom on human problems and possibilities. If I only knew more, says the disciplined nurse, about electrolyte balance, or neurological function, or sinus node activity or potassium imbalance or the dopamine theory or behavior modification or the physiological effects of prolonged stress or circadian rhythms or cognitive dissonance — if I only knew more, I could be better.

But the nature of nursing practice is not static as is an opera or a playscript or a concerto. In nursing, one never has the same words to say, nor the same notes to play or sing. The precision of discipline in nursing can never be the same as the precision of the singer who searches for and finds exactly the right interpretation of a descant which, once learned and perfected, is always there so long as the voice is. Nursing practice must change with each patient, each situation, even each heart beat. The discipline of nursing is the constant attention to difference and the regularity of unpredictability.

Choreography

To continue the musical analogy, another part of excellence is a quality that might be called **choreography**. In part, this means the graceful balancing of competing demands, attending to the tunes others play and moving in synchrony with the corps de ballet. But on another level, the excellent nurse as choreographer moves others: decides what pattern and form will make something important happen for patients, and then works so as to move people, machines, charts, forms, and decisions in what is very close to an esthetic creation. A clinical nurse specialist moves a physician consultant slightly to the left, moves the head nurse slightly to the right, moves the clinical investigations committee downstage and the director of nursing upstage behind a screen, dictates the dance they will all do to the music she has chosen, and stays out of sight or behind the proscenium.

We tend to think that nursing works by the rules of science when many of the judgments we make and the ways we cause things to happen are essentially esthetic. The movements made are intended to solve a problem, but that solution makes something that was misshapen suddenly beautiful, if only that it now makes sense. The nurse choreographer's talent is to create out of the whole cloth of moving bodies, the electricity of conflict, and the music of commitment, a piece of action that is whole and intact, smooth and integrated, subtle as a minuet, or rowdy as a Deuce Coupe. But always moving toward something, if only toward the drawing of the curtain at the close of the first act.

Responsibility

Yet another part of excellence in nursing is **responsibility**. The responsibility that the individual nurse holds, and the collective responsibility of nursing for the health care system boggles the mind. The nurse is responsible for everything from the patient's direct needs to the physician's mistakes, the housekeeping department's sloth, the dietary service's culinary disgraces, and the administration's poor management. After sundown, when everyone else has gone home to their dinner and fireplace and pipe, the nurse is literally in charge and alone and it is she who owns the hospital.

Nurses have been carrying such individual responsibility for the entire history of American nursing and much as we may feel in modern times that our turf has been invaded, that basic responsibility still exists. And we do it so well, so uncomplainingly, and so invisibly. Nurses teach the interns and residents so that they will not kill our patients. We see to it that the rooms are warm and the ice is cold, and the bathroom is clean and the chart is buffed and when we catch hell for a small slight, our rage at the ungrateful system is damped to some small corner of the duodenum. We float through darkened halls in the silence of the night, tending to a fever here, a nightmare there, a backache, a sore, a worry and we do it with the same sense of utter normalcy that an alpinist explains his conquest of Everest: because it's there.

Caring

Much has been written about the **caring** function of nursing. Most of what has been written has been...an attempt to explain that special brand of work that makes nursing something different from medicine's curing. Not much has been said about caring as an aspect of excellence in nursing.

In the first place, it is not easy to care for people, any people, any time, any where. It is especially difficult when there are no ties of blood or common interest that bind the nurse and the patient. Even in personal relationships where there are ties, caring takes hard work and constant attention, lest it curdle. In nursing, caring requires authentic altruism that must be titrated precisely so that it not overwhelm on the one hand, and so that it not be lost on the other. Caring takes enormous energy even when genuine liking is present, for it is impossible to care equally about or for everyone, yet that is exactly nursing's assignment. To care and continue to care about a patient who flaunts his irresponsibility wrings one's spirit. To care about and for the ugly, mutilated or pasty draws the serum from one's soul. Caring is neither easily done nor automatic for we know that the belief in the value of others in all their naked humanity is not inborn.

Caring cannot be forced. It may be built through the luck of a happy childhood, fostered through friends and family and teachers, nurtured by directed learning, and crafted, finally, through application. One's quantum of caring is diluted and then replenished but must always be there for excellence in nursing to happen. The nurse must find it in herself if it has drained away in the pressures of an unrewarding position, in a corrupting institution, in a bleak and confusing world. When the spark of caring is gone, the nurse is truly burnt out.

On-the-spot caring is not enough, difficult though it sometimes is. There ought also to be in excellent nursing the memory of caring. Nurses take their nursing home with them. On the ward and in the clinic we fashion a mosaic of personal caring. Now we must remember the day, too. Not hacks who pocket our pay checks and forget our calling in the parking lot, nurses bear the burden and yet have the exquisite privilege of peering through the swarm of sensations that composed the day to find in them patterns and generalities to help structure tomorrow. We later experience, like Wordsworth, "emotion recollected in tranquility." We explore with ourselves a scheduled AKA on an adolescent so we better understand this youth. We live out that mutilation within ourselves and may cry at odd moments, the horror driven home. Fingering utensils beside the stove, we are struck by a new way to handle the woman with homonymous hemianopsia. We linger in department stores, tinkering with infant car seats, cataloguing the ways parents tell their three-year-old he can't have that model of R2D2. We query the pharmacist about something to use "for my child's cold sores" just to see what she'll say. All of nature and personal experience becomes an opportunity to be a nurse and to learn about nursing, for nurses remember always what we are. The memory of caring reveals in the end that nursing is not simply a way of acting like a nurse or of knowing, however deeply, the content, but it is also a way of being — 24 hours a day. The only thing a nurse can be is a primary nurse, with timeless responsibility.

Skepticism

Another part of excellence that is rarely discussed in nursing is **skepticism** — the proper distance from the truth. Only when one keeps one's mind open to new information can new information get in. Skepticism is not cynicism, which discards all forms of information. Rather, the skeptical nurse lets knowledge in but retains in some corner of the frontal lobe the capacity to mull it over, discard it, or believe in it as further insight blooms. The skeptical nurse knows that truth is rare beyond price, that everything in the real world of health and sickness and people is subject to change, interpretation, and sheer error. Yet one must do, so the nurse keeps the mind open and free yet uses the best of the data that come to him.

In skepticism there is also idealism. For skepticism implies there is still a search for truth, even if the search is never-ending. To be skeptical does not deny that one might find truth, if, like Dorothy, one believes hard enough and long enough that one can return from Oz. To be skeptical simply keeps one alert always to the possibility of incompleteness, or bias, or misinformation, or carelessness on one's own part or others. But one hangs onto the faith in oneself to tell the difference between truth and everything else, and one acts with courage in the face of the unknown.

Perseverance

And we **persevere**, for that too is a part of excellence. From the slave labor of student nurses which created the modern hospital through the daily crises of the coronary care unit, nurses have always been there, always persevered. Collectively, we have endured the vast changes in the practice of medicine and surgery, adapted, changed, and grown. We have fought the hundred-year crusade of others to trivialize our work. We have extinguished the tunnel vision of academics and physicians who thought that nursing had no place in higher education. We have intruded deliberately and with aggression aforethought into the lacunae of medical practice as our roles have expanded to take on what was formerly medicine, obstetrics, pediatrics, psychiatry, and all the rest. We have worked alone in war zones, in ghettos, and on city streets, courting mugging or worse. We have survived miserly decisions of federal officials, state agencies, and hospital administrators, and have prevailed and organized to protect our rights and exercise our obligations. And ever and always we have been there, inching our way toward a vision of a world made better for our presence and perseverance. We have been dependable and depended upon, and when we were not there, the system came to a grinding halt.

Passion

But we have so often turned our eyes outside our practice for gratitude and evaluation and have felt saddened and undermined by the lack of professional and public response. We might more appropriately turn inward and glory in what is finally the essence of excellence: **passion**.

Excellent nurses are inflamed by nursing. The flesh may fail. The spirit may momentarily sink. But in the inner reaches of ourselves as nurses, we hunger and thirst after nursing. Far down in our centers there burns this flame that needs the constant breath of nursing contact to keep ablaze. What, then, about nursing satisfies this craving?

We are often inflamed by the new power and politics of nursing, [by] its expanded roles, its FNP's, PNP's and clinicians of assorted letters and ranks, by its lobbyists and its movers and shakers in high places. We are justly excited by these, for their work is timely, useful, necessary. Still, we ought to be more inflamed by the simple passion of nursing. Indeed, on those personal Sunday afternoons, when the sun streaks through the dust and the refrigerator buzzes and the nurse is quite alone, this above all may be the truth: to be an excellent nurse is to be suffused with a deep and almost inexpressible passion for humankind.

There is, first of all, the **passion for detail**. Even in the most supposedly menial of nursing tasks there resides a kaleidoscope of detail and texture whose observation ought to be approached with passionate energy. Such is the richness of nursing.

But there is, too, a **passion for individuality**. Every pulse bounds differently; every skin is creased and scented apart. Voices tremble, resonate, or trumpet in their particular rhythms. There are no Abbott pumps or I.V.s hanging, no Cantor, Levine, or Blakemore tubes; there are only these hollow lines entering people. In a haunting irony, a nurse realized that this country's first execution against a person's will in over a decade occurred at exactly the same hour that he was helping a young mother give birth to her first child, whom she named Oliver Wendell Holmes. Later that same day, some 273 other individuals were extinguished in a Chicago plane crash. Anguished by the fateful extinction of so many, he was nevertheless priviledged to participate in the inauguration of a new uniqueness in the world. That participation, if it is well done, is a passionate experience.

More importantly, there is the **passion toward humility**. A nurse cared for Amy, a 13-year-old girl with marked scoliosis, from the beginning of her hospitalization. He taught her about a spinal fusion with Harrington rod insertion. He medicated her. Both afraid, they comforted one another in the cool hallways of the OR: "You really didn't hurt me with the needles" she sobbed, filling the tremulous spaces in their talk. He gaped at her spine lying open like some prehistoric mammal on the table as the processes were crudely clipped off, the bone grafts thumped out of her hip, and the glinting rod inserted. Then later, the obligatory Demerol injected to calm the searing pain, he stood beside the bed as her mother leaned over Amy, vulnerable and fragile in her half cast. He yearned to enter that twosome, to feel their pain and their unity. He saw only their profiles in the dim light, so alike and so close. But the communion was sacred. If there was a passion in his involvement with this family, there was also a passion in keeping his distance. Benevolently rejected, the nurse needed the humility to appreciate that. It took deep energy — passion — to do that.

This passion undergirds all of the other qualities of excellence and animates them. Passion, for example, without perseverance yields mere flashes in the pan, nurses here and gone overnight. But perseverance without passion is truly lifeless. Likewise, passion without choreography is artless, forging no new order out of the unattractively chaotic. Choreography without passion in nursing, though, is art for art's sake, guided by no underlying spirit.

Passion as a part of excellence has a final, overreaching meaning: passion unifies us and makes us spiritual and professional equals. Rubbing someone's skin with modulated strokes is as profound an experience as delivering a thunderous appeal for restitution before a Senate Sub-committee. If we think about this passion in nursing, then perhaps we can understand our own frustration at others' views that most of nursing is menial and often meaningless drudgery, as if it were some prison sentence we dutifully endure while we grope, pilgrim-like, toward the freer air of teaching, administration, or an expanded role.

Nonsense. To be an excellent nurse is not to be serving time; it is more to be making love.

REFERENCES

Gardner, John W., **Excellence**. New York: Harper and Row (Perennial Library), 1961.

Leadership and the caring role

MURIEL A. POULIN, RN, EdD, FAAN

MUCH IS WRITTEN in the popular media about the demise of the work ethic. It is said that the "baby boom generation" is less motivated and generally less committed than earlier generations who molded the social fabric of American society. Much of the concern arises from corporate officers who see a lack of drive toward leadership positions on the part of younger managers.

The thesis of this article is that leadership is more than a matter of seeking higher levels in the organizational hierarchy. Rather than leadership as a function of corporate position, leadership is viewed as a requisite to the *caring* role which is the heart of nursing. It is a critical role in meeting accountability to clients. It is fundamental to functioning as a professional practitioner.

Accountability and the professional role

Whether nursing is truly professional continues to be debated....Rather than fitting the model of professionalism as portrayed in literature, and incidentally developed by men for male professions, nursing should assert its professionalism based on its service orientation, on the *caring* and on its accountability to clients....

What is meant by this accountability? There is general agreement that accountability is being *answerable* for what one has done. It is more than responsibility. While responsibility relates to what we are expected to do and what we have said we will do, accountability is concerned with the *answerability* for what we have done. We are dealing with the answerability for one's acts and for the outcomes, or consequences, of those acts.

The focus of accountability is a matter of concern in assessing our leadership role as professionals. Assuming accountability to one's self, accountability in a professional context is to the client/patient, the profession, and the employing organization in that order of priority.

Increasingly, society is recognizing nursing's critical role in health care delivery. People look to nurses to help meet their health care needs and nurses must function as true patient advocates. Patients' needs are nursing's primary focus. Next is one's accountability to nursing and the profession. Professional nurses belong to the professional organization, i.e., the American Nurses Association, identify with the profession, and accept its code of practice.[1] Determination of standards rests with the profession and control of practice on the basis of these standards is the responsibility of practitioners, whether for a specific patient or for nursing in a particular setting. Practitioners are also accountable to their employing agency. Having accepted responsibility for a given position as a nurse, carrying out these responsibilities according to the standards and code of practice of the profession is being accountable to the organization.

If nurses are to be truly accountable to clients, they must assume responsibility for insuring a system which allows for care according to the standards and code of practice of the profession. To achieve such practice everyone must assume leadership responsibilities in settings where care is delivered.

The specifics of the leadership role may vary but the goal orientation to *caring* remains constant.

Leadership in caring

In the present era of cost containment, high technology, and changing values, the restructuring of organizations and services often may be based on priorities of expediency and efficiency rather than on needs of patients. Nurses, individually and collectively, must participate in the decision-making process to insure representation of the interests of patients. This requires an identification with a leadership role on the part of every member of the profession.

The role is as an ideological leader. It is my belief that all professional nurses should dedicate themselves to the goals of nursing care for patients based on the values explicated in our code of practice. Leadership in this sphere rests with each of us.

According to Burns, "ideological leaders dedicate themselves to explicit goals that require substantial social change and to organizing and leading political movements to pursue these goals."[2] Nurses must be in the forefront of such political activism in shaping effective organizations and the health care systems as a whole.

In this context we must be clear about our goals, our roles as individual nurses, and the role of nursing as a profession. Our central "goal" is the *caring* of and for people, the "social change" desired is a system of health care based on the needs and human dignity of our citizens, and the political movement will be those individual and collective actions required to protect the health rights of our populations.

Rather than ideology as "doctrinaire, abstract, opinionated, rigid, and unrealistic," we are concerned with "the crucial quality of ideology...it combines both *what* one believes ...one's belief system, value structure...and *how* one came to hold such beliefs, the lenses through which one regards the world, the ideas and experience and motivation on brings to the process of sorting out and evaluating the stream of phenomena that one perceives."[3] Such an ideology, combining our values, our heritage, and our professional orientation cries out for commitment to involvement. I believe it will be operationalized in a patient advocacy role.

The nurse as patient advocate

In today's dynamic and challenging health care environments, patients' needs may be subordinated to the needs of the organization and to the larger needs of society. One need only consider the impact of Diagnostic Related Groups. Intended as a means of controlling costs of hospitalization, a valid socioeconomic goal, it has nevertheless frequently resulted in outcomes less than favorable to individual patients. Health professionals are caught up in the economic maelstrom while complaints of early discharges, inadequate home care services, and increasing costs continue.

Nurses must become proactive in dealing with the situation. A moral commitment to the public commonwealth demands an advocacy role in influencing the direction of change. Nurses and nursing should be protectors of their clients. Patients need someone to help them ensure their rights; indeed, they may at times need assistance in fighting for their rights.

While the advocacy role for nurses has become well recognized, less well developed are the actions related to the role. It is in this sphere that leadership must be exercised. In *caring*, the advocacy role requires initiating action to protect the rights and welfare of patients in the midst of conflicting organizational and interprofessional factors. The willingness of nurses to face controversy, exercise autonomy, and deal with adversity [is] necessary to the enhancement of patients' rights.

The initiation of measures to protect the rights of patients will depend on values and beliefs that transcend the economic and survival mentality currently prevalent. Leaders in health care will be those who maintain a focus on *caring* and on patients' right to care. I believe this is a central responsibility of nurses.

Conclusion

At a minimum, we must:

Withstand the movement toward greater and finite specialization and resulting fragmentation of patients' care.

Seek a balance between the scientific knowledge available to us and our values and beliefs about rights and dignity of patients.

Develop a commitment to the protection of the patient, the advocacy role, in our collaboration with intra- and inter-professional colleagues.

Function as true patient advocates in the midst of increasing emphasis on corporate and economic approaches to care.

Ultimately, the professionalism of nursing will be tested by the degree of its commitment to its *caring* function. It is a function which resides in every practitioner of nursing. It is a function that requires leadership on the part of each and every one of us. In essence it is the *ethos* of nursing.

REFERENCES

1. American Nurses' Association, *Code for Nurses and Interpretive Statement.* Kansas City, MO 1976.

2. **Burns, James McGugn**. *Leadership.* New York: Harper Torchbooks, 1978, p. 248.

3. Ibid. p. 249.

BIBLIOGRAPHY

Chinn, Peggy. *Ethical Issues in Nursing*. Rockville, Maryland: Aspen Publications. 1986.

Noddings, N. Caring: *A Feminist Approach to Ethics and Moral Education.* Berkeley: University of California Press. 1984.

Leadership in practice

JAN L. LEE, RN, MN, CS

TREMENDOUS CHALLENGES FACE nurses today: provision of safe care in a cost-containment environment, increasing numbers of elderly requiring broader and more expert nursing services, and a rise in consumerism and self-responsibility for health care decisions and outcomes. Rising to these challenges requires the concerted efforts of both nursing organizations and individual nurses. As Margretta Styles reminds us, "we are authors of the future of nursing together."[1] As such, each of us has a responsibility to contribute to that future.

The clearest and most direct route to influencing the future of nursing is through the power of practice. The power of practice is both potential and actual. The potential power is present whenever nurses nurse clients; the actual power exists when nurses strive for ultimacy in the professional performance, is articulated through "new" leadership, and is developed in stages from novice to expert.

Ultimacy of professional performance

Ultimacy...is an attitude, an intense driving force. It requires a nurse to be well-prepared, and it leads to the best achievable outcome for the client. Ultimacy does not lead to perfectionism, nor does it seek supremacy. Ultimacy does demand that we take charge of our professional selves, participate in the advancement of nursing science and practice, maintain ourselves in mind and spirit at the forefront of that practice, and accept no impediments to the fullest use of our talents.[2]

The "new" leadership

Ultimacy of professional performance is highly compatible with the development of the "new" leadership, as described by Bennis and Nanus in *Leadership: The Strategies for Taking Charge*. Five myths differentiate "old" leaders from "new" leaders.[3]

Myth 1: Leadership is a rare skill.

Not true. While great leaders may be rare, everyone has some leadership potential. In truth, leadership opportunities are plentiful and within the reach of most people. However, leaders must be groomed, leadership skills, developed.

Myth 2: Leaders are born, not made.

In fact, the major capacities and competencies of leadership can be learned. Further, natural endowments can be enhanced. As Bennis and Nanus have stated: "nurture is far more important than nature in determining who becomes a successful leader."[4]

Myth 3: Leaders are charismatic.

Most leaders aren't. Remember, leaders are just ordinary people, like you and me, who happen to be fulfilling leadership roles. Charisma, contrary to popular opinion, is the result of effective leadership, not the other way around.

Myth 4: Leadership exists only at the top of the organization.

Leadership opportunities exist at each level of an organization. The larger the organization, the more leadership roles exist.

Myth 5: The leader controls, directs, prods and manipulates.

Again to quote Bennis and Nanus, "Leadership is not so much the exercise of power as the empowerment of others."[5]

The new leader empowers others by pulling, not pushing, by inspiring, not ordering. New leaders create achievable, though challenging goals, expectations and reward systems.

From novice to expert

The power of nursing practice is best exemplified by excellence in practice. But expertise and excellence are not developed overnight. With guided practice, experience, peer insight and evaluation a nurse may move from a beginner, a novice, to an expert practitioner. Patricia Benner describes this process as being composed of five stages: novice, advanced beginner, competent, proficient, and expert.[6] Although experience is necessary for movement, movement is not automatic. [7]

Concrete suggestions

The suggestions which follow are meant to help novice nurses assess and develop their leadership potential and begin the career-long process of unleashing the power of practice.

1. Begin with self-assessment. Ask yourself the following questions.

a. How compatible is my philosophy of nursing with the concept of ultimacy? Which aspects can I buy into? Which are troublesome and require further reflection on my part?

b. What basic leadership skills do I already possess? (For instance, strong communication skills....) What skills do I need to develop? (For instance, task delegation and conflict resolution.)

c. Realistically, at what stage of Benner's model am I now? To what stage do I aspire?

2. Recognize your own potential. Based on your self-assessment, identify realistic goals. A management-by-objectives structure helps to quantify fuzzy goals.

a. Verbalize your career goals. What is your ultimate career goal in nursing?

b. Outline a five-year or ten-year plan as stepping stones to achieving your ultimate goal.

3. Implement your practice.

a. Systematically study your practice. Document common nursing diagnoses for a select patient population of interest. Own up to deficiencies and errors in your practice. Seek advice and sustenance from more advanced nurses. Emulate their admirable professional qualities.

b. Get involved in the organization which employs you. Volunteer for staff nurse governing council. Assist with the updating of standards of care. Accept peer review.

c. Develop and use professional and personal support systems. Protect yourself.

4. Above all, remember that excellence in practice is the overriding goal. Professional recognition, self-satisfaction, advanced education, and increasing expertise in practice, although ends in themselves, are made even more significant because ultimately they are means to improve nursing care.

Conclusion

Application of Styles' concept [of] ultimacy, development and enlistment of new leadership skills, and systematic study of one's own nursing practice (a la Benner) can unleash the power inherent in nursing practice itself. As you empower clients and peers, you will find yourself replenished.

Each of us shares responsibility for the future of nursing. As we move toward the twenty-first century, develop and exercise leadership potential in your nursing practice. Help move nursing toward an intentional, preferred future.

REFERENCES

1. **Styles, M.M.** *On Nursing: Toward a New Endowment.* St. Louis, Mosby, 1982, p. 6.

2. *Ibid.* pp. 128-136.

3. **Bennis, W. and Nanus, B.** *Leaders: The Strategies for Taking Charge.* New York, Harper & Row, 1985, pp. 222-225.

4. *Ibid.* p. 223.

5. *Ibid.* pp. 224-225.

6. **Benner, P.** *From Novice to Expert.* Menlo Park, CA, Addison-Wesley, 1984, p. 13.

7. *Ibid* p. 178.

The challenge for innovation: a new leadership

SHEILA A. RYAN, RN, PhD, FAAN; PATRICIA HINTON WALKER, RN, PhD

ORGANIZATIONS IN TRANSITION — the challenge is managing complex change in complex organizations. Putting new ideas into action is not a new, liberal, humanistic dream; it is a hard, cold necessity. Miller identified several conditions that are presently confronting all organizations to change. [1] We live in a society with shifting social values and demographics; our labor force values are undergoing change. Rapid technological advances and the evolution of an information era add to the pace of change in an increasingly competitive environment.

The challenge for today's leaders/administrators is to maintain stability within the organization, while providing the opportunity, mechanisms, incentives, and support for change. One priority is to develop a climate that fosters innovation in the workplace. Drucker defines innovation as "the systematic sloughing off of yesterday...the systematic search for innovative opportunities." [2] Attempts at innovation need to be seen as learning events allowing for bold moves in new directions, even if all are not guaranteed to be successful. Release of energy and freedom to experiment are keys to energizing an organization. Bold new leaders provide excitement, stimulation, and momentum for change.

To facilitate change, new leaders need abilities and understandings different from those traditionally used by managers/administrators. The central trait is an ability to grasp and seize opportunities presented by "...the nature of work in an information age, nature of culture and what it takes to change it in an organization, the art of balancing stability and change." [3]

Brandt suggests that the challenge is to shape or reshape relationships and foster increased interaction among members. He describes four principles for future organizations: structural compression that shifts authority, power, and decision making to the lowest level possible; a fluid structure without barriers between departments or units, allowing talented people to move more freely within the organization; tailoring the system to individuals rather than to organizational units, which liberates members rather than limiting them; and encouraging the sharing of resources instead of dividing them. [3]

An initial agenda item is to analyze the shape of the organization by examining needs of consumers, members, and leaders. To identify the concerns and ideas of groups of individuals in the organization, the new leader may arrange a series of "listening/learning meetings." Rather than focusing on solving problems, the leader acts as facilitator/communicator, shifting resources where possible to assist members of the organization in solving their own problems. The new leader helps members with choices about whether to change (sometimes not an option), and more often focuses on how to change. It is important to study the current organizational culture and identify the desired culture necessary for survival.

Culture reflects the integrity of the organization. It cannot be delegated. The new leader sets and influences the culture by his/her behavior, in effect, role-modeling. Brandt indicates that vocabulary, how time is spent, how meetings are conducted, the way decisions are made, and the daily habits of the leader are opportunities to affect culture. "From dress to dining to phone habits and party attendance, the personal habits...add up to a message received."[3] Successful leaders also recognize the need for humor and laughter.

It is an accepted notion that leaders need to articulate the mission, goals, and direction of an organization. The new leader examines and shapes future direction for the organization. The key is to provide opportunities for members to help define and shape the future and to fit themselves into that scenario. To maintain momentum, the new leader must articulate midpoint, achievable goals between the current state and the desired state.

The new leader focuses on processes of planning, energizing, and team building while delegating the detail work of management rituals (budget, personnel, policy) to competent middle managers. This does not mean abdicating accountability for such processes. Brandt stresses that "planning is probably the best signal ritual in a company for stimulating change...for making people more responsive to change."[3] It is the challenge of the leader to use current systems and, when necessary, to bypass those systems to get deep penetration and participation at all levels in the planning process.

The importance of effective communication cannot be understated. The new leader as a communicator values an informed membership from which new ideas, issues, and solutions to problems bubble up through the organization. This will happen only in a trusting environment. Effective leaders enhance trust by asking for help when needed, being honest with individuals, and being willing to work through difficult situations.

Team development is another process of energizing and revitalizing an organization. Fostering team building is an old notion with a new urgency. Dyer contends that team development does not mean management by committee, but a cohesive group of people who need the resources and support of one another to get the job done.[4] When members and units of an organization see themselves as helpful to each other, interdependent relationships are fostered and internal organizational support is increased.

The new leader, as described by Levinson and Rosenthal, is "wise...willing to propose, attempt, initiate...ready to act when others are still confused, afraid and indecisive. Leaders test their powers and expand their horizons, generating a life creativity activity.[5] The new leader inspires, energizes, and infuses the organization with a spirit of hope for a new tomorrow.

REFERENCES

1. Miller WC: The Creative Edge. Menlo Park, Addison-Wesley, 1986

2. Drucker. PF: Managing in Turbulent Times. New York, Harper & Row, 1980

3. Brandt SC: Entrepreneuring in Established Companies. New York, Dow Jones-Irwin, 1986

4. Dyer WG: Team Building. Menlo Park, Addison-Wesley, 1987

5. Levinson H, Rosenthal S. CEO Corporate Leadership in Action. New York, Basic Books, 1984

SECTION TWO

Conflict, cooperation, and politics in leadership

STRAINED CO-WORKER RELATIONSHIPS, unequal allocation of resources, and disagreements over preferred treatment methods are just three of the myriad sources of conflict the nurse may encounter at work. Section Two explores these and other barriers to effective leadership and explains how the astute nurse can overcome them.

In "Competition vs. Cooperation Among Nurses," Minard first reveals why nurses compete, what they compete for, and how they compete. The author then reviews the detrimental effects of such competition — patients who are often caught in the middle of the conflict and nursing staffs fraught with anger, frustration, stress, low morale, and diminished productivity. Although competition among nurses is inevitable (and, as Minard points out, sometimes beneficial), the effective leader can counter unhealthy competition and foster a cooperative spirit among nurses by using the strategies outlined in the article.

Another potential barrier to effective nursing leadership is intimidation, usually in the form of verbal abuse from doctors, patients, or other nurses. In "Taming a Tyrant," Montgomery shows how intimidation is seldom a one-time occurrence but a pattern that requires the victim's passive participation to reinforce the behavior. Interestingly, the verbal abuser rarely intends to hurt the feelings of the person he has intimidated, and the victim contributes to the problem not only by passively accepting the situation but also by unfairly categorizing the abuser as a tyrant to be avoided rather than an individual who can help solve a problem. The informed victim, claims Montgomery, can take the initiative and resolve the conflict.

The final article, "Politics, Nursing, and You," demonstrates how nurses can positively influence the welfare of patients and the status of nursing through political action in the workplace, the government, professional organizations, and the community. Mason provides six concrete steps that student nurses can take to become actively involved in politics. Such participation, the author maintains, helps promote the student nurse's leadership potential, without which the nursing profession may cease to exist as a vital, independent component of the health care system.

Competition vs. cooperation among nurses

FAITH MINARD, RN, MSN

IN TODAY'S HIGHLY competitive health care system, it may be difficult to separate corporate competition from intracorporate personal competition. Although competition is in an integral part of human relationships, personal competition among nurses often is discouraged. While competition can foster maximum effort and lead to beneficial results for individuals, groups, and entire organizations, it also can become a destructive force which contributes to conflict. Competition is rivalry between and among individuals in a group. It occurs when two or more units (either individuals or subgroups) engage in pursuing the same rewards, and when, if rewards are attained by one, there are fewer rewards for the others. Competition implies a winner and a loser. Competition is the opposite of cooperation. In a cooperative endeavor everyone either sinks or swims; in a competitive endeavor one swims and the other sinks. Deutsch [1] described the differences between competitive and cooperative efforts [as] outlined in Table 1.

For what do nurses compete?

Competitiveness is one way to enhance status. A person competes to raise or maintain self-esteem and social status. In a hospital system, promotions for nurses are proportionately few, and nurses have relatively little formal power within the organization. Thus, staff nurses often find themselves competing for "intangibles" such as recognition, acknowledgement, respect, and unofficial power and control. Nurses may seek physician or supervisor approval and friendship and seek social affiliation with those in more "powerful" or prestigious positions than their own. Others may find themselves in a contest for the unofficial title of "Super Nurse." One head nurse noted that staff rivalry on her unit increased when primary nursing was initiated and individual nurses began comparing themselves with one another. One measure of success was the number of times a nurse was requested by name. Still other nurses may vie either consciously or unconsciously for leadership of a clique or subgroup on a unit. They compete among themselves for control over who has the final say about patient care.

With the new cost cutbacks and fiscal restraints, first-line managers are very likely to have to compete with their peers for new equipment, unit renovations, additional staff, and unit publicity and recognition. Clinical nurse specialists and nurse educators may find themselves competing with each other for patient referrals and audiences at educational programs and groups. With added hospital cutbacks nurses may find themselves competing for jobs within the system. Of course, competition extends beyond the boundaries of the nursing system. Nurses may compete with other departments and disciplines, and turf issues are common. Recently, nurses have even begun to compete with physicians for referrals and control....

Strategies to deal with competition

While competition occurs whenever there are highly motivated achievers working within the same system, there are, nonetheless, some ways to minimize the negative aspects of competition and facilitate cooperation:

1. ***Recognize and address the presence of competition:***

The first step in dealing with competition is

TABLE 1. Comparison of cooperation and competition

	COOPERATION	COMPETITION
Task orientation	Mutual interests are highlighted; coordinated effort with division of labor and specialization functions; the enhancement of mutual power becomes an objective; higher productivity	Emphasis on antagonistic interests; duplication of efforts; the minimization of other's power becomes an objective; lower productivity
Attitudes	Trusting, friendly with a positive interest in the other's welfare and a readiness to respond helpfully to the other's needs and requests; wish to win respect of others	Suspicious, hostile; readiness to exploit the other's needs and weaknesses; negative responsiveness to the other's requests
Perception	Greater sensitivity to common interests while minimizing the salience of opposed interests; a sense of shared beliefs and values	Greater sensitivity to opposed interests, to threats, and to power differences; similarities are minimized
Communication	Open, honest communication of relevant information; interest in accurately informing as well as being informed; communication is persuasive rather than coercive	Little communication or misleading communication; use of espionage or other techniques to obtain information the other is unwilling to give; each seeks to obtain accurate information about the other but to mislead, discourage, or intimidate the other; communication is coercive

to acknowledge that it exists. In evaluating a nursing system for the presence of competition, it is worthwhile to ask the following questions:

- Which individuals or subgroups are rivals?
- How is this rivalry manifested?
- What is the fundamental dispute?
- How does this affect the overall functioning of the system?
- What qualities are rewarded in the system?
- For what rewards do individuals compete (money? advancement? popularity? attention? educational benefits? social advancement?)

The presence of competitiveness on a personal level should be assessed as well:

- With whom do I feel most competitive?
- What is the fundamental dispute?
- How is this rivalry manifested?
- How does this rivalry affect me personally?
- What impact does this rivalry have on others?
- What rewards are important to me?
- How do I obtain these rewards?
- How does the system reward?
- How does the system promote the competition?

2. ***Promote open and honest communication:*** Open communication promotes an exchange of information, prevents misunderstanding and mistrust, and allows for the correction of misperceptions. Problems and conflicts become accurately defined. The use of weekly staff meetings, for example, often is helpful in addressing interpersonal competition while promoting cooperation and joint problem solving. Third-party mediation may

be necessary when individuals or groups become polarized and defensive.

3. ***Encourage collaborative efforts and group projects:*** A relationship is said to be collaborative if different individuals work together and cooperate on a specific task or goal. Groups should be encouraged to identify common goals and work towards achieving these goals. Likewise, members should be aware of each other's perspectives, and the needs of all involved should be addressed. The nurse manager can facilitate collaborative efforts by assigning staff members to work groups and task forces. In doing this the manager must give these groups the time, the space, the resources and the authority to operate successfully. It also is most helpful, whenever possible, to avoid disrupting the groups by introducing temporary members and/or floating permanent ones.

4. ***Reward team efforts:*** While participation on a team often is a reward in itself, the manager should plan to reward positive group efforts. Plans developed by sanctioned work groups should be adopted. Individuals should be cited for their participation in the group efforts in performance appraisals as well as through verbal and written acknowledgement. It is important to recognize all members of a work group. Rewarding only the leader of such a group serves to divide membership, cause resentment, and promote competition within the group.

5. ***Encourage everyone to become an expert in something:*** Delegating different responsibilities to different staff members serves to increase professional autonomy, raise self-esteem and productivity, and minimize the staff's needs to compete at the same things. A head nurse on a medical-surgical unit, for example, may appoint different nurses to chair various task forces and committees (Quality Assurance, Policy and Procedure, and Physician-Nurse committee). Other nurses may be asked to become unit teachers and experts in clinical areas such as diabetes, chemotherapy, nursing diagnosis, or therapeutic touch.

6. ***Beware of splitters:*** It is important to recognize the presence and actions of "splitters" in a system. A "splitter" may be a member of the nursing staff or an individual from outside the group (a physician, a patient, an administrator). The " splitter" may sense vulnerability in a system and play on it — usually for his or her own benefit. For example, one physician tried to undermine cooperative relationships in the nursing department by attacking nursing administration in his comments to a number of staff nurses: "Nursing administrators flaunt their expensive clothes and push papers....Give me your good hard working nurses anyday....I don't see why you girls bother to put up with your supervisors." In this circumstance the staff nurses responded to the physician in this manner, "We like our jobs and we like the way our nursing department operates...it sounds as if you might have some problems with the administrators...they're very open and easy to talk to...perhaps you should speak with them...." With this, the physician shrugged his shoulders and walked away. He had not succeeded in splitting the nursing department — this time.

7. ***Clarify roles:*** With role confusion comes role blurring and confusion. It is not uncommon, for example, for head nurses and off-shift supervisors to engage in power struggles for control of a unit. Responsibilities often overlap, and lines of authority and accountability often are unclear. Individuals should know the responsibilities of others as well as their own. Forums for discussing role similarities and differences should be routine.

8. ***Minimize differences in status among group members:*** A manager who repeatedly gives preferential treatment to certain people fosters competition and resentment among other staff members. On one nursing unit the head nurse's best friend was one of her staff members. Other members of the staff resented

the fact that the head nurse allowed her friend to take longer coffee breaks and frequent sick days. They also noted that the "friend" was scheduled to work fewer weekends. Preferential treatment is to be avoided — full stop. Managers may choose to reward staff appropriately for superior performance through raises, promotions, educational opportunities, and the like. However, if they do so, it must be clear that these are the rewards of achievements, not personal friendship.

9. ***Recognize and reward definable goals:*** While competition can become a destructive force in a hospital system, it can also serve to foster maximum effort among individuals and groups. When goals are objective, concrete and obtainable, individuals may strive to excel and improve upon both their own and other's accomplishments. Rewarding academic advancement, committee work, community involvement, and clinical certification promote achievement and foster healthy competition. All can participate in such competition; the rules are measurable and apply to all. It is unfortunate that "negative" behaviors often are rewarded more frequently than positive behaviors. Chronic complainers and those who resent change, for example, often succeed in gaining more attention (albeit negative) than their peers. Similarly, these individuals frequently succeed in blocking the more forward efforts of their coworkers.

Finally, managers should evaluate staff according to measurable clinical standards. Clearly, it is important to recognize individual achievement. However, the individual's contributions to her peers and her willingness to work cooperatively for the improvement of patient care also should be recognized and evaluated.

REFERENCES

1. Deutsch, Mortin, *The Resolution of Conflict: Constructive and Destructive Processes*. New Haven: Yale University Press, 1973.

BIBLIOGRAPHY

Biddle, Bruce. *Role Theory: Expectations, Identities and Behaviors*. New York: Academic Press, 1979.

Lewis, Anita and Levy, Joyce. *Psychiatric Liaison Nursing*. Reston, Virginia: Reston Publishing Company, Inc., 1982.

Smith, Marie. "Group and Organizational Theory," in *Comprehensive Psychiatric Nursing*. Judith Haber, Anita Leach, Sylvia Schudy, Barbara Sideleau (Eds.). New York: McGraw-Hill, Inc., 1982.

Taming a tyrant

CAROL LEPPANEN MONTGOMERY, RN, MN

WHY ISN'T TODAY's weight recorded on the chart?'' screamed Dr. Philips as he slammed the chart on the desk. "Can't you nurses read? I don't know why I even bother writing orders!" Sara, a new graduate, nervously fumbled through the chart looking for the morning weights. "I haven't got time for incompetent nurses," he barked at Sara as he stomped off the unit.

Sound familiar? Almost all nurses can recall similar situations when they were unjustly "chewed out" or yelled at in front of others. The feelings of humiliation that well up after this type of verbal abuse are not easily forgotten. Some physicians — surgeons especially — have developed a reputation for delivering irrational tirades. However, they are not the only ones; patients, nurses, or anyone in a position of power can use this type of intimidation.

Verbal abuse is rarely a one-time incident. It is a behavior pattern developed by the abuser that requires the participation of victims who reinforce the behavior. Some of us have, over time, allowed and actually encouraged this behavior pattern.

Let's look at how that has happened and what we can do about it. Verbal abusers use others as objects to vent their own frustrations and restore their own feelings of power and control.[1]

The abusive person's intent is not to hurt you. He is not "out to get you." In fact, your feelings do not usually occur to him.

In order to easily act out his frustrations, the offending person must depersonalize the situation: to recognize his target as a real person would complicate the easy discharge of tension. Therefore, he perceives you as a nameless, faceless object, or as a stereotypical nurse or woman whose role is to accept whatever he delivers.

The victim participates by acquiescing to this "nonperson" status. She passively allows herself to be dumped on. She also stereotypes the abuser by relating to him not as an individual, but as a tyrant who is to be feared and avoided.

Once we see these dynamics, we have the key for breaking the cycle. Instead of perceiving your choice of response as either passive helplessness or dangerous confrontation, consider a third and less threatening alternative: humanizing the interaction.

Take advantage of times when the offending person is not upset to establish yourself in his mind as a competent person with a strong sense of self-worth. Show interest in him as a person in a manner that communicates mutual respect rather than subservience/dominance.

When a tirade does occur and the person is yelling and carrying on irrationally, do not feel obligated to respond defensively to the criticism that precipitated the outburst. Instead, allow the person time to "run down." You can view this time as an opportunity to pull yourself together.

Rather than listening to the content of the tirade at this point, focus on yourself. Do you feel embarassed or humiliated? Why should you? You are not the one who is behaving in an embarassing manner. A temper tantrum is a temper tantrum, whether it's acted out by a two-year-old or a fifty-year-old surgeon.

A tantrum is nothing more than loss of control, not to mention bad manners. Imagine that the person is wearing diapers, if this helps to reduce your feelings of intimidation.

Now focus on your response. Again, you cannot respond to content when someone is yelling at you. Pay attention to your automatic reaction. Women will often want to cry or will smile inappropriately. Stop yourself from doing either and pretend that you feel confident and in control. No one actually feels this way, so don't expect yourself to — just act it.

Position yourself at eye level by standing back if you are shorter and standing up if you are seated. Wait for the person to run down and then acknowledge the complaint, but let him know that you can't discuss it while he is yelling. Tell him you will be in the conference room (or some other area out of public view) to discuss the problem further.

Removing the scene from public view is important because it keeps patients and visitors from witnessing it. By eliminating the audience, you also lower the emotional intensity of the situation and you eliminate the secondary gain the offending person gets from performing for others.

After stating your intent, you have the right to leave for the designated area and wait a few moments. If the offender does not comply with the request, or if it is impossible to leave the situation (such as during surgery), then it is crucial to follow up later.

Do not approach this follow-up as a confrontation. Instead, act on the assumption that you respect yourself and your relationship with the person enough to take such an encounter seriously. For example, Sara might say to Dr. Philips, "I was disturbed by what happened between us yesterday and would like to talk about it."

The person may be stunned, *not* by your insolence, but by the fact that you are appealing to him on a person-to-person level and, believe it or not, he is likely to be flattered by the attention. If you act as if you are an important person who does not deserve to be dumped on, most people will assume that you are and will treat you accordingly.

Note that we are focusing on your response, rather than on the abuser's behavior. Outwardly, you are responding reasonably to unreasonable behavior. Inwardly, you are hurt, shocked, and distressed by hurtful, shocking, and distressing behavior.

These incidents are exhausting, but with other emotional baggage they can become paralyzing. Remember, even if you erred, you did not cause the tantrum. The offending person is responsible for losing control. Your error and the tantrum are two separate issues.

Once you've realized that you're not responsible for the scene, try to let go of your moral outrage by distancing yourself emotionally and by adopting a practical problem-solving approach. By focusing your energy on how you will cope and using these strategies, you will experience feelings of control rather than powerlessness.

Finally, don't forget your sense of humor. Some of these scenes, when viewed from a safe distance, are actually quite funny. With support and camaraderie, we can turn a disaster into a situation we will later recall with humor rather than tears.

REFERENCES

1. Chenevert, Melodie, *Special Techniques in Assertiveness Training for Women in the Health Professions*. St. Louis: C.V. Mosby, 1978, p. 40.

Politics, nursing, and you

DIANA J. MASON, RN,C, PhD

YOU MAY BELIEVE that politics has little relevance for the practice of nursing but, consider the following situation:

You are one of four nurses on a 40-bed medical floor. Mr. Jones is a 34-year old man with AIDS who was admitted two weeks ago with pneumocystis carinii pneumonia. He anxiously reports that he feels his temperature is rising. He is eager to be discharged because he has no health insurance and his modest financial assets make him ineligible for Medicaid. He also wants to begin an underground medication that has not been approved by the Federal Drug Administration for research or treatment. An elevated temperature may prolong his hospitalization. You have several other critically ill patients but you want to respond promptly to his concerns. The floor has two electronic thermometers, one of which has been broken for the past two weeks. You spend 10 precious minutes searching for the working thermometer. After taking Mr. Jones' temperature and noting that it is elevated, you also note that he is dyspneic. When he was transferred from the ICU, new orders were written that did not include oxygen administration. You set him up with nasal oxygen anyway.

What does this scenario have to do with politics? Everything; for example, why there are only two electronic thermometers, how many nurses are available to care for 40 patients, what kind of medical treatment has been tested for persons with AIDS, why Mr. Jones has no health insurance, and whether it is within the scope of practice of the nurse to administer oxygen therapy without a physician's prescription. Bedside patient care is a political endeavor.[1] To recognize this requires an understanding of the meaning and nature of politics.

The nature of politics

The word "politics" often conjures up images of crooked deals, payoffs, corruption in government, and other negative portrayals — things nice people don't do. And yet, politics itself is a neutral term. It is how it is used or abused that makes it positive or negative.

Politics has been defined as influencing the allocation of scarce resources.[2] It is a process by which you can influence the decisions of others and exert control over situations and events.[3] Nurses who say that they do not want to be "political" are saying that they do not want to control or influence the events in their daily practice. Politics is a means to an end, and perhaps becomes corrupted when viewed as an end in itself.

Ehrat points out that politics is inherent in our health care system because it is made up of a variety of special interest groups who are all competing for the same pie.[4] For example, in the situation given, the nurse wasted precious time to locate the one working electronic thermometer, while this same hospital had the latest in expensive medical diagnostic equipment, such as nuclear magnetic resonators and CAT scanners. Since most patients are admitted to hospitals because they need nursing care, you would expect the hospital to ensure that there were sufficient resources for efficient bedside nursing care, particularly during the current shortage of nurses. However, such is not the case in many hospitals in this country, largely because too many nurses fail to recognize the role of politics in bedside nursing care and fail to exert their potential influence.

Other nurses have refused to accept a role of powerlessness in the health care system and have been exerting their influence in a variety of constructive ways that benefit both themselves and their patients. They are calling for hospitals to reallocate their resources so that nurses are recruited and retained in adequate numbers. The current shortage of nurses has created a "critical moment" for nursing. Many of the changes nurses have identified as necessary for many years are now being made. Nurses are seizing the critical moment.

Nurses are also building coalitions with those in other disciplines and developing other effective political strategies to ensure that adequate patient care will be delivered by qualified professionals. When nurses in several city hospital emergency rooms in New York City staged a one-day "sick-out" to protest the unsafe working conditions that were jeopardizing patient care, their physician colleagues supported the nurses' call for changes. The media responded with wide coverage, including a television interview with the chief executive officer of one of those hospitals. He told the reporter that while he did not approve of the nurses' actions, they certainly did get his attention. Changes in the work environment were quickly initiated.

Nurses are recognizing that politics is an essential component of their everyday practice.

Spheres of political action

In addition to the *workplace*, nurses must be concerned with three other spheres of political action: government, professional organizations, and community. The *government* holds particular importance to nursing because of the government's role in the delivery and financing of health care, as well as in the regulation of the health professions. In the opening situation, Mr. Jones was one of over 35 million Americans who have no health insurance.[5] The United States is one of only two industrialized nations without a national health program; the other is South Africa.[6] And yet, as one nurse has noted our country spends more money on its military than on promoting the health and welfare of its citizens. These are choices our government makes about how scarce resources will be allocated.

The federal government plays a major role in determining who gets what kind of health care; whether resources will be devoted to subsidizing affordable housing at a time when the number of homeless women and children is escalating; whether funding for nursing education will again reflect the concept that nurses are an important national resource; and how much money will be devoted to the study of drugs that might be effective against AIDS and which drugs will be studied.

While much attention is currently focused on the federal government because of the presidential elections, state and local governments play important roles in developing and implementing health policy.[8] State and local governments monitor and regulate health care and the health professions through legislation and regulations. In the opening situation, the nurse's decision to begin oxygen administration without a physician's prescription is influenced by the nurse practice act of the state in which she practices and the regulation of nursing practice by the state board for nursing. Recently in New York State, the department of health issued regulations that licensed practical nurses could administer intravenous therapy through central venous lines, a position that was contrary to that of the New York State Board for nursing. The motivation of the department of health ostensibly is to provide an immediate remedy to the shortage of nurses. The New York State Nurses Association, on behalf of several nurses who have had to confront this situation in their practice, has filed a lawsuit against the New York State Department of Health and the Board of Nursing, claiming that it is the responsibility of the New York State Board for Nursing, not the health department, to regulate nursing practice.

Professional nursing organizations provide a means for nurses to exert their collective influence on such important issues as access to health care, the development of progressive nurse practice acts, and generally promoting nursing and high quality health care. The American Nurses Association (ANA) has developed a reputation as a powerful voice for nursing in Washington. Its network of congressional district coordinators organize nurses in the various congressional districts to lobby and campaign for candidates who are supportive of nursing and high quality health care. The ANA has also been politically astute in its involvement in important health related nursing coalitions, including the Tricouncil, which consists of ANA, the National League for Nursing, the American Association of Colleges of Nursing, and the Association of Nurse Executives.

On the other hand, the agenda of these and other nursing organizations and how they operate are determined by those who choose to influence these matters. The National Student Nurses Association (NSNA) provides a mechanism for nursing students to learn about the functioning of organizations, how to influence them, and to develop networks that can be used after graduation.

Finally, the *community* can be a powerful source of influence on the health care system. For example, with the growth in the number of older adults in this country, this age group has developed into a formidable lobbying force through such groups as the American Association of Retired Persons (AARP) that can be allies of nursing as the profession fights for access to high quality health care. In fact, ANA has joined AARP and other groups in making long-term care a national campaign issue this year. Leaders, individuals or groups, in the community can thus define issues that are important for the community to address such as the rise in infant mortality, educating the public about AIDS, the drug crisis, or even the nursing shortage. A nurse's community activism can also enhance his or her power base in all spheres. One nurse became well known to the leaders in her hospital and local officials because of her visible activism to fight environmental pollution in her community.

To maximize their political effectiveness, nurses must develop their influence in all four spheres. This requires a long-term plan of action that can start during your years as a student nurse.

Developing your political skills

The following principles for effective political action are particularly important for the beginning participant in political action.[8]

1. Politics is an interpersonal endeavor. Ghandi is reported to have said that politics begins with the person next to you. Politics is an interpersonal endeavor requiring effective communication skills. Every nursing curriculum includes content on communication skills. While the focus of this content is usually the nurse-patient relationship, the skills can be applied as well to political action. Ronald Reagan has been referred to as the "great communicator" because of his ability to sway the public to support his positions on issues. Nursing students can develop effective communication skills in the clinical area with clients, peers, faculty, and other team members, as well as through other student activities.

2. Individuals are most likely to engage in political action when they are deeply committed to the issue. Students are particularly limited in resources of time and money. Decisions to mobilize a group of students to action around an issue should reflect the priorities of the group or strategies for making the issue a priority. A handful of students at Columbia

University who were deeply committed to the issue of opposing apartheid in South Africa were able to mobilize their University to divest its financial investments in that country. The students' commitment and effective strategies brought broad-based attention to the issue and led to a national anti-apartheid divestiture movement. Other students have felt so strongly about curriculum issues in their schools that they have worked with faculty and fellow students on schools' curriculum committees.

3. Effective political action is often a group effort. The old saying that "there is strength in numbers" is particularly true for nurses. Several years ago, the American Nurses' Association held a reception for federal legislators during a conference on political action. The nurses who attended were given buttons to wear that stated "1 in 44." One nurse had been trying to get her congressman to speak at a program that her local nurses' association was sponsoring in her home town. Letters and phone calls had gone unanswered for two months. When she met the congressman at the reception, she reminded him of these requests and he responded that he would look into it, although in a quite unconvincing manner. Suddenly he saw her button and asked what it meant. She replied, "One in every 44 women in this country is a registered nurse." The congressman was amazed and quickly began asking her about the details of the speaking engagement.

The congressman knew, as did the emergency room nurse in New York City, that the actions of one person can seldom compare with the actions of a multitude. Not only is political power enhanced through group action, creative thinking is stimulated and mutual energizing can occur that is important to sustaining action on an issue.

Collective action requires the development of networks and a support base ahead of time and knowledge about how to mobilize a group. Nurses frequently report that they are unable to get the support of their colleagues for action on important issues. These inactive nurses will complain endlessly but refuse to take action on their own behalf, a symptom of someone who feels powerless. It becomes important, then, to find ways to empower fellow students and nurses. Miller is one of several feminist researchers and theorists who have addressed differences in how men and women relate to power.[9] Men historically have been power-grabbers, seizing power and holding it close to themselves. The classic example of this model of power is Machiavelli's *The Prince*. Miller noted that many women are often uncomfortable with this model of power, and instead prefer power-sharing or empowering others.

While one should not draw a stereotype from these descriptions, power-sharing may be a model that is particularly appropriate for collective action in nursing. Nursing's future depends upon an empowered critical mass of nurses. From May 1986 to 1988, I was the president of the New York Counties Registered Nurses Association (District 13 of the New York State Nurses Association), one of the largest local nurses' associations in the country. As president, I needed and wanted power; however, to hold that power close to myself would have been a disservice to the organization and to the members. We needed an empowered membership and I saw one of my primary roles as encouraging and facilitating empowered action by these members.

The implications of this discussion for nursing students include encouraging mutual support among your peers; decrying chronic complaining and, instead, encouraging constructive action; finding ways for other students to "shine" or contribute publicly to an issue; thanking peers for their support; and celebrating with them in victory.

4. Effective political action requires the astute application of change theory. Those of you who have already been immersed in

Summary of registration procedures and important contacts

Registration procedures

Postcard Registration: Alaska, California, Delaware, Iowa, Kansas, Kentucky, Maryland, Michigan, Minnesota, Missouri, Montana, New Jersey, New York, Ohio, Oregon, Pennsylvania, Tennessee, Texas, Utah, Wisconsin, District of Columbia.

Branch and/or deputy registration: Arizona, Arkansas, Colorado, Connecticut, Florida, Illinois, Indiana, Maine, Massachusetts, Nevada, New Mexico, South Dakota, Virginia, Washington, West Virginia, Puerto Rico, Virgin Islands.

Election day registration: Minnesota, Oregon, Wisconsin, Wyoming.

Centralized registration: Alabama, Georgia, Hawaii, Idaho, Louisiana, Mississippi, Nebraska, New Hampshire, North Carolina, Oklahoma, Rhode Island, South Carolina, Vermont, Wyoming.

Important contacts and resources

Voter registration and absence voting information. Compiled by Frontlash Foundation, Inc., 815 16 Street, NW, Room 203, Washington, D.C. 20006 (202) 783-3993 Cost: $10.00. This manual has state by state information about registration procedures and absentee voting.

National Student Roundtable. 235 Pennsylvania Ave., SE, Suite 210, Washington, D.C. 20003. (202) 547-6771. Check on campus to see if there is a local chapter conducting a student voter registration drive.

Public interest research groups. 37 Temple Place, Boston, MA 02111 (617) 423-1796. Check on campus to see if a local PIRG is conducting a voter registration drive.

American Public Health Association. 1015 Fifteenth Street NW, Washington, D.C. 20005. (202) 789-5650. *APHA Voter Registration Manual* is available which contains comprehensive information on how to conduct a drive. Also, check your state affiliate of APHA for assistance they can provide.

Do's and Don'ts of Public Affairs Activities During an Election Campaign. Planned Parenthood Federation of America, Inc, 810 Seventh Ave., New York, New York 10019. Guidelines on what to do and not do when conducting a voter registration drive.

Human Serve Fund. National Headquarters, c/o New York Urban Coalition, 99 Hudson Street, New York, N.Y. 10013 (212) 219-4500. Literature and resources available which describe their campaign to register recipients of social welfare programs.

Power at the Polls. Published by the National Association of Social Workers. 7981 Eastern Ave., Silver Springs, MD 20910 (301) 565-0333. This organization has information about voter registration drives conducted by social workers and social work students.

COPUS. The National Coalition of Independent College and University Students, 235 Pennsylvania Ave., S.E., Washington, D.C. 20003. (202) 659-1747. Check on campus to see if local chapter is planning a student voter registration drive.

Environmental Action. 1525 New Hampshire Ave., NW, Washington, D.C. 20036 (202) 745-4870. This national political lobbying organization can provide you with information about environmental health issues which you can use to educate voters about candidate's environmental platforms.

Reprinted from the NSNA *Legislative Handbook and Voter Registration Manual.*

change theory from leadership courses know that your time has been well spent. Effective political action requires thoughtful analysis of situations, people, and issues; the setting of short- and long-term goals; and developing strategies to move an issue and counter resistance to change. Whether the setting is the workplace, a nursing organization, government, your community, or even your own school, effective political action requires thoughtful analysis of the formal and informal structures and processes, as well as brainstorming possible solutions, opportunities for compromise and negotiating, and other possible strategies. Unless viewed as a deliberate process, successful political action becomes elusive and haphazard.

Choose your issues carefully. There are many opportunities for political action. You cannot tackle them all. It becomes important, particularly for the novice, to select issues for action when the odds are in your favor. Too many losses can become discouraging to the novice. It is equally as important to find success in your losses. Although you may lose the issue, what you learned in the process may enable you to be successful the next time.

Start now

With these principles in mind, and others you will learn through continued reading and experience, there are many ways for student nurses to learn about politics. The following are a few suggestions.

1. Organize a voter registration drive on your campus. Note that the target audience would not be just fellow nursing students, but all eligible students on campus. This approach could bring visibility to nursing students in a way that the public does not necessarily expect. If it is important for your group to build coalitions with other groups on campus, you could lead in the development of a drive that is organized and sponsored by a variety of campus groups. NSNA can assist you in organizing a voter registration drive through its "Legislative Handbook and Voter Registration Manual."

2. Identify opportunities for learning about politics through your nursing curriculum. Politics and health policy should be integrated into the curriculum. Sometimes it requires a creative faculty member or student to find opportunities for actualizing this mandate.

Some schools provide opportunities for students to do projects in professional issues or leadership courses that can involve politics. Many local nurses' associations welcome having students work with their legislative or other committees to help organize a student component of their annual lobby day in the state capitol, or work on another project with members of the committee. Some local officials welcome student placements for one or more semesters, and some students have continued to work with these officials in paid and unpaid capacities during summers and after graduation. As a professor of nursing, I have taken interested students with me to work in a congressman's campaign for an evening, attend a meeting or entire convention for a nurses' association, lobby a state senator about increasing state funding for nursing education, attend meetings of boards of nurses' associations and state political action committee, and to community-based meetings on health care issues. Other students have done these and other activities on their own initiative.

Because lobbying and campaign work relies so heavily on volunteer effort, the opportunities for student involvement are endless. What is important to keep in mind is that the experiences should provide opportunities to demonstrate nurses' involvement in one of the four spheres of political action.

3. Write your legislator about a legislative issue of importance to you. Again, this may fulfill a requirement for a professional issues course. Being mindful of the above principles, select an issue that is important to you, gather information about the issue, and consult the relevant nurses' association about its position on the issue and the current status of bills that have been written. Again, NSNA's "Legislative Handbook..." provides details on letter-writing. If you are unsure of who your legislator is, you can call your local League of Women Voters or board of elections for the information. You might even organize a letter-writing campaign within your school of nursing on the topic.

4. Work for the candidate of your choice

How to write to your congressman

Street Address
City, State Zip Code
Month Day, Year

The Honorable (Full Name)
U.S. House of Representatives
Washington, D.C. 20515

Dear Mr./Mrs. (Last Name),

On behalf of the National Student Nurses' Association, I am writing to you to ask for your support of the Nursing Shortage Reduction Act of 1987, which has already passed in the Senate. This bill was created to help alleviate the severe nursing shortage. By supporting this bill you will be demonstrating to your constituents, especially to those who will need health care, commitment to a higher quality of health care.

The Nursing Shortage Reduction Act of 1987 focuses on innovative projects to develop long-term solutions as well as fostering recruitment efforts to encourage qualified people to enter nursing. Since 1983 there has been a steady decline of enrollments in nursing schools across the country. In 1986, there was a 7.8% drop in enrollments and a 25% drop in applicants to nursing programs. These figures indicate that in the near future, there will be a severe shortage of registered nurses to care for the increasing number of elderly and AIDS patients as well as all others who are in need of nursing care.

Please show your support by voting "Yea" when the Nursing Shortage Act of 1987 comes to the floor.

Thank you.

Sincerely yours,

Name
Member, NSNA
Student (Name of School)

in this year's presidential campaign (or in the local race of your choice). National politics can be exciting. Students have often been an important component of the grassroots efforts of national campaigns. Campaigns provide important opportunities for learning about politics in general and for meeting people who have strong interests or good experience in politics.

5. When school issues of importance to you arise, engage in politically astute, planned change. Gather together some of your peers for an analysis and brainstorming session to clearly delineate the issue, identify possible solutions and strategies, and formulate a plan.

6. Become actively involved in your student nurses' association. Learn from it and encourage it to become involved in important issues on campus, in nursing, and in the community. One association worked with the dean's office to invite their congresswoman to speak to the entire campus, followed by a reception. The event, sponsored by the student nurses' association and the school of nursing, got excellent coverage in the student and local press and brought nursing and health care issues to the attention of the campus.

Certainly, the association should be an important vehicle for student voices to be heard. That collective voice can make a difference in curriculum matters, school policies, and even on campus issues. If the association is not serving in this capacity, you can help to transform it. If it is, but you don't agree with its issues, you can work to change the agenda.

Summary

The current shortage of nurses provides a critical moment for you and the profession. If we seize the moment, we can lead in the effort to reform a health care system that is in crisis. Such action requires a politically empowered and informed cadre of nurses. The profession needs you as a politically astute activist. Start now!

REFERENCES

1. **Mason, D.J.** The politics of patient care. In Mason, D.J. and Talbott, S.W. *Political action handbook for nurses: Changing the workplace, government, organizations, and community.* Menlo Park, CA; Addison-Wesley, 1985.

2. Ibid.

3. **Stevens, B.J.** Power and politics for the nurse executive. *Nursing and Health Care*, 1:4:208-210, April, 1980.

4. **Ehrat, K**. A model for politically astute planning and decision making. *Journal of Nursing Administation*, 13:9:September, 1983:29-34.

5. **Jonas, S.** *Health Care Delivery in the United States* (Third Edition). New York: Springer, 1986.

6. **Dallek, G**. Six myths of American medical care. *Health Pac Bulletin*, 16:3:9-15, May-June, 1985.

7. **Moccia, P.** Are we dying for nuclear weapons? *American Journal of Nursing*, October, 1986.

8. **Mason, D.J**. From bedside to White House: The local perspective. In NLN (Eds.), *Perspectives in Nursing — 1985-1987*. New York: National League for Nursing, 1986.

9. **Miller, J.B.** *Colloquium: Women and power; Stone Center for Developmental Services and Studies.* Wellesley, MA, Wellesley College, 1982.

UNIT TEN

Study questions

1. In "Values and Professional Behaviors," the American Association of Colleges of Nursing outlines seven essential values of the professional nurse. Think of someone you consider to be a leader. Which leadership values and behaviors does this person manifest?

2. Diers and Evans, in "Excellence in Nursing," identify skepticism as an integral facet of nursing excellence. In what ways does the skeptical nurse demonstrate excellence in nursing practice?

3. Accountability to the patient is the cornerstone of nursing practice, according to Poulin in "Leadership and the Caring Role." Discuss three ways in which the nurse as patient advocate fulfills the accountability role.

4. In "Leadership in Practice," Lee offers concrete suggestions for the novice nurse who wants to develop potential and skills as a leader. Name five steps you can take as a student nurse to develop your leadership skills.

5. In "The Challenge for Innovation: A New Leadership," Ryan and Walker contend that nursing executives must be willing to shift more authority and decision making to lower levels within the organization. Discuss how such a shift would benefit nurses. How would it benefit patients?

6. Identify three distinct differences between competitive and cooperative behaviors, as outlined by Minard in "Competition vs. Cooperation Among Nurses."

7. In "Taming a Tyrant," Montgomery shows how intimidating behavior is reinforced by the victim's passivity. Discuss how intimidation can hamper effective nursing leadership.

8. "Politics, Nursing, and You" demonstrates how nurses can positively influence the welfare of patients and the status of nursing through political action. Identify five steps you can take to make political leaders aware of the needs in nursing.

Acknowledgments

Special thanks to Barbara J. Bohny, RN, DNS, for her contributions to the development and organization of this book. The publisher wishes to acknowledge the following for permission to reprint or excerpt their articles:

UNIT ONE
NURSING: THE SCIENCE OF CARING

Leininger, M. (1981). The phenomenon of caring: Importance, research questions, and theoretical considerations. In *Caring: An Essential Human Need*. Proceedings of Three National Caring Conferences, pp.3-15. Thorofare, NJ: C.B. Slack.

Fry, S. (1988). The ethic of caring: Can it survive in nursing? *Nursing Outlook,* 36(1), 48. Copyright 1988, American Journal of Nursing Co. All rights reserved.

Orlick, S., and Benner, P. (1988). The primacy of caring. *American Journal of Nursing,* 88(3), 318-319. Copyright 1988, American Journal of Nursing Co. All rights reserved.

Nelson, M. (1988). Advocacy in nursing. *Nursing Outlook,* 36(3), 136-141. Copyright 1988, American Journal of Nursing Co. All rights reserved.

Allen, J. et al. (1988). Caring for Julie. *Nursing Times,* 84(2), 25-29.

Benner, P., and Wrubel, J. (1988). Caring comes first. *American Journal of Nursing,* 88(8), 1072-1075. Copyright 1988, American Journal of Nursing Co. All rights reserved.

Larson, D. (1987). Helper secrets: Internal stressors in nursing. *Journal of Psychosocial Nursing,* 25(4), 20-27.

UNIT TWO
UNIFYING CONCEPTS BASIC TO NURSING

Arnold, E. and Boggs, K. (1989). Conceptual components of the therapeutic relationship. In Arnold, E., and Boggs, K., *Interpersonal Relationships: Professional Communications Skills for Nurses.* Philadelphia, W.B. Saunders. (pp.179-189).

Whall, A. (1986). The family as the unit of care in nursing: A historical review. *Public Health Nursing,* 3(4), 240-249.

Cox, C. et al. (1988). Social risk factors: Impact on elders' perceived health status. *Journal of Community Health Nursing,* 5(1), 59-73.

Roberson, M. (1987). Home remedies: A cultural study. *Home Health Nurse,* 5(1), 35-40.

Soeken, K., and Carson, V. (1987). Responding to the spiritual needs of the chronically ill. *Nursing Clinics of North America,* 22(3), 603-611.

UNIT THREE
NURSING AS A PROCESS

Ronsman, K. (1987). Therapy for depression. *Journal of Gerontological Nursing,* 13(12), 18-25.

Miller, J. et al. (1987). The impact of nursing diagnoses in a long-term care setting. *Nursing Clinics of North America,* 22(4), 905-915.

Burnard, P. (1987). Meaningful dialogue. *Nursing Times,* 83(20), 43-45.

Katzman, E.M., and Roberts, J.I. (1987). No longer a silent partner. *Maternal-Child Nursing Journal,* 12(Nov/Dec), 383, 386-388. Copyright 1987, American Journal of Nursing Co. All rights reserved.

Creighton, H. (1987). Legal significance of charting: Part I. *Nursing Management,* 18(9), 17-20, 22.

Creighton, H. (1987). Legal significance of charting: Part II. *Nursing Management,* 18(10), 14-15.

Ethridge, P. (1987). Nurse accountability program improves satisfaction, turnover. *Health Progress,* 68(4), 44-49.

Bunting, S., and Webb, A. (1988). An ethical model for decision making. *Nurse Practitioner,* 13(12), 31-34.

Collopy, B.J., et al. (1988). Do not feed: Is stopping artificial feeding unethical? *NursingLife,* Jan/Feb, 25-27.

UNIT FOUR
LIFE CONTINUUM IN HEALTH AND ILLNESS

Yoos, L. (1987). Chronic childhood illnesses: Developmental issues. *Pediatric Nursing,* 13(1), 25-28.

Carson, V.B. (1989). Spiritual development across the life span. In Carson, V.B., *Spiritual Dimensions of Nursing Practice* (pp. 24-51). Philadelphia: W.B. Saunders.

Stolte, K., and Myers, S.T. (1987). Nurses' responses to changes in maternity care, Part I: Family centered changes and short hospitalization. *Birth,* 14(2), 82-86.

Myers, S.T., and Stolte, K. (1987). Nurses' responses to changes in maternity care, Part II: Technologic revolution, legal climate, and economic changes. *Birth,* 14(2), 87-90.

Patterson, K.L., and Ware, L.L. (1988). Coping skills for children undergoing painful medical procedures. *Issues in Comprehensive Pediatric Nursing,* 11, 113-143.

Smith, K.L.D., et al. (1987). Health concerns of adolescents. *Pediatric Nursing,* 13(5), 311-315.

Baldwin, B.A. (1988). The stress of caring: Issues confronting mid-life caregivers. *Caring* 7(3), 16-18, 66, published by the National Association for Home Care.

Pearson, B.D., and Droessler, D. (1988). Continence through nursing care. *Geriatric Nursing,* Nov/Dec, 347-349. Copyright 1988, American Journal of Nursing Co. All rights reserved.

Kübler-Ross, E. (1971). What is it like to be dying? *American Journal of Nursing,* 71(1), 54-62. Copyright 1971, American Journal of Nursing Co. All rights reserved.

Sherman, D.W., et al. (1988). Shalom, Melissa: Comforting the terminally ill leukemia patient. *Nursing88,* June 53-57.

UNIT FIVE
DIVERSITY IN HEALTH CARE SETTINGS

Fought, S. (1988). Critical care for the multiple injured patient. *Critical Care Nursing Quarterly,* 11(2), 63-69. Copyright September 1988 Aspen Publishers, Inc.

Tisdale, S. (1988). Harvest Moon: Portrait of a nursing home. *American Journal of Nursing,* 88(3), 297-300. Copyright 1988, American Journal of Nursing Co. All rights reserved.

Humphrey, C. (1988). The home as a setting for care: Clarifying the boundaries of practice. *Nursing Clinics of North America,* 23(2), 305-314.

Zelewsky, M., and Deitrick, E. (1987). Rx for caregivers: Respite care. *Journal of Community Health Nursing,* 4(2), 77-84.

Martin, N. (1988). How nursing takes over when medicine gives up. *RN,* 51(3), 30-32.

UNIT SIX
PSYCHOSOCIAL CONCEPTS IN NURSING

Arnold, E., and Boggs, K. (1989). Self-concepts in the nurse-client relationship. In E. Arnold, *Interpersonal Relationships: Professional Communication Skills for Nurses.* Philadelphia: W.B. Saunders. (pp. 107-123).

Scott, A. (1988). Human interaction and personal boundaries. *Journal of Psychosocial Nursing,* 26(8), 23-27.

Forchuk, C., and Westwell, J. (1987). Denial. *Journal of Psychosocial Nursing,* 25(6), 9-13.

Copel, L. (1988). Loneliness: A conceptual model. *Journal of Psychosocial Nursing,* 26(1), 14-19.

Kennedy, M. (1987). AIDS: Coping with the fear. *Nursing,* 17(4), 44-46.

Archer, D., and Smith, A. (1988). Sorrow has many faces: Helping families cope with grief. *Nursing88,* 18, 43-45.

Adams, F. (1988). Drug dependency in hospital patients. *American Journal of Nursing,* 88(4), 477-481. Copyright 1988, American Journal of Nursing Co. All rights reserved.

Runyon, N. et al. (1988). The borderline patient on the med-surg unit. *American Journal of Nursing,* 88(12), 1644-1650. Copyright 1988, American Journal of Nursing Co. All rights reserved.

Bydlon-Brown, B., and Billman, R. (1988). At risk for suicide. *American Journal of Nursing,* 88(10), 1358-1360. Copyright 1988, American Journal of Nursing Co. All rights reserved.

Hradek, E. (1988). Crisis intervention and suicide. *Journal of Psychosocial Nursing,* 26(5), 24-27.

Baird, S. (1987). Helping the family through a crisis. In *Nursing Assessment and Strategies for the Family at Risk,* second edition, by Suzanne Hall Johnson. Philadelphia: J.B. Lippincott Co.

UNIT SEVEN
PHYSIOLOGIC CONCEPTS IN NURSING

Harrison, M., and Cotanch, P. (1987). Pain: Advances and issues in critical care. *Nursing Clinics of North America,* 22(3), 691-697.

Iverson-Carpenter, M., et al. (1988). Fulfilling nutritional requirements. *Journal of Gerontological Nursing,* 14(4), 16-24.

Milde, F. (1988). Impaired physical mobility. *Journal of Gerontological Nursing,* 14(3), 20-24.

Barndt-Maglio, B. (1986). Sleep pattern disturbance. *Dimensions of Critical Care Nursing,* 5(6), 342-349.

Glass, J., and Dalton, J. (1988). Sexuality in older adults: A continuing education concern. *The Journal of Continuing Education in Nursing,* 19(2), 61-64.

Worker exposure to AIDS and hepatitis B: Facts for the health care industry (pamphlet). U.S. Department of Labor, Occupational Safety and Health Administration, 1987.

Jackson, M., et al. (1987). Why not treat all body substances as infectious? *American Journal of Nursing,* 87, 1137-1139. Copyright 1987, American Journal of Nursing Co. All rights reserved.

UNIT EIGHT
PROFESSIONAL PRACTICE OF NURSING

Elliott, J.E. (1987). Nursing education and nursing practice: The need for consensus. *Journal of Professional Nursing,* 3(4), 194-198.

Sandrick, K.M. (1987). Other options: Great opportunities outside the hospital. *NursingLife,* 7(4), 33-37.

Sossong, A., et al. (1987). An expanding universe: Professional career opportunities. *Nursing Management,* 18(2), 46-48.

Dunbar, S. (1987). Entry into practice: The continuing saga. *Heart and Lung,* 16(2), 22a-27a, by the C.V. Mosby Co.

Foss, J. (1988). Continuing education requirements by state. *AORN Journal,* 47(6), 1462-1464. Copyright AORN Inc.

Dobbs, K.K. (1988). The senior preceptorship as a method for anticipatory socialization of baccalaureate nursing students. *Journal of Nursing Education,* 27(4), 167-171.

Bajnok, I. (1988). Specialization meets entry into practice. *The Canadian Nurse,* 84(6), 23-24.

Davis, G.C. (1988). Learning about nursing management. *Nursing Outlook,* 36(4), 190-192. Copyright 1988 American Journal of Nursing Co. All rights reserved.

London, F. (1987). Should men be actively recruited into nursing? *Nursing Administration Quarterly,* 12(1), 75-81. Copyright Fall 1987 Aspen Publishers, Inc.

UNIT NINE
PATTERNS OF NURSING AND HEALTH CARE

Christmyer, C.S., et al. (1988). Bridging the gap: Theory to practice—part I, clinical applications. *Nursing Management,* 19(8), 42-50.

Field, P.A. (1987). The impact of nursing theory on the clinical decision making process. *Journal of Advanced Nursing,* 12, 563-571.

Hinshaw, A.S. (1988). The National Center for Nursing Research: Challenges and initiatives. *Nursing Outlook,* 36(2), 54-56. Copyright 1988, American Journal of Nursing Co. All rights reserved.

Hinshaw, A.S. (1988). The National Center for Nursing Research: Challenges and initiatives. *Nursing Outlook,* 36(2), 54-56. Copyright 1988, American Journal of Nursing Co. All rights reserved.

Goode, C.J., et al. (1987). Use of research based knowledge in clinical practice. *Journal of Nursing Administration,* 17(12), 11-18.

Kramer, M., and Schmalenberg, C. (1987). Magnet hospitals talk about the impact of DRGs on nursing care—Part I. *Nursing Management,* 18(9), 38-42.

Kramer, M., and Schmalenberg, C. (1987). Magnet hospitals talk about the impact of DRGs on nursing care—Part II. *Nursing Management,* 18(10), 33-40.

Maas, M., and Hardy, M. (1988). A challenge for the future. *Journal of Gerontological Nursing,* 14(3), 8-13.

van Bemmel, J.H. (1987). Computer assisted care in nursing: Computers at the bedside. *Computers in Nursing,* 5(4), 132-139.

UNIT TEN
LEADERSHIP FOR CHANGE

American Association of Colleges of Nursing. (1986). Values and professional behaviors. In *Essentials of College and University Education for Professional Nursing: Final Report.* Washington, DC: American Association of Colleges of Nursing.

Diers, D., and Evans, D. (1980). Excellence in nursing. *Image,* 12(2), 27-30.

Poulin, M. (1987). Leadership and the caring role. *Imprint,* 34(6), 51, 53-54.

Lee, J. (1987). Leadership in practice. *Imprint,* 34(6), 57-58, 61.

Ryan, S., and Walker, P. (1988). The challenge for innovation: A new leadership. *Journal of Professional Nursing,* 4(3), 148, 230.

Minard, F. (1988). Competition vs. cooperation among nurses. *Nursing Management,* 19(3), 28-32.

Montgomery, C. (1987). Taming a tyrant. *American Journal of Nursing,* 87(2), 234, 238. Copyright 1987, American Journal of Nursing Co. All rights reserved.

Mason, D. (1988). Politics, nursing, and you. *Imprint,* 35(3), 47-52.

Index

t refers to a table

t refers to a table

t refers to a table

t refers to a table

t refers to a table

t refers to a table

t refers to a table

t refers to a table

t refers to a table

t refers to a table

t refers to a table